The Authors

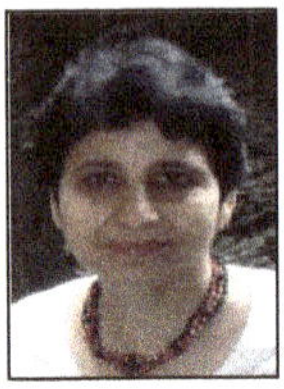

Professor Neelam Khetarpaul, former-Dean (COHS) and HOD (FN) also at CCS Haryana Agricultural University, Hisar is the recipient of many awards *viz.*, Distinguished Teacher Award, Young Investigator Award, Ms. Manju Utreja Gold Medal and cash award for doing the best research work in the University and Best Research Paper Awards by many scientific socities. She is the recipient of various Visiting Fellowships abroad funded by different national and international agencies and visited USA, Australia, UK, Hungary, Ghana, Ecuador and Netherlands for academic pursuits. She is the country Coordinator of Indo-Netherlands Tailoring Biotechnologies project programme being funded by the Department of Biotechnology, Ministry of Science and Technology, Govt. of India and the Wageningen University, The Netherlands under which 4 students are doing Ph.D from WU, the Netherlands. She has published more than 240 research papers in various journals of national and international repute, 22 books and guided 28 post graduate students in the discipline of Food Science and Human Nutrition.

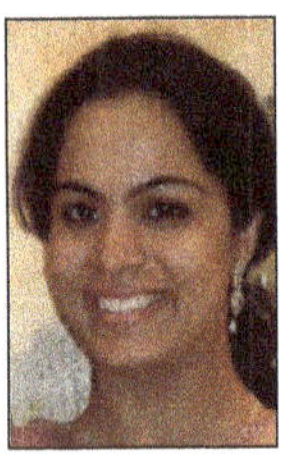

Dr. Anubha Mutneja, MD graduated from Maulana Azad Medical College, New Delhi and pursued further training in internal medicine from university of Florida in Gainesville, FL, USA. She is currently pursuing a fellowship in nephrology in Washington University in St Louis MO, USA. She has special interest in cardiology, immunology and human nutrition.

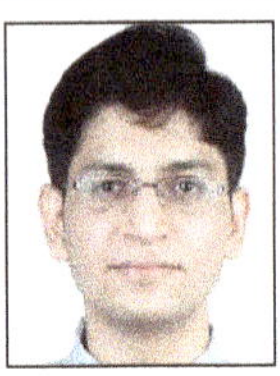

Dr. Vipul Khetarpaul graduated with distinction in the MBBS degree from Kasturba Medical College, Manipal University, Manipal, India and scored the highest marks in Manipal University. He is the recipient of gold medals, various prizes and awards including Dr. R. L. Adiga Prize, Dr.K.M.Kudva and Mrs.Gauri M.Kudva Prize for standing First in final MBBS Part 2 University Examination held during the year 2005-2006, the Bhagyamma Purushotam Prize for standing first in Obstetrics and gynecology, Dr. T. M. A. Pai Prize for standing first in final MBBS Part 2 University Examination and for good conduct. He also got certificate of Merit for Excellent Academic Performance (2004-2005). Throughout schooling, he was amongst the top 1 per cent and invariably at the 99th percentile. He has done **Basic Life Support (BLS)** provider course by American Heart Association, **Advanced Cardiac Life Support (ACLS)** provider course by American Heart Association, **ITLS** (International Trauma Life Support) Advanced Course, **and Fundamental Critical Care Support** provider course by the Society of Critical Care Medicine. He has attended a number of workshops and conferences at AIIMS, Apollo hospital, Batra hospital etc. He cleared USMLE examinations with 99 percentile and did residency in surgery from WSU, USA. Presently, he is doing fellowship in Vascular Surgery in Washington University in St Louis MO, USA. He has keen interest in human nutrition and is the Co-author of one book on 'Advances in Lipid Nutrition'.

Fats and Oils in Health and Nutrition

Neelam Khetarpaul
Anubha Mutneja
Vipul Khetarpaul

2014
Daya Publishing House®
A Division of
Astral International Pvt. Ltd.
New Delhi – 110 002

ISBN 9789351300847

Published by : **Daya Publishing House®**
A Division of
Astral International Pvt. Ltd.
– ISO 9001:2008 Certified Company –
4760-61/23, Ansari Road, Darya Ganj
New Delhi-110 002
Ph. 011-43549197, 23278134
E-mail: info@astralint.com
Website: www.astralint.com

Laser Typesetting : **Classic Computer Services**, Delhi - 110 035

Printed at : **Replika Press Pvt. Ltd.**

PRINTED IN INDIA

Preface

Fats have received a bad reputation over the last decade, resulting in a plethora of low-fat diet programs and fat-free food products. While certain types of fats or excessively high amounts can be problematic but fats in moderation are actually vital to our body. Beyond the enjoyment and satisfaction that fat adds to food, it is a critical player in human health. The essential functions of fat in the body are not breaking news, but at times they have been forgotten. Fats and components of or products of metabolism of fats are found in the wall of each cell in the human body, and are particularly critical components of the brain and nervous tissue. Our body requires fats and oils to support growth and development especially during infancy and childhood. It is no surprise that 55 per cent of the calories in breast milk come from fats, critical for the developing human body. They are essential components of all body tissues and are especially important in the development of cell membranes, the retina and brain tissue. Fats are used to make hormones that affect such bodily functions as blood pressure, blood clotting, immune function and smooth muscle contraction. Fat soluble nutrients require fat for proper absorption. Importantly, fat is not to be feared, it is a critical component of a healthful diet.

The scientific knowledge regarding the role of various types of fats and fatty acids in determining health and nutritional well- being particularly with respect to their role in neonatal and infant growth and development, health maintenance, the prevention of cardiovascular disease, diabetes, cancers and age-related functional decline etc. has expanded dramatically in the past few years. Our aim in writing this book is to provide a single concise source for all kind of recent up to date information available about role of fats and oils in human nutrition and health.

The text is organized into 21 chapters, covering a wide spectrum starting initially with definition and classification of lipids to their recommended levels, disturbances in lipid metabolism and fat substitutes. This book also provides a stimulating overview of current concepts in clear language about the role of fats and various types of fatty acids in atherosclerosis, coronary vascular disease, cancer and immune system. Focus has also been laid to provide latest information on recommendations of daily intake of various types of fats to be consumed to remain healthy. One of the most extensive chapters of this book deals with as to how and why use mix of blended oils and fats instead of single type of oil to achieve optimum ratio of recommended fatty acids in the daily diets for achieving optimum nutrition and good health. Other chapters are related to health effects of trans fats, role of omega-3 fatty acids in health and disease, hypocholesterolemic effect of fibres from cereals and legumes, fat substitutes and dietary components of therapeutic life style changes in CVD. Another section of the book is devoted to recent developments and advances in knowledge regarding trends in production and consumption of oilseed, oils and fats at the global and national level. The book has been written clearly with many illustrations to help the reader to gain an understanding of the subject thoroughly. A detailed reference list is being appended for further additional and detailed reading.

We strongly feel that this shall be a very useful reference material for nutritionists, dietitians and health professionals in teaching graduate and postgraduate students and counseling of patients. This book is truly and strongly recommended to any common reader who is interested to know which type of fat to be included or not included, how many calories to be taken from saturated and unsaturated fat, their dietary sources, which type of vegetable oils to be blended to attain optimum ratio of various types of fatty acids for prevention of degenerative diseases as most of us are health conscious now a days. We hope to get great response from our readers. We are also grateful to our friends and colleagues who have directly or indirectly helped us in writing this book. We wish to extend a special acknowledgement to the publishers, especially to Mr. Anil Mittal for his continued interest in bringing out this updated and revised edition on lipids.

Neelam Khetarpaul

Anubha Mutneja

Vipul Khetarpaul

Contents

Chapter 1

Definition and Classification of Lipids I

Definitions of Lipid

Lipids come from the Greek lipos, meaning fat. Although lipid analysts tend to have a firm understanding of what is meant by the term "lipid", there is no widely-accepted definition.

Fats and oils are classified as "lipids" which is a category that embraces a broad variety of chemical substances. In addition to triglycerides, it also includes mono- and diglycerides, phosphatides, cerebrosides, sterols, terpenes, fatty alcohols, fatty acids, fat-soluble vitamins, and other substances.

Generally, lipids are usually described as a group of naturally occurring compounds, which are hydrophobic and have in common a ready solubility in such organic solvents as hydrocarbons, chloroform, benzene, ethers and alcohols. They include a diverse range of compounds, like fatty acids and their derivatives, carotenoids, terpenes, phospholipids, steroids, bile acids and waxes. It should be apparent that many of these compounds have little by way of structure or function to relate them. In fact, a definition of this kind is positively misleading, since many of the substances that are now widely regarded as lipids may be almost as soluble in water as in organic solvents.

> Lipids are fatty acids and their derivatives, and substances related biosynthetically or functionally to these compounds.

This treats cholesterol (and plant sterols) as a lipid, and could be interpreted to include bile acids, tocopherols and certain other compounds. It also enables classification of such compounds as gangliosides as lipids, although they are more soluble in water than in organic solvents. However, it does not include such natural substances as steroidal hormones, petroleum products, some fat-soluble vitamins, carotenoids or terpenes, except in rare circumstances.

If "lipids" are defined in this way, fatty acids must be defined also. They are compounds synthesised in nature via condensation of malonyl coenzyme A units by a fatty acid synthase complex. They usually contain even numbers of carbon atoms in straight chains (commonly C_{14} to C_{24}), and may be saturated or unsaturated, and can contain a variety of substituent groups.

Fahy *et al.* (2005) as described in *J. Lipid Res.* (46, 839-862) have developed a classification system for lipids that holds promise. While their definition of a lipid is too broad, it is based on sound scientific principles, *i.e.*

Hydrophobic or amphipathic small molecules that may originate entirely or in part by carbanion-based condensations of thioesters (fatty acids, polyketides, etc.) and/or by carbocation-based condensations of isoprene units (prenols, sterols, etc.).

Functions

Fats and oils are recognized as essential nutrients in both human and animal diets. Nutritionally, they are concentrated sources of energy (9 Kcal/gram); provide essential fatty acids which are the building blocks for the hormones needed to regulate bodily systems; and are a carrier for the oil soluble vitamins A, D, E, and K. Fat is also is used in our bodies to cushion vital organs like the kidneys and serve as insulation, especially just beneath the skin.

They also enhance the foods we eat by providing texture and mouth feel, imparting flavor, and contributing to the feeling of satiety after eating. Fats and oils are also important functionally in the preparation of many food products. They act as tenderizing agents, facilitate aeration, carry flavors and colors, and provide a heating medium for food reparation. Fats and oils are present naturally in many foods, such as meats, dairy products, poultry, fish, and nuts, and in prepared foods, such as baked goods, margarines, and dressings and sauces.

Classification

The most common lipid classes in nature consist of fatty acids linked by an ester bond to the trihydric alcohol–glycerol, or to other alcohols such as cholesterol, or by amide bonds to sphingoid bases, or on occasion to other amines. In addition, they may contain alkyl moieties other than fatty acids, phosphoric acid, organic bases, carbohydrates and many more components, which can be released by various hydrolytic procedures.

There is no single, internationally accepted system of classification for the lipids. The names of these compounds, do fall into certain categories as the, component structures present are considered.

1. Simple Lipids

They are defined as those that on hydrolysis yield at most two types of primary product per mole esters of fatty acids with alcohols. Examples are fats, oils and waxes.

Triacylglycerols (Triglycerides), Neutral Fats

The triglycerides are the most abundant lipids in nature. Nearly all the commercially important fats and oils of animal and plant origin consist almost exclusively of the simple lipid class triacylglycerols (often termed "triglycerides"). A triglyceride consists of three fatty acids attached to one glycerol molecule. Since there are three fatty acids attached, these are known as triglycerides. If all three fatty acids are identical, it is a simple triglyceride. The more common forms, however, are the "mixed" triglycerides in which two or three kinds of fatty acids are present in the molecule. The names neutral fat, TG and fat are used synonymously.

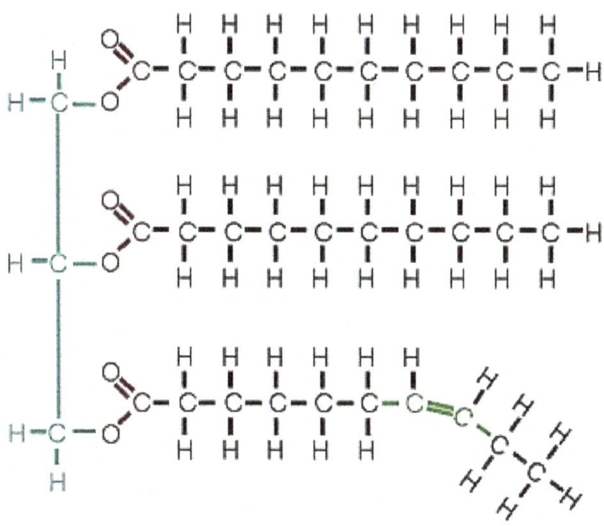

In nature, they are synthesised by enzyme systems, which determine that a centre of asymmetry is created about carbon-2 of the glycerol backbone, so they exist in enantiomeric forms, *i.e.* with different fatty acids in each position.

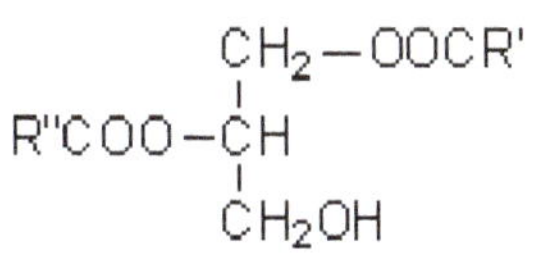

1,2-/2,3-diacylglycerol

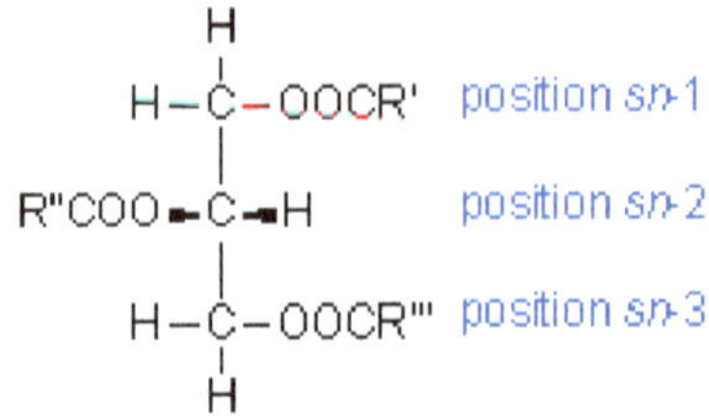

Fischer projection of a triacyl-sn-glycerol

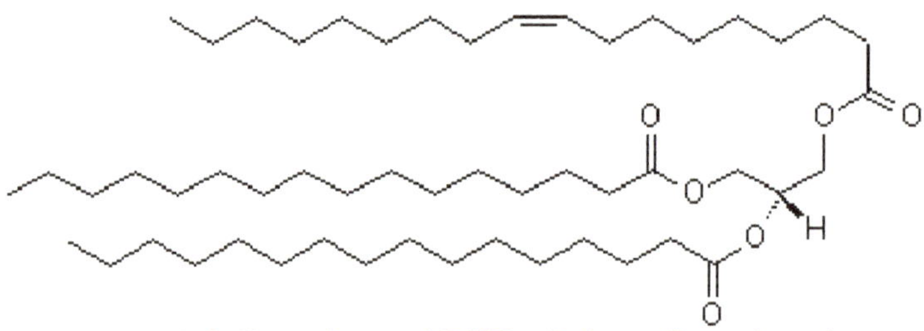

1,2-dihexadecanoyl-3-(9Z-octadecenyl)-sn-glycerol

A stereospecific numbering system has been recommended to describe these forms. In a Fischer projection of a natural L-glycerol derivative, the secondary hydroxyl group is shown to the left of C-2; the carbon atom above this then becomes C-1 and that below is C-3. The prefix *"sn"* is placed before the stem name of the compound, when the stereochemistry is defined. Their primary biological function is to serve as a store of energy. As an example, the single molecular species 1,2-dihexadecanoyl-3-(9Z-octadecenoyl)-*sn*-glycerol has been illustrated.

Diacylglycerols

Diacylglycerols (less accurately termed "diglycerides") are esters of the trihydric alcohol glycerol in which two of the hydroxyl groups are esterified with long-chain fatty acids. Diglycerides are formed in the intestinal tract as a result of the normal digestion of triglycerides. They are also present in natural fats. They can exist in three stereochemical forms.

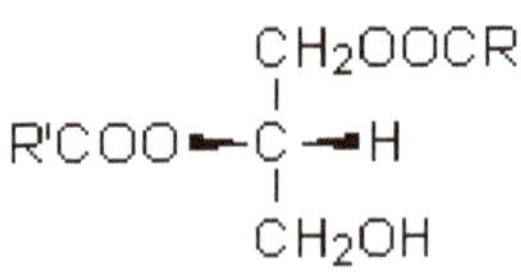

sn-1,2-diacylglycerol

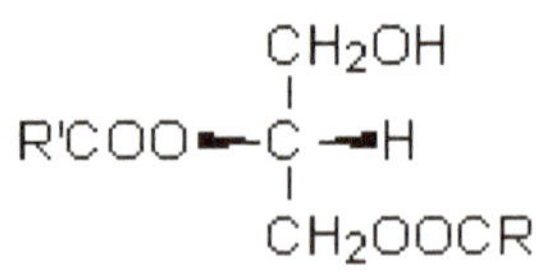

sn-2,3-diacylglycerol

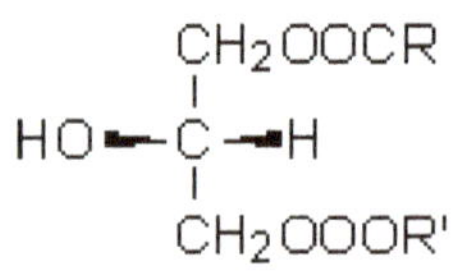

sn-1,3-diacylglycerol

1,2-diacyl-*sn*-glycerols are key intermediates in the biosynthesis of triacylglycerols and other lipids, and they are vital cellular messengers, generated on hydrolysis of phosphatidylinositol and related compounds by a specific phospholipase C.

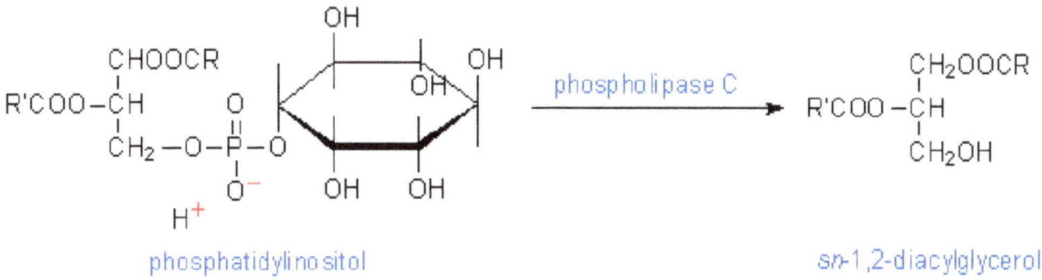

They occur naturally in very minor amounts in both animal fats and vegetable oils. Oil composed mainly of diglycerides have also been used as a replacement for oil composed of triglycerides. They are used frequently in foods as emulsifiers. They are prepared commercially by the reaction of glycerol and triglycerides or by the esterification of glycerol and fatty acids. Recently, edible oils consisting of 80 per cent 1,3-diacylglycerols have been marketed in Japan as nutritional supplements. It is claimed that they are metabolized in a different way from triacylglycerols with beneficial nutritional effects. The 1(3)-monoacylglycerols formed when they are digested are absorbed into tissues relatively poorly, apparently limiting the accumulation of fats in body tissues.

Monoacylglycerols

Monoacylglycerols (or "monoglycerides") are esters of the trihydric alcohol glycerol in which only one of the hydroxyl groups is esterified with a long-chain fatty acid, and they can also exist in three stereochemical forms.

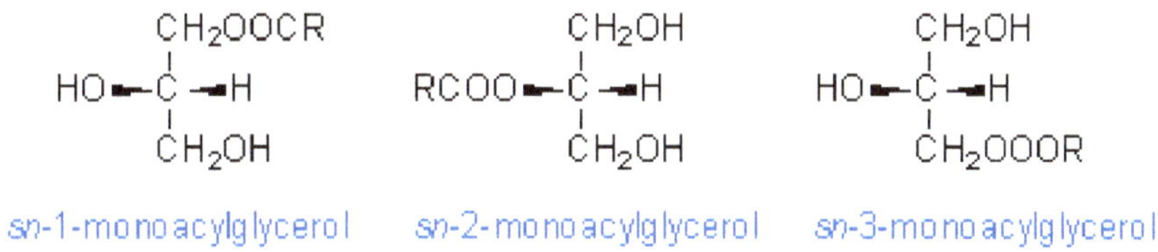

They are formed as intermediates or end-products of the enzymatic hydrolysis of triacylglycerols; these and other positional isomers are powerful surfactants. 2-Arachidonoylglycerol has important biological properties.

They tend to be minor components only of most plant and animal tissues, and indeed would not be expected to accumulate because their strong detergent properties would have a disruptive effect on membranes. 2-Monoacylglycerols are a major end product of the intestinal digestion of dietary fats in animals via the enzyme pancreatic lipase. They are taken up directly by the intestinal cells and converted to triacylglycerols via the monoacylglycerol pathway before being transported in lymph to the liver.

Tocopherols and Tocotrienols

Tocopherols [substituted benzopyranols (methyl tocols)] and tocotrienols are important minor constituents of most vegetable fats. They serve as antioxidants to retard rancidity and as sources of the essential nutrient vitamin E. Tocopherols which occur naturally in most vegetable oils are partially removed during processing. Corn and soybean oils contain the highest levels. Tocopherols are not present in appreciable amounts in animal fats. Tocotrienols are mainly present in palm oil, but can also be found in rice bran and wheat germ oils.

In the tocopherols, the C_{16} side chain is saturated, and in the tocotrienols it contains three double bonds. Different forms (α-, β-, γ- and δ-) are recognized according to the number or position of methyl groups on the aromatic ring. The four main constituents are termed–*alpha* (5, 7, 8-trimethyl), *beta* (5, 8-dimethyl), *gamma* (7,8-dimethyl) and *delta* (8-methyl). Of these, *alpha*-tocopherol is most readily absorbed from the intestines. They are all important natural antioxidants with some Vitamin E activity, but only α-tocopherol (including synthetic material) or natural mixtures containing this can be sold as 'Vitamin E'. However, the tocotrienols are more potent antioxidants, while γ-tocopherol has some specific biological properties that are distinct from those of α-tocopherol. Among tocopherols, alpha-tocopherol has the highest vitamin E activity and the lowest antioxidant activity. Delta tocopherol has the highest antioxidant activity.

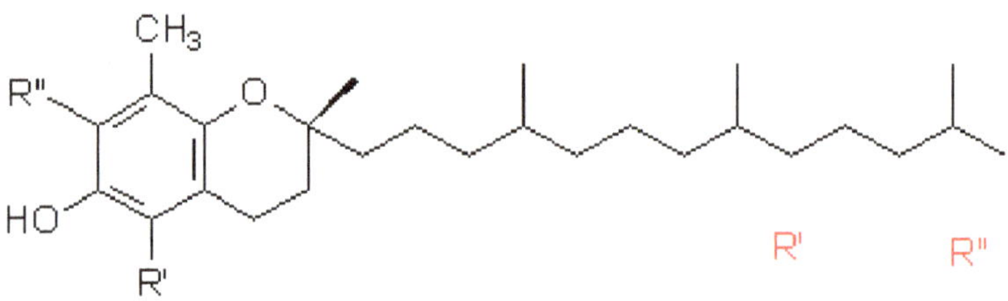

	R'	R''
alpha-tocopherol	—CH_3	—CH_3
beta-tocopherol	—CH_3	—H
gama-tocopherol	—H	—CH_3
delta-tocopherol	—H	—H

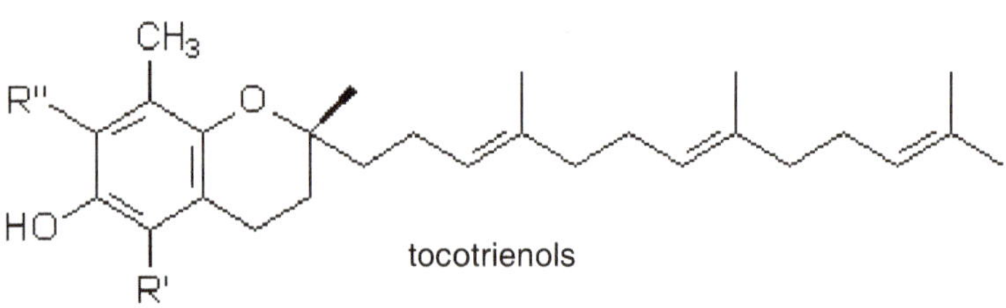

tocotrienols

Pigments

Carotenoids are yellow to deep red color materials that occur naturally in fats and oils. They consist mainly of carotenes such as lycopene, and xanthophylls such as lutein. Palm oil contains the highest concentration of carotene. Chlorophyll is the green coloring matter of plants which plays an essential role in photosynthesis. Canola oil contains the highest levels of chlorophyll among common vegetable oils.

At times, the naturally occurring level of chlorophyll in oils may cause the oils to have a green tinge. Gossypol is a pigment found only in cottonseed oil. The levels of most of these color bodies are reduced during the normal processing of oils to give them acceptable color, flavor, and stability.

Waxes

Wax is derived from the Anglo-Saxon word "weax" for beeswax, so a practical definition of a wax may therefore be "a substance similar in composition and physical properties to beeswax". Technologists use the term for a variety of commercial products of mineral, marine, plant and insect origin that contain fatty materials of various kinds. Biochemists link waxes with the thin layer of fatty constituents that cover the leaves of plants or provide a surface coating for insects or the skin of animals.

All of these tend to contain wax esters as major components, *i.e.* esters of long-chain fatty alcohols other than glycerol with long-chain fatty acids. The latter tend to be saturated or have one double bond only. Such compounds are found in animal, plant and microbial tissues and they have a variety of functions, such as acting as energy stores, waterproofing and lubrication. Long chain alcohols are of little importance in most edible fats. A small amount esterified with fatty acids is present in waxes found in some vegetable oils. Larger quantities are found in some marine oils.

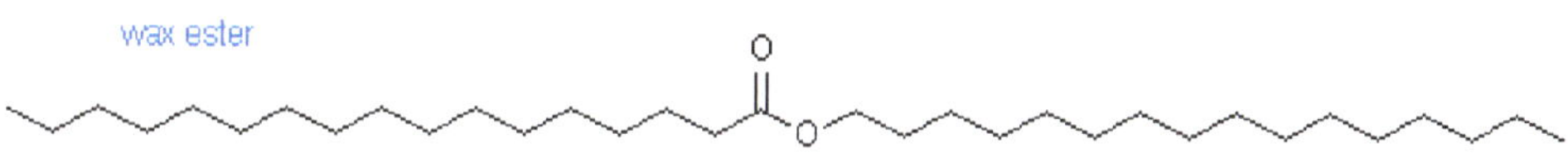

In some tissues, such as skin, avian preen glands or plant leaf surfaces, the wax components can be much more complicated in their structures and compositions. They can contain aliphatic diols, free alcohols, hydrocarbons (*e.g.* squalene), aldehydes and ketones. The nature of the other lipid constituents can vary greatly with the source of the waxy material, but they include hydrocarbons, sterol esters, aliphatic aldehydes, primary and secondary alcohols, diols, ketones, β-diketones, triacylglycerols, and many more.

Also, the chain-length and degree of unsaturation and branching of the aliphatic constituents will vary with the origin of the wax, but other than in some waxes of marine origin or from some higher animals, the aliphatic moieties tend to be saturated or monoenoic.

A number of waxes are produced commercially in large amounts for use in cosmetics, lubricants, polishes, surface coatings, inks and many other applications.

2. Compound Lipids

They are esters of fatty acids containing groups in addition to an alcohol and fatty acid. They include phospholipids, glycolipids, lipoproteins etc. They usually contain glycerol + 2 Fatty Acids + P and something. They yield three or more primary hydrolysis products per mole. Alternatively, the terms "neutral" and "polar" lipids, respectively are used to define these groups, but are less exact. The complex/

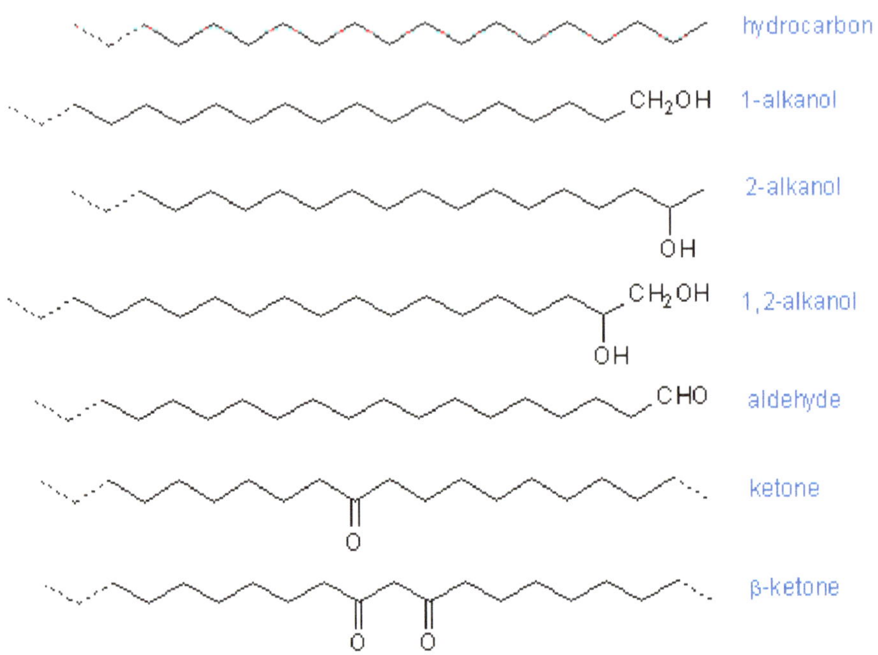

compound lipids for many purposes are best considered in terms of either the glycerophospholipids (or simply as phospholipids), which contain a polar phosphorus moiety and a glycerol backbone, or the glycolipids (both glycoglycerolipids and glycosphingolipids), which contain a polar carbohydrate moiety, since these are more easily analysed separately.

Phospholipids (Phosphatides)

They can be the derivatives of glycerophosphate and sphingosine phosphate. They are found chiefly in animal tissues. Substituted fats, consisting of phosphatidic acid; composed of glycerol, fatty acids, and phosphoric acid bound in ester linkage to a nitrogenous base. The majority of the phosphatides are removed from oil during refining. Phosphatides are an important source of natural emulsifiers marketed as lecithin.

These compounds can be separated into a variety of subgroups depending upon the structural components in the parent molecule. The following classification is an example of this grouping.

Glycerophosphatides or Phosphoglycerides

In some of the books, they are grouped as under:

A. Phosphatidyl choline (Lecithin)

B. Phosphatidyl ethanolamines (Cephalin)

C. Other substitutes attached to the phosphatidyl group

1. Nitrogenous; sering, threonine, methylethanolamine, hydroxyproline
2. Carbohydrate-like; inositol, phosphoinositol, glycerol, polyglycerol

D Phosphosphingosides or sphingomyelins

According to Lipid Library, UK, glycerophosphatides are classified as under:

- Ether lipids
- Phosphatidic acid and related lipids
- Phosphatidylglycerol and related lipids
- Diphosphatidylglycerol (cardiolipin)
- Phosphatidylinositol and related lipids
- Phosphatidylserine
- Phosphatidylethanolamine
- Phosphatidylcholine
- Mono- and digalactosyldiacylglycerols and from plants and microorganisms, etc
- Glycosyldiacylglycerols and related lipids from animals
- Glycophospholipids

These are discussed in detail in Chapter 2.

Lecithin

They are found in brain, egg yolk, and organ meats. Phosphatidyl choline or serine; phosphatide linked to choline; a lipotropic agent; important in fat metabolism and transport; used as emulsifying agent in the food industry.

Cephalin

They occur predominantly in nervous tissue. Phosphatidyl ethanolamine; phosphatide linage to serine or ethanolamine; plays a role in blood clotting.

Plasmalogen

They are found in brain, heart, and muscle. Phosphatidal ethanolamine or choline; phosphatide containing an aliphatic aldehyde.

Lipositol

Found in brain, heart, kidneys, and plant tissues together with phytic acid. Phosphatidyl inositol; phosphatide linked to inositol; rapid synthesis and degradation in brain; evidence for role in cell transport processes.

Sphingomyelin

Found in nervous tissue, brain, and red blood cells. Sphingosine-containing phosphatide; yields fatty acids, choline, sphingosine, phosphoric acid, and no glycerol; source of phosphoric acid in body tissue.

Glycolipids (Non-phosphorylated lipids)

Cerebroside

They are found in myline sheaths of nerves, brain, and other tissues. They consist of a ceramidevwith a single sugar residue at the 1-hydroxyl moiety. The sugar residue can be either glucose or galactose. The two major types are therefore called glucocerebrosides and galactocerebrosides. Galactocerebrosides are typically found in neural tissue, while glucocerebrosides are found in other tissues.

Ganglioside

It is found in brain, nerve tissue, and other selected tissues, notably spleen; contains a ceramide linked to hexose (glucose or galactose), neuraminic acid, sphingosine, and fatty acids.

Sulfolipid

It occurs in white matter of brain, liver, and testicle; also plant chloroplast. Sulfur-containing glycolipid; sulfate present in ester linkage to galactose.

Proteolipids

It occurs in brain and nerve tissue. These are complexes of protein and lipids having solubility properties of lipids.

3. Terpenoids and Steroids

a. Terpenes

They are found in essential oils, resin acids, rubber, plant pigments such as carotenoids and lycopenes, Vitamin A, and camphor. Large group of compounds are made up of repeating isoprene units; Vitamin A is of nutritional interest; fat soluble Vitamin E and K, which are also related chemically to terpenes.

b. Sterols and Sterol Esters

They are found both in animal fats and vegetable oils, but there are substantial biological differences.

i) Cholesterol

It is the primary animal fat sterol and is found in egg yolk, dairy products, and animal tissues. It is a consituent of bile acids and a precursor of Vitamin D. Cholesterol is by far the most common member of a group of steroids in animal tissues. The great French chemist Chevreul was the first to isolate it from gallstones and characterize it as a single compound as long ago as 1815. Cholesterol has an important role in membranes and in lipid metabolism in general, so is a lipid by any definition. Steroidal hormones, derived biosynthetically from cholesterol, are not lipids in the sense of definition of lipids as mentioned above.

Cholesterol has a tetracyclic ring system with a double bond in one of the rings and one free hydroxyl group. It is found both in the free state, where it has an essential role in maintaining membrane fluidity, and in esterified form, *i.e.* as cholesterol esters.

Other sterols may be found in free and esterified form in animal tissues, but at trace levels only.

Cholesterol is formed biosynthetically from squalene (or strictly speaking from mevalonate) via lanosterol by a complex sequence of reactions, as illustrated in simplified form below. The rate-limiting enzyme is HMG-CoA reductase. Synthesis occurs in the endoplasmic reticulum of liver cells primarily, and cholesterol can then be exported and transported to other tissues in the form of lipoprotein complexes for uptake via low-density lipoprotein receptors. Cholesterol synthesis or the enzyme HMG-CoA reductase specifically is inhibited by drugs known as statins, so that animal cells must then obtain their cholesterol primarily from the diet via the circulation.

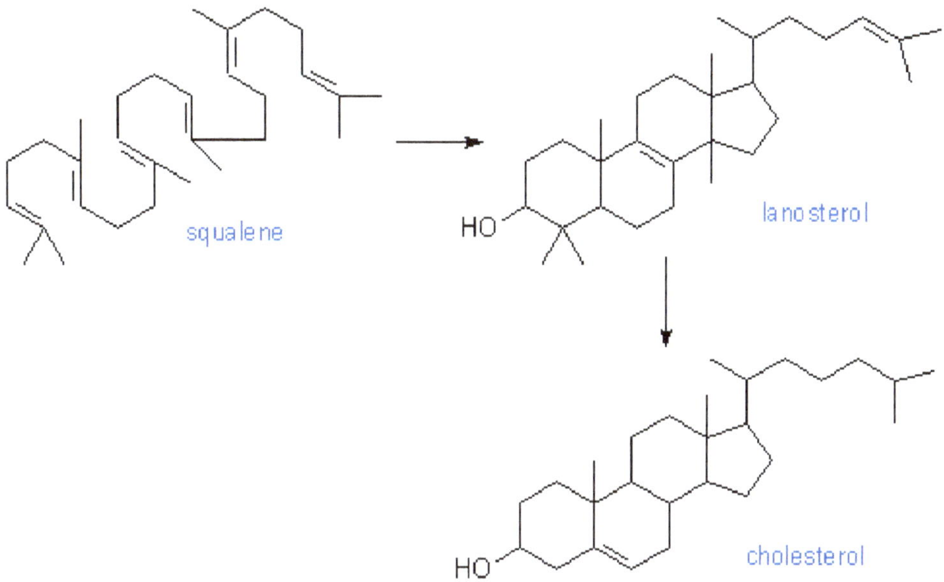

Cholesterol is a ubiquitous component of all animal tissues. It occurs in the free form and esterified to long-chain fatty acids (*cholesterol esters*) in animal tissues, including the plasma lipoproteins. Animals in general synthesise a high proportion of their cholesterol requirement, but they can also ingest and absorb appreciable amounts in their diets. Many invertebrates, including insects, cannot synthesise cholesterol and must receive it from the diet; they can also make much more use of plant sterols than do higher animals.

In plants, cholesterol is rarely present in other than small amounts, but such phytosterols as sitosterol, stigmasterol, avenasterol, campesterol and brassicasterol, and their fatty acid esters are usually found, and they perform a similar function. In plants, it tends to be a minor component only of a complex sterol fraction.

It is generally believed that the main function of cholesterol is to modulate the fluidity of membranes by interacting with their complex lipid components, specifically the phospholipids such as phosphatidylcholine and sphingomyelin, increasing the degree of order by promoting a 'liquid-ordered phase'. Cholesterol also has a key role in the lateral organization of membranes and free volume distribution, factors that control membrane protein activity. High cholesterol concentrations in membranes reduce their passive permeability to solutes. These effects permit the fine-tuning of membrane lipid composition, organization and function. There is also considerable evidence for more intimate protein-cholesterol interactions that may regulate the activities of certain membrane proteins.

Elevated cholesterol and cholesterol ester levels are associated with the pathogenesis of cardiovascular disease. It is less well known that a decrease in the concentration of cholesterol in the body can result in severe health problems, such as the autonomal recessive Smith-Lemli-Opitz syndrome in infants born with a decreased body concentration of the enzyme 7-dihydrocholesterol reductase. In animal tissues, cells can obtain the cholesterol they require either from the diet, via the circulating low-density lipoproteins (LDL)) or they can synthesise it themselves. A protein within cells that is able to sense the existing concentration of cholesterol, controls the levels.

ii) Lanosterol

It was first found in wool wax, both in free and esterified form, and this is still the main commercial source. It is found at low levels only in most other animal tissues. Similarly, other sterols may be present in tissues but almost invariably as a very small proportion of the total.

When increased levels of plasma sterols other than cholesterol are found in plasma, they usually serve as markers for abnormalities in lipid metabolism associated with disease states. For example, premature atherosclerosis and xanthomatosis occur in two rare lipid storage diseases, Cerebrotendinous xanthomatosis and sitosterolemia. In the former, cholestanol is present in all tissues, while in sitosterolemia, dietary campesterol and sitosterol accumulate in plasma and red blood cells. Inhibition of cholesterol biosynthesis may be associated with the appearance of precursor sterols in the plasma.

iii) Cholesterol Esters

Cholesterol esters, *i.e.* with long-chain fatty acids linked to the hydroxyl group, are much less polar than free cholesterol and appear to be the preferred form for transport in plasma and for storage. Those in plasma are synthesised largely by transfer of fatty acids from position sn-2 of phosphatidylcholine by the enzyme lecithin-cholesterol acyl transferase (LCAT). In other animal tissues, another enzyme acyl-CoA: cholesterol acyltransferase (ACAT,1 EC 2.3.1.26) synthesises cholesterol esters. ACAT exists in two forms, both of which are intracellular enzymes found in the endoplasmic reticulum.

Because of the action of LCAT, plasma cholesterol esters tend to contain relatively high proportions of the polyunsaturated components typical of phosphatidylcholine. Arachidonic and "adrenic" (20:4(n-6)) acids can be especially abundant in adrenal cholesterol esters.

Cholesterol esters are major constituents of the adrenal glands, where esters of steroidal hormones, may also be present at low levels. In addition, cholesterol esters accumulate in the fatty lesions of atherosclerotic plaques.

iv) Plant Sterols, Sterol Esters and Sterol Glycosides

Plants contain a rather different range of sterols from animals and some of the more common of these are illustrated below.

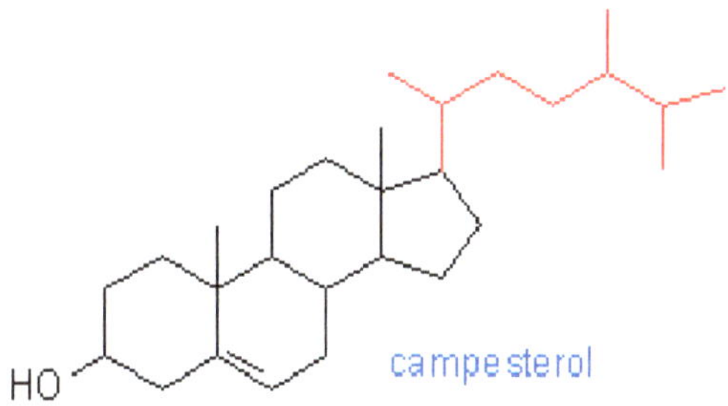

campesterol

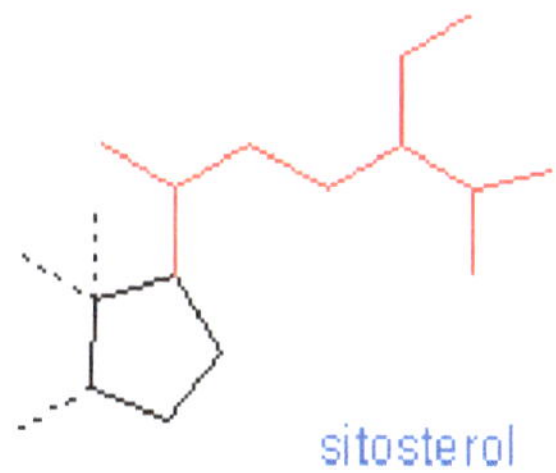

sitosterol

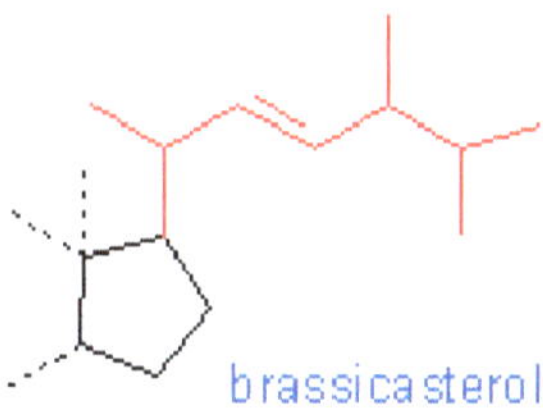

brassicasterol

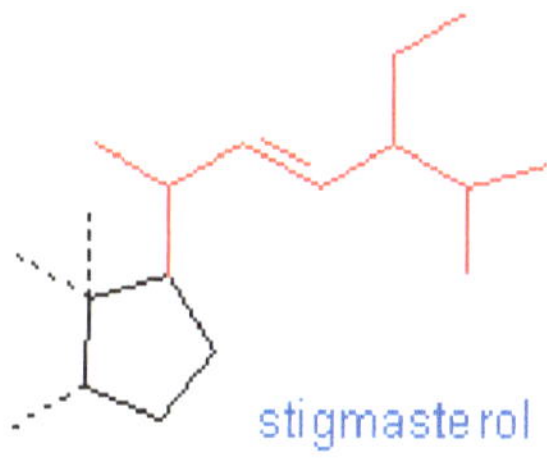

stigmasterol

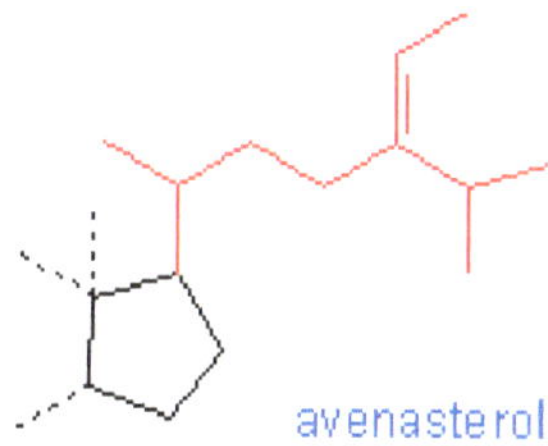

avenasterol

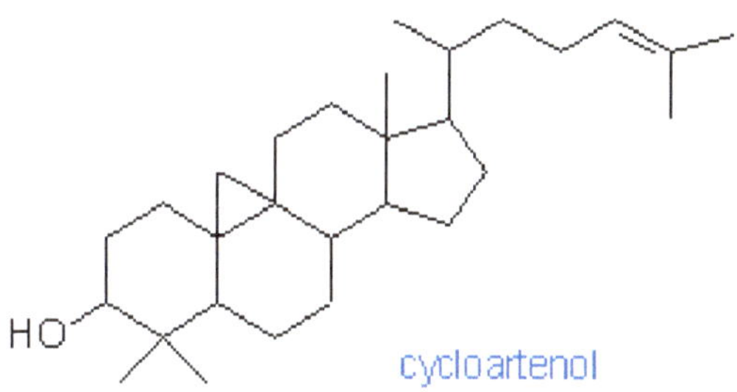

cycloartenol

Vegetable oil sterols are collectively called 'phytosterols'. These phytosterols (as opposed to zoosterols) include campesterol, β-sitosterol, stigmasterol and Δ5-avenasterol. Stigmasterol and sitosterol are the best known vegetable oil sterols. Sitosterol has been shown to reduce both serum and LDL cholesterol when incorporated into margarines and /or salad dressings. The type and amount of vegetable oil sterols vary with the source of the oil. As the name suggests, brassicasterols are found mainly in the brassica family of plants. A variety of other sterols may be present, and the amounts and relative proportions of all are dependent on the plant species. As a rough generality, a typical plant sterol mixture would be 70 per cent sitosterol, 20 per cent stigmasterol and 5 per cent campesterol.

There is increasing interest in commercial sources of plant sterols to be added as "nutraceuticals" to margarines and other foods, as it appears that they can inhibit the uptake of cholesterol from the diet. Hydrogenated phytosterols or "stanols" are also used for this purpose.

Sterol esters are also present in plant tissues, but as relatively minor components other than in waxes. Usually the sterol components of sterol esters are similar to the free sterols, although there may be relatively less of stigmasterol. The fatty acid components tend to resemble those of the other plant tissue lipids, but there can be significant differences on occasion.

The nature of the sterol and the carbohydrate moieties can vary with the plant species, and indeed the carbohydrate moiety can be quite complex with up to five hexose units linked in a linear fashion. Similarly, the nature of the fatty acid components can vary as well as the hydroxyl group to which they are linked.

The gram-negative bacterium *Helicobacter pylori*, one of the most common human pathogens, contains appreciable amounts of unique cholesterol glucosides, including cholesteryl-6-O-acyl-α-D-glucopyranoside, in its cell walls. Other than in this species, cholesteryl glucosides are rather rare in bacteria. It is known that the cholesterol of these lipids is obtained from the host and is not synthesised by bacteria.

v) Ergosterol

Ergosterol is the main sterol in fungi and yeasts, and like cholesterol is produced biosynthetically via lanosterol. Indeed some antifungal drugs are targeted against ergosterol biosynthesis. Ergosterol stabilizes the liquid-ordered phase in the same manner as cholesterol, whereas lanosterol does not. It is also evident that ergosterol has a multiplicity of functions in the regulation of yeast growth.

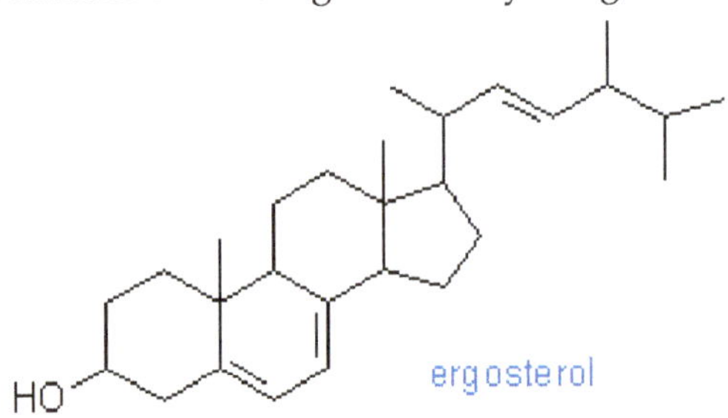

vi) Cholesterol 3-sulfate

The strongly acidic sulfate ester of cholesterol occurs in all mammalian cells, but it is especially abundant in keratinized tissue, such as skin and hooves. Although present at low levels, it can be the main sulfolipid in many cell types, but especially kidney, and reproductive and nervous tissues. Sterols sulfates have been detected occasionally in lower life forms, such as the sea star, *Asterius rubrius*, and the marine diatom, *Nitzschia alba*.

Cholesterol sulfate may have a role in ensuring the integrity and adhesion of the various skin layers, while also regulating some enzyme activities.

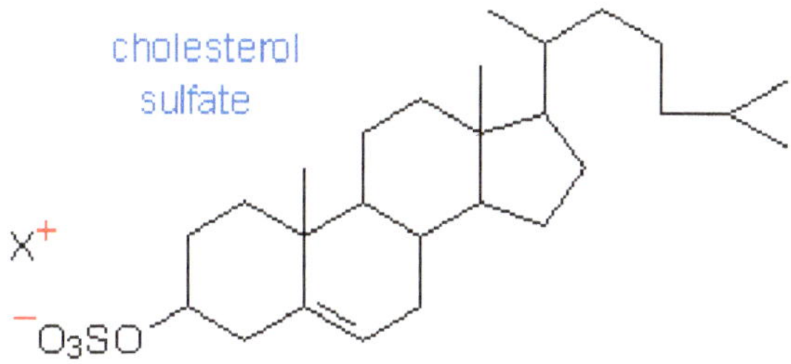

In many organs, it appears to be concentrated in epithelial cell walls or in plasma membranes. The function of this lipid is still only partly understood, but it may play a part in cell adhesion, differentiation and signal transduction. In addition, it has a stabilizing role, for example in protecting erythrocytes from osmotic lysis and regulating sperm capacitation.

vii) 7-dehydrocholesterol

It is found in animal tissues and underneath skin. It is converted to D_3 on irradiation.

c. Androgens and Estrogens (Sex Hormones)

They are found in ovaries and testes.

d. Adrenal Corticolsteroids

They occur in adrenal cortex, blood.

4. Derived Lipids

They occur in plant and animal foods; also exhibit in complex forms with other substances. They are obtained from hydrolysis of simple and complex lipids and usually contain an even number of carbon atoms and are straight chain derivatives. These lipids contain glycerol, free fatty acids and other alcohols. These are sometimes present as waste products of metabolism.

As the name suggests, free fatty acids are the unattached fatty acids present in a fat. Some unrefined oils may contain as much as several percent free fatty acids. The levels of free fatty acids are reduced in the refining process. Fully refined fats and oils usually have a free fatty acid content of less than 0.1 per cent.

Classification of fatty acids is based on the length of the carbon chain (short, medium, or long); the number of double bonds (unsaturated, mono-, or polyunsaturated); or essentiality in the diet (essential or non-essential). A current designation is based on the position of the endmost double bond, counting from the methyl (CH_3) carbon, called the omega end. The most important omega fatty acids are: Omega 6–linoleinc and arachidonic acids and Omega 3–linolenic, eicosapentaenoic, and docosahexaenoic acids.

Sample Nomenclature for Fatty Acids

Name	*Carbon Length : Number of Double Bonds*	*Position of Double Bond*
Butyric acid	4:0	–
Palmitic acid	16:0	–
Oleic acid	18:1	(9)
Linoleic acid	18:2	(9,12)
Linolenic acid	18:3	(9,12,15)
Arachidonic acid	20:4	(5,8,11,14)
Eicosapentaenoic acid	20:5	(5,8,11,14,17)
Docosahexaenoic acid	22:6	(4,7,10,13,16,19)

Saturated fatty acids have commonly straight chains and even carbon number (4-30). They have the general formula: $CH_3\,(CH)_n COOH$. They are named from the saturated hydrocarbon with the same number of carbon atoms, the final -e is changed to **-oic**. For example, the fatty acid with 18 carbon atoms is correctly termed octadecanoic acid but it has also a trivial name (as several common fatty acids), *i.e.* stearic acid. This compound may be defined also 18:0. Below, is found a list of the most common saturated fatty acids.

Saturated Fatty Acids

Systematic Name	*Trivial Name*	*Shorthand Designation*	*Molecular Wt.*	*Melting Point (°C)*
Butanoic	Butyric	4:0	88.1	–7.9
Pentanoic	Valeric	5:0		
Hexanoic	Caproic	6:0	116.1	–3.4
Octanoic	Caprylic	8:0	144.2	16.7
Nonanoic	Pelargonic	9:0	158.2	12.5
Decanoic	Capric	10:0	172.3	31.6
Dodecanoic	Lauric	12:0	200.3	44.2
Tetradecanoic	Myristic	14:0	228.4	53.9
Hexadecanoic	Palmitic	16:0	256.4	63.1
Heptadecanoic	Margaric (Daturic)	17:0	270.4	61.3
Octadecanoic	Stearic	18:0	284.4	69.6
Eicosanoic	Arachidic	20:0	312.5	75.3
Docosanoic	Behenic	22:0	340.5	79.9
Tetracosanoic	Lignoceric	24:0	368.6	84.2
Hexacosanoic	Cerotic	26:0	396.7	88
Heptacosanoic	Carboceric	27:0	410.7	
Octacosanoic	Montanic	28:0	424.8	

Contd...

Contd...

Systematic Name	*Trivial Name*	*Shorthand Designation*	*Molecular Wt.*	*Melting Point (°C)*
Triacontanoic	Melissic	30:0	452.9	
Dotriacontanoic	Lacceroic	32:0	481	
Tritriacontanoic	Ceromelissic (Psyllic)	33:0	495	
Tetratriacontanoic	Geddic	34:0	509.1	
Pentatriacontanoic	Ceroplastic	35:0	523.1	

Unsaturated Fatty Acids

This group of fatty acids is characterized by having one or more double bonds or ethylenic groups. They can be monoethenoic, dienoic, trienoic and polyenoic depending on the number of double bonds present.

Common name	*Chemical structure*	*D^x*	*C:D*	*n–x*
Myristoleic acid	$CH_3(CH_2)_3$**CH=CH**$(CH_2)_7COOH$	*cis*-Δ^9	14:1	*n*–5
Palmitoleic acid	$CH_3(CH_2)_5$**CH=CH**$(CH_2)_7COOH$	*cis*-Δ^9	16:1	*n*–7
Sapienic acid		*cis*-Δ^6	16:1	*n*–10
Oleic acid	$CH_3(CH_2)_7$**CH=CH**$(CH_2)_7COOH$	*cis*-Δ^9	18:1	*n*–9
Linoleic acid	$CH_3(CH_2)_4$**CH=CH**CH_2**CH=CH**$(CH_2)_7$ COOH	*cis,cis*-Δ^9,Δ^{12}	18:2	*n*–6
α-Linolenic acid	CH_3CH_2**CH=CH**CH_2**CH=CH**CH_2 **CH=CH**$(CH_2)_7COOH$	*cis,cis,cis*-$\Delta^9,\Delta^{12},\Delta^{15}$	18:3	*n*–3
Arachidonic acid	$CH_3(CH_2)_4$**CH=CH**CH_2**CH=CH**CH_2 **CH=CH**CH_2**CH=CH**$(CH_2)_3COOH^{NIST}$	*cis,cis,cis,cis*-$\Delta^5\Delta^8,\Delta^{11},\Delta^{14}$	20:4	*n*–6
Eicosapentaenoic acid	CH_3CH_2**CH=CH**CH_2**CH=CH**CH_2 **CH=CH**CH_2**CH=CH**CH_2**CH=CH** $(CH_2)_3COOH$	*cis,cis,cis,cis,cis*-$\Delta^5,\Delta^8,\Delta^{11},\Delta^{14},\Delta^{17}$	20:5	*n*–3
Erucic acid	$CH_3(CH_2)_7$**CH=CH**$(CH_2)_{11}COOH$	*cis*-Δ^{13}	22:1	*n*–9
Docosahexaenoic acid	CH_3CH_2**CH=CH**CH_2**CH=CH**CH_2 **CH=CH**CH_2**CH=CH**CH_2**CH=** **CH**CH_2**CH=CH**$(CH_2)_2COOH$	*cis,cis,cis,cis, cis,cis*-$\Delta^4,\Delta^7,\Delta^{10},\Delta^{13},\Delta^{16},\Delta^{19}$	22:6	*n*–3

Classification of Lipids According to Lipid Library, UK

According to lipid library, UK, the classification of lipids is dicussed in detail as under..

Simple Lipids:

- ☆ Triacylglycerols
- ☆ Di- and monoacylglycerols
- ☆ Sterols and sterol esters
- ☆ Tocopherols and other isoprenoids

Free (unesterified) fatty acids:

- ☆ Cyanolipids
- ☆ Waxes

Complex Glycerolipids:

- ☆ Ether lipids
- ☆ Phosphatidic acid and related lipids
- ☆ Phosphatidylglycerol and related lipids
- ☆ Diphosphatidylglycerol (cardiolipin)
- ☆ Phosphatidylinositol and related lipids
- ☆ Phosphatidylserine
- ☆ Phosphatidylethanolamine
- ☆ Phosphatidylcholine
- ☆ Mono- and digalactosyldiacylglycerols and from plants and microorganisms, etc.
- ☆ Glycosyldiacylglycerols and related lipids from animals
- ☆ Glycophospholipids

Some Miscellaneous Lipids:

- ☆ Phosphonolipids
- ☆ Carnitine and acylcarnitines
- ☆ Coenzyme A esters
- ☆ Proteolipids
- ☆ Anandamide, oleamide and other fatty amides
- ☆ Lipid A and bacterial lipopolysaccharides
- ☆ Sulfonolipids
- ☆ Betaine lipids

Sphingolipids:

- ☆ Introduction + rafts
- ☆ Long-chain or sphingoid bases
- ☆ Ceramides
- ☆ Sphingomyelin and related lipids

Sphingosine-1-phosphate:

- ☆ Monoglycosylceramides (cerebrosides)
- ☆ Oligoglycosylceramides (neutral)
- ☆ Gangliosides
- ☆ Sulfoglycosphingolipids

Fatty acids:

- ☆ Saturated straight-chain
- ☆ Monoenoic straight-chain
- ☆ Methylene-interrupted polyenoic
- ☆ Conjugated and multimethylene-interrupted polyenoic
- ☆ Branched-chain
- ☆ Cyclic (natural)
- ☆ Hydroxy, epoxy and furanoid

Eicosanoids and related lipids:

- ☆ Introduction–structures and key enzymes
- ☆ Isoprostanes
- ☆ Prostaglandins, prostacyclins and thromboxanes
- ☆ Hydroxyeicosatetraenoic acids and related compounds
- ☆ Leukotrienes and lipoxins
- ☆ Resolvins and neuroprotectins
- ☆ Plant oxylipins

Lipid Classification Scheme- LIPID MAPS Structure Database (LMSD)

Lipids are produced, transported, and recognized by the concerted actions of numerous enzymes, binding proteins, and receptors. A comprehensive analysis of lipid molecules, lipidomics, in the context of genomics and proteomics is crucial to understanding cellular physiology and pathology; consequently, lipid biology has become a major research target of the postgenomic revolution and systems biology. To facilitate international communication about lipids, a comprehensive classification of lipids with a common platform that is compatible with informatics requirements have been developed to deal with the massive amounts of datas that has been generated by lipid community (Fahy *et al.*, 2005, 2009).

The new system is part of an effort by the Lipid Metabolites and Pathways Strategy (LIPID MAPS) consortium to produce a detailed understanding of the structure and function of all the lipids within a cell. The consortium is a large collaborative effort led by the University of California, San Diego. More than 30 researchers at 18 universities, medical research institutes and companies across the United States participated in this research.

The LIPID MAPS Lipid Classification System developed by Fahy *et al.* (2009) is comprised of eight lipid categories, each with its own subclassification hierarchy. They have devised a common manner of representing the chemical structures of individual lipids and their derivatives, and provided a 12 digit identifier for each unique lipid molecule and it is called as LMSD. All lipids in the LIPID MAPS Structure Database (LMSD) have been classified using this system and have been assigned LIPID MAPS ID's (LM_ID) which reflects their position in the classification hierarchy. Starting from a lipid category, one can drill down through the hierarchy to the LMSD record for an individual lipid, where one will find an image of the molecular structure, common and systematic names, links to external databases, other annotations and links to structure viewing tools.

This lipid classification scheme is chemically based and driven by the distinct hydrophobic and hydrophilic elements that compose the lipid. This structured vocabulary will facilitate the systematization of lipid biology and enable the cataloguing of lipids and their properties in a way that is compatible with other macromolecular databases.

Eight Major Categories of Lipids according to LMSD

1. Fatty Acyls
2. Glycerolipids
3. Glycerophospholipids
4. Sphingolipids
5. Sterol lipids
6. Phenol lipids
7. Saccharolipids
8. Polyketides

Sub-classification is as under:

Fatty Acyls (FA)

- ✰ Fatty Acids and Conjugates **[FA01]**
- ✰ Straight chain fatty acids **[FA0101]**

- ☆ Methyl branched fatty acids **[FA0102]**
- ☆ Unsaturated fatty acids **[FA0103]**
- ☆ Hydroperoxy fatty acids **[FA0104]**
- ☆ Hydroxy fatty acids **[FA0105]**
- ☆ Oxo fatty acids **[FA0106]**
- ☆ Epoxy fatty acids **[FA0107]**
- ☆ Methoxy fatty acids **[FA0108]**
- ☆ Halogenated fatty acids **[FA0109]**
- ☆ Amino fatty acids **[FA0110]**
- ☆ Cyano fatty acids **[FA0111]**
- ☆ Nitro fatty acids **[FA0112]**
- ☆ Thia fatty acids **[FA0113]**
- ☆ Carbocyclic fatty acids **[FA0114]**
- ☆ Heterocyclic fatty acids **[FA0115]**
- ☆ Mycolic acids **[FA0116]**
- ☆ Dicarboxylic acids **[FA0117]**
- ☆ ⊞Octadecanoids **[FA02]**
- ☆ 12-oxophytodienoic acid metabolites **[FA0201]**
- ☆ Jasmonic acids **[FA0202]**
- ☆ Other Octadecanoids **[FA0200]**
- ☆ ⊞Eicosanoids **[FA03]**
- ☆ Prostaglandins **[FA0301]**
- ☆ Leukotrienes **[FA0302]**
- ☆ Thromboxanes **[FA0303]**
- ☆ Lipoxins **[FA0304]**
- ☆ Hydroxy/hydroperoxyeicosatrienoic acids **[FA0305]**
- ☆ Hydroxy/hydroperoxyeicosatetraenoic acids **[FA0306]**
- ☆ Hydroxy/hydroperoxyeicosapentaenoic acids **[FA0307]**
- ☆ Epoxyeicosatrienoic acids **[FA0308]**
- ☆ Hepoxilins **[FA0309]**
- ☆ Levuglandins **[FA0310]**
- ☆ Isoprostanes **[FA0311]**
- ☆ Clavulones and derivatives **[FA0312]**
- ☆ Other Eicosanoids **[FA0300]**
- ☆ Docosanoids **[FA04]**
- ☆ Fatty alcohols **[FA05]**
- ☆ Fatty aldehydes **[FA06]**

- ☆ ⊞Fatty esters **[FA07]**
- ☆ Wax monoesters **[FA0701]**
- ☆ Wax diesters **[FA0702]**
- ☆ Cyano esters **[FA0703]**
- ☆ Lactones **[FA0704]**
- ☆ Fatty acyl CoAs **[FA0705]**
- ☆ Fatty acyl ACPs **[FA0706]**
- ☆ Fatty acyl carnitines **[FA0707]**
- ☆ Fatty acyl adenylates **[FA0708]**
- ☆ ⊞Fatty amides **[FA08]**
- ☆ Primary amides **[FA0801]**
- ☆ N-acyl amines **[FA0802]**
- ☆ Fatty acyl homoserine lactones **[FA0803]**
- ☆ N-acyl ethanolamines (endocannabinoids) **[FA0804]**
- ☆ Fatty nitriles **[FA09]**
- ☆ Fatty ethers **[FA10]**
- ☆ Hydrocarbons **[FA11]**
- ☆ Oxygenated hydrocarbons **[FA12]**
- ☆ ⊞Fatty acyl glycosides **[FA13]**
- ☆ Fatty acyl glycosides of mono- and disaccharides **[FA1301]**
- ☆ Sophorolipids **[FA1302]**
- ☆ Rhamnolipids **[FA1303]**
- ☆ Other Fatty acyl glycosides **[FA1300]**
- ☆ Other Fatty Acyls **[FA00]**

Glycerolipids [GL]

- ☆ Monoradylglycerols **[GL01]**
- ☆ Monoacylglycerols **[GL0101]**
- ☆ Monoalkylglycerols **[GL0102]**
- ☆ Mono-(1Z-alkenyl)-glycerols **[GL0103]**
- ☆ ⊞Diradylglycerols **[GL02]**
- ☆ Diacylglycerols **[GL0201]**
- ☆ 1-alkyl,2-acylglycerols **[GL0202]**
- ☆ 1-acyl,2-alkylglycerols **[GL0207]**
- ☆ Dialkylglycerols **[GL0203]**
- ☆ 1Z-alkenylacylglycerols **[GL0204]**
- ☆ Di-glycerol tetraethers **[GL0205]**

- ☆ Di-glycerol tetraether glycans **[GL0206]**
- ☆ Triradylglycerols **[GL03]**
- ☆ Triacylglycerols **[GL0301]**
- ☆ Alkyldiacylglycerols **[GL0302]**
- ☆ Dialkylmonoacylglycerols **[GL0303]**
- ☆ 1Z-alkenyldiacylglycerols **[GL0304]**
- ☆ Estolides **[GL0305]**
- ☆ ⊞Glycosylmonoradylglycerols **[GL04]**
- ☆ Glycosylmonoacylglycerols **[GL0401]**
- ☆ Glycosylmonoalkylglycerols **[GL0402]**
- ☆ ⊞Glycosyldiradylglycerols **[GL05]**
- ☆ Glycosyldiacylglycerols **[GL0501]**
- ☆ Glycosylalkylacylglycerols **[GL0502]**
- ☆ Glycosyldialkylglycerols **[GL0503]**
- ☆ Other Glycerolipids **[GL00]**

Glycerophospholipids [GP]

- ☆ ⊞Glycerophosphocholines **[GP01]**
- ☆ Diacylglycerophosphocholines **[GP0101]**
- ☆ 1-alkyl,2-acylglycerophosphocholines **[GP0102]**
- ☆ 1-acyl,2-alkylglycerophosphocholines **[GP0108]**
- ☆ 1Z-alkenyl,2-acylglycerophosphocholines **[GP0103]**
- ☆ Dialkylglycerophosphocholines **[GP0104]**
- ☆ Monoacylglycerophosphocholines **[GP0105]**
- ☆ Monoalkylglycerophosphocholines **[GP0106]**
- ☆ 1Z-alkenylglycerophosphocholines **[GP0107]**
- ☆ ⊞Glycerophosphoethanolamines **[GP02]**
- ☆ Diacylglycerophosphoethanolamines **[GP0201]**
- ☆ 1-alkyl,2-acylglycerophosphoethanolamines **[GP0202]**
- ☆ 1-acyl,2-alkylglycerophosphoethanolamines **[GP0208]**
- ☆ 1Z-alkenyl,2-acylglycerophosphoethanolamines **[GP0203]**
- ☆ Dialkylglycerophosphoethanolamines **[GP0204]**
- ☆ Monoacylglycerophosphoethanolamines **[GP0205]**
- ☆ Monoalkylglycerophosphoethanolamines **[GP0206]**
- ☆ 1Z-alkenylglycerophosphoethanolamines **[GP0207]**
- ☆ ⊞Glycerophosphoserines **[GP03]**
- ☆ Diacylglycerophosphoserines **[GP0301]**

- ☆ 1-alkyl,2-acylglycerophosphoserines **[GP0302]**
- ☆ 1Z-alkenyl,2-acylglycerophosphoserines **[GP0303]**
- ☆ Dialkylglycerophosphoserines **[GP0304]**
- ☆ Monoacylglycerophosphoserines **[GP0305]**
- ☆ Monoalkylglycerophosphoserines **[GP0306]**
- ☆ 1Z-alkenylglycerophosphoserines **[GP0307]**
- ☆ ⊞Glycerophosphoglycerols **[GP04]**
- ☆ Diacylglycerophosphoglycerols **[GP0401]**
- ☆ 1-alkyl,2-acylglycerophosphoglycerols **[GP0402]**
- ☆ 1-acyl,2-alkylglycerophosphoglycerols **[GP0411]**
- ☆ 1Z-alkenyl,2-acylglycerophosphoglycerols **[GP0403]**
- ☆ Dialkylglycerophosphoglycerols **[GP0404]**
- ☆ Monoacylglycerophosphoglycerols **[GP0405]**
- ☆ Monoalkylglycerophosphoglycerols **[GP0406]**
- ☆ 1Z-alkenylglycerophosphoglycerols **[GP0407]**
- ☆ Diacylglycerophosphodiradylglycerols **[GP0408]**
- ☆ Diacylglycerophosphomonoradylglycerols **[GP0409]**
- ☆ Monoacylglycerophosphomonoradylglycerols **[GP0410]**
- ☆ ⊞Glycerophosphoglycerophosphates **[GP05]**
- ☆ Diacylglycerophosphoglycerophosphates **[GP0501]**
- ☆ 1-alkyl,2-acylglycerophosphoglycerophosphates **[GP0502]**
- ☆ 1Z-alkenyl,2-acylglycerophosphoglycerophosphates **[GP0503]**
- ☆ Dialkylglycerophosphoglycerophosphates **[GP0504]**
- ☆ Monoacylglycerophosphoglycerophosphates **[GP0505]**
- ☆ Monoalkylglycerophosphoglycerophosphates **[GP0506]**
- ☆ 1Z-alkenylglycerophosphoglycerophosphates **[GP0507]**
- ☆ ⊞Glycerophosphoinositols **[GP06]**
- ☆ Diacylglycerophosphoinositols **[GP0601]**
- ☆ 1-alkyl,2-acylglycerophosphoinositols **[GP0602]**
- ☆ 1Z-alkenyl,2-acylglycerophosphoinositols **[GP0603]**
- ☆ Dialkylglycerophosphoinositols **[GP0604]**
- ☆ Monoacylglycerophosphoinositols **[GP0605]**
- ☆ Monoalkylglycerophosphoinositols **[GP0606]**
- ☆ 1Z-alkenylglycerophosphoinositols **[GP0607]**
- ☆ ⊞Glycerophosphoinositol monophosphates **[GP07]**
- ☆ Diacylglycerophosphoinositol monophosphates **[GP0701]**
- ☆ 1-alkyl,2-acylglycerophosphoinositol monophosphates **[GP0702]**

- ☆ 1Z-alkenyl,2-acylglycerophosphoinositol monophosphates **[GP0703]**
- ☆ Dialkylglycerophosphoinositol monophosphates **[GP0704]**
- ☆ Monoacylglycerophosphoinositol monophosphates **[GP0705]**
- ☆ Monoalkylglycerophosphoinositol monophosphates **[GP0706]**
- ☆ 1Z-alkenylglycerophosphoinositol monophosphates **[GP0707]**
- ☆ ⊞Glycerophosphoinositol bisphosphates **[GP08]**
- ☆ Diacylglycerophosphoinositol bisphosphates **[GP0801]**
- ☆ 1-alkyl,2-acylglycerophosphoinositol bisphosphates **[GP0802]**
- ☆ 1Z-alkenyl,2-acylglycerophosphoinositol bisphosphates **[GP0803]**
- ☆ Monoacylglycerophosphoinositol bisphosphates **[GP0804]**
- ☆ Monoalkylglycerophosphoinositol bisphosphates **[GP0805]**
- ☆ 1Z-alkenylglycerophosphoinositol bisphosphates **[GP0806]**
- ☆ ⊞Glycerophosphoinositol trisphosphates **[GP09]**
- ☆ Diacylglycerophosphoinositol trisphosphates **[GP0901]**
- ☆ 1-alkyl,2-acylglycerophosphoinositol trisphosphates **[GP0902]**
- ☆ 1Z-alkenyl,2-acylglycerophosphoinositol trisphosphates **[GP0903]**
- ☆ Monoacylglycerophosphoinositol trisphosphates **[GP0904]**
- ☆ Monoalkylglycerophosphoinositol trisphosphates **[GP0905]**
- ☆ 1Z-alkenylglycerophosphoinositol trisphosphates **[GP0906]**
- ☆ ⊞Glycerophosphates **[GP10]**
- ☆ Diacylglycerophosphates **[GP1001]**
- ☆ 1-alkyl,2-acylglycerophosphates **[GP1002]**
- ☆ 1Z-alkenyl,2-acylglycerophosphates **[GP1003]**
- ☆ Dialkylglycerophosphates **[GP1004]**
- ☆ Monoacylglycerophosphates **[GP1005]**
- ☆ Monoalkylglycerophosphates **[GP1006]**
- ☆ 1Z-alkenylglycerophosphates **[GP1007]**
- ☆ ⊞Glyceropyrophosphates **[GP11]**
- ☆ Diacylglyceropyrophosphates **[GP1101]**
- ☆ Monoacylglyceropyrophosphates **[GP1102]**
- ☆ ⊞Glycerophosphoglycerophosphoglycerols **[GP12]**
- ☆ Diacylglycerophosphoglycerophosphodiradylglycerols **[GP1201]**
- ☆ Diacylglycerophosphoglycerophosphomonoradylglycerols **[GP1202]**
- ☆ 1-alkyl,2-acylglycerophosphoglycerophosphodiradylglycerols **[GP1203]**
- ☆ 1-alkyl,2-acylglycerophosphoglycerophosphomonoradylglycerols **[GP1204]**
- ☆ 1Z-alkenyl,2-acylglycerophosphoglycerophosphodiradylglycerols **[GP1205]**

- ☆ 1Z-alkenyl,2-acylglycerophosphoglycerophosphomonoradylglycerols **[GP1206]**
- ☆ Dialkylglycerophosphoglycerophosphodiradylglycerols **[GP1212]**
- ☆ Dialkylglycerophosphoglycerophosphomonoradylglycerols **[GP1213]**
- ☆ Monoacylglycerophosphoglycerophosphomonoradylglycerols **[GP1207]**
- ☆ Monoalkylglycerophosphoglycerophosphodiradylglycerols **[GP1208]**
- ☆ Monoalkylglycerophosphoglycerophosphomonoradylglycerols **[GP1209]**
- ☆ 1Z-alkenylglycerophosphoglycerophosphodiradylglycerols **[GP1210]**
- ☆ 1Z-alkenylglycerophosphoglycerophosphomonoradylglycerols **[GP1211]**
- ☆ ⊞CDP-Glycerols **[GP13]**
- ☆ CDP-diacylglycerols **[GP1301]**
- ☆ CDP-1-alkyl,2-acylglycerols **[GP1302]**
- ☆ CDP-1Z-alkenyl,2-acylglycerols **[GP1303]**
- ☆ CDP-Dialkylglycerols **[GP1304]**
- ☆ CDP-Monoacylglycerols **[GP1305]**
- ☆ CDP-Monoalkylglycerols **[GP1306]**
- ☆ CDP-1Z-alkenylglycerols **[GP1307]**
- ☆ ⊞Glycosylglycerophospholipids **[GP14]**
- ☆ Diacylglycosylglycerophospholipids **[GP1401]**
- ☆ 1-alkyl,2-acylglycosylglycerophospholipids **[GP1402]**
- ☆ 1Z-alkenyl,2-acylglycosylglycerophospholipids **[GP1403]**
- ☆ Dialkylglycosylglycerophospholipids **[GP1407]**
- ☆ Monoacylglycosylglycerophospholipids **[GP1404]**
- ☆ Monoalkylglycosylglycerophospholipids **[GP1405]**
- ☆ 1Z-alkenylglycosylglycerophospholipids **[GP1406]**
- ☆ ⊞Glycerophosphoinositolglycans **[GP15]**
- ☆ Diacylglycerophosphoinositolglycans **[GP1501]**
- ☆ 1-alkyl,2-acylglycerophosphoinositolglycans **[GP1502]**
- ☆ 1Z-alkenyl,2-acylglycerophosphoinositolglycans **[GP1503]**
- ☆ Monoacylglycerophosphoinositolglycans **[GP1504]**
- ☆ Monoalkylglycerophosphoinositolglycans **[GP1505]**
- ☆ 1Z-alkenylglycerophosphoinositolglycans **[GP1506]**
- ☆ ⊞Glycerophosphonocholines **[GP16]**
- ☆ Diacylglycerophosphonocholines **[GP1601]**
- ☆ 1-alkyl,2-acylglycerophosphonocholines **[GP1602]**
- ☆ 1Z-alkenyl,2-acylglycerophosphonocholines **[GP1603]**
- ☆ Dialkylglycerophosphonocholines **[GP1604]**

- ☆ Monoacylglycerophosphonocholines **[GP1605]**
- ☆ Monoalkylglycerophosphonocholines **[GP1606]**
- ☆ 1Z-alkenylglycerophosphonocholines **[GP1607]**
- ☆ ⊞Glycerophosphonoethanolamines **[GP17]**
- ☆ Diacylglycerophosphonoethanolamines **[GP1701]**
- ☆ 1-alkyl,2-acylglycerophosphonoethanolamines **[GP1702]**
- ☆ 1Z-alkenyl,2-acylglycerophosphonoethanolamines **[GP1703]**
- ☆ Dialkylglycerophosphonoethanolamines **[GP1704]**
- ☆ Monoacylglycerophosphonoethanolamines **[GP1705]**
- ☆ Monoalkylglycerophosphonoethanolamines **[GP1706]**
- ☆ 1Z-alkenylglycerophosphonoethanolamines **[GP1707]**
- ☆ Di-glycerol tetraether phospholipids (caldarchaeols) **[GP18]**
- ☆ Glycerol-nonitol tetraether phospholipids **[GP19]**
- ☆ Oxidized glycerophospholipids **[GP20]**
- ☆ Other Glycerophospholipids **[GP00]**

Sphingolipids [SP]

- ☆ Sphingoid bases **[SP01]**
- ☆ Sphing-4-enines (Sphingosines) **[SP0101]**
- ☆ Sphinganines **[SP0102]**
- ☆ 4-Hydroxysphinganines (Phytosphingosines) **[SP0103]**
- ☆ Sphingoid base homologs and variants **[SP0104]**
- ☆ Sphingoid base 1-phosphates **[SP0105]**
- ☆ Lysosphingomyelins and lysoglycosphingolipids **[SP0106]**
- ☆ N-methylated sphingoid bases **[SP0107]**
- ☆ Sphingoid base analogs **[SP0108]**
- ☆ Ceramides **[SP02]**
- ☆ N-acylsphingosines (ceramides) **[SP0201]**
- ☆ N-acylsphinganines (dihydroceramides) **[SP0202]**
- ☆ N-acyl-4-hydroxysphinganines (phytoceramides) **[SP0203]**
- ☆ Acylceramides **[SP0204]**
- ☆ Ceramide 1-phosphates **[SP0205]**
- ☆ Phosphosphingolipids **[SP03]**
- ☆ Ceramide phosphocholines (sphingomyelins) **[SP0301]**
- ☆ Ceramide phosphoethanolamines **[SP0302]**
- ☆ Ceramide phosphoinositols **[SP0303]**
- ☆ Phosphonosphingolipids **[SP04]**

- ☆ GalNAcβ1-4GlcNAcβ1-3Manβ1-4Glc- (Arthro series) **[SP0508]**
- ☆ Gal- (Gala series) **[SP0509]**
- ☆ Other Neutral glycosphingolipids **[SP0500]**
- ☆ Neutral glycosphingolipids **[SP05]**
- ☆ Simple Glc series **[SP0501]**
- ☆ GalNAcβ1-3Galα1-4Galβ1-4Glc- (Globo series) **[SP0502]**
- ☆ GalNAcβ1-4Galβ1-4Glc- (Ganglio series) **[SP0503]**
- ☆ Galβ1-3GlcNAcβ1-3Galβ1-4Glc- (Lacto series) **[SP0504]**
- ☆ Galβ1-4GlcNAcβ1-3Galβ1-4Glc- (Neolacto series) **[SP0505]**
- ☆ GalNAcβ1-3Galα1-3Galβ1-4Glc- (Isoglobo series) **[SP0506]**
- ☆ GlcNAcβ1-2Manα1-3Manβ1-4Glc- (Mollu series) **[SP0507]**
- ☆ Acidic glycosphingolipids **[SP06]**
- ☆ Gangliosides **[SP0601]**
- ☆ Sulfoglycosphingolipids (sulfatides) **[SP0602]**
- ☆ Glucuronosphingolipids **[SP0603]**
- ☆ Phosphoglycosphingolipids **[SP0604]**
- ☆ Other Acidic glycosphingolipids **[SP0600]**
- ☆ Basic glycosphingolipids **[SP07]**
- ☆ Amphoteric glycosphingolipids **[SP08]**
- ☆ Arsenosphingolipids **[SP09]**
- ☆ Other Sphingolipids **[SP00]**

Sterol Lipids [ST]

- ☆ Sterols **[ST01]**
- ☆ Cholesterol and derivatives **[ST0101]**
- ☆ Cholesteryl esters **[ST0102]**
- ☆ Ergosterols and C24-methyl derivatives **[ST0103]**
- ☆ Stigmasterols and C24-ethyl derivatives **[ST0104]**
- ☆ C24-propyl sterols and derivatives **[ST0105]**
- ☆ Gorgosterols and derivatives **[ST0106]**
- ☆ Furostanols and derivatives **[ST0107]**
- ☆ Spirostanols and derivatives **[ST0108]**
- ☆ Furospirostanols and derivatives **[ST0109]**
- ☆ Cycloartanols and derivatives **[ST0110]**
- ☆ Calysterols and derivatives **[ST0111]**
- ☆ Cardanolides and derivatives **[ST0112]**
- ☆ Bufanolides and derivatives **[ST0113]**

- ☆ Brassinolides and derivatives **[ST0114]**
- ☆ Solanidines and alkaloid derivatives **[ST0115]**
- ☆ Steroids **[ST02]**
- ☆ C18 steroids (estrogens) and derivatives **[ST0201]**
- ☆ C19 steroids (androgens) and derivatives **[ST0202]**
- ☆ C21 steroids (gluco/mineralocorticoids, progestogins) and derivatives **[ST0203]**
- ☆ Secosteroids **[ST03]**
- ☆ Vitamin D2 and derivatives **[ST0301]**
- ☆ Vitamin D3 and derivatives **[ST0302]**
- ☆ Vitamin D4 and derivatives **[ST0303]**
- ☆ Vitamin D5 and derivatives **[ST0304]**
- ☆ Vitamin D6 and derivatives **[ST0305]**
- ☆ Vitamin D7 and derivatives **[ST0306]**
- ☆ Bile acids and derivatives **[ST04]**
- ☆ C24 bile acids, alcohols, and derivatives **[ST0401]**
- ☆ C26 bile acids, alcohols, and derivatives **[ST0402]**
- ☆ C27 bile acids, alcohols, and derivatives **[ST0403]**
- ☆ C28 bile acids, alcohols, and derivatives **[ST0404]**
- ☆ C22 bile acids, alcohols, and derivatives **[ST0405]**
- ☆ C23 bile acids, alcohols, and derivatives **[ST0406]**
- ☆ C25 bile acids, alcohols, and derivatives **[ST0407]**
- ☆ C29 bile acids, alcohols, and derivatives **[ST0408]**
- ☆ Steroid conjugates **[ST05]**
- ☆ Glucuronides **[ST0501]**
- ☆ Sulfates **[ST0502]**
- ☆ Glycine conjugates **[ST0503]**
- ☆ Taurine conjugates **[ST0504]**
- ☆ Other Sterol lipids **[ST00]**

Prenol Lipids [PR]

- ☆ Isoprenoids **[PR01]**
- ☆ C5 isoprenoids (hemiterpenes) **[PR0101]**
- ☆ C10 isoprenoids (monoterpenes) **[PR0102]**
- ☆ Acyclic monoterpenoids **[PR010201]**
- ☆ Irregular acyclic monoterpenoids **[PR010202]**
- ☆ Halogenated dimethyloctane monoterpenoids **[PR010203]**

- ☆ Ochtodane monoterpenoids **[PR010204]**
- ☆ Ethyl,dimethylcyclohexane monoterpenoids **[PR010205]**
- ☆ Cyclopropane and cyclobutane monoterpenoids **[PR010206]**
- ☆ Iridoid, 10-alkyliridoid and secoiridoid monoterpenoids **[PR010207]**
- ☆ Other cyclopentane monoterpenoids **[PR010208]**
- ☆ Menthane monoterpenoids **[PR010209]**
- ☆ Other cyclohexane monoterpenoids **[PR010210]**
- ☆ Cycloheptane monoterpenoids **[PR010211]**
- ☆ Bicyclic monoterpenoids **[PR010212]**
- ☆ Tricyclic monoterpenoids **[PR010213]**
- ☆ Other monoterpenoids **[PR010214]**
- ☆ C15 isoprenoids (sesquiterpenes) **[PR0103]**
- ☆ Acyclic farnesane sesquiterpenoids **[PR010301]**
- ☆ Furanoid farnesane sesquiterpenoids **[PR010302]**
- ☆ Irregular acyclic sesquiterpenoids **[PR010303]**
- ☆ Cyclobutane and cyclopentane sesquiterpenoids **[PR010304]**
- ☆ Cyclofarnesane sesquiterpenoids **[PR010305]**
- ☆ Bisabolane sesquiterpenoids **[PR010306]**
- ☆ Cyclobisabolane sesquiterpenoids **[PR010307]**
- ☆ Elemane sesquiterpenoids **[PR010308]**
- ☆ Germacrane sesquiterpenoids **[PR010309]**
- ☆ Lepidozanes and bicyclogermacrane sesquiterpenoids **[PR010310]**
- ☆ Humulane sesquiterpenoids **[PR010311]**
- ☆ Caryophyllane sesquiterpenoids **[PR010312]**
- ☆ Bicyclohumulane sesquiterpenoids **[PR010313]**
- ☆ Cuparane sesquiterpenoids **[PR010314]**
- ☆ Cyclolaurane sesquiterpenoids **[PR010315]**
- ☆ Herbertane sesquiterpenoids **[PR010316]**
- ☆ Laurane sesquiterpenoids **[PR010317]**
- ☆ Trichothecane sesquiterpenoids **[PR010318]**
- ☆ Eudesmane sesquiterpenoids **[PR010319]**
- ☆ Emmotin sesquiterpenoids **[PR010320]**
- ☆ Oppositane sesquiterpenoids **[PR010321]**
- ☆ Farfugin sesquiterpenoids **[PR010322]**
- ☆ Cycloeudesmane sesquiterpenoids **[PR010323]**
- ☆ Gorgonane sesquiterpenoids **[PR010324]**
- ☆ Eremophilane sesquiterpenoids **[PR010325]**

- ☆ Chiloscyphane sesquiterpenoids **[PR010326]**
- ☆ Aristolane sesquiterpenoids **[PR010327]**
- ☆ Nardosinane sesquiterpenoids **[PR010328]**
- ☆ Brasilane sesquiterpenoids **[PR010329]**
- ☆ Cacalol sesquiterpenoids **[PR010330]**
- ☆ Valerane sesquiterpenoids **[PR010331]**
- ☆ Rearranged eudesmane sesquiterpenoids **[PR010332]**
- ☆ Cadinane sesquiterpenoids **[PR010333]**
- ☆ Alliacane sesquiterpenoids **[PR010334]**
- ☆ Oplopane sesquiterpenoids **[PR010335]**
- ☆ Mutisianthol sesquiterpenoids **[PR010336]**
- ☆ Drimane sesquiterpenoids **[PR010337]**
- ☆ Coloratane sesquiterpenoids **[PR010338]**
- ☆ Xanthane sesquiterpenoids **[PR010339]**
- ☆ Carabrane sesquiterpenoids **[PR010340]**
- ☆ Guaiane sesquiterpenoids **[PR010341]**
- ☆ Pseudoguaiane sesquiterpenoids **[PR010342]**
- ☆ Aromadendrane sesquiterpenoids **[PR010343]**
- ☆ Cubebane and ivaxillarane sesquiterpenoids **[PR010344]**
- ☆ Patchoulane sesquiterpenoids **[PR010345]**
- ☆ Valerenane sesquiterpenoids **[PR010346]**
- ☆ Africanane sesquiterpenoids **[PR010347]**
- ☆ Lippifoliane and himachalane sesquiterpenoids **[PR010348]**
- ☆ Longipinane sesquiterpenoids **[PR010349]**
- ☆ Longifolane sesquiterpenoids **[PR010350]**
- ☆ Longibornane sesquiterpenoids **[PR010351]**
- ☆ Pinguisane sesquiterpenoids **[PR010352]**
- ☆ Thapsane and fukinane sesquiterpenoids **[PR010353]**
- ☆ Picrotoxane sesquiterpenoids **[PR010354]**
- ☆ Daucane sesquiterpenoids **[PR010355]**
- ☆ Isodaucane sesquiterpenoids **[PR010356]**
- ☆ Perforane and pacifigorgiane sesquiterpenoids **[PR010357]**
- ☆ Asteriscane sesquiterpenoids **[PR010358]**
- ☆ Illudane and protoilludane sesquiterpenoids **[PR010359]**
- ☆ Sterpurane sesquiterpenoids **[PR010360]**
- ☆ Illudalane sesquiterpenoids **[PR010361]**

- ☆ Isolactarane, merulane, lactarane and marasmane sesquiterpenoids **[PR010362]**
- ☆ Furodysin and furodysinin sesquiterpenoids **[PR010363]**
- ☆ Botrydial sesquiterpenoids **[PR010364]**
- ☆ Spirovetivane sesquiterpenoids **[PR010365]**
- ☆ Acorane sesquiterpenoids **[PR010366]**
- ☆ Chamigrane sesquiterpenoids **[PR010367]**
- ☆ Spirosesquiterpenoids **[PR010368]**
- ☆ Cedrane and isocedrane sesquiterpenoids **[PR010369]**
- ☆ Zizaane and prezizaane sesquiterpenoids **[PR010370]**
- ☆ Clovane sesquiterpenoids **[PR010371]**
- ☆ Precapnellane and capnellane sesquiterpenoids **[PR010372]**
- ☆ Hirsutane and rearranged hisutane sesquiterpenoids **[PR010373]**
- ☆ Pentalenane sesquiterpenoids **[PR010374]**
- ☆ Silphinane, silphiperfoliane and presilphiperfoliane sesquiterpenoids **[PR010375]**
- ☆ Isocomane sesquiterpenoids **[PR010376]**
- ☆ Panasinsane sesquiterpenoids **[PR010377]**
- ☆ Modhephane sesquiterpenoids **[PR010378]**
- ☆ Quadrane sesquiterpenoids **[PR010379]**
- ☆ Campherenane and santalane sesquiterpenoids **[PR010380]**
- ☆ Sativane sesquiterpenoids **[PR010381]**
- ☆ Copacamphane and sinularane sesquiterpenoids **[PR010382]**
- ☆ Copaane sesquiterpenoids **[PR010383]**
- ☆ Ishwarane sesquiterpenoids **[PR010384]**
- ☆ Rotundane sesquiterpenoids **[PR010385]**
- ☆ Thujopsane sesquiterpenoids **[PR010386]**
- ☆ Bourbonane sesquiterpenoids **[PR010387]**
- ☆ Gymnomitrane sesquiterpenoids **[PR010388]**
- ☆ Other sesquiterpenoids **[PR010389]**
- ☆ C20 isoprenoids (diterpenes) **[PR0104]**
- ☆ Acyclic diterpenoids **[PR010401]**
- ☆ Prenylbisabolane and cyclophytane diterpenoids **[PR010402]**
- ☆ Labdane and halimane diterpenoids **[PR010403]**
- ☆ Colensane and clerodane diterpenoids **[PR010404]**
- ☆ Abietane diterpenoids **[PR010405]**
- ☆ Cycloaibetiane and Abeoabietaine diterpenoids **[PR010406]**

- ✰ Totarane and nagilactone diterpenoids **[PR010407]**
- ✰ Pimarane diterpenoids **[PR010408]**
- ✰ Cassane and vouacapane diterpenoids **[PR010409]**
- ✰ Cleistanthane and isocleistanthane diterpenoids **[PR010410]**
- ✰ Isocopalane and spongiane diterpenoids **[PR010411]**
- ✰ Podocarpane diterpenoids **[PR010412]**
- ✰ Kaurane and phyllocladane diterpenoids **[PR010413]**
- ✰ Beyerane diterpenoids **[PR010414]**
- ✰ Villanovane, atisane, trachylobane and helvifulvane diterpenoids **[PR010415]**
- ✰ Aphidicolane diterpenoids **[PR010416]**
- ✰ Gibberellins **[PR010417]**
- ✰ Leucothol and grayanotoxane diterpenoids **[PR010418]**
- ✰ Cembrane diterpenoids **[PR010419]**
- ✰ Rearranged cembrane diterpenoids **[PR010420]**
- ✰ Eunicellane and asbestinane diterpenoids **[PR010421]**
- ✰ Sphaerane diterpenoids **[PR010422]**
- ✰ Briarane diterpenoids **[PR010423]**
- ✰ Dolabellane and modified dolabellane diterpenoids **[PR010424]**
- ✰ Dolastane and modified dolastane diterpenoids **[PR010425]**
- ✰ Cyathane diterpenoids **[PR010426]**
- ✰ Sphaeroane diterpenoids **[PR010427]**
- ✰ Verrucosane and modified verrucosane diterpenoids **[PR010428]**
- ✰ Casbane diterpenoids **[PR010429]**
- ✰ Jatrophane and cyclojatrophane diterpenoids **[PR010430]**
- ✰ Lathyrane diterpenoids **[PR010431]**
- ✰ Rhamnofolane and daphnane diterpenoids **[PR010432]**
- ✰ Tigliane and ingenane diterpenoids **[PR010433]**
- ✰ Jatropholane and secojatropholane diterpenoids **[PR010434]**
- ✰ Fusicoccane diterpenoids **[PR010435]**
- ✰ Valparane and mulinane diterpenoids **[PR010436]**
- ✰ Spatane diterpenoids **[PR010437]**
- ✰ Verticillane diterpenoids **[PR010438]**
- ✰ Taxane and Abeotaxane diterpenoids **[PR010439]**
- ✰ Trinervitane and kempane diterpenoids **[PR010440]**
- ✰ Amphilectane, cycloamphilectane, adociane and neoamphilectane diterpenoids **[PR010441]**

- ☆ Xenicane and xeniaphyllane diterpenoids **[PR010442]**
- ☆ Viscidane diterpenoids **[PR010443]**
- ☆ Eremane diterpenoids **[PR010444]**
- ☆ Prenyleudesmane, prenylgermacrane and prenylbicyclogermacrane diterpenoids **[PR010445]**
- ☆ Lobane diterpenoids **[PR010446]**
- ☆ Pachydictyane and cneorubin diterpenoids **[PR010447]**
- ☆ Serrulatane and biflorane diterpenoids **[PR010448]**
- ☆ Decipiane diterpenoids **[PR010449]**
- ☆ Sacculatane diterpenoids **[PR010450]**
- ☆ Obtusane diterpenoids **[PR010451]**
- ☆ Irieol diterpenoids **[PR010452]**
- ☆ Sphenolobane diterpenoids **[PR010453]**
- ☆ Ginkgolides and Bilobalides **[PR010454]**
- ☆ Other diterpenoids **[PR010455]**
- ☆ C25 isoprenoids (sesterterpenes) **[PR0105]**
- ☆ Acyclic sesterterpenoids **[PR010501]**
- ☆ Cyclohexane sesterterpenoids **[PR010502]**
- ☆ Cericerane sesterterpenoids **[PR010503]**
- ☆ Bicyclic sesterterpenoids **[PR010504]**
- ☆ Cheilanthane and ophiobolane sesterterpenoids **[PR010505]**
- ☆ Scalarane sesterterpenoids **[PR010506]**
- ☆ Other sesterterpenoids **[PR010507]**
- ☆ C30 isoprenoids (triterpenes) **[PR0106]**
- ☆ Acyclic triterpenoids **[PR010601]**
- ☆ Cyclohexane triterpenoids **[PR010602]**
- ☆ Botryococcene triterpenoids **[PR010603]**
- ☆ Prostostane and fusidane triterpenoids **[PR010604]**
- ☆ Lanostane triterpenoids **[PR010605]**
- ☆ Cucurbitane triterpenoids **[PR010607]**
- ☆ Dammarane triterpenoids **[PR010608]**
- ☆ Tirucallane/euphane triterpenoids **[PR010609]**
- ☆ Apotirucallane triterpenoids **[PR010610]**
- ☆ Nortriterpenoids **[PR010611]**
- ☆ Quassinoid nortriterpenoids **[PR010612]**
- ☆ Baccharane triterpenoids **[PR010613]**
- ☆ Lupane triterpenoids **[PR010614]**

- ☆ Oleanane triterpenoids **[PR010615]**
- ☆ Taraxerane, multiflorane, glutinane and friedelane triterpenoids **[PR010616]**
- ☆ Pachysanane triterpenoids **[PR010617]**
- ☆ Taraxastane, ursane and bauerane triterpenoids **[PR010618]**
- ☆ Hopane triterpenoids **[PR010619]**
- ☆ Neohopane, fernane, adianane and filicane triterpenoids **[PR010620]**
- ☆ Arborinane and stictane triterpenoids **[PR010621]**
- ☆ Gammacerane triterpenoids **[PR010622]**
- ☆ Serratane and onocerane triterpenoids **[PR010623]**
- ☆ Polypodane, malabaricane and podiodane triterpenoids **[PR010624]**
- ☆ Other triterpenoids **[PR010625]**
- ☆ C40 isoprenoids (tetraterpenes) **[PR0107]**
- ☆ Polyterpenes **[PR0108]**
- ☆ Retinoids **[PR0109]**
- ☆ Quinones and hydroquinones **[PR02]**
- ☆ Ubiquinones **[PR0201]**
- ☆ Vitamin E **[PR0202]**
- ☆ Vitamin K **[PR0203]**
- ☆ Polyprenols **[PR03]**
- ☆ Bactoprenols **[PR0301]**
- ☆ Bactoprenol monophosphates **[PR0302]**
- ☆ Bactoprenol diphosphates **[PR0303]**
- ☆ Phytoprenols **[PR0304]**
- ☆ Phytoprenol monophosphates **[PR0305]**
- ☆ Phytoprenol diphosphates **[PR0306]**
- ☆ Dolichols **[PR0307]**
- ☆ Dolichol monophosphates **[PR0308]**
- ☆ Dolichol diphosphates **[PR0309]**
- ☆ Hopanoids **[PR04]**
- ☆ Other Prenol lipids **[PR00]**

Saccharolipids [SL]

- ☆ Acylaminosugars **[SL01]**
- ☆ Monoacylaminosugars **[SL0101]**
- ☆ Diacylaminosugars **[SL0102]**
- ☆ Triacylaminosugars **[SL0103]**
- ☆ Tetraacylaminosugars **[SL0104]**

- ☆ Pentaacylaminosugars **[SL0105]**
- ☆ Hexaacylaminosugars **[SL0106]**
- ☆ Heptaacylaminosugars **[SL0107]**
- ☆ Acylaminosugar glycans **[SL02]**
- ☆ Acyltrehaloses **[SL03]**
- ☆ Acyltrehalose glycans **[SL04]**
- ☆ Other acyl sugars **[SL05]**
- ☆ Other Saccharolipids **[SL00]**

Polyketides [PK]

- ☆ Linear polyketides **[PK01]**
- ☆ Halogenated acetogenins **[PK02]**
- ☆ Annonaceae acetogenins **[PK03]**
- ☆ Macrolides and lactone polyketides **[PK04]**
- ☆ Ansamycins and related polyketides **[PK05]**
- ☆ Polyenes **[PK06]**
- ☆ Linear tetracyclines **[PK07]**
- ☆ Angucyclines **[PK08]**
- ☆ Polyether antibiotics **[PK09]**
- ☆ Aflatoxins and related substances **[PK10]**
- ☆ Cytochalasins **[PK11]**
- ☆ Flavonoids [PK12]
- ☆ Anthocyanidins **[PK1201]**
- ☆ Flavans, Flavanols and Leucoanthocyanidins **[PK1202]**
- ☆ Proanthocyanidins **[PK1203]**
- ☆ Biflavonoids and polyflavonoids **[PK1204]**
- ☆ Isoflavonoids **[PK1205]**
- ☆ Rotenoid flavonoids **[PK1206]**
- ☆ Pterocarpans **[PK1207]**
- ☆ Isoflavans **[PK1208]**
- ☆ Coumestan flavonoids **[PK1209]**
- ☆ Neoflavonoids **[PK1210]**
- ☆ Flavones and Flavonols **[PK1211]**
- ☆ Chalcones and dihydrochalcones **[PK1212]**
- ☆ Aurone flavonoids **[PK1213]**
- ☆ Flavanones **[PK1214]**
- ☆ Dihydroflavonols **[PK1215]**
- ☆ Other Flavonoids **[PK1216]**

- ☆ Aromatic polyketides **[PK13]**
- ☆ Monocyclic aromatic polyketides **[PK1301]**
- ☆ Naphthalenes and naphthoquinones **[PK1302]**
- ☆ Benzoisochromanquinones **[PK1303]**
- ☆ Anthracenes and phenanthrenes **[PK1304]**
- ☆ Anthracyclinones **[PK1305]**
- ☆ Dibenzofurans, griseofulvins, dibenzopyrans and xanthones **[PK1306]**
- ☆ Diphenylmethanes, acylphloroglucinols and benzophenones **[PK1307]**
- ☆ Depsides and depsidones **[PK1308]**
- ☆ Diphenyl ethers, biphenyls, dibenzyls and stilbenes **[PK1309]**
- ☆ Benzofuranoids **[PK1310]**
- ☆ Benzopyranoids **[PK1311]**
- ☆ Other aromatic polyketides **[PK1312]**
- ☆ Non-ribosomal peptide/polyketide hybrids **[PK14]**
- ☆ Other Polyketides **[PK00]**

The new classification system has already been implemented and Dr. Dennis, Dr. Fahy and their collaborators from Europe, Asia and across the US hope that it will eventually gain widespread acceptance. Interactive access to this classification scheme can be viewed at http://www.lipidmaps.org

Chapter 2

Definition and Classification of Lipids II

II. Complex Glycerolipids

They are classified and discussed in detail as under:

- ☆ Ether lipids
- ☆ Phosphatidic acid and related lipids
- ☆ Phosphatidylglycerol and related lipids
- ☆ Diphosphatidylglycerol (cardiolipin)
- ☆ Phosphatidylinositol and related lipids
- ☆ Phosphatidylserine
- ☆ Phosphatidylethanolamine
- ☆ Phosphatidylcholine
- ☆ Mono- and digalactosyldiacylglycerols and from plants and microorganisms, etc
- ☆ Glycosyldiacylglycerols and related lipids from animals
- ☆ Glycophospholipids

Ether Lipids

Lipids with ether bonds to long-chain alkyl moieties in addition to having ester bonds to fatty acids are not important constituents of many lipids of commercial value, but they are very common in nature, especially as membrane constituents.

Usually the ether bond is to position sn-1 of a glycerol moiety, which may be part of a non-polar lipid or a phospholipid in animal tissues or in micro-organisms. At one time, they were considered little more than a biological novelty. However, findings of elevated levels of ether lipids in cancer tissues, followed by the discovery of distinctive ether lipids, such as platelet-activating factor, with important biological activities greatly stimulated the interest in these compounds. Two main types of ether bonds exist in natural lipids–ether and vinyl ether as illustrated. The double bond adjacent to the oxygen atom in the latter has the Z or cis configuration.

$$R-O-(CH_2)_nCH_3 \qquad \text{ether}$$

$$R-O-CH=CH-(CH_2)_mCH_3 \qquad \text{vinyl ether}$$

Ether bonds are stable to both alkaline and acidic hydrolysis under most practical conditions, but vinyl ether bonds open readily under acidic conditions to form aldehydes.

'Platelet-activating factor' or 1-alkyl-2-acetyl-sn-glycerophosphorylcholine is an ether-containing phospholipid that is presently being studied intensively because it can exert profound biological effects at minute concentrations. For example, it affects aggregation of platelets at concentrations as low as 10^{-11} M, and it induces a hypertensive response at very low levels. Also, it is a mediator of inflammation and has messenger functions.

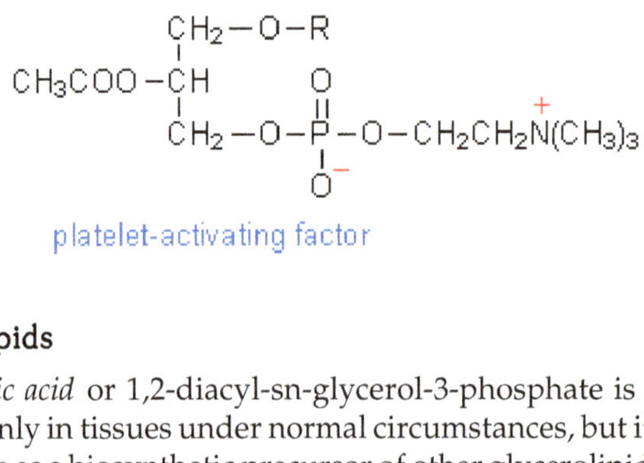

platelet-activating factor

Glycerophospholipids

1. *Phosphatidic acid* or 1,2-diacyl-sn-glycerol-3-phosphate is found in trace amounts only in tissues under normal circumstances, but it has metabolic importance as a biosynthetic precursor of other glycerolipids. It is strongly acidic and is usually isolated as a mixed salt. One specific isomer is illustrated as an example.

   Lysophosphatidic acid with one mole of fatty acid per mole of lipid (in position sn-1) is a marker for ovarian cancer, and is a key cellular messenger.

2. *Phosphatidylglycerol* or 1,2-diacyl-sn-glycerol-3-phosphoryl-1'-sn-glycerol tends to be a trace constituent of most tissues, but it is often the main component of some bacterial membranes. *Escherichia coli*, has up to 20 per cent phosphatidylglycerol in its membranes (phosphatidylethanolamine makes up much of the rest with a little diphosphatidylglycerol). In many

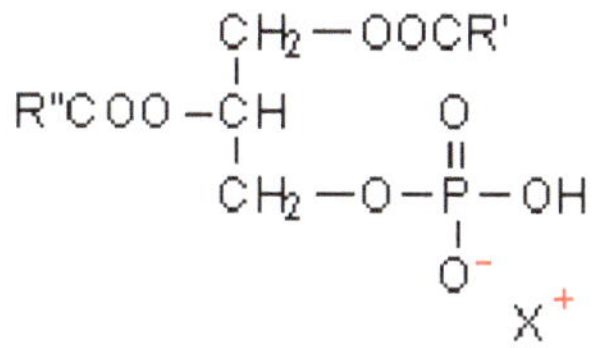

where, X = Na, K, H, Ca, etc.

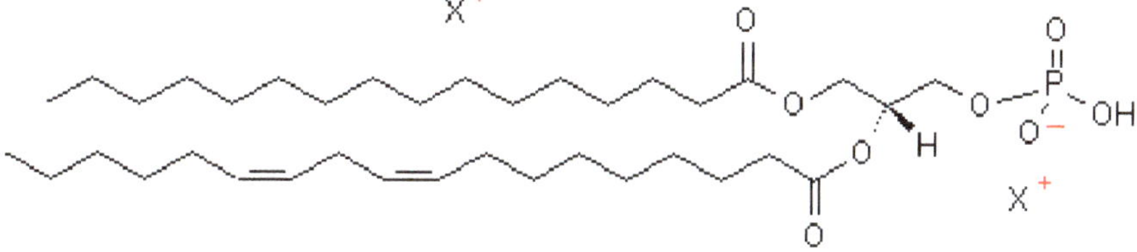

1-hexadecanoyl, 2-(9Z,12Z-octadecadienoyl)-*sn*-glycero-3-phosphate
(phosphatidic acid)

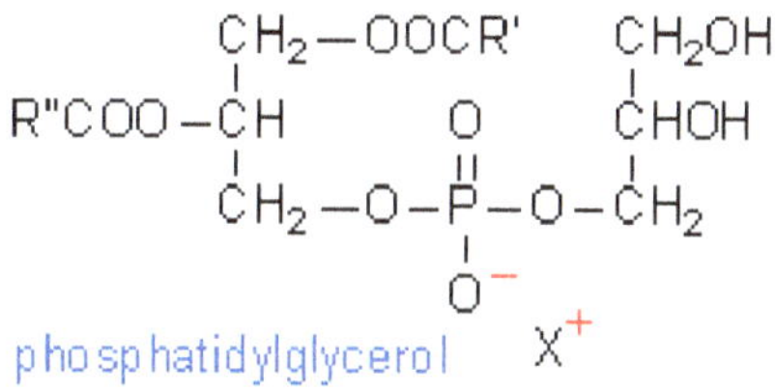

phosphatidylglycerol

bacteria, the diacyl form of the lipid predominates, but in others the alkylacyl- and alkenylacyl forms are more abundant. There is clear evidence that *E. coli* has an absolute requirement for phosphatidylglycerol in its membranes, and that this has a multiplicity of functions. In plants, phosphatidylglycerol is found in all cellular membranes, but it appears to be especially important in the thylakoid membrane where it can comprise 10 per cent of the total lipids with a high proportion (up to 70 per cent) in the outer monolayer. In cereals such as oats, a form with an additional fatty acid linked to the 3'-hydroxyl of the glycerol moiety has been found. Phosphatidylglycerol is also present in most animal tissues as a minor constituent, but it is an essential functional component of the lung surfactant. It has important functions in lung surfactant, where its physical properties are significant, and in plant chloroplasts, where it appears to have an essential role in photosynthesis. Also, it is the biosynthetic precursor of cardiolipin.

3. *Cardiolipin* (or diphosphatidylglycerol more precisely 1,3-bis(sn-3'-phosphatidyl)-sn-glycerol) is a unique phospholipid with in essence a dimeric structure, having four acyl groups and potentially carrying two negative charges (and is thus an acidic lipid). The trivial name 'cardiolipin' is derived from the fact that it was first found in animal hearts, where it is especially abundant, but it can be found in mitochondria of all animal tissues and indeed of the eukaryotic kingdom, *i.e.* those whose function is

to generate an electrochemical potential for substrate transport and ATP synthesis. For example, it amounts to about 10 per cent of the phospholipids of bovine heart muscle, and 20 per cent of the phospholipids of the mitochondrial membrane.

It is an important constituent of mitochondrial lipids especially, so heart muscle is a rich source. Amongst other functions, it plays a key role in modifying the activities of the enzymes concerned with oxidative phosphorylation.

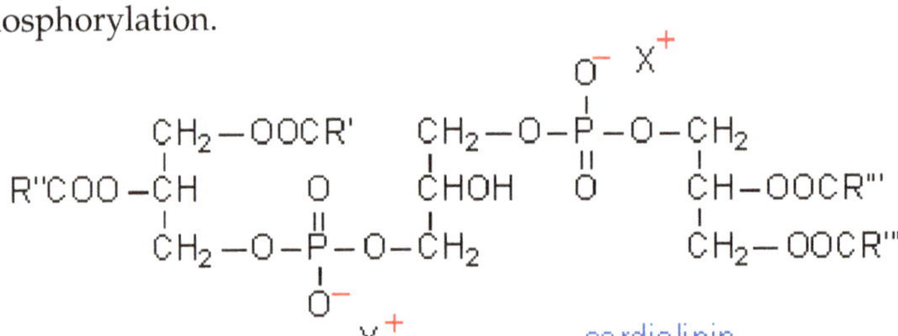

As there are four distinct fatty acyl groups in cardiolipin, the potential for complexity in the distribution within molecular species is enormous. However, the compositions can be remarkably simple, very different from those of other phospholipids, and in animals resistant to dietary manipulation. For example, in animal tissues, diphosphatidylglycerol contains almost exclusively 18 carbon fatty acids, and 80 per cent of this is typically linoleic acid (18:2(n-6)). This appears to be true of higher plants also. Yeast diphosphatidylglycerol can differ in having more 16:1 and 18:1 fatty acids, while the bacterial lipid contains saturated and monoenoic fatty acids with 14 to18 carbons. In some marine species, cardiolipin contains only docosahexaenoic acid, while lymphoblast cardiolipin contains only monoenoic fatty acids.

Glycoglycerolipids

a. Mono- and Digalactosyldiacylglycerols from Plants and Microorganisms

In plants, especially the photosynthetic tissues, a substantial proportion of the lipids consists of 1, 2-diacyl-sn-glycerols joined by a glycosidic linkage at position sn-3 to a carbohydrate moiety. The main components are the mono- and digalactosyldiacylglycerols, but related compounds have been found with up to four galactose units, or in which one or more of these is replaced by glucose moieties. It is clear that these have an important role in photosynthesis, but many of the details have still to be worked out.

Bacterial Glycosyldiacylglycerols

A wide variety of glycosyldiacylglycerols are found in Eubacteria; those with one to three glycosyl units linked to sn-1,2-diacylglycerol are most common, although others with up to five glycosyl units are found. These tend to be very different from the plant glycosyl diacylglycerols, in that glucose is much more common than galactose,

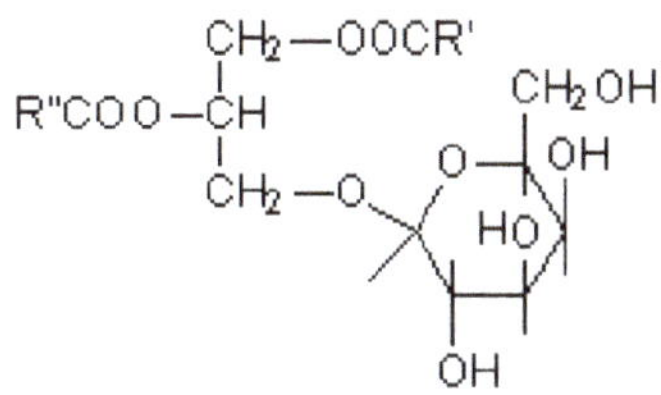

monogalactosyldiacylglycerol

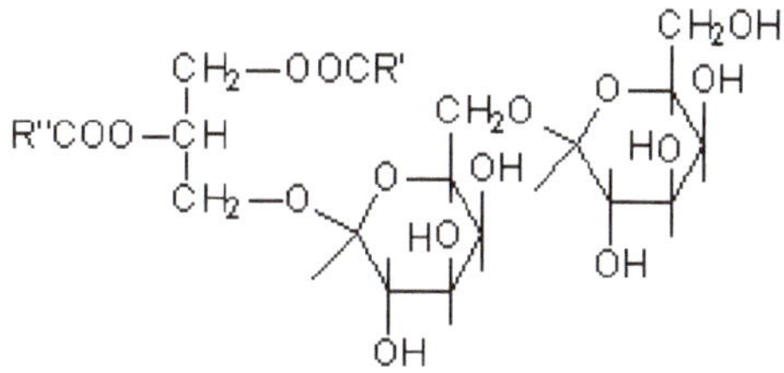

digalactosyldiacylglycerol

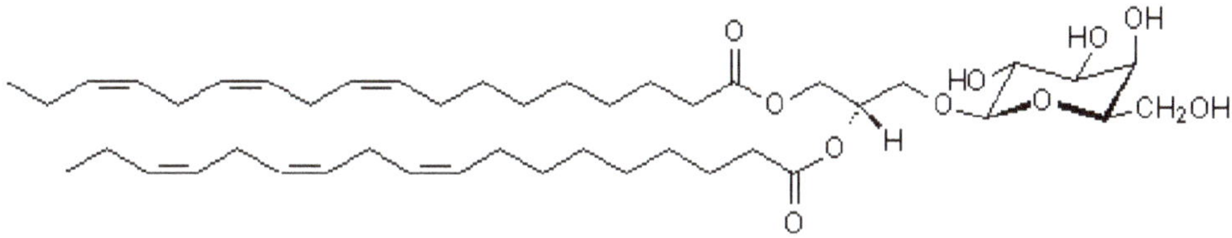

1,2-di-(9Z,12Z,15Z)-octadecatrienoyl-3-O-β-D-galactosyl-sn-glycerol

while the fatty acid components are mainly saturated, monoenoic and branched-chain or cyclopropanoid. For example, some Streptococcus species contain mono- and diglucosyldiacylglycerols, with the diglucoside unit having a α-(1!2) linkage as in kojibiose, and so can be termed 'kojibiosyldiacylglycerols', and a galactosylglucosyldiacylglycerol is also known, as are various lipids of this type with a fatty acyl group attached to a carbohydrate moiety (usually in position 3 or 6). Some microorganisms accumulate galactofuranosyl-diacylglycerols rather than the galactopyranosyl form, and a variety of unusual glycosyldiacylglycerols with differing carbohydrate moieties, or with differences in the glycosidic bonds from those in higher plants, have been found. For example, *Micrococcus luteus* synthesises mono- and dimannosyldiacylglycerols. Other bacteria have glycosyldiacylglycerols with a glycerophosphate group linked to a carbohydrate moiety ('**glycophospholipids**'). *Bacillus megaterium* contains N-acetylgalactosamine linked to a diacylglycerol.

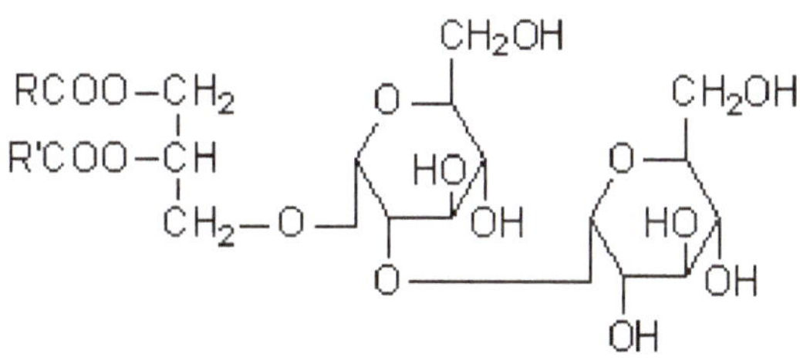

1,2-diacyl-3-O-α-D-kojibiosyl-sn-glycerol

Sulfoquinovosyldiacylglycerol

Sulfoquinovosyldiacylglycerol or 1,2-di-O-acyl-3-O-(6'-deoxy-6'-sulfo-α-D-glucopyranosyl)-sn-glycerol (quinovose = 6-deoxyglucose) is the single glycolipid most characteristic of photosynthetic organisms.

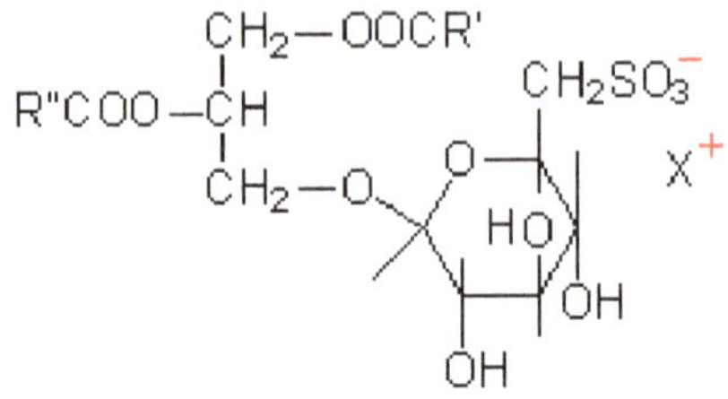

sulfoquinovosyldiacylglycerol

In many species of higher plants, the sn-1 position is reportedly enriched in 16:0 and the sn-2 position in 18:3 and 18:2. Other than in active photosynthetic organisms, this lipid has only been found in a few bacterial species, mainly of the genus Rhizobium, which have a symbiotic relationship with plants in root nodule.

b. Glycosyldiacylglycerols and Related Lipids from Animals

i) *Mono- and diglycosyldiacylglycerols*

Following the discovery of mono- and digalactosyldiacylglycerols in plants, a search began for similar lipids in animal tissues. They are now known to be ubiquitous if minor components of brain and other nervous tissues, usually amounting to only 0.1 to 0.6 per cent of the total lipids, and they can occur in trace amounts in other tissues. They exist in both diacyl and alkyl acyl forms, and contain mainly saturated and monoenoic fatty acid components, with 16:0, 18:0 and 18:1 comprising 90 per cent or more of the total. The alkyl moieties consist of 70 per cent or more of 16:0. The monogalactosyldiacylglycerol of mammalian brain is similar to that of plants, *i.e.* it is 1,2-di-O-acyl-3-O-β-D-galactopyranosyl-sn-glycerol (and the 1-alkyl,2-acyl form).

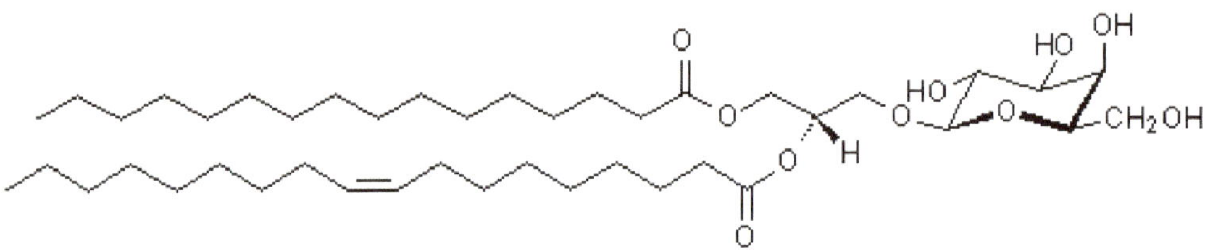

1-hexadecanoyl,2-9Z-octadecenoyl-3-O-β-*D*-galactosyl-*sn*-glycerol

In fish brain, only the diacyl form is found, and it can be accompanied by related lipids in which the position 6 of the galactose unit is acylated, or in which an aldehyde is linked to the carbohydrate moiety via an acetal linkage. Galactolipids probably have a role in myelination, and may also have a function in cell differentiation and intracellular signalling. The glucolipids in saliva and related secretions may be involved in a defense mechanism against microbial attack.

ii) *Seminolipid*

As the name suggests, seminolipid or 1-O-hexadecyl-2-O-hexadecanoyl-3-O-β-D-(3'-sulfo)-galactopyranosyl-sn-glycerol was first found in mammalian spermatozoa and testes, where it can amount to 3 per cent of the total lipids and 90 per cent of the glycolipids. There are abundant evidences that seminolipid is essential for spermatogenesis.

c) Lysobisphosphatidic Acid

Lysobisphosphatidic acid or bis(monoacylglycerol) phosphate is an interesting lipid as its stereochemical configuration differs from that of other animal glycerophospholipids in that the phosphodiester moiety is linked to positions sn-1 and sn-1′ of glycerol, rather than to position sn-3, to which the fatty acids are esterified. It is usually a rather minor component of animal tissues, but is enriched in the lysosomes of liver and appears to be a marker for this organelle.

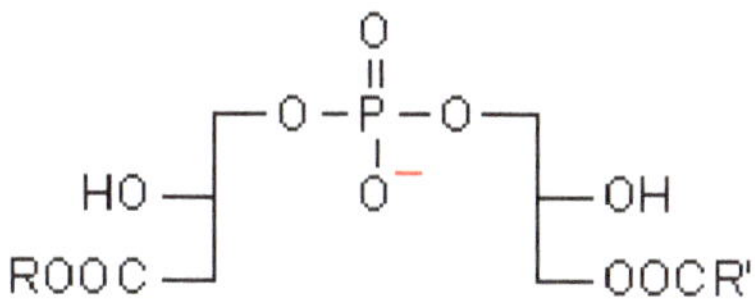

lysobisphosphatidic acid

d) Phosphatidylcholine

Phosphatidylcholine or 1,2-diacyl-sn-glycerol-3-phosphorylcholine (or "lecithin", although the term is now used more frequently for the mixed phospholipid by-products of seed oil refining) is usually the most abundant lipid in the membranes of animal tissues, and it is often a major lipid component of plant membranes, but only rarely of bacteria. With the other choline-containing phospholipid, sphingomyelin, it constitutes most of the lipid in the external monolayer of the plasma membrane of animal cells.

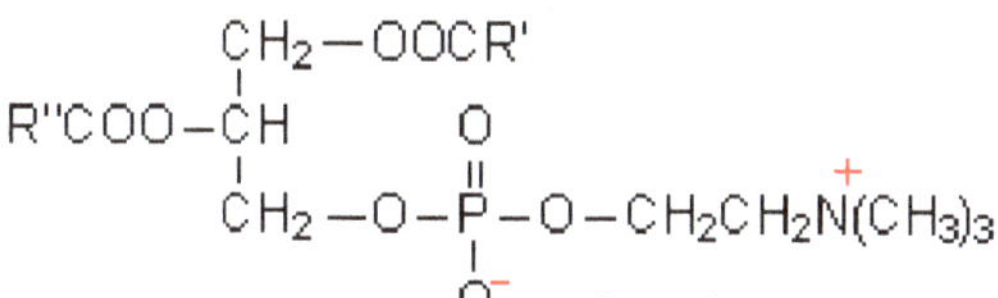

phosphatidylcholine

e) Phosphatidylethanolamine

Phosphatidylethanolamine (once given the trivial name "cephalin") is usually the second most abundant phospholipid class in animal and plant tissues, and can be the major lipid class in microorganisms. As part of an important cellular process, the amine group can be methylated enzymically to yield first phosphatidyl-N-monomethylethanolamine and then phosphatidyl-N,N-dimethyl-ethanolamine, but

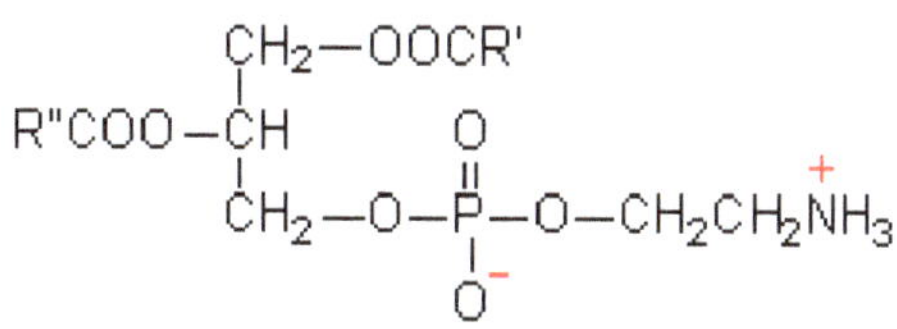

phosphatidylethanolamine

these never accumulate in significant amounts; the eventual product is phosphatidylcholine. N-Acyl-phosphatidylethanolamine is a minor component of some plant tissues, especially cereals, and it is occasionally found in animal tissues, where it is the precursor of some biologically active amides. Lysophosphatidylethanolamine contains only one mole of fatty acid per mole of lipid.

f) Phosphatidylserine

It is a weakly acidic lipid phospholipid with three ionizable groups, *i.e.* the phosphate moiety, the amino group and the carboxyl function. As with other acidic lipids, it exists in nature in salt form. The 1-octadecanoyl-2-arachidonoyl molecular species is illustrated here.

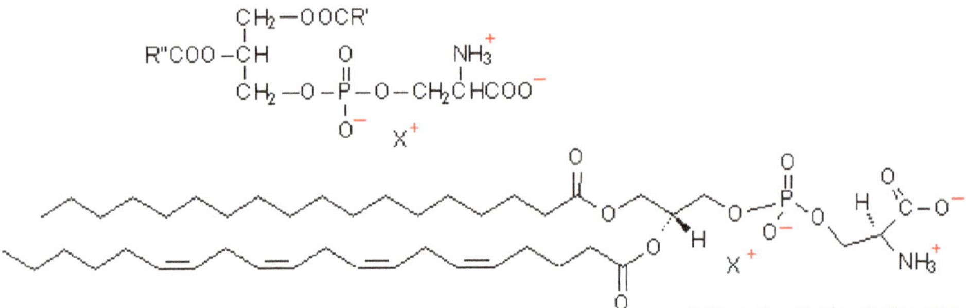

(where X = H, Na, K, Ca, etc)

1-octadecanoyl, 2-(5Z,8Z,11Z,14Z-eicosatetraenoyl)-*sn*-glycero-3-phosphoserine

Although phosphatidylserine or 1,2-diacyl-sn-glycero-3-phospho-L-serine is distributed widely among animals, plants and microorganisms, it is usually less than 10 per cent of the total phospholipids, the greatest concentration being in myelin from brain tissue. However, it may comprise 10 to 20 mol per cent of the total phospholipid in the plasma membrane and endoplasmic reticulum of the cell. In yeasts, such as *S. cerevisiae*, it is a minor component of most cellular organelles other than the plasma membrane, where it can amount to more than 30 per cent of the total lipids. N-Acylphosphatidylserine has been detected in some animal tissues.

It is located entirely on the inner monolayer surface of the plasma membrane and other cellular membranes. Phosphatidylserine is an essential cofactor for the activation of protein kinase C, and it is involved in the blood coagulation process in platelets. It is believed to have an important role in the regulation of apoptosis. There is currently great interest in the use of phosphatidylserine as a nutritional supplement for the elderly, as there is evidence from clinical trials that it improves brain function, and in particular reduces the risk or intensity of cognitive dysfunction and of dementia. There are also suggestions that it may be a valuable nutrient for sportsmen by reducing the level of stress hormones.

g) Phosphatidylthreonine

Phosphatidyl-L-threonine, which is closely related structurally and metabolically to phosphatidylserine, was first characterized as a minor component of polyoma virus-transformed embryo fibroblasts in hamsters and more recently in cultured hippocampal neurons.

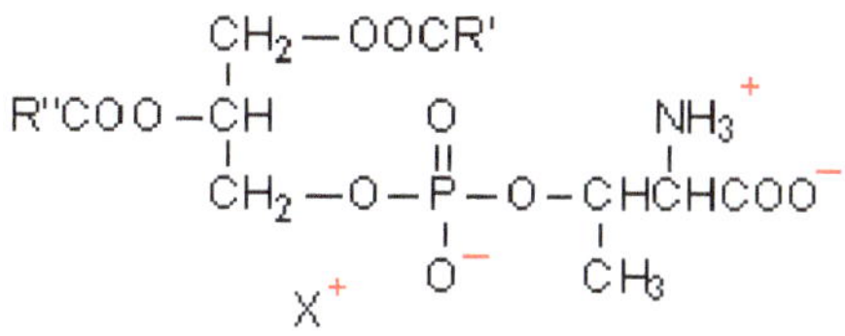

phosphatidyl-L-threonine

Biosynthetic studies with microsomes from rat brain suggest that it is synthesised by the same base exchange enzyme involved in phosphatidylserine synthesis but with much lower activity.

h) Phosphatidylinositol

Phosphatidylinositol is an important lipid, both as a key membrane constituent and as a participant in essential metabolic processes in all plants and animals (and in some bacteria (actinomycetes)), both directly and via a number of metabolites. It is an acidic (anionic) phospholipid that in essence consists of a phosphatidic acid backbone, linked via the phosphate group to inositol (hexahydroxycyclohexane). As with most other phospholipids, phosphatidylinositol is formed biosynthetically from the precursor CDP-diacylglycerol by reaction with inositol, catalysed by the enzyme CDP-diacylglycerol inositol phosphatidyltransferase. This is located in the endoplasmic reticulum mainly, although it may also occur in the plasma membrane in yeasts, and almost entirely on the cytosolic side of the bilayer. Phosphatidylinositol is especially abundant in brain tissue, where it can amount to 10 per cent of the phospholipids, but it is present in all tissues and cell types.

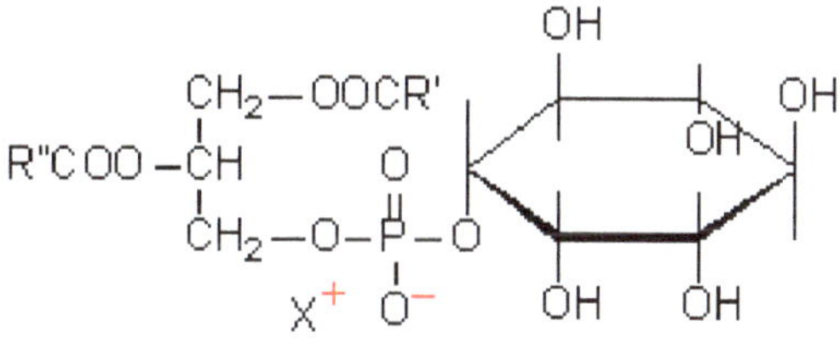

phosphatidylinositol

In most organisms, the stereochemical form of the last is myo-D-inositol (with one axial hydroxyl in position 2 with the remainder equatorial), although other forms (scyllo- and chiro-) have been found on occasion in plants. The 1-stearoyl,2-

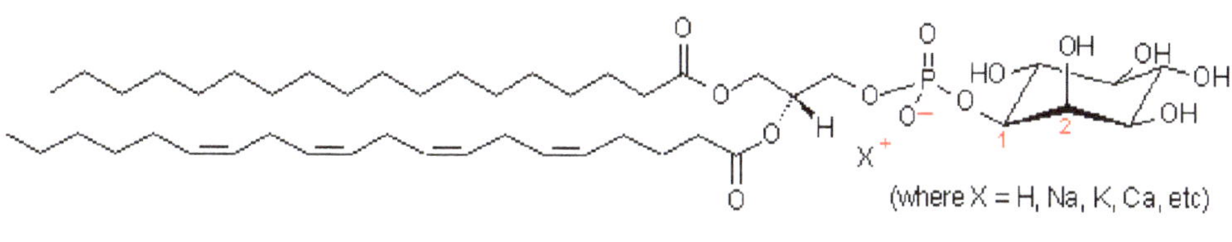

1-octadecanoyl, 2-(5Z,8Z,11Z,14Z-eicosatetraenoyl)-*sn*-glycero-3-phospho-(1'-*myo*-inositol)

arachidonoyl molecular species, which is of considerable biological importance, is illustrated.

In animal tissues especially, it may be accompanied by small amounts of phosphatidylinositol 4-phosphate and phosphatidylinositol 4,5-bisphosphate (poly-phosphoinositides). These compounds have a rapid rate of metabolism in animal cells, and are converted to metabolites such as diacylglycerols and inositol phosphates, which are important in regulating vital processes. For example, diacylglycerols regulate the activity of a group of enzymes known as protein kinase C, which in turn control many key cellular functions, including differentiation, proliferation, metabolism and apoptosis.

In animal tissues, phosphatidylinositol is the primary source of the arachidonic acid required for biosynthesis of eicosanoids, including prostaglandins, via the action of the enzyme phospholipase A_2, which releases the fatty acids from position sn-2.

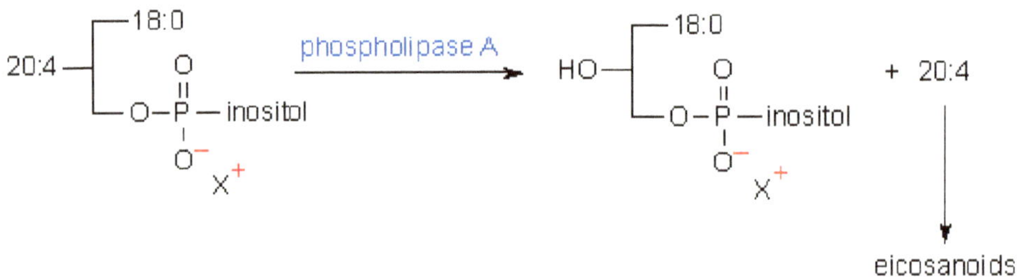

i) Lipophosphoglycans

In addition to the GPI-anchor molecules, carbohydrates attached to phosphatidylinositol play a role in the surface antigenicity of prokaryotic organisms, especially those of actinomycetes or coryneform bacteria. Such lipophosphoglycans are present on the external cell surface, where they are intimately involved in host-pathogen interactions. Key lipids are phosphatidylinositol mannosides, with the first mannose residue attached to the 2-hydroxyl group and the second to the 6-hydroxyl of myo-inositol, which are found in the cell walls of Mycobacteria and related bacterial species. These range in structure from simple monomannosides in

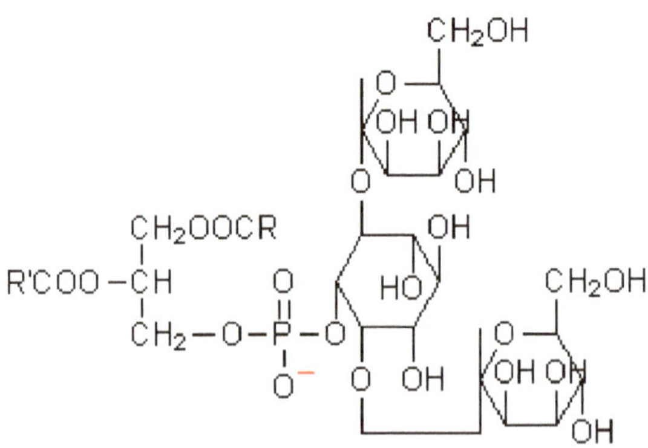

phosphatidylinositol dimannoside

some Streptomyces, Mycobacterium species and in propionibacteria to molecules with 40 or more hexose units. In addition, several fatty acyl groups can be linked to the inositol-mannose chain.

Glycero-Glycophospholipids

As the name suggests, glycophospholipids are lipid molecules that contain both phosphate and carbohydrate as integral structural components. There are two main types of glycophospholipid based on a glycerol backbone. One type is derived biosynthetically from glycosyldiacylglycerols, in which the sugar moiety is phosphorylated, *i.e.* in which the carbohydrate moiety is linked to a diacylglycerol. The second group comprises more conventional phospholipids, with a phosphate moiety attached to a diacylglycerol, *i.e.* in which the phosphate is further glycosylated. The stereochemistry of the glycerophosphate unit can then often be a distinguishing feature, as this is dependent on the biosynthetic origin. A suggestion that the first group be termed 'phosphoglycolipids' and the second 'glycophospholipids' does not appear to have been widely adopted. However, they are used below for practical convenience. In addition, there are some lipids that at first glance appear to have features of both groups. It appears that most of these lipids occur in relatively small amounts in bacteria, and it has been suggested that they do not have an important role in membranes but may have some metabolic importance that has yet to be defined. Glycophospholipids are also found among the sphingolipids.

Phosphoglycolipids

One of the first phosphoglycolipids to have its structure fully elucidated was found in Streptococcus and related bacterial species, *i.e.* 1,2-diacyl-3-[6″-(sn-glycero-1-phospho-)-α-D-kojibiosyl]-sn-glycerol. It is derived from a diglucosyldiacylglycerol, with the diglucoside unit equivalent to kojibiose in that it has a -(1!2) linkage. The other distinctive feature is the stereochemistry of the glycerophosphate moiety attached to position 6 of the second glucose unit; this is linked via position sn-1 of glycerol rather than the sn-3 position as in most other phospholipids. Subsequently, an analogous lipid with a single glucose moiety was characterized from this organism, and a related lipid with a phosphorylated galactofuranosyl residue has been found in *Bifidobacterium bifidum*. Similar triglycosyl lipids or diglycosyl analogues with the sn-glycerol-1-phosphate residue in different positions from that illustrated or with more than one such substituent are also known. In some species, there is an alkenyl ether moiety in position sn-1 of the lipid component rather than a fatty acid.

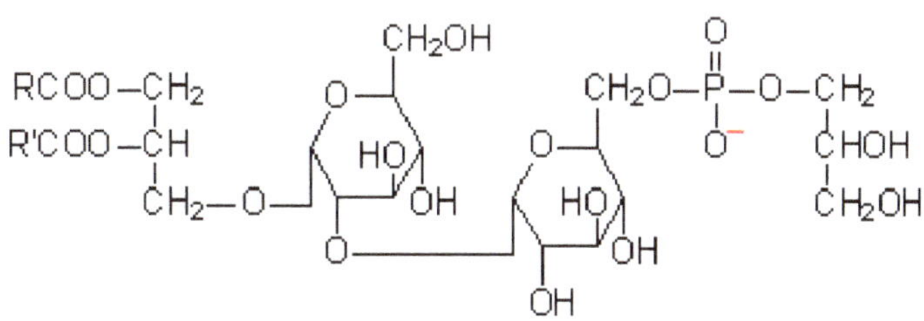

1,2-diacyl-3-[6″-(*sn*-glycero-1-phospho-)-α-D-kojibiosyl]-*sn*-glycerol

Some lipids occur with both a glycosyldiacyl moiety and a phosphatidyl group within a single molecule. For example, phosphatidylglucosyldiacylglycerol or 3-O-[6′-O-(1″,2″-diacyl-3′-phospho-sn-glycerol)-α-D-glucopyranosyl]-1,2-diacyl-sn-glycerol and the analogous diglycosyl phosphatidylkojibiosyldiacylglycerol have been found in some Streptococcus species and in *Pseudomonas diminuta*.

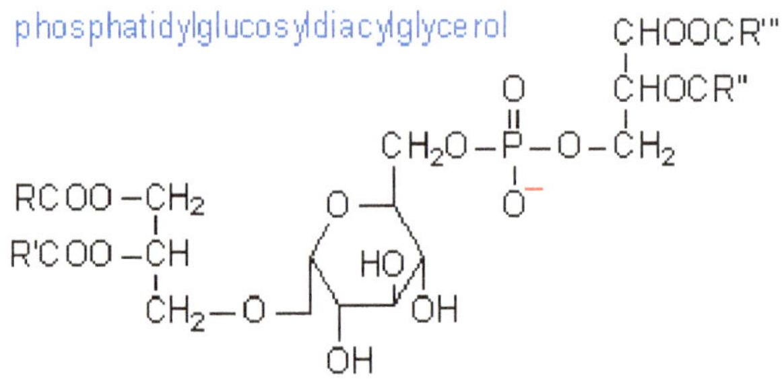

The key to the classification of these lipids within this first type of phosphoglycolipids has come from biosynthetic studies, which have shown that they are synthesised by an enzyme-catalysed transphosphatidylation of monoglucosyldiacylglycerols with phosphatidylglycerol as donor of the phosphatidyl group, rather than by a glycosylation reaction, for example.

monoglucosyldiacylglycerol + phosphatidylglycerol ⟶ phosphatidylmonoglucosyldiacylglycerol + glycerol

Glycosyldiacylglycerols are the lipid unit at the terminal end of the lipoteichoic acids, which are complex phospho-polysaccharides associated with the cell walls of Gram-positive and some Gram-negative bacteria, the lipid components are linked to a polymer of sn-glycerol-1-phosphate residues, which may be substituted with glycosyl (often N-acetylglucosamine) or alanyl residues.

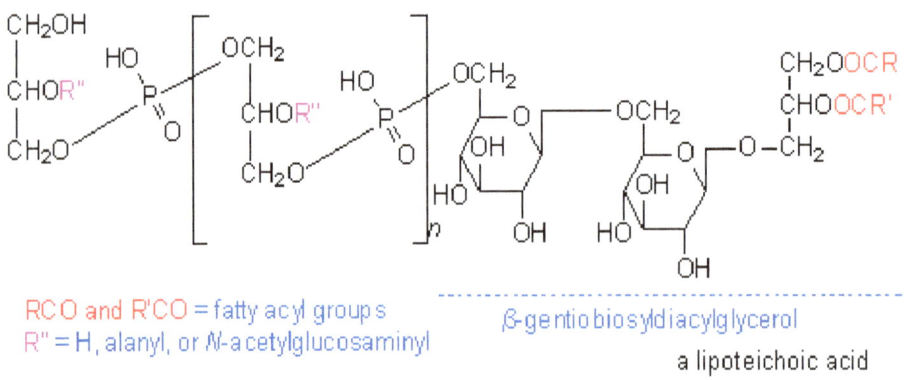

The diacylglycerol unit serves as an anchor to hold the molecule in the membrane of the cell wall by hydrophobic interactions. While this is believed to be the main type of lipoteichoic acid, exceptions are known to exist with poly (digalactosylglycerophosphate), or ribitol or choline phosphate in place of the glycerophosphate residues.

A choline-containing phosphoglycolipid, *i.e.* 6'-O-phosphocholine-α-glucopyranosyl-(1→3)-1,2-diacyl-sn-glycerol, from the human pathogenic bacterium *Mycoplasma fermentans* is distinctive for a number of reasons. In structural terms, it differs from most of the other phosphoglycolipids described here in that the phosphate moiety on position 6′ of glucose is linked to a choline moiety, rather than to glycerol. In biological terms, it has been suspected of involvement in the pathogenesis of rheumatoid arthritis and of acquired immunodeficiency syndrome (AIDS), as it is a major immunological determinant for the organism in infected tissues.

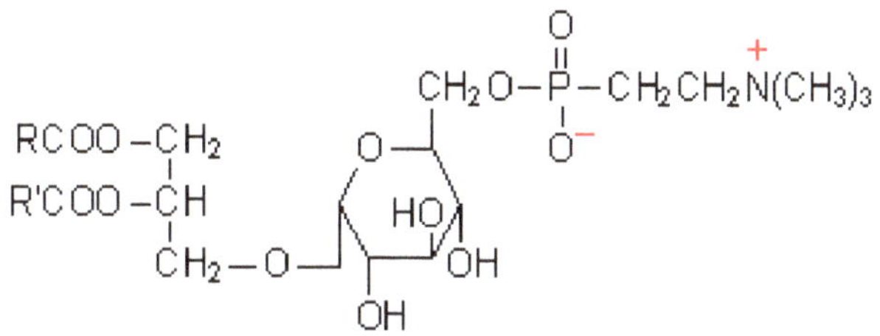

a choline-containing glycophospholipid

Glycophospholipids

Some of the lipids in the second group of glycerol-containing glycophospholipids defined above, *i.e.* with a phosphatidyl backbone, are discussed in relation to the parent phospholipids. They include the glycosyl-phosphatidylinositols, which are ubiquitous lipids that serve to anchor proteins in membranes. For some time, these were erroneously thought to be the only glycophospholipids found in higher organisms.

Phosphatidylglucose was first described from the bacterium *Staphylococcus aureus* in 1970, but doubts have been cast on the identification. The first definitive isolation and characterization of this lipid was as recently as 2001, when surprisingly it was found in mammalian cell types rather than in a microorganism. Phosphatidyl-β-D-glucopyranoside was found first in human cord red cells with a fatty acid composition and distribution similar to the other phospholipids. Subsequently, it was characterized from an erythroblastic leukemia cell line, and most recently from developing astroglial membranes of HL60 cells (together with phosphatidyl-β-D-(6-O-acetyl)-glucopyranoside).

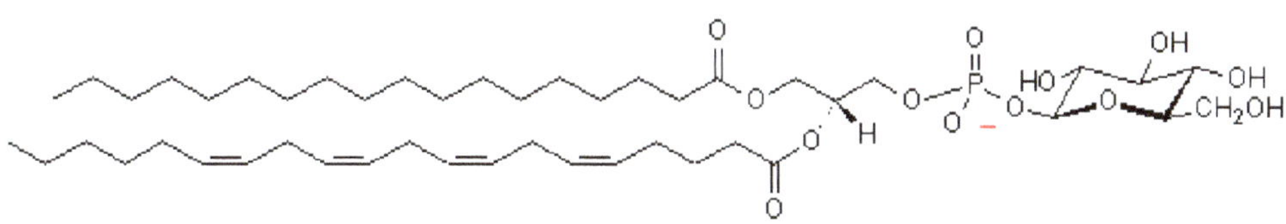

phosphatidyl-β-D-glucopyranoside

III. Sphingolipids

They are classified and discussed in detail as under:

- ☆ Sphingolipids:
- ☆ Introduction + rafts
- ☆ Long-chain or sphingoid bases
- ☆ Ceramides
- ☆ Sphingomyelin and related lipids
- ☆ Sphingosine-1-phosphate
- ☆ Monoglycosylceramides (cerebrosides)
- ☆ Oligoglycosylceramides (neutral)
- ☆ Gangliosides
- ☆ Sulfoglycosphingolipids
- ☆ Complex Glycerolipids

Sphingolipids consist of long-chain bases, linked by an amide bond to a fatty acid and via the terminal hydroxyl group to complex carbohydrate or phosphorus-containing moieties. The root term "sphingo-" was first coined by J.L.W. Thudichum in 1884 because the enigmatic nature of the molecules reminded him of the riddle of the sphinx.

Long-chain bases (sphingoids or sphingoid bases) are the characteristic structural unit of sphingolipids. They are long-chain (12 to 22 carbon atoms) aliphatic

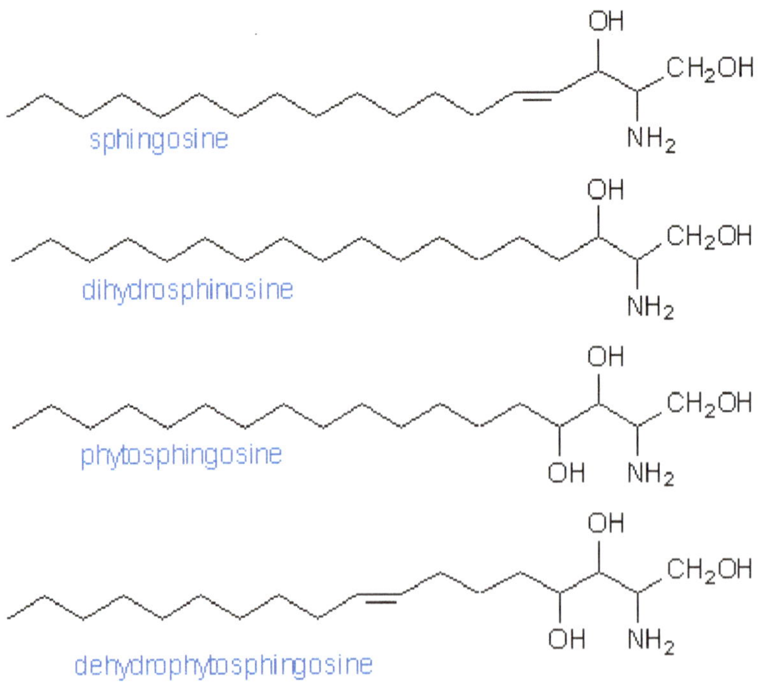

amines, containing two or three hydroxyl groups, and often a distinctive trans-double bond in position 4. The commonest or most abundant of these in animal tissues is sphingosine, ((2S,3R,4E)-2-amino-4-octadecen-1,3-diol). More than 60 long-chain bases have been found in animals, plants and microorganisms, and many of these may occur in a single tissue, but almost always as part of a complex lipid as opposed to in the free form. The aliphatic chains can be saturated, monounsaturated and diunsaturated, with double bonds of either the cis or trans configuration, and they may sometimes have methyl substituents. In addition, saturated and monoenoic straight- and branched-chain trihydroxy bases are found. The aliphatic moiety is similar to that of a fatty acid in its physical properties.

Phytosphingosine ((2S,3S,4R)-2-amino-octadecanetriol) is the most common long-chain base of plant origin.

For shorthand purposes, a nomenclature similar to that for fatty acids can be used, *i.e.* the chain-length and number of double bonds are denoted in the same manner with the prefix "d" or "t" to designate di- and trihydroxy bases, respectively. Thus, sphingosine is d18:1 and phytosphingosine is t18:0. Phytosphingosine also is found in significant amounts in intestinal cells of animals, with much smaller relative proportions in kidney and skin, having entered via the food chain. Sphingoid bases are unusual amongst lipids in that they bear a small positive charge at neutral pH, a consequence of intra-molecular hydrogen bonding. This enables them to cross membranes or move between membranes with relative ease. Most the sphingoid base is linked via the amine group to a fatty acid, *i.e.* to form a ceramide, while a polar head group is attached to the primary hydroxyl moiety. An important exception is sphingosine-1-phosphate which has signalling functions in cells akin to those of lysophospholipids.

$$CH_3(CH_2)_{13}.CHOH.CHOH.CHNH_2.CH_2OH$$

phytosphingosine

Ceramides consist of a long-chain or sphingoid base linked to a fatty acid via an amide bond. In general, they are present at low levels only in tissues, but they are key intermediates in the biosynthesis of the complex sphingolipids. In addition, they have important functions in cellular signalling, and especially in the regulation of apoptosis, and cell differentiation, transformation and proliferation.

Unusual ceramides have been located in the epidermis of the pig and humans; the fatty acids linked to the sphingoid base consist of C_{30} and C_{32} (omega-hydroxylated components, with predominantly the essential fatty acid, linoleic acid, esterified to the terminal hydroxyl group. They are believed to have a special role in preventing the loss of moisture through the skin.

R.CHOH.CH.CH₂OH
        |
        NHOC.R'

ceramide

Depending on the particular layer of the skin (epidermis, stratum corneum, etc.), the lipid composition can vary. These lipids have an obvious role in the barrier properties of the skin, limiting loss of water and solutes and at the same time preventing ingress of harmful substances.

It is now recognized that ceramides have an important role in cellular signalling, and especially in the regulation of apoptosis, and cell differentiation, transformation and proliferation. Indeed, they appear to be formed under all conditions of cellular stress in eukaryotic organisms. Failure to properly regulate apoptosis can have catastrophic consequences, and many disease states including cancer, diabetes, neuropathies, Alzheimer's disease, Parkinson's disease, and atherosclerosis, are thought to arise from deregulation of apoptosis. In addition, ceramides appear to be involved in many aspects of the biology of aging and of male and female fertility.

Sphingomyelin is a sphingophospholipid and consists of a ceramide unit linked at position 1 to phosphorylcholine; it is found as a major component of the complex lipids of all animal tissues but not of plants or micro-organisms.

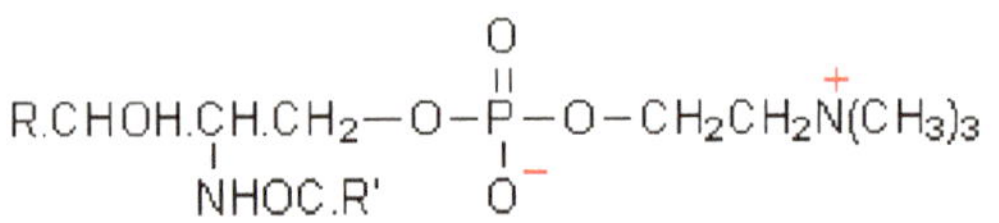

sphingomyelin

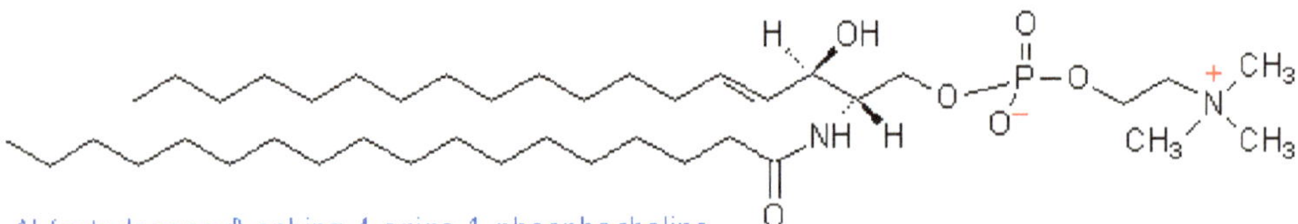

N-(octadecanoyl)-sphing-4-enine-1-phosphocholine

It is a ubiquitous component of animal cell membranes, where it is by far the most abundant sphingolipid. Indeed, it can comprise as much as 50 per cent of the lipids in certain tissues, though it is usually less abundant than phosphatidylcholine. For example, it makes up about 10 per cent of the lipids of brain. It is the single most abundant lipid in erythrocytes of most ruminant animals, where it replaces phosphatidylcholine entirely. In this instance, there is known to be a highly active phospholipase A that breaks down the glycerophospholipids, but not sphingomyelin. Like phosphatidylcholine, sphingomyelin tends to be most abundant in the plasma membrane, and especially in the outer leaflet, of cells.

It resembles phosphatidylcholine in many of its physical properties, and can apparently substitute in part for this in membranes although it also has its own unique role. For example, it is a major constituent of the plasma membrane of cells, where it is concentrated together with sphingoglycolipids and cholesterol in tightly organized sub-domains termed 'rafts'. Sphingosine tends to be the most abundant long-chain base constituent, and it is usually accompanied by sphinganine and C_{20} homologues.

Sphingomyelin is a precursor for a number of sphingolipid metabolites that have important functions in cellular signalling, including sphingosine-1-phosphate, as part of the 'sphingomyelin cycle'. A correct balance between the various metabolites is vital for good health. Niemann-Pick disease is a rare lipid storage disorder that results from of a deficiency in the enzyme responsible for the degradation of sphingomyelin.

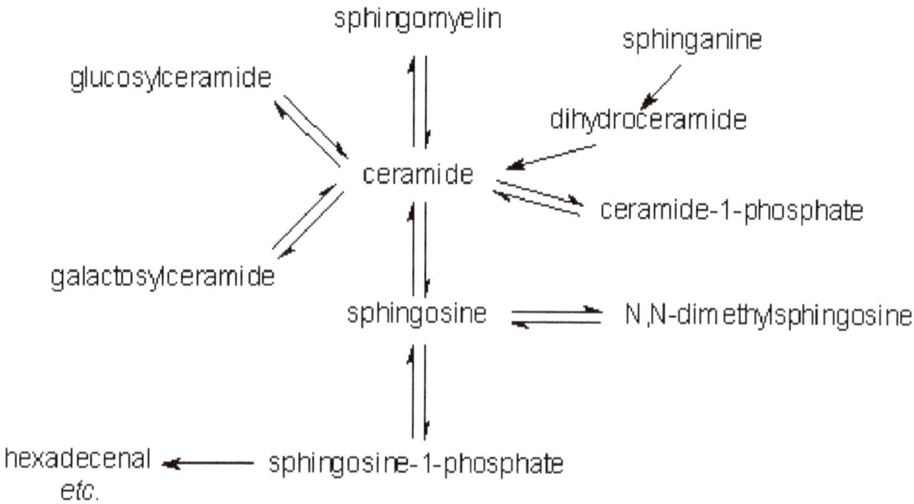

The 'sphingomyelin cycle'

About 60 per cent of the fatty acids of the sphingomyelin of the grey matter of human brain consist of stearic acid (18:0), while lignoceric (24:0) and nervonic (24:1) acids make up 60 per cent of the corresponding lipid of white matter. Polyunsaturated fatty acids such as arachidonic acid are rarely present, although they have sometimes been mistakenly identified in the literature. Exceptions are the sphingomyelins of testes and spermatozoa, which contain very-long-chain polyunsaturated fatty acids (up to 34 carbon atoms), a proportion of which have hydroxyl groups in position 2.

Although there is no known nutritional requirement for sphingolipids, such as sphingomyelin, they are a component of any meat diet. Sphingomyelin in the diet is hydrolysed by an intestinal alkaline sphingomyelinase and neutral ceramidase to free fatty acids and sphingosine. The latter is absorbed, converted to palmitic acid and acylated into the triacylglycerol component of chylomicrons. The alkaline sphingomyelinase in particular is unusual in that is very different in its structure and other properties from intracellular enzymes with a related function. It is believed to have a role in the production of sphingolipid metabolites within the intestines and colon, especially, that may influence a number of disease states. From animal experiments, there is evidence that feeding sphingolipids inhibits colon carcinogenesis, reduces serum LDL cholesterol but elevates HDL concentrations, and may alleviate some of the symptoms of inflammatory bowel disease.

The apparent similarity between phosphatidylcholine and sphingomyelin is superficial, and there are great differences in the hydrogen bonding capacities and physical properties of the two lipids. For example, sphingomyelin has an amide bond at position 2 and a hydroxyl on position 3 of the sphingoid base that can both participate in hydrogen bonding, while the trans double bond appears to assist intermolecular interactions in membranes. With phosphatidylcholine, in contrast, the two ester carbonyl groups can only act as hydrogen acceptors. The degree of unsaturation of the alkyl moieties in each lipid is very different, and this gives them very different packing properties in membranes. It is now recognized that sphingomyelin (and other sphingolipids) and cholesterol may be located together in specific sub-domains.

Sphingolipids closely related to sphingomyelin. An unusual sphingolipid, 3-O-acyl-D-erythro-sphingomyelin, has been found in plasma of the newborn pig and infant (but not in that of adults). In this instance, position 3 of the sphingosine residue is linked to an additional fatty acid (C_{16} or C_{18}) via an ester bond (alkali-labile).

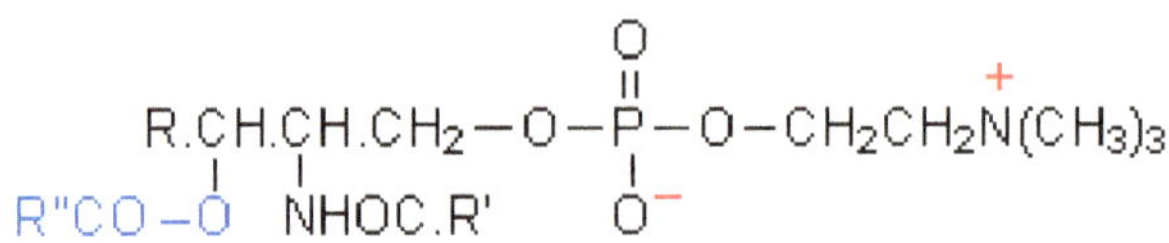

3-*O*-acyl-*D*-*erythro*-sphingomyelin

A further novel sphingomyelin, isolated from a cyanobacterium, *Scytonema julianum*, contains fatty acids in an estolide linkage, *i.e.* with an acetyl group esterified to an ?-1 hydroxyl of a long-chain fatty acid.

Sphingosine phosphorylcholine, or lyso-sphingomyelin, is found at trace levels only in tissues, but again appears to be involved in many cellular processes. It is produced under physiological and pathological conditions, and interacts with specific cell receptors (coupled to G proteins). It has many similar functions to sphingosine-1-phosphate.

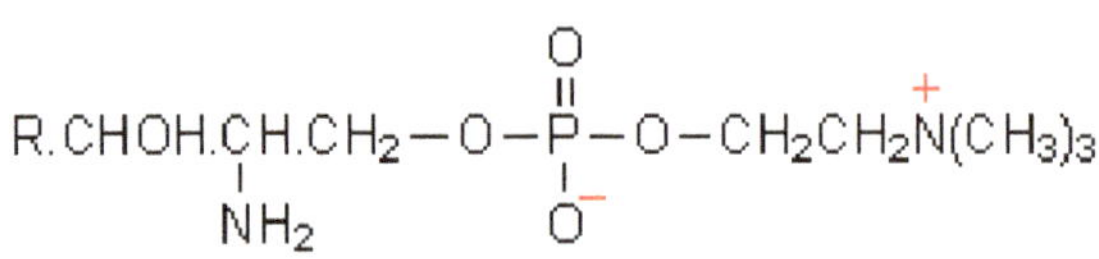

sphingosine phosphorylcholine

In addition, sphingolipids have been found in a species of earthworm with phosphorylcholine linked to the carbohydrate moiety of mono- and digalactosylceramides.

Ceramide phosphorylethanolamine, the sphingolipid analogue of phosphatidylethanolamine, is a component of the lipids of insects, some fresh water invertebrates and many species of bacteria (where it is often accompanied by ceramide phosphorylglycerol). Recently, it has been characterized comprehensively in three species of plant fungal pathogens (Oomycetes). The fatty acid and long-chain bases components vary with species, and for example one contains phytosphingosine and another unusual branched-trienoic base.

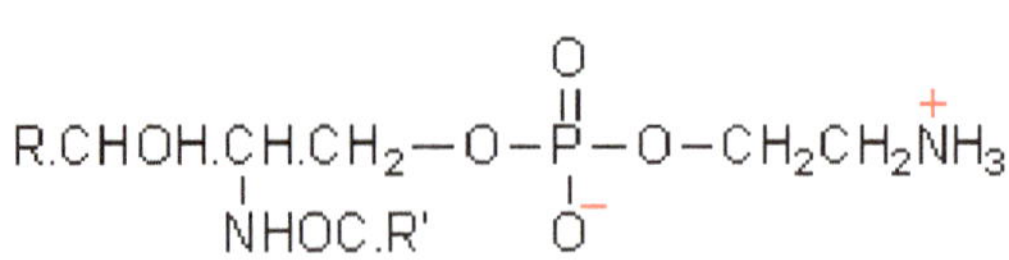

ceramide phosphorylethanolamine

It is synthesised by a similar mechanism to sphingomyelin, *i.e.* by transfer of phosphorylethanolamine from phosphatidylethanolamine to ceramide. A phosphonolipid analogue of ceramide phosphorylethanolamine is found in certain organisms.

Ceramide phosphorylinositol or myo-inositol-(1-O)-phosphoryl-(O-1)-ceramide, the sphingolipid analogue of phosphatidylinositol, is a major component of sphingolipids in yeasts, such as *Saccharomyces cerevisiae*, where it is accompanied by the inositol-containing sphingolipids, mannosylinositolphosphorylceramide and mannosyldiinositolphosphorylceramide. In addition, ceramide phosphorylinositol and glycosylated forms of this are components of the membranes of higher plants.

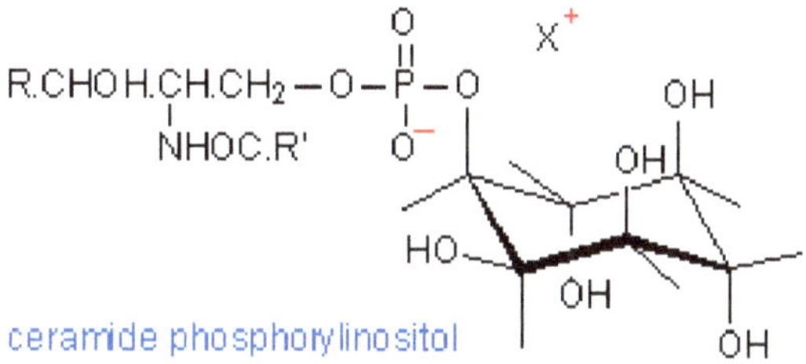

ceramide phosphorylinositol

Some bacteria and parasitic organisms also contain ceramide phosphorylinositol, and it is present in many species of fungi, sometimes together with glycosylated forms (usually mannose). In addition, higher plants contain a number of distinctive lipids with ceramide phosphorylinositol as the backbone with carbohydrate moieties linked to inositol, and they have been termed 'phytoglycosphingolipids'.

Ceramide phosphorylmannose has recently been identified and characterized for the first time in the lipids of Sphingobacterium spiritivorum.

Ceramide-1-phosphate, a sphingoid analogue of phosphatidic acid or lysophosphatidic acid, is one of the metabolites in the 'sphingomyelin cycle' but is only indirectly related to sphingomyelin as it is formed from ceramide by the action of a specific ceramide kinase. It has been detected in human leukaemia (HL 60) cells and in bone marrow from mice, but the ceramide kinase is present in many other cell types.

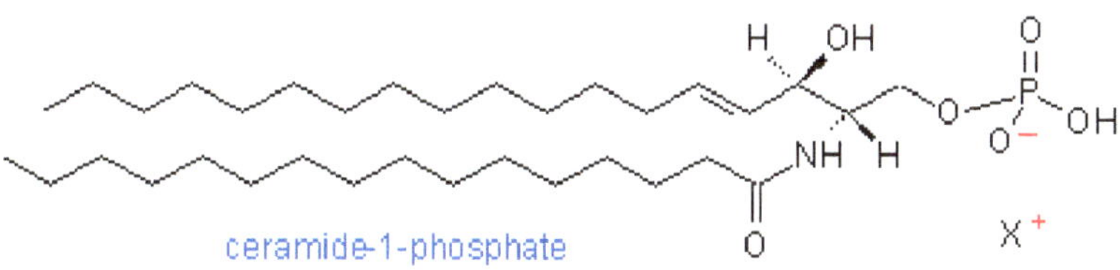

ceramide-1-phosphate

It is now known to have a number of biological functions, some of which are confined to specific cell types. For example, it is mitogenic for fibroblasts and blocks apoptosis in macrophages. In addition, it is believed to be an important mediator of the inflammatory response, by stimulating the release of arachidonic acid by activating a specific phospholipase A_2, *i.e.* the initial rate-limiting step of eicosanoid synthesis.

Neutral Glycosylceramides

The most widespread glycosphingolipids are the monoglycosylceramides (or cerebrosides), and they consist of a basic ceramide unit linked by a glycosidic bond at carbon 1 of the long-chain base to glucose or galactose. They were first found in brain lipids, where the principal form is galactosylceramide, but they are now known to be ubiquitous constituents of animal tissues. Glucosylceramide is also found in animal tissues, and especially in skin, where it functions as part of the water permeability barrier. It is the biosynthetic precursor of lactosylceramide, and thence of the complex oligoglycolipids and gangliosides. In addition, glucosylceramide is found in plants, where the main long-chain base is phytosphingosine.

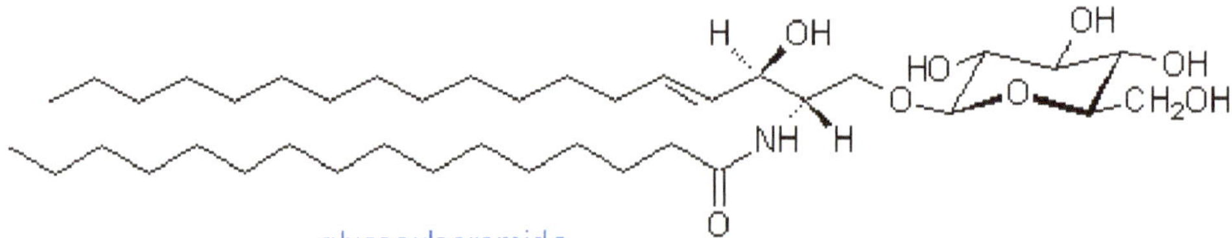

O-Acyl-glycosylceramides have been detected in small amounts in some tissues, as have cerebrosides with monosaccharides such as xylose, mannose and fucose.

Di-, tri- and tetraglycosylceramides (**oligoglycosylceramides**) are present also in most animal tissues at low levels. The most common diglycosyl form is lactosylceramide, and it can be accompanied by related compounds containing further galactose or galactosamine residues. Tri- and tetraglycosylceramides with a terminal galactosamine residue are sometimes termed "globosides", while glycolipids containing fucose are known as "fucolipids". Lactosylceramide is the biosynthetic precursor of most of these with further monosaccharide residues being added to the end of the carbohydrate chain. Oligoglycosylceramides with more than 20 carbohydrate residues have been isolated from animal tissues, and those from intestinal cells are of special interest. They are an important element of the immune response system.

Sulfate esters of galactosylceramide and lactosylceramide (sulfoglycosphingolipids–often referred to as "sulfatides" or "lipid sulfates"), with the sulfate group linked to position 3 of the galactosyl moiety, are major components of brain lipids and they are found in trace amounts in other tissues.

Complex plant sphingolipids, phytoglycosphingolipids, containing glucosamine, glucuronic acid and mannose linked to the ceramide via phosphorylinositol, were isolated and characterized from seeds initially, but related compounds are also known to be present in other plant tissues and in fungi.

Gangliosides are highly complex oligoglycosylceramides, which contain one or more sialic acid groups (N-acyl, especially acetyl, derivatives of neuraminic acid, abbreviated to "NANA") in addition to glucose, galactose and galactosamine.

The polar and ionic nature of these lipids renders them soluble in water (contrary to some definitions of a lipid). They were first found in the ganglion cells of the

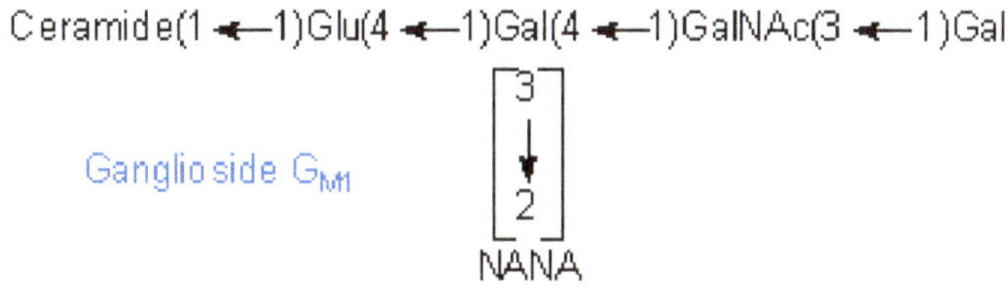

Ganglioside G_{M1}

central nervous system, hence the name, but are now known to be present in most animal tissues. Gangliosides have been shown to control growth and differentiation of cells, and they have important roles in the immune defence systems. Also, they bind specifically to various bacterial toxins, such as those from botulinum, tetanus and cholera.

Sphingosine 1-phosphate is one of the simplest sphingolipids structurally. Sphingosine-1-phosphate is an important cellular metabolite, derived from ceramide that is synthesized de novo or as part of the sphingomyelin cycle (in animal cells). It has also been found in insects, yeasts and plants. It is present at low levels only in animal tissues, but it is a pivotal lipid in many cellular signalling pathways.

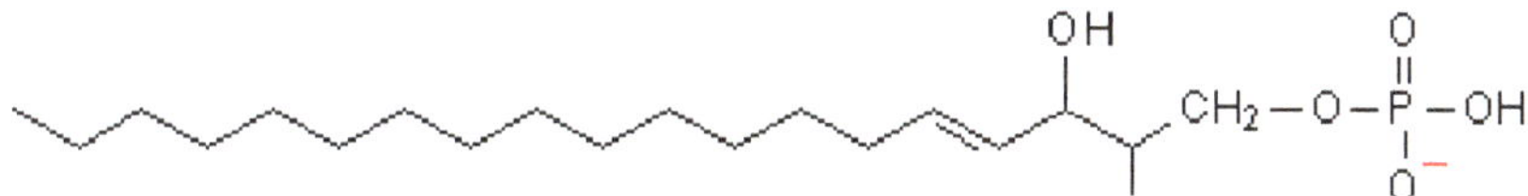

sphingosine-1-phosphate

Intracellularly, sphingosine-1-phosphate functions also to regulate calcium mobilization and cell growth in response to a variety of extracellular stimuli. Current opinion appears to suggest that the balance between sphingosine-1-phosphate and ceramide and/or sphingosine levels in cells is critical for their viability. These are important for the growth of new blood vessels, vascular maturation, cardiac development and immunity, and for directed cell movement.

Monoglycosylceramides (Cerebrosides)

Galactosylceramide (Galß1-1'Cer) is the principal glycosphingolipid in brain tissue, hence the trivial name "cerebroside", which was first conferred on it in 1874,

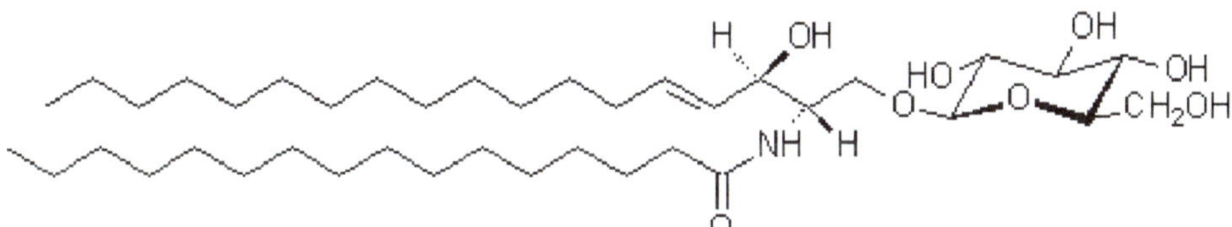

glucosylceramide

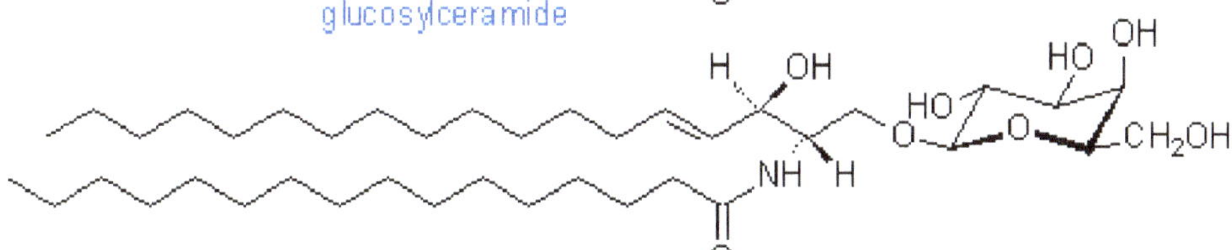

galactosylceramide

although it was much later before it was properly characterized. In fact, galactosylceramides are found in all nervous tissues, but they can amount to 2 per cent of the dry weight of grey matter and 12 per cent of white matter.

Glucosylceramide (Glcß1-1'Cer) is also found at low levels in animal tissues, such as spleen and erythrocytes, as well as in nervous tissues. The d18:1/16:0 molecular species are illustrated above. It is a major constituent of skin lipids. Glucosylceramide is usually considered to be the principal glycosphingolipid in plants, although this may be because the more polar complex glycosphingolipids are not easily extracted and are missed in conventional analyses. Nonetheless, glucosylceramide is abundant in photosynthetic tissues.

Harmful quantities of glucosylceramide accumulate in the spleen, liver, lungs, bone marrow, and, in rare cases, the brain of patients with Gaucher's disease, the most common of the inherited metabolic disorders involving storage of excessive amounts of complex lipids.

Psychosine

Psychosine is the trivial name for a monoglycosylsphingoid, *i.e.* it is the non-acylated or lyso form of a cerebroside, normally galactosylsphingosine.

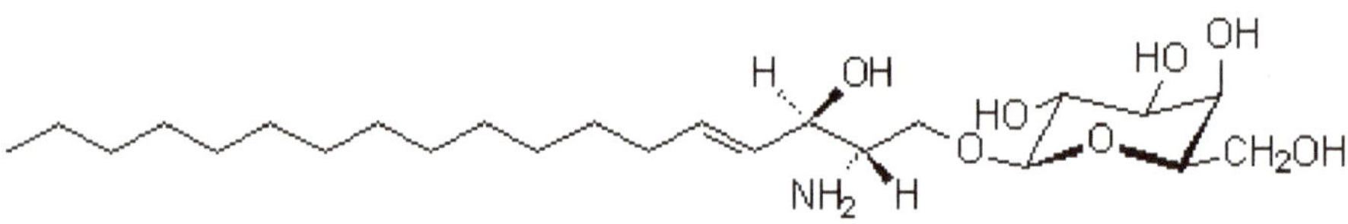

galactosylsphingosine (psychosine)

It is a minor intermediate in the catabolism of monoglycosylceramides, and is normally present in tissues at very low concentrations. However, it may have some specific function in animal cells, for example in pathophysiology or in signalling since specific receptors have been found. It accumulates in tissues in the genetic disorder, Krabbe's disease, and to a certain extent also in Gaucher's disease. It is believed to inhibit cytokinesis, *i.e.* the last stage in the process by which a single cell divides to produce two daughter cells, with production of multinucleate cells instead.

Carnitine and Acylcarnitines

Carnitine (L-3-hydroxy-4-aminobutyrobetaine or L-3-hydroxy-4-N-trimethylaminobutanoic acid), and its acyl esters (acylcarnitines) are essential compounds for the metabolism of fatty acids. They are present in animals, plants and some microorganisms. In animal tissues, carnitine concentrations are relatively high, typically between 0.2 and 6mmol/kg, with most in the heart and skeletal muscle.

Carnitine can be synthesised de novo in animal cells, with lysine and methionine as the primary precursors and butyrobetaine as an intermediate, but it is believed that most comes from the diet. In humans, the major sources of carnitine are meat, fish and dairy products, which can supply 2 to 12 ìmol per day per kg of body weight, as opposed to 1.2 ìmol per day per kg of body weight of endogenous carnitine. The latter

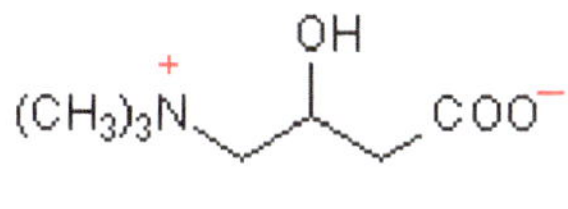

carnitine

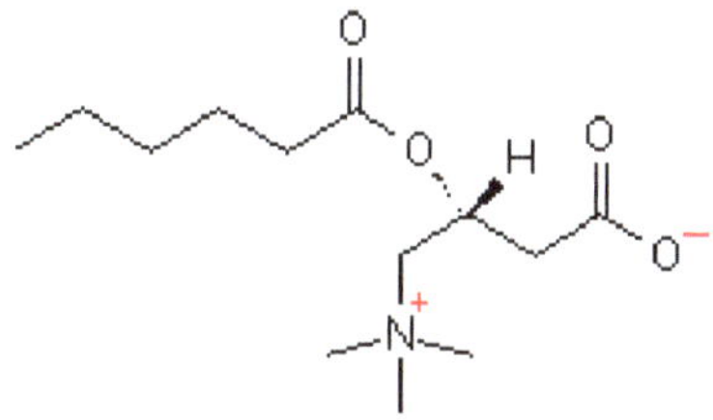

O-hexanoyl-(*R*)-carnitine

is synthesised in the kidney, liver and brain and is transported to other tissues in the circulation. In the kidney, carnitine and butyrobetaine are reabsorbed efficiently so urinary loss is minimized.

The main function of carnitine is to assist the transport and metabolism of fatty acids into mitochondria, where they are oxidized for energy production. In so doing, carnitine maintains a balance between free and esterified coenzyme A, since an excess of acyl-CoA intermediates is potentially toxic to cells. In addition, carnitine is required to remove any surplus of acyl groups from mitochondria.

Oligoglycosylceramides (Neutral)

i) Lactosylceramide and Other Diosylceramides

Non-acidic di- and oligoglycosphingolipids, *i.e.* with two or more carbohydrate moieties attached to a ceramide unit, are vital components of cellular membranes of most eukaryotic organisms and some bacteria. Their abundance relative to other lipids is usually low other than in epithelial and neuronal cells, while the nature and proportions of the different glycolipid classes vary with the type of cell and the stage of growth. However, they are extremely important for the function of cells.

The most important and abundant of the diosylceramides is ß-D-galactosyl-(1-4)-ß-D-glucosyl-(1-1')-ceramide, more conveniently termed lactosylceramide (LacCer), using the trivial name of the disaccharide.

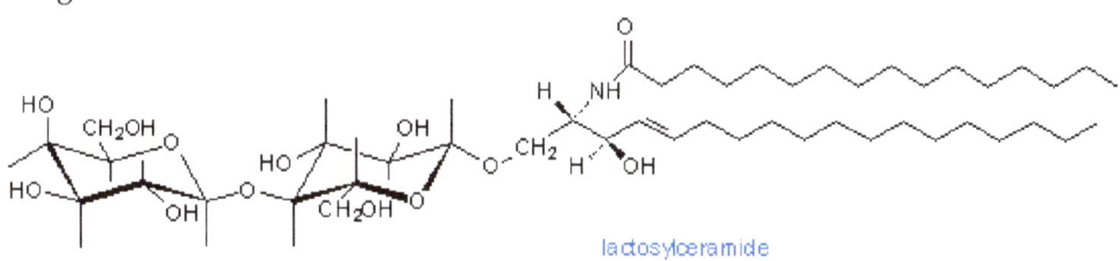

lactosylceramide

It is found in small amounts in most animal tissues. Galabiosylceramide (Galα 1-4Galß1-1'Cer) has also been found in small amounts in kidney and pancreas, for example, and it is one of the lipids that accumulates in excessive amounts in Fabry's disease. Lactosylceramide may assist in stabilizing the plasma membrane and activating receptor molecules in the special micro-domains as with the cerebrosides. There are suggestions that it plays a role in the pathogenesis of atherosclerosis. However, it is especially important as the biosynthetic precursor of most of the neutral oligoglycosylceramides and gangliosides.

ii) Oligoglycosylceramides of Animal Tissues

Neutral oligoglycosylceramides with from three to more than twenty monosaccharide units in the chain have been detected in animal tissues ('megaloglycolipids' with up to 50 carbohydrate groups occur in erythrocytes). Of these, tri- to pentaglycosylceramides are often the most abundant or at least are most intensively studied.

Fucolipids are oligoglycolipids in any of the above series in which a fucose (Fuc) residue substitutes for one of the usual carbohydrate residues. In addition, certain of the oligoglycolipids exist as lipid sulphates, and others are linked to sialic acid residues, *i.e.* gangliosides.

Literally hundreds of different neutral oligoglycosphingolipids have been found in various organs and species of animals, with further complexity being added by the nature of the ceramide unit. In addition, there is a body of evidence to suggest that the composition of the ceramide unit is biologically important. As with the other sphingolipids, the oligoglycosylceramides are concentrated together with cholesterol in the specific region of membranes. In any given cell type, the number of different glycosylceramides may be relatively small, but their nature and compositions may be characteristic and in some way related to the function of the cell. This composition tends to change substantially as an animal develops.

iii) Oligoglycosylceramides of Plants

In plants, elongation of glucosylceramide (mainly) and mannosylceramide occurs with either mannosyl or glucosyl units, via ß1-4 linkages, by mechanisms that are presumably related to those in animals. Addition of a further glucose unit terminates the elongation step, but further mannose units may continue to be added. The consequence is that series of di-, tri- and tetraglycosylceramides occur, terminating in either a glucose or mannose unit. Little is known of their functions.

Coenzyme A Esters

Before a fatty acid can be metabolized in tissues, for example by being esterified, oxidized or subjected to synthetic modification, it must usually be activated by conversion to a Coenzyme A ester or acyl-CoA, with the fatty acid group linked to the terminal thiol moiety. The thiol ester is a highly energetic bond that permits a facile transfer of the acyl group to receptor molecules. This is true for the simplest fatty acid of all, acetic acid (*i.e.* as acetyl-CoA), as well as for long-chain fatty acids.

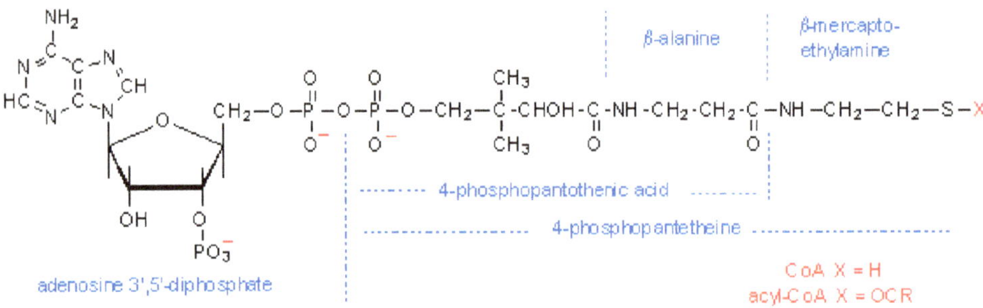

Coenzyme A (CoASH) itself is a highly polar molecule, consisting of adenosine 3',5'-diphosphate linked to 4-phosphopantethenic acid (Vitamin B_5) and thence to β-mercaptoethylamine. Not only is it intimately associated with most reactions of fatty acids, but it is also a key molecule in the catabolism of carbohydrates via the citric acid cycle in which acetyl-CoA is a major end-product.

In addition to their role in lipid biosynthesis and catabolism, CoA esters have been shown to regulate the activities of a variety of enzymes, including that of acetyl-CoA carboxylase, an essential enzyme in fatty acid synthesis. Long-chain acyl-CoA esters also bind to certain hormone receptors and have a signalling function.

Phosphonolipids

Phosphonolipids consist of aminoethylphosphonic acid residues, *i.e.* with a phosphorus-carbon bond, attached to a lipid backbone, which can be either a ceramide or diacylglycerol. The first of the sphingolipids to be discovered was ceramide 2-aminoethylphosphonate, which was found in sea anemones. Subsequently, it was detected in a variety of molluscs, protozoa, bacteria, and even bovine brain tissue, sometimes accompanied by an N-methylethanolamine analogue.

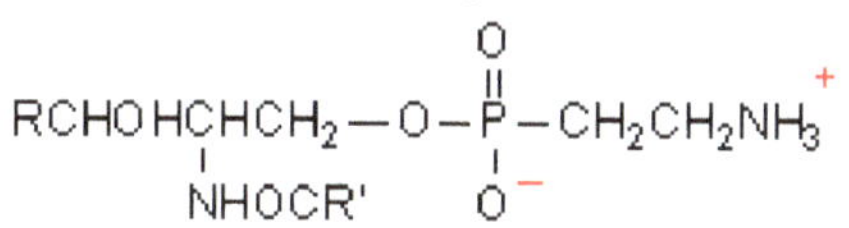

ceramide 2-aminoethylphosphonate

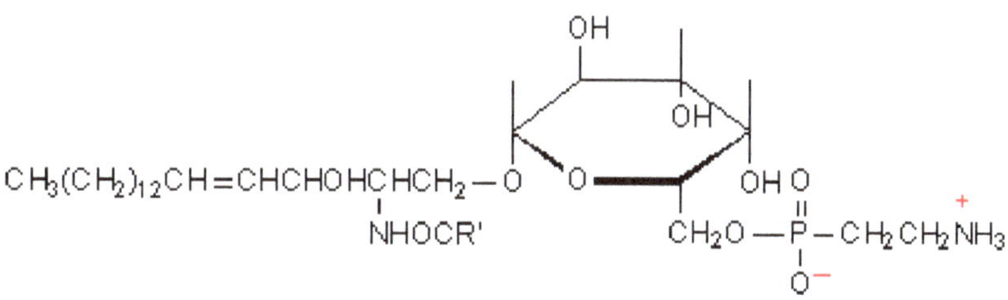

6-O-(aminoethylphosphono)-galactopyranosylceramide

It is sometimes accompanied by small amounts of ceramide 2-methylaminoethylphosphonate. In addition, phosphonoglycosphingolipids, such as 6-O-(aminoethylphosphono)galactosyl ceramide and its N-methylethanolamine analogue, related oligoglycosphingolipids, and a triphosphonoglycosphingolipid have been found in marine invertebrates.

Proteolipids

In 1951, proteins that were soluble in organic solvents such as chloroform-methanol were found in rat brain myelin, although it was another twenty years before it was shown that they contained covalently bound fatty acids and so differed from the lipoproteins. Such proteins are now known to be widespread in nature with a variety of important functions. The term proteolipid is used to define all proteins containing covalently bound lipid moieties, including fatty acids, isoprenoids, cholesterol and glycosylphosphatidylinositol.

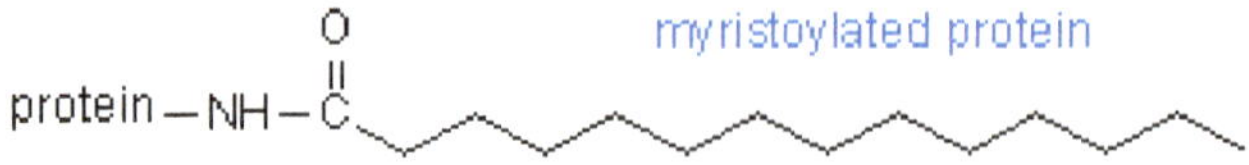

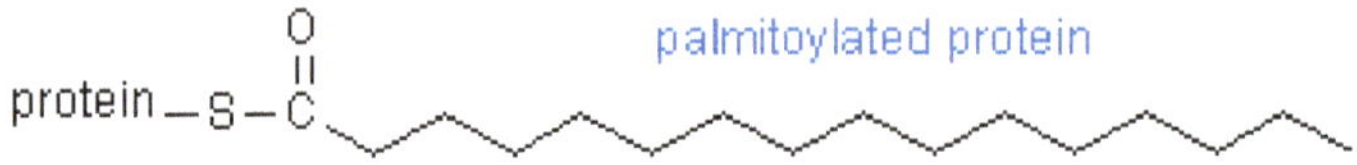

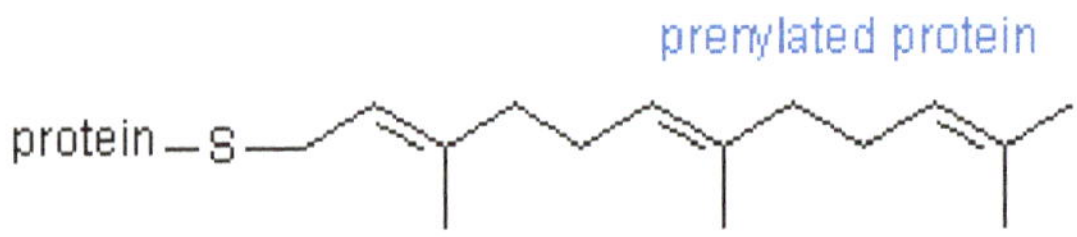

i) N-Myristoylated Proteins

In the N-myristoylated proteins, myristic acid (14:0) specifically, which is a ubiquitous but usually minor component of cellular lipids, is bound to the amino-terminal glycine residue (of a relatively conserved sequence of the protein) via an amide linkage that is relatively stable to hydrolysis. These constitute a large family of essential eukaryotic and viral proteins presumably with many different functions, and they are located either in the cytosol or in the cytosolic (inner) membrane of cells, or both. The acyl group anchors the protein to the membrane, although simultaneous binding to phospholipids or other membrane constituents is necessary to increase the strength of the interaction.

ii) Palmitoylated Proteins

In the palmitoylated proteins, palmitic acid (16:0) is linked to one or more (up to four) internal cysteine (or occasionally threonine or serine) residues via labile thioester bonds. The name is something of a misnomer in this instance, as other fatty acids are often present, including 16:1, 18:0 and 18:1. Some N-myristoylated proteins may also be palmitoylated internally. The thio-acylated residues can be in many different regions of the proteins, either cytoplasmic or within a predicted trans-membrane domain.

iii) Prenylated Proteins

Prenylated proteins are formed by attachment of isoprenoid lipid units, farnesyl (C_{15}) or geranylgeranyl (C_{20}), via cysteine thio-ether bonds at or near the carboxyl

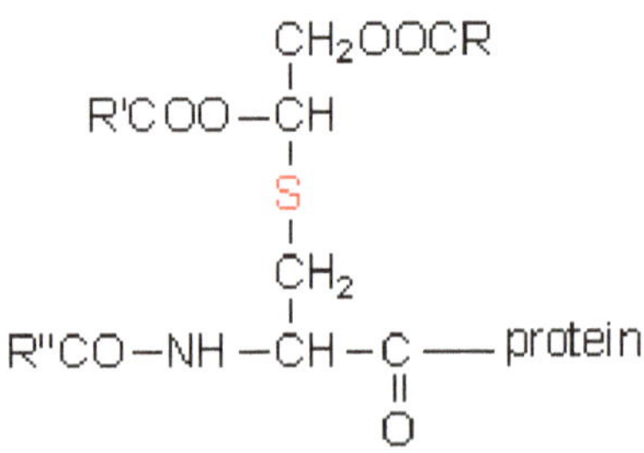

bacterial proteolipid

terminus. Such proteins are ubiquitous in mammalian cells, where they can amount to up to 2 per cent of the total proteins, and they are increasingly being found in plants.

iv) Proteins Linked Covalently to Cholesterol

Relatively recently, it was discovered that cholesterol can be found in covalent linkage to specific proteins, known as the "hedgehog" signalling family. These are formed post-translationally by attachment of cholesterol via an ester bond to glycine in a highly conserved region of the protein. They were first found and studied in insects, but they are now known to occur in higher organisms, including vertebrates from fish to humans.

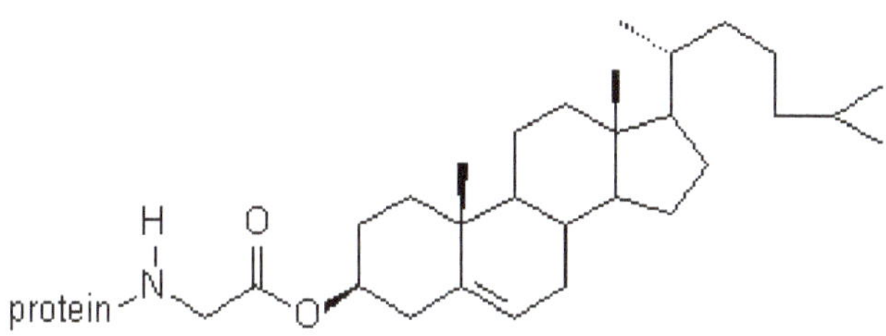

cholesterol-linked protein

These proteolipids are believed to have a major role in signalling during the differentiation of cells in the development of embryos. Indeed, they are required for a considerable range of processes, from the control of left-right asymmetry of the body to the specification of individual cell types within the brain. If further confirmation is needed, this illustrates once more the vital importance of cholesterol in animal tissues.

v) Bacterial proteolipids

All bacteria contain large numbers of proteins (more than 2000 have been identified) with a unique and distinctive post-translational lipid modification that appears to be essential for their efficient function, and even for their pathogenesis via host-pathogen interactions. The lipid moiety consists of an N-acyl-S-diacylglycerol group attached to an N-terminal cysteine, *i.e.* it contains a thio ether bond. As with other proteolipids, the lipid moiety acts as an anchor to hold the protein tightly to a hydrophobic cellular membrane while permitting it to operate in an aqueous environment in such important activities as transport, signalling adhesion, digestion and growth.

Chapter 3

Gastrointestinal Digestion and Absorption of Lipid

I. General Aspects of Intestinal Lipid Digestion and Absorption

Most of the dietary fat, whether plant or animal in origin, consists of triglyceride. Triglycerides (TG) are triesters of glycerol. Long-chain fatty acids, such as oleate (18:1) and palmitate (16:0), are the major fatty acids (FA) present in dietary TG. Traces of medium-chain FA are also present. The small intestine is presented daily with other lipids such as phospholipid (PL), cholesterol and other sterols. Both phospholipid and cholesterol are major components of bile. Biliary PL is a more important source of PL than dietary PL. In man, it has been calculated that the daily biliary secretion of PL into the small intestine is 11-12 g, whereas the dietary contribution is 1-2 g. Over 90 per cent of the biliary phospholipid is lecithin (phosphatidylcholine). Although the predominant sterol in the diet is cholesterol, but there are also plant sterols which account for 20-25 per cent of the total dietary sterol.

Intraluminal Digestion of Triglyceride

Although the majority of TG digestion is completed in the small intestinal lumen, the digestion starts in the stomach. The presence of gastric lipase has been reported in human gastric juice. The major source of gastric lipase is from the secretion of a group of serous glands beneath the circumvallate papillae. The gastric lipase is similar to the pancreatic lipase in that they both have the ability to cleave the ester bond at the sn-1 and sn-3 positions of the TG. However, the gastric lipase preferentially cleaves the sn-3 position relative to the sn-1 position, regardless of the FA present. Furthermore, the digestion products of gastric lipase are diglyceride and FA, whereas those of pancreatic lipase are 2-monoglyceride (2-MG) and FA. The lingual lipase plays an important role in the digestion of fat in the newborn. Partly this is due to the abundant presence of short and medium-chain TG in milk fat. These are readily hydrolyzed by lingual lipase. Furthermore, the infant's pancreatic lipase activity not being fully developed is compensated for by the lingual lipase. Even in adults, the lingual lipase aids in the digestion and absorption of TG both in normal and in diseased states. The action of lingual lipase aids the digestion of TG and partial glycerides by pancreatic lipase in the intestinal lumen in various ways.

The lipid emulsion enters the small intestinal lumen as fine lipid droplets < 0.5 mm in diameter. The combined action of the bile and the pancreatic juice brings about a marked change in the chemical and physical form of the ingested lipid emulsion. Most of the digestion of TG is brought about by pancreatic lipase in the upper part of the intestinal lumen. The pancreatic lipase works at the interface between the oil and the aqueous phases.

Pancreatic lipase acts mainly on the 1- and 3-ester bonds of the TG to release 2-MG and free FA. Although 1-MG is sometimes derived from 2-MG through isomerization in an aqueous medium, it probably occurs slowly in the gut. Further hydrolysis of the 1- or 2-MG results in the formation of glycerol and FA. A pancreatic esterase has been demonstrated to catalyze such processes. Researchers also found that it worked more efficiently with the I-isomer than with the 2-isomer.

The activity of purified pancreatic lipase is very much inhibited in the presence of bile salts with concentrations above the critical micellar concentration. However, the inhibition can be overcome by the presence of another protein from the pancreatic juice which has been purified and identified as colipase. Colipase acts by attaching to the ester bond, region of the TG molecule. In turn, the lipase binds strongly to the colipase by electrostatic interactions, thereby allowing the hydrolysis of the TG by the lipase molecule.

The lipolytic products then distribute themselves between aqueous and oil phases. Calcium ions have been shown to aid in the desorption of the lipolytic products from the oil/water interface. In the aqueous phase, the TG lipolytic products exist mainly as part of the mixed bile salt micelle, although some exist in very low concentrations as monomolecular species in classical solution.

Digestion of Phospholipid

The majority of the intraluminal PL is lecithin (PC). The PC entering the intestinal lumen is derived predominantly from the bile, but with a small portion from the diet. Upon exposure to the pancreatic phospholipase A, the PC is hydrolyzed to form lysolecithin and FA. As the name of the enzyme indicates, it attacks the FA at the 2-position. Both the enzyme and its anionic zymogen have been purified from porcine pancreas. Bile salt and Ca^{2+} are required for the proper functioning of the phospholipase. Although it is generally accepted that bile PC is only absorbed after hydrolysis by pancreatic phospholipase A_2 to form 1-lysolecithin, it has been proposed that bile PC is resistant to the action of phospholipase A_2, there being an enterohepatic circulation of bile PC.

Sphingomyelin, another luminal PL, is probably not broken down appreciably in the intestinal lumen. It is absorbed mainly as intact molecules.

Cholesterol Digestion

Cholesterol enters the small intestine both as free cholesterol and as cholesterol esterified with FA. The esterified cholesterol first has to be hydrolyzled by the pancreatic cholesterol esterase to the free sterol prior to its absorption.

II. Permeation of the Digested Fat into the Enterocyte

There is now a concensus that the lipid digestion products (FA, 2-monoglyceride, lysolecithin, and free cholesterol) pass into the absorptive cell membrane from aqueous dispersion by passive diffusion.

Whether lipid molecules penetrate the cell membrane to any extent in the form of micelle aggregates is still open to debate. There is evidence from several groups that lipid molecules penetrate as monomers. Penetration is a passive process.

III. Absorption of Digested Lipids

The question of intestinal absorption of lipids has been a challenging problem for a very long time. Until very recently, it was not well understood as to how the animal organism, which operates its metabolic activities in an aqueous environment, can deal with lipids, which are inherently insoluble in water, and yet are required for its survival. Even though the concept of lipoproteins had partly answered this point, the baffling question still remained is that, lipoproteins can't exist during digestion of lipids in the intestine. Eventually, we learnt that in order to circumvent such difficulties higher organisms have evolved two important secretions, namely, the pancreatic and biliary secretions. The importance of these two secretions in the absorption of lipids was clearly established when it was demonstrated that the MG and FFA produced in the intestinal lumen by the action of pancreatic lipase on TG appear along with bile salts in a water-clear micellar solution. Ultimately, this observation led to the concept of micellar solubilisation of lipids, according to which lipids are absorbed from a finely dispersed and molecularly defined micellar state. It is now generally assumed that from such micellar solutions lipids penetrate the microceillus membranes and enter the mucosal cell, presumably by a process of difference. The concept of micellar solubilisation, though mainly developed for understanding the absorption of TG, seems to be important in the absorption of other classes of lipids also, like cholesteryl and retinyl esters and phospholipids.

Although it is now widely accepted that during absorption TG are broken down to 2-MG and FFA, which in turn are reacylated to TG in the cell, an important missing link in this picture was unequivocal demonstration that the 2-MG is absorbed intact during this process. While 86 per cent of the hydrolysed TG is present as 2-MG in the lumen, only the remaining 14 per cent is hydrolysed to glycerol and FFA. About 80 per cent of the absorbed 2-MG maintains its positional intestine during reacylation to TG in the mucosal cell.

The bile salts, so essential for micellar formation, are not absorbed along with the lipids. During absorption, the bile salts are left behind in the interlumen. In the mucosal cell, long chain fatty acids with 14 carbon atoms or more are converted to acyl COA derivatives and acylate the mono- and diglycerides to form triglycerides. The TG then combine with small amounts of phospholipid and protein to form chylomicrons which enter the blood circulation via the lacteals and thoracic duct. Glycerol being water soluble readily enters the mucosal cell. Part of it is phosphorylated and used for phospholipid synthesis. The rest of the glycerol and short chain fatty acids with 12 or less carbon atoms are transported to the liver via the portal route.

One common feature in the absorption of these lipids thus appears to be their partial or complete hydrolysis in the lumen so as to make the products more soluble in the aqueous environment. Another common feature is reesterification of such products inside the cell. Such seemingly wasteful processes of hydrolysis followed by resynthesis to the parent compounds appear to serve two important purposes. Firstly, the hydrolytic products are more soluble than the parent compounds. Secondly, through such processes the mucosal cell can exert its selectivity, so that only a particular molecular species is synthesized and transported through the lymph. The latter is well supported by the observations that, while the FA composition of the lymph TG closely resembles that of the dietary TG, the FA composition of the lymph retinyl esters is similar to that at the α-position of the lymph lecithin. It was therefore, suggested that the FAs at the α-position of lymph lecithin and of retinyl esters originate from the same acyl donor.

There are certain differences also in the overall process of absorption of these lipids, *e.g.* in reesterification in the cell. Thus, resynthesis of retinyl and cholesteryl esters is independent of ATP and COA, and therefore, it seems possible that they are formed by means of transesterification; probably the fatty acids are derived from the α- and the β-positions of the lecithin molecule, respectively. The acylation of 2-MG and lysolecithin (LL) on the other hand is dependent on ATP and COA and takes place in the smooth endoplasmic reticulum of the cell.

Though both retinyl and cholesteryl esters have only one ester group, they differ markedly in their mechanisms of absorption in that, the retinyl esters are partially hydrolysed in the lumen with the result that both the ester and the free alcohol are found in the micelle. Probably small amounts of the micellar esters are taken up by the mucosal cell. Cholesteryl esters on the other hand are completely hydrolysed during the digestive phase so that only free cholesterol could be detected in the micelle as well as in the brush-border during its absorption.

Phospholipid is another important class of lipids. No doubt, that these compounds are relatively more soluble in water than TG, but the solubility of their lyso-derivatives is even more pronounced. While the pancreatic secretion is known to contain a very powerful phospholipase A which can rapidly hydrolyse lecithin to lysolecithin, attempts of earlier workers to demonstrate direct acylation of lysolecithin to lecithin with cell free preparations from rat intestinal mucosa had failed. But, by using a brush-border free particulate fraction of rat intestinal mucosa, the presence of highly active enzyme in this tissue has been demonstrated. Dietary lecithin hydorlysed to its lysoderivative in the intestinal lumen is taken up by mucosa cell and is reacylated to lecithin. Therefore, it would appear that lysolecithin is the preferred form for micellar solubilisation. Even though lysolecithin might be the preferred species, but it is a strong cytolytic agent. Following an intake of large amount of lecithin, a situation might arise where the mucosa may have to face a large concentration of its lysoderivative. But the mucosal cell is rather unique in that, nature has endowed it with a soluble machinery (in the form of enzyme systems) for effectively dealing with such a situation. Thus, lysolecithin can be converted to lecithin by direct acylation with fatty acyl COA. It can be hydolysed to GPC and FFA. Finally, it can be converted to GPC and lecithin by intermolecular transesterification. While all the three enzymes are active in this tissue, the extent to which lysolecithin is metabolized through any of the three pathways can be determined by several factors. One such factor is the concentration of lysolecithin itself. Under these conditions where the concentration of lysolecithin in the cell is low, the acyltransferase reaction would predominate, while the lysolecithinase and dismutase would become more effective when lysolecithin concentration becomes higher. On the other hand, their relative specific activities indicate that, of all the three reactions, lysolecithinase is the most active, thereby suggesting that under normal physiological conditions hydrolysis of lysolecithin is the most predominant pathway in this tissue.

Finally, absorption of retinoic acid is rather unusual as it is absorbed through the portal system and is quickly exerted through the bile, in contrast to the behaviour of the common long-chain FA's which are absorbed through the lymphatic system. The reasons for such behaviour of retinoic acid are not clear. It is possible that it is conjugated in the intestine with glucoronic acid, which prevents its esterification with glycerol or other alcohols and consequently leads to its transport through the portal system.

Impaired Absorption

In certain diseased conditions, intestinal absorption of lipids is impaired leading to the loss of hydrolysed or unhydrolysed fat in the stools and this condition is called steatorrhea. Steatorrhea is either due to defective secretion of bile or pancreatic juice into the intestine or due to defective absorption across the mucosal cell. Severe liver dysfunction, extra hepatic biliary obstruction or biliary fistula, affect the flow of bile into intestine. Similarly, pancreatectomy or pancreatic fibrosis disturbs the flow of pancreatic juice into the intestine. Failure of active absorption occurs in celiac disease in children or in sprue in adults. In all the diseased conditions where lipid absorption is impaired, fat soluble substances are also poorly absorbed.

IV. Intracellular Metabolism of Absorbed Lipids

Once the digestion products have penetrated the cell membrane, they must be transported through the cytoplasmic matrix to the site where complex lipid resynthesis occurs. The major site of absorbed lipid metabolism is in the endoplasmic reticulum. However, how the FA and the other absorbed lipids are transported that is unknown. Presence of a fatty acid-binding protein (FABP) was noticed in the intestinal mucosa. This protein has been characterized. It has a molecular weight of 12,000 and is present in intestinal mucosa, the liver, the myocardium, adipose tissue, and the kidney. As determined by quantitative radio immuno-diffusion, the supernatant FABP concentration in mucosa was higher in the proximal and middle intestines than in the distal intestine. Some scientists have suggested a possible role of FABP in regulating TG biosynthesis by adjustings the amount of FA made available for activation and incorporation into TG. Although we may explain that FA is transported to the endoplasmic reticulum (ER) by binding to FABP, we have yet to explain how the other digested lipids get to the ER.

A. Intracellular Metabolism of Absorbed Monoglyceride and Fatty Acid

1. Monoglyceride Pathway

The absorbed MG and FA are reconstituted into TG through the MG pathway. The enzymes involved are acyl-CoA synthetase, MG transacylase and diglyceride (DG) transacylase. The three enzymes are present together as an enzyme complex called "triglyceride synthetase". The acyl-CoA synthetase activates FA to form acyl-CoA in the presence of CoA. The acyl-CoA is then used for the reacylation of MG to DG and subsequently to TG. The enzymes involved in the MG pathway have been demonstrated to be present in the intestinal mucosa of numerous mammals studied. The substrate for MG transacylase can be 1-MG, 2-MG, or ether analogs of the MG. However, the 2-MG is preferred substrate. The intracellular locations of the enzymes for the MG pathway have not been completely defined. The enzymes are located in the microsomal fraction, while other fractions could contain some of the enzymes as a result of contaminations.

2. α-Glycerophosphate Pathway

The other pathway involved in TG biosynthesis is the α-glycerophosphate pathway. This pathway involves five major reactions. These reactions are as follows:

i. Activation of FA to form acyl-CoA (catalyzed by acyl-CoA synthetase)
ii. Formation of L-α-glycerophosphate from glycerol (glycerol kinase)
iii. Conversion of L-α-glycerophosphate to phosphatidic acid (glycerophosphate acyltransferase)
iv. Conversion of phosphatidic acid to DG (phosphatidate phosphohydrolase)
v. Acylation of DG to form TG (diglyceride transacylase)

The enzymes responsible for the α-glycerophosphate pathway are mainly found in the microsomal fraction of intestinal mucosal fraction. Steps 1 and 5 of the α-glycerophosphate pathway are also involved in the monoglyceride pathway.

3. Interaction between the MG and the α-glycerophosphate Pathways

The relative importance of the two pathways depends on the lipid mixture absorbed. The α-glycerophosphate pathway becomes important when long-chain FA alone are absorbed. When MG and FA are absorbed together, the MG pathway plays a more important role.

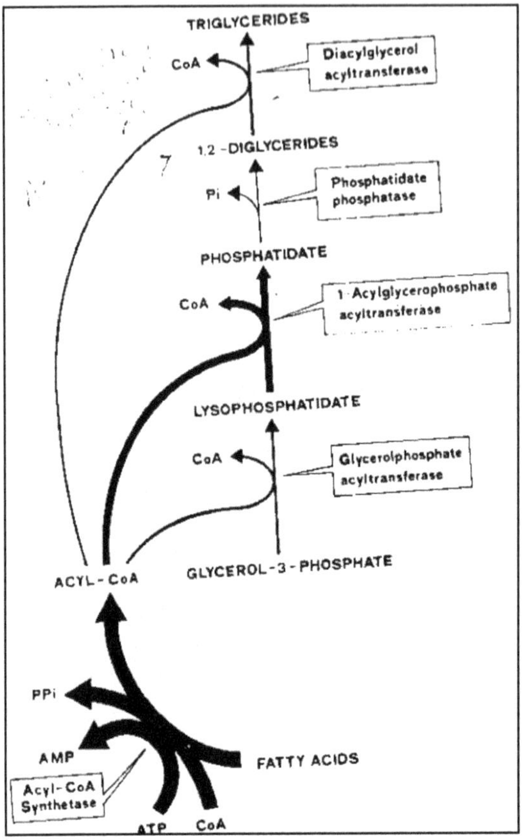

Figure 3.1: Enzymes Involved in the Glycerol-3-phosphate Pathway of TG Synthesis

While TGs are the major products of the two pathways, the DG and TG derived from these pathways seem to enter separate intracellular pools. For instance, the DG from the α-glycerophosphate pathway, not the MG pathway, is used in the *de novo* synthesis of PC via the Kennedy pathway. This would imply the presence of two DG pools in the intestinal mucosal cells, only one of the being available for the biosynthesis of PC. The exact mechanism and the functional role of this phenomenon are unclear. A difference in the distribution of the enzyme activities of the two pathways between the tip enterocytes as compared to the crypt enterocytes has been proposed as an explanation for the existence of more than one DG pool. Another feasible explanation for the existence of two DG pools is offered by the fact that the enzymes involved with the MG pathway are associated mainly with the smooth ER, whereas those involved with the α-glycerophosphate pathway are associated mainly with the rough ER. However, the problem is far from being resolved.

An evidence for the existence of two mucosal TG pools has also been provided by some workers. The TG pool which derives its glyceride-glycerol from luminal TG is rapidly transported into lymph as chylomicrons. The other TG pool which derives its glyceride-glycerol largely from endogenous sources is slowly transported into lymph. It is the second TG pool that seems to efflux back into the small bowel lumen. This efflux of mucosal TG back into the intestinal lumen might be increased during a disease state, thereby causing steatorrhoea. Furthermore, there is a MG hydrolase present in the intestinal mucosa which hydrolyses both the 1-MG as well as the 2-MG. It has been suggested that the MG hydrolase provides a means to metabolize excess MG if there are not enough FA to esterify it to form TG. In summary, it is evident that both the MG-pathway and the α-glycerophosphate pathway are important in the biosynthesis of TG in the intestinal mucosa, depending on the lipid absorbed.

B. Intracellular Metabolism of Absorbed Phospholipids

Phospholipid is another important class of lipids. The small intestine receives considerable amounts of these compounds from the biliary and dietary sources. No doubt these compounds are relatively more soluble in water that TG, but the solubility of their lyso-derivatives is even more pronounced. While the pancreatic secretion is known to contain a very powerful phospholipase A which can rapidly hydrolyse lecithin to lysolecithimn, attempts of earlier workers to demonstrate direct acylation of lysolecithin to lecithin with cell free preparations from rat intestinal mucosa had failed. But, by using a brush-border free particulate fraction of rat intestinal mucosa, the presence of a highly active enzyme in this tissue has been demonstrated. Dietary lecithin is hydrolysed to its lyso derivative in the intestinal lumen which is then taken up by the mucosal cell and is reacylated to lecithin. Therefore, it would appear that lysolecithin is the preferred form for micellar solubilisation.

Even though lysolecithin might be the preferred species, but it is a strong cytolytic agent. Following an intake of large amounts of lecithin a situation might arise where the mucosa may have to face a large concentration of its lyso derivate. But the mucosal cell is rather unique in that, nature has endowed it with suitable machinery (in the form of three enzyme systems) for effectively dealing with such a situation. Thus, lysolecithin can be converted to lecithin by direct acylation with fatty acyl COA. The enzyme responsible for this acylation is found mainly in the microsomal fraction of the rat intestinal mucosa. However, a considerable amount of the absorbed lysolecithin is hydrolyzed by lysolecithinase. The glycerylphosphorylcholine (GPC) released can be transported in blood and the FA released can be used for the synthesis of TG. Finally, in the liver, two molecules of lysolecithin react to form a molecule of GPC and lecithin by intermolecular transesterification. The enzyme responsible for this reaction has been found in the rat intestinal mucosa. Thus, the intestinal cells are well equipped with various enzyme systems to ensure the rapid disposition of absorbed lysolecithin.

While all the three enzymes are active in this tissue, the extent to which lysolecithin (LL) is metabolized through any of the three pathways can be determined by several factors. One such factor is the concentration of lysolecithin itself. Under those conditions where the concentration of LL in the cell is low, the acyltransferase reaction would premominate, while the lysolecithinase and dismutase would become more effective when LL concentration becomes higher. On the other hand, their relative specific activities indicate that, of all the three reactions lysolecithinase is the most active, thereby suggesting that under normal physiological conditions hydrolysis of LL is the most predominant pathway in this tissue.

Sphingomyelin (SPH) is absorbed intact. The real breakdown of the molecule occurs in the mucosal cell. The brush borders have been reported to have high sphingomyelinase activity. SPH is broken down to ceramide and phosphorylcholine. The phosphorylcholine can be used for PC biosynthesis or split to form phosphate and choline. The ceramide is degraded to form FA and sphingosine by ceramidase. The sphingosine can be used for the resynthesis of cerebroside and SPH or it can be further degraded to FA.

C. Intracellular Metabolism of Absorbed Cholesterol

Cholesterol absorbed by the enterocytes enters a free cholesterol pool. This free cholesterol pool in the enterocyte contains cholesterol from endogenous sources as well. The endogenous cholesterol is derived both from non-dietary cholesterol absorbed from the lumen and cholesterol synthesized. Cholesterol synthesized *de novo* also makes an important contribution to endogenous lymphatic cholesterol output.

Both endogenous and absorbed dietary cholesterol are transported in chylomicrons (CM) and very low-density lipoproteins (VLDL) as free and esterified cholesterol. Oleic acid is the preferred fatty acid for the esterification of cholesterol. It has not been demonstrated conclusively whether the esterification of cholesterol is rate limiting for lymphatic transport of cholesterol. However, the esterified cholesterol fraction is usually the one that is most altered if there is a change in cholesterol transport into lymph. Thus, it would seem that the efficiency of cholesterol esterification is a factor in overall absorption of cholesterol into lymph. It was generally held that the esterification of cholesterol was catalyzed by a cholesteryl ester hydrolase, an enzyme of pancreatic origin. Following either pancreatectomy or pancreatic diversion in rats, the intestinal mucosal cholesterol esterifying activity disappeared. It was later confirmed that the mucosal cholesterol ester hydrolase was derived from the pancreatic cholesterol esterase.

In addition, there have been studies showing the presence of another mucosal enzyme important in the esterification of cholesterol. The enzyme is called the acyl-CoA: cholesterol acyltransferase (ACAT). A severalfold increase was observed in the intestinal esterifying activity following an increase in the dietary cholesterol intake, yet pancreatic activity remained unchanged. This suggests that the mucosal cholesterol esterifying activity does not originate exclusively from the pancreatic juice. Mucosal ACAT plays an important role in the esterification and lymphatic transport of cholesterol.

V. The Intracellular Assembly of Intestinal Lipoproteins

Transport of Lipids through the Blood

Blood is the effective vehicle of transport of lipids between tissues. In the humans, postabsorptive blood plasma normally appears clear and it contains about 500 mg of total lipid per 100 ml. The plasma lipid is made up of about 25 per cent TGs, 40 per cent cholesterol (mostly esterified), and the remaining is phospholipid. During active absorption of lipids, plasma shows a milky opalescence, a condition described as absorptive lipemia and is due to the discharge of chyle rich in chylomicron into the venous blood. Any increase in the blood lipids is known as lipemia and this could occur in some pathological conditions such as diabetes and glycogen storage disease.

In addition to chylomicron, a blood plasma contains several water soluble macromolecular lipid-protein complexes, the lipoproteins, which play an important role in the transport of lipids to tissues. These are characterized as very low-density, low density, high density and very high density lipoproteins depending on their density. The low and high density components are also called α and β lipoproteins, respectively. Because of their low density, the lipoproteins float on centrifugation and can also be characterized by their Svedberg floatation constants, S_f values. The very low density and low density proteins have sf values of 12-400 and 0-12, respectively. The very high density and low density lipoproteins are the predominant species in plasma. However, the blood LP profile varies with age, sex, as well as disease. For example, patients with nephrotic syndrome or those surviving a myocardial infarction show an elevated level of low density lipoproteins in plasma.

Blood plasma contains a lipoprotein lipase (clearing factor) which appears during lipemia. This enzyme hydrolyses TG bound to proteins, that is, those present in chylomicron and lipoproteins. The liberated free fatty acids combine with serum albumin and the fatty acid albumin complexes are transported to tissues. The lipoprotein lipase is activated by heparin.

A. Lipoproteins Secreted by the Small Intestine

The intestine secretes two major types of lipoproteins, chylomicrons (CM) and very low density lipoproteins (VLDL). Both CM and VLDL are TG-rich lipoproteins. Havel (1980) also called the intestinal VLDL 'small chylomicron'.

During fasting, VLDL are the major lipoproteins secreted by the small intestine. Following fat feeding, VLDL secretion continues but CM become the major lipoproteins secreted by the small intestine. The small intestine also secretes high-density lipoprotein-like (HDL-like) lipoproteins into lymph, but the significance of intestinal HDL to the metabolism of plasma HDL has yet to be elucidated. Since CM are the major lipoproteins produced by the small intestine during fat absorption, most of the discussion of the assembly process of intestinal lipoproteins will involve CM.

B. Assembly and Secretion of Chylomicrons

The term "chylomicron" was first introduced by Gage (1920) when he observed under dark-field illumination that the blood taken after a fatty meal was filled with dancing particles which were called chylomicrons. With the advent of the ultracentrifuge, CMs have been defined as those lipoproteins with Svedberg floatation (S_f) rate exceeding 400.

There was a difference in the chemical composition of the CMs collected from lymph as compared to the intracellular lipid droplets harvested from the same animals. Intracellular droplets were called as "prechylomicrons" (pre-cm) to distinguish them from the CM in the lymph and plasma. The prechylomicrons contained more free FA, more free cholesterol, more protein and different phospholipid composition from CM.

i) Biosynthesis of CM Components

The process of assembly in the enterocytes is poorly understood. Certain aspects of the process, however, are now well documented. Mucosal TG biosynthesis is carried out mainly in the endoplasmic reticulum (ER). This is supported by both biochemical and morphological data. Biochemically, all the enzymes involved in the MG and the α-glycerophosphate pathways have been isolated from the microsomal fraction of the intestinal mucosa. Morphological studies employing cytochemical techniques showed that the MG pathway aceyltransferases were located mainly on the inner surface of smooth ER, whereas the α-glycerophosphate pathway aceyltransferases were located mainly on the rough ER. Acyltransferase activities from both pathways are also found on the outside cisternae of the Golgi membranes. Using [^{14}Cloleate [^{3}H] leucine, and [^{14}C] glucosamine, it was found that the lipid, protein and sugar of the pre-CM particles are synthesized in the smooth ER, rough ER, and Golgi apparatus, respectively. It is important to remember that the biosynthesis of these pre-CM components does not occur exclusively in one subcellular organellie. Rather, it involves all of them. The three organelles (rough ER smooth ER, and the Golgi apparatus), involved in the packaging of pre-CM are closely linked to each other, forming the endomembrane system. For instance, the addition of carbohydrates to the newly synthesized protein occurs both at the ER and the Golgi apparatus.

Our current concept of intestinal formation and secretion is largely derived from morphological studies. After fat feeding, osmosphilic droplets in great quantities occupy the smooth ER cisternae. The oil droplets contain predominantly TG but also present are PL, cholesterol, and cholesteryl ester. The PL coating of these lipid droplets within the smooth ER is derived from the acylation of the absorbed lysolecithin as well as PC synthesized *de novo*. The enzyme involved in the reacylation of lysolecithin (lysolecithin acyltransferase) is distributed evenly between the smooth and the rough ER, whereas those enzymes involved in the synthesis of PC *de novo* are located predominantly at the rough ER.

ii) Apolipoprotein Composition of CM

Proteins occupy only 1-2 per cent by weight of the CM mass. There is a close similarity between the rat and the human CM apolipoproteins. The major apolipoproteins are A-I, E (ARP), A-IV, C, and B. The apolipoprotein B (apoB) present in CM is what is commonly known as the small apoB, which has a molecular weight (MW) of 240,000 in the rat and 260,000 in the human. Apolipoprotein A-II, a minor apolipoprotein in the rat, is present in human CM. Some scientists have detected little difference in the apolipoprotein composition between intestinal lymph CMs and VLDLs.

iii) Apolipoprotein B and Pre-CM Assembly

As yet, we have little knowledge regarding the addition of apolipoproteins to the pre-CM. For instance, we do not know whether all the apolipoproteins are added at the same time or precisely where the association of lipid and protein occurs. However, we do know that certain apolipoproteins, in particular apoB, play an important role in the formation and secretion of CMs by the enterocytes.

iv) Other Apolipoproteins and CM Assembly

There are apolipoproteins other than apoB produced by the enterocytes. These are ApoA-1, apoA-IV, a small amount of C apolipoproteins, and possibly trace amounts of apoE. ApoA-1 is produced in substantial quantities by the enterocytes, 130-140 mg/hour of apoA-1 secreted into mesenteric lymph of glucose-fed rats. The cellular A-1 content and also the secretion of apoA-1 into lymph increase severalfold after fat feeding. Although apoA-1 production by the small intestine is stimulated by fat feeding, apoA-1 does not seem to play an important part in the secretion of intestinal CM. This is supported by the fact that patients carrying defective apoA-1 genes seem to have normal plasma TG levels, although the plasma HDL levels are much reduced. These patients have either a complete lack of circulating apoA-1 or defective apoA-1. The other major apolipoprotein secreted by the enterocytes is apoA-IV. This is supported by the increase in the output of apoA-IV into lymph during intraduodenal infusion of a lipid emulsion. Whether apoA-IV plays a role in intestinal secretion is unknown. The enterocyte also produces a small quantity of apoA-II and the C apolipoproteins. As yet we have little knowledge of where and how these apolipoproteins become associated with the intestinal lipoproteins.

v) Role of Golgi Apparatus

The Golgi apparatus is a part of the endomembrane system. The endomembrane system is the functional continuum of cellular membrane consisting of nuclear envelope, ER, and the Golgi apparatus.

Two mechanisms have been proposed for the transport of maturing pre-CM from the smooth ER to the Golgi apparatus. First, it has been proposed that vesicles containing these lipid droplets bud off from the tubules of the smooth ER and then merge with the Golgi apparatus. According to another mechanism, the smooth ER and the Golgi apparatus are connected by tubules called "Boulevard Peripherique" which transport the lipid droplets between these two organelles. Further experiments are needed to study the two mechanisms proposed. It is not inconceivable that both processes are involved.

Both the ER and the Golgi apparatus have been shown to carry out glycosylation of both proteins and lipids. Although the addition of carbohydrate moieties to the newly formed apolipoprotein starts at the ER, the terminal glycosylation takes place in the Golgi apparatus. The terminal position is often occupied by monosaccharides such as sialic acid, fucose, galactose, and N-acetylgalactosamine. ApoB, a protein intimately involved in intestinal lipid transport, contains 5-9 per cent by weight of carbohydrate moieties. Whether the glycosylation of apoB is in any way involved in the formation and transport of intestinal TG-rich lipoproteins is unknown.

vi) Exocytosis of Intestinal Chylomicrons

During active lipid absorption, the Golgi cisternae become distended with the pre-CM droplets. These then pinch off from the Golgi apparatus to become the Golgi-derived pre-CM-containing vesicles. These pre-CM-filled Golgi vesicles can be easily visualized within the enterocytes using electron microscopy. The vesicle containing pre-CM migrates toward the plasma membrane and then releases its contents into the intercellular space by exocytosis. After exocytosis, the Golgi vesicle membrane presumably becomes part of the plasma membrane.

C. Secretion of Intestinal Very Low-Density Lipoproteins

Lipoproteins with a Svedberg flotation (S_f) rate of 20-400 are defined as very low-density lipoproteins (VLDL). As mentioned previously, the intestinal VLDL have also been called "small chylomicrons". Whether intestinal CM and VLDL represent two separate populations of TG-rich lipoproteins assembled by the enterocytes is not yet resolved. Studies suggesting that CM and VLDL are two distinct populations of lipoproteins are as follows:

1. The infusion of palmitate resulted in a marked increase in VLDL transport. With the infusion of oleate and linoleate, VLDL output into lymph remained unchanged. Furthermore, the FA composition of the TG from VLDL was different from the TG of CM, therefore, suggesting different assembly for the VLDL and CM particles.
2. Golgi's vesicles contained either CM or VLDL with little mixing of particle sizes.
3. Cholesterol and TG differentially affect the particle size of intestinal lymph lipoproteins. With increasing cholesterol absorption, more lipid was carried by CMs.
4. A hydrophobic surfactant, Pluronic L-81 preferentially inhibits the formation and secretion of CM- but not of VLDL-sized particles. This hydrophobic surfactant is obviously a useful tool for the investigation of the pathways of intestinal lipoprotein synthesis, assembly, and secretion.

Although this evidence seems to support the separate assembly of intestinal CM and VLDL by the enterocytes, this question is far from being resolved. For instance, it has been reported that lymph from fat-fed rats contains a continuous spectrum of TG-rich lipoproteins ranging in size from 300-4300°A, suggesting the presence of one population of TG-rich lipoproteins varying in size according to the amount of core lipid and surface coating material the lipoprotein is carrying.

VI. Factors Affecting the Intestinal Chylomicron Secretion

A. Synthesis of Apolipoprotein

Under normal physiological conditions, the supply of apolipoprotein for the coating of the pre-CM is probably abundant. Using immunofluorescence, it has been demonstrated that there is pool of apoB present in the enterocytes during fasting. This pool of apoB is probably used to coat the pre-CM during the initial period after lipid ingestion. Shortly after the ingestion of lipid (≈ 15 minutes), the cellular apoB content as measured by radioimmunoassay increased. ApoB production probably continues as long as lipid transport is occurring. It is not known whether the production of apoB in the enterocyte is regulated by the amount of lipid accumulated inside the cell.

B. Role of Luminal Lecithin in Lipid Transport

As pointed out earlier, the majority of luminal phospholipid is contributed by the bile. In a 70-kg man, about 11-12 g of biliary phospholipid enters the intestinal lumen, whereas only 1-2 g of luminal phospholipid is contributed by the diet. The two major functions of the luminal phospholipid in the secretion of intestinal TG-rich lipoproteins are to provide membrane phospholipid for the maintenance of normal membrane functioning of the enterocyte and to provide the surface phospholipid coat of the newly formed intestinal lipoproteins.

i) Maintenance of Enterocyte Membrane Function by Luminal Lecithin

It has been demonstrated that bile diversion in rats produced a reduction in the lipid reesterifying enzymes of the intestinal mucosa. This deficiency in enzyme activity was restored by infusing sodium taurocholate and phosphatidylcholine (PC) at concentrations of 7.5 and 2 mM, respectively. Infusion of sodium taurocholate alone resulted in partial restoration of enzyme activity. Thus, it would seem that the activity of the membrane-bound reesterifying enzyme may be affected by the alteration in phospholipid composition and the phospholipid content of the enterocytes sub-cellular organelle membrane. The role of luminal phospholipid, in particular the biliary PC, is therefore, to maintain both the phospholipid composition and phospholipid content of the enterocytes.

The rate of protein biosynthesis as measured by leucine incorporation was much lower in the everted sacs prepared from bile fistula rats as compared to the bile duct-intact rats. This deficiency in protein biosynthesis in bile fistula rats can be greatly improved by the presence of either PC or choline in the incubating medium. It is concluded that the presence of luminal PC is important for the maintenance of normal protein biosynthesis in the intestinal mucosa. As apolipoproteins are part of the numerous proteins synthesized by the gut, presumably their biosynthesis is influenced by the presence and absence of luminal PC.

Supply of Lecithin for CM Surface Coat

Phospholipid, especially, PC is major component of the surface coat of chylomicron. Chemical composition of chylomicron has been described. In most mammals, phospholipid comprised 5-7 per cent of the particle weight. Of the phospholipid present in chylomicron, about 80 per cent is phosphatidylcholine.

During fat absorption, PC showed the greatest increase in specific activity as compared to other phospholipids. Phospholipids in the enterocytes, to be used both for the surface coat of TG-rich lipoproteins and for structural lipids, can be derived from the acylation of lysolecithin from the lumen (biliary or dietary), from the plasma, or by *de novo* synthesis via the Kennedy pathway. It is now generally accepted that PC is absorbed as lysolecithin by the small intestine. The lysolecithin can be reacylated intracellularly to form PC. Much evidence has indicated that luminal PC is an important contributor to the TG-rich lipoprotein coating. There is good evidence that there is a preferential incorporation of biliary PC over dietary PC into cylomicron PC. Using lymph fistula rats, it has been demonstrated that bile diversion resulted in a decrease in the lipid transported by the small intestine when a high dose of fat (180 mmol/hour of fatty acid) was infused. This deficiency in the ability of the bile fistula rat to transport lipid was restored to normal by merely adding 10 mmol/hour of biliary PC to the lipid emulsion fed to the rat. Thus, it was concluded that biliary PC plays an important role in the translocation of a large amount of absorbed fat into lymph. This observation supported the earlier claim that luminal PC is important for normal intestinal transport of lipid.

The other source of intracellualar PC that can be used for the chylomicron coat is *de novo* synthesis via the Kennedy pathway. In the bile-diverted rats, the Kennedy pathway becomes the major pathway used to generate the PC required both for the coating of pre-CM and for the increased membrane turnover during fat absorption. Apparently, this pathway alone is insufficient to provide the PC required during the absorption of a large dose of fat in bile-diverted rats, causing an impairment in lymphatic TG and phospholipid output.

Although the enterocyte acquires PC from the circulation, it has been demonstrated recently that serum PC is only poorly incorporated into chylomicron PC even in the bile-diverted rats. Under normal physiological conditions, the contribution of plasma PC to the chylomicron PC is minimal.

A luminal supply of PC, whether biliary or dietary, is important in sustaining a normal lymphatic fat transport of a large amount of absorbed fat.

The Role of Ca^{2+}

The specific role of calcium in intestinal absorption remains to be clearly defined. Its importance can only be assumed from the fact that it is present in relatively high concentrations in both biliary and pancreatic juices. Its obligatory presence was demonstrated in what have been assumed to be some of the key steps in the processes of lipolysis and absorption of fats.

Calcium is necessary for the formation and release of chylomicron-like particles. It is undoubtedly necessary for the lipase-colipase system, exactly how it works is still uncertain. Calcium also appears to be necessary intracellularly. However, this has only been shown in *in vitro* systems. Unfortunately, studies in intact animals are lacking. Much work remains to be done.

VII. Regional Differences in Lymphatic Lipid Transport

A difference in the abilities of the proximal and the distal intestines to transport absorbed fat has been observed. Not only was the distal intestine much less efficient in chylomicron production than the proximal intestine, but also the chylomicrons produced by the distal intestine were larger. It has been suggested that this difference between intestinal segments could be due to the availability of phospholipid or altered intracellular membrane lipid composition. The rationale for this difference between the proximal and the distal intestine is still unknown.

Researchers have highlighted the importance of luminal PC in maintaining the normal lymphatic transport of lipid when the animal is absorbing a large amount of fat. Normally, most of the ingested phospholipid is absorbed in the proximal intestine, leaving the distal intestine poorly nourished with phospholipid. Whether this lack of phospholipid supply in the distal intestine has anything to do with its ability to produce chylomicron is unclear.

VIII. Portal Transport of Long-Chain Fatty Acids

The majority of absorbed fatty acid (FA) is transported by intestinal lymph as chylomicron and VLDL. However, there is evidence for increased portal transport of the long-chain FAs when there is a defect in the reesterification of FA to form TG or an important with chylomicron formation. For instance, in the bile fistula rats, there is an increased portal transport of absorbed FA as a result of deficient reesterification in the absence of bile acids. There is also evidence of increased FA transport in the portal vein when chylomicron formation is impaired, without necessarily a deficiency in esterification, in puromycin treated rats. In abetalipoproteinemia in man, 75-90 per cent of fat may be absorbed in the virtual absence of chylomicron formation.

In a research study, at low lipid infusion rates, 0.3 mmol/hour of long-chain FA, a substantial amount of the absorbed FA (58 per cent for linoleic acid C 18: 2) was transported in the portal blood. Physiologically, it is unlikely to have such low FA concentration in the intestinal lumen. However, in humans with bile or lipase deficiency this condition may prevail and the portal route may become important in FA transport by the intestinal mucosa.

IX. Storage and Mobilization of Lipids

Though lipid is found in all tissues, the lipid absorbed from the intestine, as well as that synthesized from excess energy of other foodstuffs, is primarily stored as depot fat in the adipose tissue. In the adipose tissue, the stored lipid appears as droplets in the cytoplasm. In mammals, most of lipid is located subcutaneously and acts as an insulator against heat loss and thus, helps homoisotherms in maintaining the body temperature. Generally the adipose tissue appears white and comprises of mainly of TG composed of fatty acids, as saturated as possible, yet in a fluid state at body temperature. However, the adipose tissue FA composition may be altered by dietary manipulation and may be made unsaturated by unsaturated fats. In some mammals, certain areas of adipose tissue, as for example, the interscapular depots of the fat appear which is due to presence of brown pigment and large amounts of glycogen. This is called brown adipose tissue. The brown appearance is believed to be given by the cytochromes of a large number of mitochondria that surround the lipid vacuoles. The brown fat may have a special function in the production of heat.

The adipose tissue fat increases in quantity on excess energy intake and is utilized as the primary source of energy under conditions of saturation and inanition. However, in animals that are in caloric balance, adipose tissue lipid undergoes continuous metabolic flux. It assimilates fatty acids, TGs, as well as CH_2O intermediates necessary for the synthesis of lipids. While there are several modes of input into the adipose tissue, mobilization of lipid occurs exclusively as the free fatty acids. A lipase present in the adipose tissue hydrolyses the TGs to free fatty acids (FFAs), which then bind to serum albumin and are thus, transported to tissues for oxidation. The adipose tissue lipase is sensitive to hormones, and therefore, mobilization of depot fat is under neuro endocrine control. In addition, some hepatic poisons such as CCl_4, and certain chronic infectious diseases like tuberculosis also cause mobilization of lipids from the adipose tissue and increase the content of liver lipid.

Effects of Hormones on Lipid Mobilization

A number of hormones affect the mobilization of depot fat. The mechanism of action is not completely understood, but several possibilities may be considered. Hormones may:

1. Increase lipolysis of adipose tissue TG by the lipase
2. Increase release of FFA, or
3. Alter membrane permeability to glucose and other CH_2O intermediates and thus, increase TG synthesis in the adipose tissue.

Several hormones, like epinephrine, norepinephrine (and also serotonin), adrenal steroids, glucagon, prolactin, ACTH, TSH, Growth hormone, lipotropic hormones and vasopression stimulate lipolysis in the adipose tissue and cause release of free fatty acids. Prostaglandins inhibit release of free fatty acids from adipose tissue and counteract the effect of epinephrine and norepinephrine. Insulin inhibits FFA release from adipose tissue and stimulates lipogenesis in this tissue from CH_2O sources.

Significance of Blood Lipids and Lipoproteins in Health and Disease

Before discussing the significance of lipids and lipoproteins, it would be better to define them which is as under:

Lipoproteins

a) *VLDL or pre β-lipoproteins*: These are synthesized in the liver and transport endogenously produced TG which is derived from circulating CH_2Os and FFAs generally mobilized from the tissues.
b) *LDL or β-lipoprotein*: This accounts for most of the cholesterol in the plasma. It has a short half life of three days and mostly a metabolic product of VLDL after the dissociation of the TG from the VLDL aggregate. It has the highest atherogenic potential.
c) *HDL or alpha-LP*: Carry the remaining cholesterol in the plasma, besides phospholipids. However, its major component is apoprotein A. HDL probably has the least disease producing potential.
d) *Chylomicrons*: Chylomicrons are the lipoproteins of intestinal origin. These consist almost entirely of dietary TGs with small amounts of cholesterol, phospholipids and proteins. Chylomicrons are present in the plasma for 1-4 h after a meal. The enzyme LP lipase by its action dissociates TG from chylomicron with the resulting FFA being transported to adipose tissue,

heart and skeletal muscles for utilization. The glycerol is removed by the liver.

The protein part of the lipoprotein is named apo-lipoprotein. At least three different apolipoproteins (A, B and C) have been demonstrated.

The different physical and chemical characteristics of the lipid protein aggregates allow classification of hyperlipoproteinemias.

Hyperlipoproteinemia

One or more of the LP carrying cholesterol and TGs are present in excess.

Secondary Hyperlipoproteinemia

When excess of lipoproteins and their components is on the basis of some other disease disorder. Several such diseases have been identified and include uncontrolled diabetes mellitus, hypothyroidism, nephrotic syndrome, inappropriate dietary habits, biliary tract destructive disease, pancreatitis etc.

Primary Hyperlipoproteinemia

When the existing elevated serum levels of lipoproteins are not due to one of the many causes. These are genetically determined defects in lipid or lipoprotein metabolism which are exaggerated by environmental factors through poorly understood mechanisms.

Such a classification allows a general finding of elevated cholesterol and/or TGs to be related to a specified class. This in turn gives useful additional clues to the understanding of underlying metabolic abnormalities and their prognostic and therapeutic implication.

Hyperlipidemia refers to excess cholesterol or TG or both are present in the plasma and it is of concern to physicians for several reasons. It is generally accepted as a coronary risk factor. Its presence increases the risk of developing atherosclerotic coronary artery disease. In some familial lipid metabolic disorders, pancreatitis may occur. Skin rashes or xanthomotas may appear acutely or be chronically present needing management. Its presence on the other hand, may indicate many factors like unsuitable diet, excessive alcohol intake, stress or disorders causing secondary fat metabolism abnormalities like hypothyroidism, diabetes mellitus, nephrotic syndrome, biliary obstructive disease, or pancreatitis may be existing unsuspected, requiring evaluation and management.

Chapter 4

Disturbances in Lipid Metabolism

Normally, various kinds of lipids of various tissues are synthesized, deposited, mobilized, and catabolised at rates that tend to maintain a relatively steady state. The most common disturbances in lipid metabolism involve the deposition and mobilization of triglycerides in the fat depots, leading to obesity when deposition exceeds mobilization, and ultimately to caexexia when mobilization exceeds deposition.

The term 'lipidosis' is used for a group of inherited metabolic disorders in which the lipid content of tissues and plasma is elevated. Accumulation of lipids inside the cells results in large foamy cells. The organs in which these foam cells are present become pale, firm and heavy. The liver, spleen, lungs and bone marrow are commonly involved. In some types of lipidoses, neurological functions are markedly impaired, either due to the abnormal deposition of the lipids or other related metabolic defects.

1. Obesity

The amount of fat in the storage depots is determined by the balance between the rates of deposition and mobilization. An animal becomes fat when the rate of deposition exceeds the rate of deposit mobilization and lean when the processes are reversed. It has been established that obesity results purely from the ingestion of more food that is necessary to meet energy requirements; in other words, it is a question of appetite being improperly balanced (controlled) with energy needs. Alteration in energy demand or an animal without simultaneous change in appetite may occur for various reasons. This may be true with decreased muscular activity. Also, endocrine disturbance may decrease activity and lead to obesity. Castration is often associated with obesity because of lowered activity, as is hypothyroidism, which depresses the rate of food oxidation. In some cases neither of these conditions causes obesity because appetite is proportionately lowered. Certain pituitary deficiencies may lead to abnormal distribution of body fat without changing the total quantity. Some cases of hyperinsulinism become obese because of greatly stimulated appetite. It has been demonstrated that hypothalamus region of the brain is concerned with regulation of appetite. Injuries to this region in experimental animals may lead to great obesity due to appetite stimulation. Many experiments have shown that the processes of fat metabolism in obese individuals are normal.

2. Cachexia

There are a number of conditions that lead to abnormally high rates of mobilization from fat depots relative to the rates of deposition, causing, in severe cases, disappearance of most of the adipose tissue. Such situation may be observed in carcinoma, malnutrition, certain chronic infectious diseases, hyperthyroidism, and severe uncontrolled diabetes. The greater increased mobilization of body fat to supply the increased energy demand is the primary cause of the wasting away or cachexia of hyperthyroidism. Two processes operate to cause the cachexia of severe uncontrolled diabetes. In the first place due to inability to utilize appreciable CH_2O, energy is supplied through the mobilization and utilization of excessive amounts of depot fat. In the second place, the capacity of the diabetic to synthesize fat for deposit is drastically reduced. Severe thiamine deficiency leads to decreased capacity to convert CH_2O to fat and also decreased appetite with depletion of fat depots. Of course, in the plain starvation, the net effect is fat mobilization to supply energy without deposition.

3. Sphingolipidosis

Sphingolipids are fatty acid esters of the base sphingosine and other chemical moieties. The sphingolipidosis are recessively inherited disorders in which there is a deficiency of a specific lysosomal hydrolytic enzyme and consequent deposition of complex lipids in various tissues (Tables 4.1 and 4.2). They are almost all degenerative diseases with mental retardation and early demise. Lipid storage disease exhibit several constant features such as:

- ✰ In various tissues, there is an accumulation of complex lipids that have a portion of their structure in common-ceramide.
- ✰ The rate of synthesis of the stored lipid is comparable to that in normal humans.
- ✰ The enzymatic defect in each of these diseases is a deficiency due to gene mutation of a specific lysosomal hydrolytic enzyme necessary to breakdown the lipid or of a key activator protein of the enzyme.
- ✰ The extent to which the activity of the affected enzyme is decreased is similar in all of the tissues of the affected individuals.

Several clinical syndromes due to accumulation of different sphingolipids have been described in detail.

Table 4.1: Sphingolipidosis

Disease	Signs and Symptoms	Enzyme Defect	Lipid Accumulating
Farber's Disease	Hoarseness, dermatitis, skeletal deformation, mental retardation, fatal in early life	Ceramidase sphingosine	Ceramide
Gaucher's Disease	Spleen and liver enlargement, erosion of long bones and pelvis, mental retardation only in infantile form	β-glucosidase	Glucosylceramide
Niemann-Pick Disease	Liver and spleen enlargement, mental retardation, about 30% with red spot in retina, fatal in early life.	Sphingomyelinase	Sphingomyelin
Krabbe's Disease (globoid)	Mental retardation, almost total absence of myelin	β-galactosidase	Galacto-sylceramide
Metachromatic leukodystrophy	Mental retardation, psychological disturbances in adult form, nerves stain yellow-brown with cresyl violet dye, demyelination	Arylsulfatase A	3-Sulfogalacto-sylceramide
Fabry's Disease	Reddish purple skin rash, kidney failure, pain in lower extremities	α-galactosidase	Globotriaosyl-ceramide
Tay-Sachs Diseasae	Mental retardation, red spot in retina, blindness, muscular weakness	Hexosaminidase A	G_{M2} Ganglioside
Tay-Sach variant or Sandhoff's Disease	Same as in Tay-Sach, but progresses more rapidly	Hexosaminidase A and B	Globoside Plus G_{M2}Ganglioside
Generalized gangliosidosis	Mental retardation, liver enlarge-ment, skeletal deformities	ß-Galactosidase	G_{M1} Ganglioside
Fucosidosis	Cerebral degeneration, muscle spasticity, thick skin	α -Fucosidase	H-isoantigen
Ceramide lactoside lipidosis	Progressing brain damage, liver and spleen enlargement	ß-Galactosidase	Ceramide lactoside

i) Gaucher's Disease

Gauther first observed this hereditary disease in a patient in whom the splenic pulp had been replaced entirely by large pale cells, known as Gaucher cells. The Gaucher cells are found particularly in spleen, brain, and bone marrow. Gaucher cells have been known to contain abnormally large amounts of (a) a cerebroside composed of galactose, sphingosine and lignoceric acid (keracin); (b) a cerebroside containing glucose instead of galactose, and (c) a water soluble glycolipid made up of sphingosine and or a sphingosine like base, long chain saturated fatty acids, and one or more hexose groups. This substance has been known as 'polycerebroside'. In Gaucher's disease, there is an imbalance between the rates of cerebroside formation and catabolism leading to the accumulation of cerebrosides in certain cells to form Gaucher cells.

Table 4.2: Summary of Basic Metabolic Defects in Lipid Disorders

Disorder	*Accumulated Sphingolipid*	*Chemical Composition*	*Deficient Enzyme*
Gaucher's	Cerebroside	Ceramide + glu	Glucocerebrosidase
Krabbe's	Galactosyl ceramide	Ceramide + gal	Galacto-cerebroside-β-galactosidase
Niemann pick	Sphingomyelin	Ceramide + phosphoryl choline	Sphingomyelinase (tyupes A and B), lyso somal hydrolase
Metachromatic leukodystrophy	Sulphatide	Cer + gal + sulphate	Cerebroside sulphatase and larylsuephatase
Fabry's	Glycosphingolipid	Cer + 2 gal + glu	Ceramide galactosyl hydrolase
Tay-Sachs	GM_2 ganglioside	Cer + sialic acid + 2 gal + glu	GM_2 ganglioside hexosaminidase
GM_1 gangliosidosis	GM_1 ganglioside	Cer + sialic acid + 3 gal + glu	β-galactosidase

The cerebroside-laden cells are large and have an eccentric nucleus. Their cytoplasm appears like crumbled silk. The spleen is markedly enlarged, and there are signs of hypersplenism like anemia, leukopenia, and thrombocytopenia. The liver is enlarged and the narrow cavity is widened due to Gaucher cell deposits.

Three clinical variants are described. In type I (chronic or adult form), the disease is chronic, visceral involvement is prominent but there are no neurological signs. The disease may be detected in older people. In type II (early infantile form), the disease starts early and death occurs before the age of two years. Neurological symptoms are usually present. In type III, the onset is in the second year, the course is subacute and both visceral and neurological manifestations occur.

ii) Niemann Pick Disease

This disease has many clinical features in common with Gaucher's disease. It is characterized by a very generalized distribution of large pale cells (Niemann Pick Cells) having a foamy appearing vacuolated cytoplasm. The spleen, lung, lymph nodes, liver, and bone marrow are primarily involved, though organs in general are infiltered. The ganglion cells of the CNS and elsewhere undergo degeneration. There is an immense accumulation of lipid in the Niemann Pick Cells, of which sphingomycelin is the major component. Conversion of ceramide (acylsphingosine) to sphingomyelin is normal, but the reverse process is defective. Cholesterol deposits in the tissues are increased. Five clinical variants are known. In type A, onset is early, the course of disease is acute, neurological damage is severe and death occurs before the child is 4 years old. In type B, visceral involvement is more pronounced than the neurological involvement. The disease is mild. Type C has a chronic course. Type D is a mild variant of type C. Type E does not have neurological involvement.

A hereditary condition of infants which in many respects resembles Niemann Pick disease is Tay-Sachs disease. In both the conditions there is a cherry red spot in the macula and macular degeneration. The histological conditions in brain are similar in both conditions and cases of Niemann-Pick and Tay-Sachs disease have been observed in siblings of the same families. In Tay-Sachs disease, the chief pathology is related to degeneration of ganglion cells of the CNS and retina. Apparently this degeneration is caused by the accumulation of lipid in the cells. However, sphingomyelin does not appear to be prominent component of this lipid. In Tay-Sachs disease, the neuronal cells are distended with 'membranous cytoplasmic bodies' which originate from lysosomes. There is a deficiency of an enzyme which catalyzes the cleavage of the molecule of N-acetyl galactosamine from Tay-Sachs ganglioside (GM_2).

iii) Krabbe's Disease

Patients with globoid leukodystrophy (Krabbe's disease) exhibit the usual signs of severe mental retardation, blindness and deafness. There is nearly a total absence of myelin in the nervous system. It is replaced by a severe gliosis and 'globoid bodies' appear in the white matter. The metabolic defect in this disorder is a deficiency of a β-galactosidase which catalyses the hydrolysis of galactocerebroside.

$$\text{Galactocerebroside} + H_2O \xrightarrow{\text{Galactocerebrosidase}} \text{Ceramide} + \text{Galactose}$$

Galactocerebroside is one of the chief lipid components of myelin and its accumulation is presumed to arise from the turn over and restructuring of the myelin sheath during development of the nervous system. The lipids are engulfed by phagocytic cells, and because of the attenuated catalytic activity of galactocerebrosidase, lipid accumulates and is accompanied by distension and proliferation of these cells. The heterozygous carriers of globoid leukodystrophy are said to be identifiable through galactocerebrosidase assay performed on serum samples. The disease is fatal before six months of age.

iv) Metachromatic Leukodystrophy (MLD)

Sulphated cerebrosides accumulate in the nervous tissue, peripheral nerves, liver and kidney. Myelin degenerates but neuronal cells are affected to a lesser degree. Granular masses accumulate in the white matter. The substance which accumulates in tissues of patients with MLD is sulphatide, the 3′-O-sulphate ester of galctocerebroside. The enzymatic lesion is a deficiency of sulphatidase.

$$\text{Sulphatide} + H_2O \xrightarrow{\text{Sulphatidase}} \text{Galactocerebroside} + H_2SO_4$$

There is a decrease in nerve conduction time in these patients, and nerve biopsies show brownish-yellow metachromatic granules when stained with cresyl voilet dye. This metachromatic staining gives the name to the disease. Early clinical manifestations of disturbances of gait, lack of coordination and progressive mental deterioration appear in the second year. Death occurs before the age of 10 years.

v) Fabry's Disease

Patients with this disease have a reddish purple, maculopurple rash in the umbilical, inguinal and scrotal areas. They also have severe renal impairment, corneal opacities, peripheral neuralgias, and electro-cardiogram changes. The enzymatic effect is a deficiency of ceramide trihexoside-α-galactosidase.

$$\text{Ceramide-glu-gel-gal} + H_2O \xrightarrow[\alpha\text{-galactosidase}]{} \text{Ceramide-glu-gal} + \text{gal}$$

The principal source of the accumulating ceramide trihexoside is red cell globoside. The tissue distribution of trihexoside in the tissues of patients with the disease is quite interesting. It accumulates in the endothelial lining of blood vessels, and it is deposited extensively in kidney glomeruli. The degradation of globoside occurs primarily in the reticuloendothelial cells of the liver and spleen (and perhaps bone marrow) and then the trihexoside is carried in the blood and deposited in other tissues, especially the kidney.

vi) Ceramide Lactoside Lipodosis

This is an extremely rare disorder. The patient had slowly progressing CMS impairment, hepatosplenomegaly, foam cells in the bone marrow, increased serum acid phosphatase and mild anemia. The metabolic defect is a deficiency of a β-galactosidase required for the hydrolytic cleavage of lactosylceramide.

$$\text{Ceramide-glu-gal} \xrightarrow[\beta\text{-galactosidase}]{\text{Ceramide lactoside}} \text{Ceramide-glu} + \text{gel}$$

vii) Generalized (GM_1) Gangliosidosis

The clinical manifestations of this disorder include mental retardation, hepatospslenomegaly, foam cells in bone marrow, rarefaction of bones and skeletal deformation. Approximate 50 per cent of these infants have a cherry red spot in the macula. The disease is caused by a deficiency of GM_1–ganglio-side-β-galactosidase.

Ceramide-glu-gal-NANA-N-acetyl galactosamine-gal+H_2O

↓ GM1-gangliosidase

gal+cer-glu-gal-NANA-N-acetyl galactosamine

Galactocerebroside and ceramide lactoside metabolism is not impaired. The accumulating ganglioside may arise from the turnover of plasma membrane components of various cells since gangliosides are selectively concentrated in these structures.

viii) Fucosidosis

The children suffering from this disorder show progressive cerebral degeneration, weakness, spasticity, emaciation, thickening of the skin, and cardiomegaly. The enzymatic defect is complete deficiency of α-L-fucosidase activity in the tissues of these patients. The natural substrate(s) of this enzyme are still not completely known. However, it is known that intestinal tissue, red blood cells, and some other tissues such as human adenocaxinoma contain fucoglycolipids. A very large increase of a pentahexosyl-fucoglycolipid has been observed in the liver tissue obtained from a patient with fucosidosis.

ix) Tangier's Disease (Anal phalipoproteinemia)

During this disorder, the normal high density α-lipoproteins are absent in the plasma. Instead, small quantities of abnormal high density lipoprotein may be present. Plasma cholesterol is low but there is extensive deposition of cholesterol esters in the tonsils, liver, spleen, lymph nodes and skin. This explains the characteristic clinical features of orange yellow enlargement of tonsils, hepato-plenomegaly and lymph node enlargement.

4. Idiopathic Hyperlipemia (Buerger-Griitz Disease)

This hereditary disease is characterized by very high serum lipid levels. Total fatty acids largely as fat, may be ten times the normal. Also, there are marked elevations of cholesterol and phospholipids. The fasting serum is milky white. Widely distributed cutaneous xanthomas, consisting of soft yellow papules and nodules, are, a prominent feature of the disease. The principal complications are episodes of relapsing pancreatitis and atherosclerosis. Many patients in teens and twenties suffer from angina pectoris or myocardial infarction.

Little is known about the disease, but there is some evidence that the turnover of plasma fatty acids is decreased and that blood lipase is deficient.

5. Disorders of Lipoprotein Metabolism

Inherited defects in lipoprotein metabolism lead to primary condition of either hypo or hyper lipoproteinemia associated with lipoproteins of abnormal composition or distribution of the normal lipoprotein classes. Diseases such as diabetes mellitus, hypothyroidism, kidney disease and atherosclerosis show abnormal lipoprotein patterns that are very similar to one or another of the primary inherited conditions. All of these primary conditions are due to a defect at a stage in lipoprotein formation, transport or destruction. Primary disorders of plasma lipoproteins are summarized in the Table 4.3.

In abetalipoproteinemia, possible genetic defects may be either (i) deficient synthesis of apoprotein of low density β-lipoproteins, (ii) increased utilization of apoproteins or (iii) difficulty in incorporation of apoprotein into the lipoprotein. β-lipoproteins and chylomicrons in the plasma are absent. Plasma cholesterol and TG levels are low. Betalipoproteins are necessary for the chylomicron formation. As beta lipoproteins are not available, chylomicron formation is deficient. The fats are normally digested and assimilated in the intestinal mucosa, but these can't be transported adequately in the form of chylomicrons from these cells to plasma. Thus, these patients suffer from malabsorption. Lipoproteins may be necessary for transport of some essential nutrients to erythrocytes and their absence may therefore, interfere with the synthesis of the red cell membrane. The erythrocytes appear abnormally crenated and thorny (acanthocytosis). The patients may have retinitis pigmentosa and neurological signs of ataxia, tremors, athetosis, loss of vibration and position senses. Pathogenesis of the eye and brain changes is not clear.

Table 4.3: Disorders of Lipoprotein Metabolism

Name	*Defect*
Hypolipoproteinemias	
Abetalipoproteinemia	Absence of chylomicrons, VLDL, or LDL are formed because of defect in triacylglycerol transfer protein (MTP), which prevents the loading of apo B with lipid
Familial hypobetalipoproteinemia	LDL concentration is 10-60 per cent of normal.
Familial alpha-lipoprotein deficiency Tangier disease Fish-eye disease Apo-A-I deficiencies	Low or near absence of HDL in all.
Hyperlipoproteinemias Familial lipoprotein lipase LPL or apo-C-II deficiency (type I)	Deficiency of LPL, or production of abnormal LPL or apo-C-II deficiency
Familial hypercholesterolemia (type II)	Type IIa: Defective LDL receptors or mutation in ligand region of apo B-100. Type IIb: Tendency for VLDL to be elevated in addition.
Wolman's disease (cholesteryl ester storage disease)	Deficiency of cholesteryl ester hydrolase in lysosomes.
Familial type III hyper-lipoproteinemia (broad beta disease, remnant removal disease, familial dysbetalipoproteinemia)	Deficiency in remnant clearance by the liver is due to abnormality in apo E, which is normally present in 3 isoforms: E2, E3, and E4. Patients have only E2, which does not react with the E receptor.Truncated apo B species present.
Familial hypertriacylglycerolemia (type IV)	Overproduction of VLDL often associated with glucose intolerance and hyperinsulinemia.
Familial type V hyperlipoproteinemia	Elevated levels of chylomicrons and VLDL, cause unknown.
Familial hyperalphalipoproteinemia	Increased concentrations of HDL.
Hepatic lipase deficiency	Deficiency of the enzyme leads to accumulation of large triacylglycerol-rich HDL and VLDL remnants.
Familial lecithin: cholesterol acyltrans-ferase (LCAT) deficiency	Absence of LCAT leads to block in reverse cholesterol transport. HDL incapable of taking up and esterifying cholesterol.
Familial lipoprotein (a) excess	Lp(a) consists of 1 mol of LDL attached to 1 mol of apo(a). Apo(a) shows structural homologies to plasminogen.

6. Atherosclerosis

Atherosclerosis is a type of arteriosclerosis characterized by plaques, as a result of which there is a variable combination of changes in the intima of arteries and blood products, fibrous tissue and calcium. Atherosclerosis occurs in the aorta, coronary, cerebral, renal, iliac, and femoral arteries. There is a gradual narrowing of the artery leading to a reduction in blood supply, and there may be a sudden occlusion of a vessel due to superimposition of a thrombus on the atherosclerotic lesion. In the earliest stages of disease, there is a focal accumulation of fat-laden cells under the endothelium. Subsequently, fibrous tissue is added, and there are ulceration and other changes.

Atherosclerosis does not appear to be caused by any single agent or condition but lipids are always associated as a causative agent. The blood lipids being the prime suspect as the causative agent, much attention is now being focused on cholesterol, lipoproteins, neutral fat, and total dietary calories.

The earliest studies were concerned with cholesterol induced atherosclerosis in rabbits fed a diet containing 1-3 percent cholesterol. Although very extensive lipid deposits in the aorta and other vessels can be produced, there is not a good correlation between the amount of cholesterol fed and the severity of the disease produced.

The amount of cholesterol in the body is the sum of the following tissue contents: brain 25 g, RBC 5-6 g, aorta 0.03-0.2 g, skin 13 g, muscle 30 g, plasma 5-6 g, liver 305 g etc. Not all of these tissue pools of cholesterol are in dynamic equilibrium with plasma cholesterol or with aorta cholesterol.

The amount and type of fat in the diet determines the production of atherosclerosis. The protein content of the cholesterol fed diet is another limiting variable. It represents not pure lipids but mixtures of fat, cholesterol, phospholipid and protein in the form of chylomicrons and lipoproteins. It is the circulating lipid complexes than that are in direct contact with the intima, so that it seems likely that changes in the lipoprotein of plasma would be correlated best with the disease.

Chapter 5

Types of Fats Consumed in Diet and their Relation to Health

Dietary fat encompasses all the sources of lipids in foods, including those in plant and animal cellular membranes, as well as the readily recognized fats and oils. Technically called lipids, fats and oils are made up of many different types of fatty acids. Fatty acids are the same whether they come from plants or animals. Oleic acid that is found in olive oil is exactly the same as the oleic acid found in lard (pig fat). It is the proportion of fatty acids that will vary from plant to plant, from animal to animal, and from plant to animal.

A fatty acid is a molecule that is made up of a chain of carbon atoms. These chains can vary in length from 1 – 24 carbons. Fatty acids are given their names based of how long the chain is and at what position the "unsaturation" occurs. If the fatty acid is saturated, the carbon chain length determines the name. Depending upon the composition of fatty acids, fats are of two types:

1. Saturated fat
2. Unsaturated fat

These are described in detail as under:

1. Saturated Fat

Each carbon atom in the fatty acid chain has room for two hydrogen molecules, except at the end, where it has room for three. A fatty acid possessing two hydrogen atoms for every carbon atom in the chain is said to be saturated. Butyric (4:0), myristic

(14:0), palmitic (16:0), and stearic (18.0) acids are examples of saturated fatty acids. Beef tallow (fat), dairy, palm oil, coconut oil, vanaspati, ghee etc. are the examples of saturated fats. Their roles in the body include:

- ☆ They constitute at least 50 per cent of our cell membranes and give our cells integrity.
- ☆ They play a vital role in the health of our bones.
- ☆ They lower Lp(a), a substance in the blood that is said to indicate proneness to heart disease.
- ☆ They protect the liver from alcohol and other toxins like tylenol (Acetaminophen).
- ☆ They enhance the immune system.
- ☆ They are needed for proper utilization of essential fatty acids.
- ☆ Stearic acid and palmitic acid, both saturated fats, are the preferred energy source of the heart. This is why the fat around the heart muscle is mainly saturated. The best sources for palmitic acid are beef, butter and palm oil.
- ☆ Short and medium chain saturated fatty acids have strong antimicrobial properties. They help to protect us from harmful microorganisms. The best sources are tropical oils such as coconut oil and palm oil.

Because the carbon atoms are saturated with hydrogen atoms, saturated fats are very stable and generally do not go rancid. These fats are the best sources for cooking because of their stability and positive functions that they play in our bodies.

2. Unsaturated Fat

A fatty acid missing two or more hydrogen atoms along the chain, which causes double bonds between carbon atoms, is said to be unsaturated. Unsaturated fats have at least one unsaturated bond that is, at least one place that hydrogen can be added to the molecule. They're often found in liquid oils of vegetable origin.

Unsaturated fats such as liquid oils have a greater tendency than saturated fats to become rancid when exposed to air.

Unsaturated fatty acids can be described in shorthand with a notation depicting first the chain length, and then the number of double bonds. For example, linoleic acid, which has 18 carbon atoms and two double bonds, is described as 18:2. Almost all naturally occurring unsaturated fatty acids have a 'cis' configuration, meaning that the two hydrogen atoms attached to the double-bonded carbon atoms are on the same side of the chain.

There are several kinds of polyunsaturated fatty acids (PUFAs); two that are nutritionally important are linoleic acid and linolenic acid. They are also referred as essential fatty acids because the body cannot produce them; they have to be obtained from food. Certain forms of PUFAs, called omega-3 fatty acids, have gained special attention because of their positive health effects. Studies have shown that eicosapentaenoic acid (EPA) and docosahexaenoic acid (DHA) from fish and fish oils may reduce coronary heart disease (CHD) risk. In fact, the Food and Drug administration has recently allowed foods with omega-3 fatty acids to carry a qualified health claim on the label about their role in reducing the risk of heart disease.

Unsaturated fatted acids can be further of two types:

i) Monounsaturated Fatty Acids

If there is one double bond, the fatty acid is referred to as monounsaturated. The predominant monounsaturated fatty acid is oleic acid (18:1). *Sources of these fatty acids are chicken fat, duck fat, goose fat, turkey fat, olive oil, canola oil, peanut oil, hazel nuts, almonds, cashews, brazil nuts, avocados etc.* Although olive oil is the best vegetable monounsaturated fat to use in cooking because of its high oxidation threshold, it is not recommended for repeated use or deep frying. Purchasing extra virgin olive oil ensures that it has not been extracted with heat or detergents. Olive oil that is not labelled "Extra Virgin" comes to stores already denatured and containing high amounts of free radicals from the extraction process. Rapeseed oil also contains a relatively high proportion of monounsaturated fat. In avocados, 60-70 per cent of the fat is monounsaturated. In meat, poultry, eggs, milk, butter, lard, nuts, and other vegetable oils and margarines, 10-50 per cent of the fat is monounsaturated. Recent research has shown that monounsaturated fats may also help reduce blood cholesterol as long as the diet is very low in saturated fat.

ii) Polyunsaturated Fatty Acids

If there are two or more double bonds found along the chain, the fatty acid is referred to as polyunsaturated. They are liquid at room temperature and in the refrigerator. They easily combine with oxygen in the air to become rancid.

Polyunsaturated fatty acids are divided into the omega-3 (ù3) and omega-6 (ù6) series according to the distance of their first double bond from the methyl end of the carbon chain. These fatty acids are also termed as 'Essential Fatty Acids' as need to be included in the diet because the human metabolism cannot create them other fatty acids. Since these fatty acids are polyunsaturated, the terms n-3 PUFAs and n-6 PUFAs are also applied to omega-3 and omega-6 fatty acids, respectively. These fatty acids use the Greek alphabet (α,β,γ,.,ù) to identify the location of the double bonds. The "alpha" carbon is the carbon closest to the carboxyl group (carbon number 2), and the "omega" is the last carbon of the chain because omega is the last letter of the Greek alphabet. Linoleic acid is an omega-6 fatty acid because it has a double bond six carbons away from the "omega" carbon. Alpha-linolenic acid is an omega-3 fatty acid because it has a double bond three carbons away from the "omega" carbon. By subtracting the highest double-bond located in the scientific name from the number of carbons in the fatty acid we can obtain its classification. For arachidonic acid, we subtract 14 from 20 to obtain 6; therefore, it is an omega-6 fatty acid. This type of terminology is sometimes applied to oleic acid which is an omega-9 fatty acid. Linoleic (18:2) and arachadonic (20:4) acids are omega-6 fatty acids, whereas eicosopentanoic (20:5), decosahexanoic (22:6), and alpha-linolenic (18:3) acids are omega-3 fatty acids.

DHA (docosahexaenoic acid) and AA (arachidonic acid) are both crucial to the optimal development of the brain and eyes. The importance of DHA and AA in infant nutrition is well established, and both substances are routinely added to infant formulas. Excessive amounts of omega-6 polyunsaturated fatty acids and a very high omega-6/omega-3 ratio have been linked with pathogenesis of many diseases, including cardiovascular disease, cancer, and inflammatory and autoimmune diseases. The ratio of omega-6 to omega-3 in modern diets is approximately 15:1, whereas ratios of 2:1 to 4:1 have been associated with reduced mortality from cardiovascular disease, suppressed inflammation in patients with rheumatoid arthritis, and decreased risk of breast cancer.

Sources of PUFAs are corn oil, soy oil, safflower oil, sunflower oil, cotton seed oil, walnuts, flax oil, hemp oil, herring, salmon, sardines, mackerel etc. Safflower, corn, sunflower, soybean and cottonseed oils all contain over 50 per cent of the highly unstable fatty acid omega-6 and should never be used in cooking, frying or baking. Heating these oils causes oxidation and produces large amounts of free radicals.

Doctors generally advise heart patients to consume polyunsaturated fats as they are good for health. Polyunsaturated fats tend to help the body to get rid of newly formed cholesterol. Thus, they keep the blood cholesterol level down and reduce cholesterol deposits in artery walls. Unfortunately, over consumption of polyunsaturated fats causes many health problems too. One of the biggest reasons polyunsaturated fats are so unhealthy is because they are very susceptible to becoming oxidized or rancid when exposed to heat and light. The extraction process is the problem:

- Throughout the entire process, these oils are exposed to oxygen.
- The oil is extracted with mechanical pressing and heated to 230 degrees.
- Then a chemical solvent is used to get what oil is left.
- The solvent is then boiled off. Again exposing the oils to heat.
- Because these oils become rancid, they are treated with deodorizers to get rid of the horrible smell.
- Finally, most oils are then bleached to give them eye appeal. Consumers like the light golden color.

Now, the consumer goes to the store to purchase soy oil, which has been touted as super healthy, not knowing that what he or she actually purchasing is a free radical cocktail that over time causes serious health problems. Free radicals, or "chemical marauders" as some scientists refer to them, wreak havoc on our bodies. Some of the problems they can cause to us include:

- Attack cell membranes
- Cause damage to DNA/RNA strands, triggering mutations in tissues throughout the body
- Cause wrinkles and premature aging
- Damage to tissues and organs sets the stage for tumors
- Damage to blood vessels initiates plaque buildup
- Linked to autoimmune diseases like arthritis

☆ Linked to Alzheimer's disease

☆ Linked to cataracts

Table 5.1: Fatty Acid Composition of Common Fats and Oils

Fats and Oils (g/100 g.)	*Saturated*	*Mono-unsaturated*	*Linoleic*	*Alpha Linolenic*	*Predominant Fatty Acids*
Coconut	91	7	2	< 0.5	Saturated
Palm kernel	82	15	2	< 0.5	Saturated
Ghee[a,b]	65	32	2	< 1.0	Saturated
Vanaspati[b]	24	19	3	< 0.5	Saturated
Red Palm Oil (raw)	50	40	9	< 0.5	Saturated + Monounsaturated
Palm Oil	45	44	10	< 0.5	Saturated + Monounsaturated
Olive	13	76	10	< 0.5	Monounsaturated
Groundnut	24	50	25	< 0.5	Monounsaturated
Rape/Mustard[c,d]	8	70	12	10	Monounsaturated
Sesame	15	42	42	1.0	Mono and Polyunsaturated
Rice bran	22	41	35	1.5	Mono and Polyunsaturated
Cotton seed	22	25	52	1.0	Polyunsaturated
Corn	12	32	55	1.0	Polyunsaturated
Sunflower	13	27	6	<0.5	Polyunsaturated
Safflower	13	17	70	<0.5	Polyunsaturated
Soybean	15	27	53	5.0	Polyunsaturated

a. Mainly short and medium chain fatty acids (Coconut 77 per cent, Ghee 25 per cent)

b. Trans fatty acids (Ghee 2 per cent, Vanaspati 53 per cent).

c. Long chain monounsaturated fatty acids (50 per cent erucic acid and 5 per cent eicosenoic acid).

d. Good source of alpha-linoleic acid.

Trans Fats

At one time, tropical oils with anti-microbial properties like coconut and palm oils were the fats used in thousands of food products. Oils like coconut oil and palm kernel oil are the best sources of lauric acid. Lauric acid has anti-microbial properties that inactivate viruses like HIV, measles, herpes simplex-1, vesicular stomatitis, visna and cytomeglovirus. To increase the shelf-life and stability of these unusually healthy oils, they are often hydrogenated.

Hydrogenation is the process of making oils more solid through the addition of hydrogen atoms, thus breaking the double bonds, as in the case of shortening. Complete hydrogenation converts unsaturated fats into saturated fats. Because they are saturated with hydrogen atoms, fully hydrogenated fats contain no *trans* fatty acids. Partial hydrogenation creates *trans fatty acids*. Foods containing "shortening," "partially hydrogenated vegetable oil" or "hydrogenated vegetable oil" in the ingredients list contain *trans* fats. These manmade fats are literally toxins to our bodies.

To produce *trans* fat, manufacturers begin with the cheapest oils, including soy, corn, cottonseed and canola, which are already rancid from the extraction process. The oil is mixed with metal particles, usually nickel oxide, and is then subjected to hydrogen gas in a high-pressure, high-temperature container. Next, emulsifiers and starch are added to the oil/metal mixture to give it a better consistency. It is the base for margarine, only it smells bad because it's rancid and it's gray from the metallic additive. Who would buy a spread like this? Nobody, that's why it is then steam cleaned to get rid of the smell, and colors and flavors are added to make it resemble butter. This junk has actually been pushed onto us by the food industries.

Hydrogenation serves two main purposes. First, the process causes the hydrogen atoms to rearrange and makes a normally curved molecule straighter. The straighter the fat molecules are, the easier they pack. The unnaturally straighter molecules allow a fat that is normally liquid at room temperature, like soy oil, to be solid. Second, hydrogenation makes the naturally unstable polyunsaturated molecules more stable by destroying most of the omega-3 and omega-6 fatty acids, both essential for good health. Being unnaturally more stable, these fats extend the shelf life of processed foods.

Trans fat is toxic to our bodies, and as early as the 1940s, researchers found a strong correlation between cancer, heart disease and the consumption of hydrogenated fats, although the results were presented as though the culprit was saturated fats. In fact, until recently, saturated fats were usually lumped together with *trans* fat in the various data bases that researchers use to correlate dietary trends with disease conditions. Because the FDA has turned a blind eye to the unreported levels of *trans* fat in foods, the consumer is being misled about the fat composition of the foods he eats.

Effects of *Trans* Fats on Health

- ☆ Lowers high density lipoproteins (HDL), otherwise known as the "good cholesterol."
- ☆ Raises low density lipoproteins (LDL), otherwise known as the "bad cholesterol."
- ☆ Raises C-reactive protein, a substance in the blood that indicates arterial inflammation and is said to indicate proneness to heart disease.
- ☆ Raises Lipoprotein (a) (Lp(a)), a substance in the blood that indicates arterial inflammation and is said to indicate proneness to heart disease.
- ☆ Promotes improper management of blood sugar, thus having detrimental effects in diabetics.
- ☆ Interferes with the function of the immune system.
- ☆ Decreases the body's ability to utilize and decreases the amount of the healthy omega-3 fatty acids in our tissues.

Decades of research show the consumption of *trans* fats to be detrimental to health. The latest studies confirm that *trans* fat is directly related with heart disease, increases LDL cholesterol and reduces HDL cholesterol. Because of that, the Institute of Medicine, a branch of the National Academy of Sciences, declared there is no safe amount of *trans* fat in the diet. "There should be a warning on food made with this stuff like there is on nicotine products. It's that bad for you", says Dr. Jeffery Aron, Professor of medicine, University of California at San Francisco and one of the US leading experts on fatty acids and their effect on the body.

Dietary Intake of Saturated Fat and *Trans* Fatty Acids and their ill Health Effects

The intake of dietary fat is generally high in developed countries and low in developing countries. Although both the quantity and the quality of fat can influence the risk of cardiovascular disease, saturated fatty acids are in general hypercholesterolaemic. The various saturated fatty acids, however, behave differently. Evidence in 1991 showed that myristic acid had a greater effect in raising cholesterol levels than did palmitic acid (Hegsted, 1991). On the basis of experiments in which the triacylglycerols were structurally modified, regression equations predicting the response of plasma cholesterol to dietary fatty acids indicated that total saturated fatty acids were twice as effective in raising cholesterol as polyunsaturated fatty acids were in decreasing cholesterol, and that monounsaturated fatty acids were neutral. Confounding effects came from the different species of triacylglycerol and the minor components in the fat or oil.

Several human clinical trials suggest that palm oil and palm olein do not raise total cholesterol and LDL cholesterol to the extent predicted from the fatty acid composition. In a normocholesterolaemic Malaysian population obtaining approximately 30 per cent of their energy from fat, palm olein and soybean oil had similar effects on plasma levels of total cholesterol and LDL cholesterol (Marzuli *et al.*, 1991). A switch from coconut oil (containing predominantly lauric and myristic acids) to palm olein (containing predominantly palmitic and oleic acids) lowered total cholesterol and LDL cholesterol; the switch to corn oil (containing predominantly linoleic acid) lowered it further (Ng TKW *et al.*, 1991). Current evidence indicates that the cholesterolaemic effects of the various saturated fatty acids are not equal and that myristic acid is the most potent in raising plasma cholesterol (Khosla and Sundram, 1998). This is of public health relevance, especially in populations in which coconut oil is the principal fat consumed.

In an Indian population obtaining 27 per cent of its energy from fat, partial replacement of groundnut (peanut) oil by palm olein did not affect total cholesterol or lipo-protein cholesterol levels (Ghafoorunissa *et al.*, 1995). Australian men and women obtaining 30 per cent of their energy from fat and ingesting less than 200 mg of cholesterol per day showed no difference in their plasma and lipoprotein levels resulting from a 5 per cent exchange of energy between palm oil and olive oil (Choudhury *et al.*, 1995). These investigators also reported similar results from a human study comparing palm olein and canola oil (Truswell *et al.*, 1993). Also, diets containing palm olein and canola oil, and the step 1 diet of the American Heart

Association, all of which provide about 31 per cent of their energy as fat and less than 200 mg cholesterol per day, had similar effects on levels of total cholesterol, very low-density lipoprotein (VLDL) cholesterol, and LDL cholesterol; only the step 1 diet increased HDL cholesterol and altered the LDL/HDL ratio beneficially (Sundram *et al.*, 1995). The studies conducted in humans obtaining about 30 per cent of their energy from fat in a mixed diet showed that vegetable oils, such as palm oil, palm olein, olive oil, canola oil, and soybean oil, behave similarly with respect to blood cholesterol and lipoproteins.

Partial hydrogenation of vegetable oils results in the formation of isomers of monounsaturated fatty acids and sometimes polyunsaturated fatty acids. *Trans* monounsaturated fatty acids are the most common of these isomers, and their physico-chemical properties are similar to those of saturated fatty acids. Their effects on blood cholesterol and lipoproteins, however, are different when compared to the most common *cis* monounsaturated fatty acids. Relative to oleic acid, *trans* fatty acids raise the atherogenic LDL and probably lipoprotein (a) and lower the beneficial HDL (Mensink and Katan, 1990; Zock and Katan, 1992; Nestel *et al.*, 1992; Judd *et al.*, 1994).

In a comparison between two diets providing 32 per cent to 34 per cent of their energy as fat, one with 8.7 per cent of total energy from *trans* monounsaturated fatty acids and the other with 9.3 per cent of total energy from stearic acid, the diet containing *trans* monounsaturated fatty acids had a more adverse effect on lipoproteins (Aro A 1997). As compared with the other diet, the diet containing stearic acid lowered LDL levels, and the diet containing *trans* monounsaturated fatty acids lowered HDL levels and also significantly increased lipoprotein (a) levels. These studies were conducted in industrialized countries where the fat intake was high (providing 36 per cent -40 per cent of total energy), but a study conducted in Malaysia (with 32 per cent of total energy from fat) showed that *trans* fatty acids had a greater adverse effect than saturated fatty acids (Sundram,1997). Generally, *trans* fatty acids tend to worsen the LDL/HDL ratio.

Food products requiring a solid or semi-solid consistency have traditionally been formulated with saturated and/or *trans* fatty acids. In view of the growing knowledge of *trans* fatty acids and their health implications, formulations should aim to reduce or eliminate the use of partially hydrogenated fats. Saturated fatty acids on their own could fulfil the same functional requirements. This may be an important consideration in some developing countries where the consumption of solid fats containing *trans* fatty acids is high. Although stearic acid has been reported to be neutral with respect to its effects on blood cholesterol and lipoproteins, questions remain about its possible thrombogenicity. In any case, it is best to avoid high levels of *trans* fatty acids in the diet.

Fats and Oils as Sources of Vitamin A and Carotenoids

Palm oil is by far the most important source of carotenoids. Total carotenoid levels have been reported between 300 and 3,000 ppm. On average palm oil contains 500 to 700 ppm of carotenoids (Trujillo, 1990). Corn oil (90 ppm), rapeseed oil (<100 ppm), and olive oil (5 ppm) have been reported as having lower carotenoid levels.

The purpose of refining palm oil is to remove undesirable odour and colour compounds, but at the same time refining removes all carotenoids. It has been observed that heating can transform carotenoids completely into hydrocarbon-type derivatives. These compounds will not have the physiological effects of carotenoids. Refining of the world production of palm oil (13.5 million tons in 1996) destroys approximately 6.8 tons of carotenoids. Improved technologies are being developed to preserve the carotenoids in palm oil.

Vitamin A values (retinol equivalents or RE) for palm oil between 3,600 and 21,700 RE/100 g have been reported, using the NAS-NRC conversion factor of 1 RE to 6 mg *trans* -carotene. This makes palm oil a very significant contributor to vitamin A needs, especially in developing countries.

Fat-based products may contain beta-carotene (*e.g.*, for colour in spreads) or be fortified with vitamin A. The latter is a legal obligation in a considerable number of countries. Most developing countries do not have such legislation, but when fat is fortified in developing countries, the range is 5 to 10 mg/kg. Both vitamin A and carotenes are well absorbed from fat-based products.

MUFA Rich Mediterranean Diet-Healthy for Humans

Epidemiological studies of ethnic groups living in some parts of Asia and Europe particularly in the Mediterranean region suggest protective health effects from consuming traditional diets that include food sources rich in MUFAs and PUFAs. Consumption of these unsaturated fats as part of a healthful diet may improve blood cholesterol levels, lower the risk for heart disease and even certain cancers. Today, these cultures remain among some of the world's healthiest populations. Here are some examples of traditional food patterns and lessons learned concerning MUFA and PUFA consumption:

- ☆ Olive oil is rich in MUFA and is a major ingredient of the Greek, Southern Italian, and Spanish culinary traditions.
- ☆ When consumed as a substitute for butter or lard, olive oil appears to lower blood LDL ("bad") cholesterol levels, increase HDL ("good") cholesterol, and reduce the risk of heart attack.
- ☆ This may also help explain why CHD death rates are lower among Mediterranean populations.
- ☆ Their diets are higher in vegetables, fruits, and whole grain products than the typical western diet.
- ☆ Furthermore, antioxidants in olive oil, fruits, and vegetables may protect body cells and tissues from damage by oxidation, a process that could set the stage for heart disease.

MUFA may also have other health benefits. In a study of 3,442 Italian women's dietary habits, those who ate large amounts of olive oil (about 1.5 tablespoons) daily reduced their risk for ovarian cancer by 30 percent. A survey of 5,632 elderly participants called the Italian Longitudinal Study on Aging (ILSA) showed that the higher an individual's MUFA consumption is, the lower the likelihood for developing age-related cognitive decline, a mild deterioration in memory. However, these results are preliminary. It is currently recommended that MUFA and PUFA sources should be eaten more frequently than foods rich in saturated fat, *trans fat*, and cholesterol but within the parameters of 25 to 35 per cent of total calories.

Types of Dietary Fats Consumed in the World

The quantity and quality of fat consumed varies greatly in different parts of the world. As a general rule, consumption of total fat and of saturated fat increases with economic development. This is because people in developed countries generally eat more meat, meat products, dairy products, table fat, and baked goods, such as biscuits, pastries and cakes, which contain hydrogenated fats and oils. In low- and middle-income Asia, fat supplied less than 15-22 per cent total energy. In the developed countries of Europe and North America, fat supplied from 30 per cent to 45 per cent total energy.

In the richer developed countries, fat consumption as a percentage of total energy is now decreasing. This is a result partly of dietary advice to consume less fat, largely in the context of cardiovascular disease, and more recently cancer. This is turn has led to changes in packaged and prepared foods. In the USA, for example, estimated average fat intake had dropped from 41 per cent total energy in 1977, to 34 per cent in 1993-94.

Consumption of saturated/animal fat is the lowest in Africa and low income Asia, at 5-7 per cent total energy, and the highest in Europe and Australia, at 15 per cent or more. Consumption of polyunsaturated/vegetable fat as a percentage of total energy intake is the lowest in sub-Saharan Africa and the Pacific Islands and the highest in North America and Europe.

Fat consumption has changed markedly in the twentieth century in many areas of the world. In Japan since the 1950s, and in China and Korea since the 1970s, intake of meat and, thereby, of total fat, has increased markedly, particularly in large cities and urban areas. In areas of the developing world that are now rapidly becoming urbanized, intakes of total and saturated fat are increasing rapidly.

The intake of total and saturated/animal fat in the diets of developed countries generally increases as the availability and consumption of fatty meat, dairy products, added fats and oils increases. Fats and oils are extracted from a variety of plant and animal sources. Vegetable oils are derived from the storage lipids in plant seeds or nuts. Animal-fat products include butter and ghee made from milk fat, as well as lard (from pigs), tallow or suet (from cattle or sheep) and drippings (from cooked meat).

Since the early twentieth century, the hydrogenation process has been used to convert oils of vegetable and animal origin into hardened, variably saturated fats for use as table fats (margarine) and in commercially baked goods and many processed foods. Hydrogenation increases the amount and proportion of saturated/animal fat and trans-fatty acids in the diets of people living in industrialized parts of the world.

Added fats and oils account for 10-15 per cent total energy in the Middle East and North Africa, 10 per cent in central and South America, and 5-10 per cent in Asia and sub-Saharan Africa. In all these regions, vegetable oils predominate over animal fats. In Europe and North America, added fats and oils contribute 15-20 per cent total energy. In Europe, vegetable oils and animal fats contribute equally, with the exception of the Mediterranean region where olive oil predominates. In North America, soya bean and corn oil are the predominant types of added fats.

On average, worldwide, added fats and oils make up around 40 per cent total dietary fat, with the remainder derived from fats in meat, fish, poultry, milk and milk products. Worldwide, the intake of added fats and oils (as well as total fat intake) contributed 50 per cent more to total energy intake in the mid -1990s than it did in 1961. This trend has been most marked in areas with previously low or moderate dietary fat intake, such as parts of Asia, Africa and South America, where consumption of added fats has typically increased by 50-100 per cent. A 100-200 per cent increase in the contribution to total energy intake made by added fat has been recorded in some sub-Saharan African nations and several high-income East Asian countries, including Malaysia and Japan. Consumption of added fat has recently increased only modestly, from a high baseline, in Europe and North America.

Types of Dietary Fats Consumed in India

The major nutritional problem of India, a country of more than one billion, is chronic energy deficiency associated with low fat intake. The urban affluent and middle-income groups are increasing in number, with a corresponding increase in the prevalence of obesity, diabetes, and coronary heart disease in that segment of the population. Fat intake in India is income dependent and highly skewed.

Visible Fat

The vegetable oils used in cooking represent 80 per cent of the visible fat consumed in India. A single oil is generally chosen for cooking, especially in rural areas. Groundnut oil predominates in the western and southern states, whereas mustard seed oil predominates in the northern and eastern states. In Karnataka and South Maharashtra, safflower oil is preferred. Sesame oil is produced and used all over India, but mostly as a second rather than the main oil. Coconut oil is popular in Kerala. Sunflower and rice bran oils have been introduced, and sunflower oil has become popular. Palm oil, used over the last 15 years, is available through the public distribution system and is likely to become important indigenous oil because of the introduction of palm cultivation. Vegetable ghee (*vanaspati*), popular in the northern states, is used in confectionery, bakery, and ready-to-eat foods. Ghee, made from milk in the home or purchased, contributes to the high intake of fat in the urban affluent and middle-income groups. Farming community in Punjab and Haryana generally consumes desi ghee.

The fatty acids in commonly occurring visible fats vary according to the source. In safflower, sunflower, soybean, and cottonseed oils, linoleic acid constitutes more than half of the total fatty acids. In sesame, rice bran, groundnut, and mustard oils, linoleic acid accounts for 20 per cent to 40 per cent of the total fatty acids; in palm oil it accounts for about 10 per cent. Coconut and palm kernel oils have a high proportion of short- and medium-chain-length saturated fatty acids. Rapeseed, mustard, and soybean oils contain *n-3* linolenic acid and the first two also have long-chain eicosanoic (20:1) and erucic acids (22:1). Ghee, which has the fatty acids of milk fat, is high in saturated fatty acids, of which 40 per cent are of short or medium chain length. *Vanaspati* contains long-chain saturated fatty acids and up to 55 per cent *trans* fatty acids.

Invisible Fat

Invisible fat in animal and plant foods was once poorly analysed because structural and tightly bound lipids were not extracted. Although cereal and millet contain only 1 per cent to 3 per cent fat, of which linoleic is a major fatty acid, as bulk items in the Indian diet they contribute significantly to the total fat intake.

Dietary data from national surveys of the rural poor (an estimated 80 per cent of the population) show that the average daily intake of cereal and millet is about 500 g, whereas the intake of visible fats and oils is less than 10 g per person. By using data on invisible fat and fatty acids in Indian foods and information on dietary intake of the rural population, it has been found that cereal and millet alone furnish about 70 per cent of the total invisible fat in the diet. Pulses, milk, fresh coconut, whole oil seeds, and spices constitute the rest. The daily intake of cereal, millet, pulses, and milk contains an average of about 16 g (7 en per cent) fat, 5 g (2 en per cent) linoleic acid, and 0.6 g (0.2 en per cent) n-3 linolenic acid. Thus, invisible fat from cereal and pulses alone furnishes two thirds of the requirement for linoleic acid. Diets of urban high-income groups are low in cereal (200-300 g per person per day) but contain more legumes, pulses, vegetables, and milk (and also, for non-vegetarians, eggs and animal foods). Therefore, the invisible fat contributes 30 g (12 en per cent) to the diet. The average daily intake of visible fat in the urban population is about 13 g in slum dwellers, 23 g in industrial labourers and low-income groups, 35 g in middle-income groups, 6-22 g (13g/cu) in rural areas and 46 g in high-income groups, but it is much higher in the top affluent group. In the rural population, the lower limit of visible fat in Indian diets is about 20 g per person per day. Since chronic energy deficiency is a major problem in low-income groups, increasing dietary fat could help to remedy this situation.

In the urban high-income group, a daily intake of about 50 g per person (18 en per cent) would be the upper limit of visible fat (*e.g.*, oil, ghee, *vanaspati*, and butter) (ICMR, 2010). It was estimated that one third of all the fat in India was consumed by the 5 per cent of the population who constituted the urban rich (Singh and Mulukuntia, 1996). This segment of the population, which has a high prevalence of obesity and cardiovascular disease, could lower the consumption of fat and ease the pressure on the supply of edible oil elsewhere in the country.

During pregnancy and lactation, when the requirements of total fats and essential fatty acids are high, the invisible fat of cereals, pulses, and milk in Indian diets can meet 42 per cent and 30 per cent of the recommended level for linoleic acid of 3 en per cent as proposed by FAO/WHO (1978) (4.5 en per cent in pregnancy and 6 en per cent in lactation). To furnish the additional amounts of linoleic acid recommended, the visible fat intake should be about 30 g in pregnant and lactating women (ICMR, 2010).

In meeting the energy needs of children over two years of age by cereal-pulse diets, excess bulk is a problem. To prevent this, diets should contain a minimum of 25 en per cent fat. Widespread dietary energy deficiency in young children of low-income groups was attributed to an insufficient quantity of food (Gopalan *et al.*, 1973), but re-examination of the intakes of energy and fat by preschool children belonging to different socio-economic groups in both rural and urban areas showed that increased energy intake was closely associated with increased intake of visible fat (Susheela and Narasinga Rao, 1983). The data also showed that when the intake of visible fat was 15 en per cent, the energy intake was judged to be adequate (Narasinga Rao, 1983). These observations reinforce the importance of increasing the energy density of diets for young children.

In diets of the rural poor, invisible fat furnishes about 5 g of saturated fatty acids, 4 g of monounsaturated fatty acids, 8 g of *n-6* linoleic acid, and 0.3 g of *n-3* linolenic acid; the ratios of polyunsaturated fatty acids to saturated fatty acids and *n-6* to *n-3* are about 1 and 13, respectively. In the urban high-income group, invisible fat furnishes about 13 g of saturated fatty acids, 6 g of monounsaturated fatty acids, 4 g of linoleic acid, and 0.6 g of *n-3* linolenic acid; the ratios of polyunsaturated fatty acids to saturated fatty acids and *n-6* to *n-3* are 0.3 and 6, respectively (Ghafoorunissa, 1989).

Degenerative Disease Related to Fat intake among Indians

Heart disease is rising on an epidemic scale in Indian men and women, vegetarians and non vegetarians, whether they are living in India or abroad. Compared to Whites, Blacks and Latinos, Indian women suffered the highest all cause mortality and the highest cardiovascular mortality in the U.S. Women transmit heart disease related genes to their offspring more efficiently than men. 'Like mother like son!' Used to be 'like father like son'.

Risk Factors for CVD more Common in Indians!

- Sedentary life style.
- Meager intake of fresh fruits and vegetables.
- High consumption of simple sugars, dairy products, fried foods and desserts.
- Central obesity (Increased waist line)
- High Insulin levels and high blood sugar levels. (Insulin Resistance)
- Low HDL (good cholesterol)
- High triglycerides (bad fat)
- High blood pressure
- Metabolic Syndrome: when three or more of the above conditions are present!
- Diabetes= heart disease
- Borderline high LDL (bad cholesterol)
- High Lp (a), promotes plaque and blood clots in the arteries

Indian women have similar rates of heart attacks as Indian men although smoking is rare among Indian women. Indian women have much higher prevalence of diabetes and therefore diabetes related complications. Results from AAPI sponsored Indo-US study showed a very high incidence of metabolic syndrome (35 per cent) and type 2 diabetes (18 per cent) among Indian men and women. Half of the people diagnosed to have diabetes in this study did not even know that they were walking around with untreated diabetes with increasing risk of heart attack, stroke, kidney failure, blindness and loss of limb. In fact, metabolic syndrome and diabetes are likely to account for most of the heart disease prevalent among Indian population. Due to more intake of total fat especially saturated fat, obesity occurs which leads to insulin resistance and ultimately to diabetes and other degenerative diseases including heart diseases.

Childhood obesity is rising at an alarming rate due to changing life style and eating patterns. Over thirty percent of children are obese. This trend is only going to get worse unless we address these problems seriously and offer and provide effective life style solutions and early medical attention (Heart disease update, 2006).

Problem and Scope of Heart Disease among Indians

- ✰ The NIH program 'Healthy People 2010' designated the Asian Indian Immigrant Population in the United States as a "high risk group for heart disease."
- ✰ The World Health Report of 2002 projects Cardio Vascular Disease (**CVD=heart disease and stroke**) to be the largest cause of death and disability in India by 2020.
- ✰ Cardiovascular disease will account for 33.5 per cent of total deaths by the year 2015, would replace infectious diseases, as the number one killer in Indian population.
- ✰ The death rate due to heart attack will be 295 per 1,00,000 population in 2015.
- ✰ The World Health Report of 2004 states that every year, more women than men die of CVD and that CVD leads to more deaths in women than cancer, HIV/AIDS and Malaria combined. CVD is the largest cause of death in women and the risk for CVD rises with age.
- ✰ More women than men died of cardiovascular disease (CVD- heart disease and stroke) in the United States since 1984. Women represent 53.1 percent of all deaths from CVD.
- ✰ Women are under investigated, under diagnosed, under treated for heart disease and they are also under represented in clinical research studies.

Scope for Improvement in Quality of Fat Intake in Indian Diets

Estimates of the various fatty acids in the total diet indicate that the levels of linoleic acid are generally adequate because of its high levels in cereals and many vegetable oils in Indian diets. The levels of *n-3* linolenic acid, however, are low. To correct the quality of fat in Indian diets, *n-3* polyunsaturated fatty acids should be increased (Ghafoorunissa, 1996). Saturated and/or *trans* fatty acids are often needed in food products where a solid or semi-solid fat is desired. On their own, saturated fatty acids could fulfil the same functional requirements. Therefore, in countries where the consumption of *trans* fatty acids is high, solid fat formulations could be based on saturated fatty acids. In the high-income group, use of oils such as safflower, sunflower, sesame, or groundnut provides high ratios of n-6 to n-3 (Ghafoorunissa *et al.*, 1995). The levels of *n-3* linolenic acid will be in the desirable range only when mustard, rapeseed, or soya bean oils are used. Analyses of commonly consumed fish in India indicate that fish with high fat (>5 g/100 g), medium fat (1-5 g/100 g), and low fat (<1 g/100 g), respectively, furnish an average of about 1.2,0.4, and 0.1 g of long-chain n-3 polyunsaturated fatty acids per 100 g of muscle. The use of any single oil does not ensure the quality of fat (individual fatty acid levels, polyunsaturated fatty acids/saturated fatty acids, and n-6/n-3 ratios), as recommended for the prevention of cardiovascular disease (Ghafoorunissa, 1996).

The habitual diets of Indians contain a number of factors that are known to reduce the risk of coronary heart disease (Ashwell, 1993), including low fat intake (except in urban high-income and affluent groups, whose fat intake may exceed 30 en per cent), provision of essential fatty acids by invisible fat, high fibre, and provision of more than 60 per cent of total energy intake by complex carbohydrates (Vinodini *et al.*, 1993; Gopalan, 1994). Indian diets are also rich in spices and condiments, which may have antioxidant properties.

A series of metabolic studies were conducted in Indian subjects to determine the possible atherogenic effects of changing the cooking fat from groundnut oil to palmolein (Ghafoorunissa, 1995), ghee, canola oil (Indu and Ghafoorunissa *et al.*, 1992), or mustard oil. The results showed that canola oil decreased LDL cholesterol, and mustard oil, with its high level of erucic acid, increased LDL cholesterol and triacylglycerol.

Improvements to the dietary fat in India could best be accomplished by:

- ☆ Using oils with moderate levels of linoleic acid, such as groundnut, rice bran, or sesame oil;
- ☆ Adding an oil or fat with a low level of linoleic acid, such as palm oil, to an oil with a high level of linoleic acid, such as safflower, sunflower, cottonseed, or soybean oil;
- ☆ Using a preferred oil along with mustard oil to increase the *n-3* fatty acid content and moderate the intake of erucic acid from the mustard oil;
- ☆ Combining soybean oil with palm oil in equal proportions;
- ☆ Using oils with minor components, such as antioxidants, which contribute to their nutritional benefits;
- ☆ Consuming foods rich in *n-3* linolenic acid, such as some vegetable oils and green leafy vegetables, and (for non-vegetarians) eating fish.

Since the requirements for *n-3* polyunsaturated fatty acids increase with increased intake of *n-6* polyunsaturated fatty acids, it is important to moderate linoleic acid and to increase the intake of *n-3* polyunsaturated fatty acids. Use of more than one source of oil gives the added advantage of providing a greater variety of the minor components in the diet.

Interpretation of Studies on Dietary Fat Intake: Limitations

The intake of total fat is correlated with the intake of other components of diet. There is a possible inverse relationship between the intake of fat and that of vegetables and fruits (Ziegler *et al.*, 1992), and a strong direct relationship with consumption of meat, meat products and dairy products.

In developed societies, a substantial amount of fat from meat and table fats and oils may be discarded, so that house-hold or supply data may overestimate fat intake, particularly that of total fat and saturated/animal fat. However, weight-conscious and food-conscious individuals may underestimate their fat intake in answers to dietary questionnaires. These opposite tendencies bias estimates of fat in different directions in different types of study.

Individual-level epidemiological studies vary in their ability to quantify total fat intake. Some studies have attempted to assess diet as a whole, whereas others have included only a short list of relevant foods. Various studies have examined different types of dietary fat in ways that also make comparison among studies problematic. For example, studies have investigated some or all of the following categories: total fat, saturated and unsaturated fat; monounsaturated and polyunsaturated fat; omega-3 and trans-fatty acids; oleic, linoleic, and other individual fatty acids; animal and vegetable fat; and meat, fish, and dairy fat.

Within the populations of most cohort and case-control studies, variation in fat intake is not broad enough to allow comparison of extremes of intake. Thus, if fat intakes below 20-25 per cent total energy are protective against cancer, few of the studies conducted so far in Europe or North America would produce findings to this effect as not enough individuals with this level of intake are in the studies.

Despite the fact that diets consumed in developed countries typically contain 30-45 per cent total energy as fat, and that a high proportion of fats and oils in these diets are extracted or hydrogenated, there are no reliable data specifically on the effects of these food processes on cancer risk.

The relationship between the risk of cancer and fat intake is often adjusted for total energy intake, so that fat is assessed not absolutely but as a proportion of total dietary energy (Willett *et al.*, 1997).

Adjustment for total energy intake may also better simulate many dietary intervention studies, when such studies alter the composition of the diet while holding total energy intake constant. However, data from experimental studies are complicated by this relationship between total energy and fat intake. If the treatment diet is high-fat, then the low-fat control diet may be isocaloric, and therefore necessarily higher in other energy-providing macroconstituents that may themselves be relevant to cancer risk. Alternatively, the control diet may be equivalent in carbohydrate and protein, and therefore, lower in total energy content and in the proportion of total energy from fat. Although isocaloric models have generally been preferred, these may not be the appropriate model for humans in real life. The rise of body mass with age, and the prevalence of overweight and obesity in sedentary populations consuming high-fat diets, suggest a general tendency for such populations to be in positive energy balance.

The grouping of saturated with animal fat, and polyunsaturated with plant fat allows a reasonable assessment of the evidence without excessive fragmentation of the data. Most epidemiological studies that have reported on saturated fat have not reported on animal fat; the converse is also true. While saturated and animal fat are neither interchangeable nor synonymous, they can be viewed as markers for one another. The majority of saturated fat in most diets comes from animal foods, although a significant portion may come from tropical oils in some diets. Also, while saturated fat is a key component of animal fat, between one- and two-thirds of the fat in most animal foods is unsaturated. Polyunsaturated and plant fat are similarly not synonymous. While many plant oils are made up pre-dominantly of polyunsaturated fat, some oils are very high in monounsaturated fat (for example olive oil) or saturated fat (for example coconut and palm oils).

Summary and Recommendations

- ☆ Data on the composition and intake of dietary fat are scarce in developing countries. Collection of reliable data should be encouraged.
- ☆ Updated knowledge on dietary fat should be available. Analysts and local analytical capacity are needed to examine these constituents of the diet.
- ☆ In determining the intake of dietary fat, the sometimes large differences between population groups have to be taken into account.
- ☆ Energy deficiency is normally associated with a low-fat diet. To reach FAO/ WHO recommendations, an increased fat intake may be necessary. In most cases, for the general population the fatty acid composition is less critical than the amount of total fat.
- ☆ In general, dietary guidelines should not be automatically adopted from industrial countries but should take into account local health issues and positive features of the local dietary situation.
- ☆ For groups in developing countries who have a high-fat intake, dietary guidelines similar to those of industrialized countries are applicable.
- ☆ Where *n-3* fatty acids are in short supply, consideration should be given to the *n-6/n-3* balance of fatty acids. Special attention should be given to women of reproductive age, infants, and children.
- ☆ High concentrations of *trans* fatty acids in food products should be avoided.
- ☆ Infants should be breastfed. Complementary foods, produced locally whenever possible, should contain more energy from fat and provide essential fatty acids with a balanced n-6/n-3 ratio.
- ☆ Fortification with vitamin A through concerted efforts of governments, international organizations, and industry is recommended to overcome critical vitamin A deficiency. Where unrefined palm oil is used, its continued use should be encouraged. Alternatively, red palm oil rich in carotenoids should be included in the total dietary fat to enhance vitamin A activity.

Chapter 6

Health Effects of *Trans* Fatty Acids

History

The story of trans fats begins with the 20th century. Nobel laureate Paul Sabatier worked in the 1890s towards developing the chemistry of hydrogenation to advance the margarine, oil hydrogenation, and synthetic methanol industries. While Sabatier only considered hydrogenation of vapours, the German chemist Wilhelm Normann showed in 1901 that liquid oils could be hydrogenated, and patented the process in 1902. In 1909 Procter and Gamble in Cincinnati acquired the US rights to the Normann patent and in 1911 they began marketing Crisco, the first hydrogenated shortening, which contained a large amount of partially hydrogenated cottonseed oil. Further success came from the marketing technique of giving away free cookbooks with every recipe calling for Crisco. Hydrogenation strongly stimulated whaling, as it made it possible to stabilize whale oil for human consumption.

In the 1950s, advocates said that the *trans* fats of margarine were healthier than the saturated fats of butter, but this has been proven incorrect. One example of the effects of *trans* fats vs saturated fats came from the "Walter Willett Nurses Study" (Professor of Medicine, Harvard Medical School). The 14-year study of 80,082 women who were 34 to 59 years of age concluded that a 2 per cent increase in *trans* fats, compared to the same increase in carbohydrates, increased a woman's risk of heart disease by 19.3 per cent, while the same study found that a 5 per cent increase in saturated fats increased heart disease risk by 17 per cent compared with the same increase in carbohydrates.

The Center for Science in the Public Interest (CSPI) campaigned against fast foods using saturated fats starting in 1984. When fast food companies replaced the saturated fat with *trans* fat, CSPI's campaign against them ended. CSPI defended *trans* fats in their 1987 Nutrition Action newsletter. However, by 1992, CSPI began to speak against *trans* fats and is currently strongly against their use.

Meaning of *Trans* Fat

Naturally occurring unsaturated fats contain double bonds that are nearly all in the *cis* configuration, and these occur most commonly in certain positions in the aliphatic chain. Enzymes involved in fatty acids synthesis have evolved to recognize these natural fatty acids with a high degree of specificity. Changes in the fatty acid composition of the diet can have major effects on several critical physiologic processes because the number and position of double bonds influence the function and metabolism of fatty acids, including their incorporation into phospholipids and transformation into prostaglandins and other eicosanoids. Through human evolution, oleic acid, linoleic acid, linolenic acid, and the long-chain n-3 fatty acids from fish oils constituted almost all of the unsaturated fat in the food supply. The only appreciable sources of *trans* isomers were dairy fat and the meat of ruminants, whose stomachs contain bacterial isomerases capable of converting the double bonds of polyunsaturated fats in plants to *trans* configuration.

Meaning of *Trans* Fat

- ☆ A type of fat created when oils are hydrogenated, which chemically transforms them from their normal liquid state (at room temperature) into solids.
- ☆ During the hydrogenation procedure extra hydrogen atoms are pumped into unsaturated fat, thereby creating *trans* fatty acids.
- ☆ This process converts the mixture into a saturated fat, which obliterates its polyunsaturate benefits.
- ☆ Chemically speaking, *trans* fats are made of the same building blocks as non-*trans* fats, but are a slightly different shape. From a molecular perspective, the different shape is caused by double bonds between carbon atoms being in the *trans* rather than the cis configuration. *Trans* fats are more of a straight shape, while the cis shape is more kinked.
- ☆ *Trans* fatty acids can be found in a wide array of processed foods including cookies and margarines.
- ☆ Any food with "hydrogenated oils" or "partially hydrogenated oils" on the label contains *trans* fatty acids.
- ☆ Some researchers believe such foods may actually be more damaging than regular saturated fats to those watching their cholesterol, saying *trans* fatty acids decrease the good (HDL) cholesterol and increase the bad LDLs.
- ☆ Other scientists argue that the evidence is inconclusive and that *trans* fatty acids are no worse than butter. In either case, it would seem that "moderation" is the watchword when consuming foods containing *trans* fatty acids.

At the turn of the century, a dramatic change in the fatty acid composition of the food supply of industrialized countries occurred when a process was discovered to convert liquid oils into solid or semisolid fats. In this process, known as partial hydrogenation, oils are heated in the presence of nickel or other metal catalysts and exposed to hydrogen gas. This process causes some double bonds to be saturated while others are changed to a *trans* configuration (geometric isolerism) or are shifted to a new position in the aliphatic chain (positional isomerism). The end products of partial hydrogenation typically contain > 20 new isomers of oleic and linoleic acids; these artificial fatty acids may make up to 40 per cent or more of the total fat. Altering the conditions of partial hydrogenation allows the creation of different fats that are used in the manufacture of margarine, fats for deep frying, or shortenings for baking.

Chemistry

In a natural fatty acid, the hydrogen atoms are usually on the same side of the double bonds of the carbon chain. However, partial hydrogenation reconfigures most of the double bonds that do not become chemically saturated, twisting them so that the hydrogen atoms end up on different sides of the chain. This type of configuration is called *trans*, which means "across" in Latin. It is not just a swapping of the position of the single hydrogen atom, rather it is a twisting of the whole molecule from that point on that creates the *trans* alignment; the arrangement of the red oxygen atoms in the diagram below to see this effect.)

Oleic Acid	*Elaidic Acid*
Oleic acid is a *cis* unsaturated fat that comprises 55-80 per cent of olive oil. To visualize the reason for the different shape, count the carbon atoms on the "top" vs. the "bottom" of both molecules.	Elaidic acid is a *trans* unsaturated fat and a major *trans* fat found in hydrogenated vegetable oils. It is a geometric isomer of Oleic acid (chemically identical except for the arrangement of the double bond).

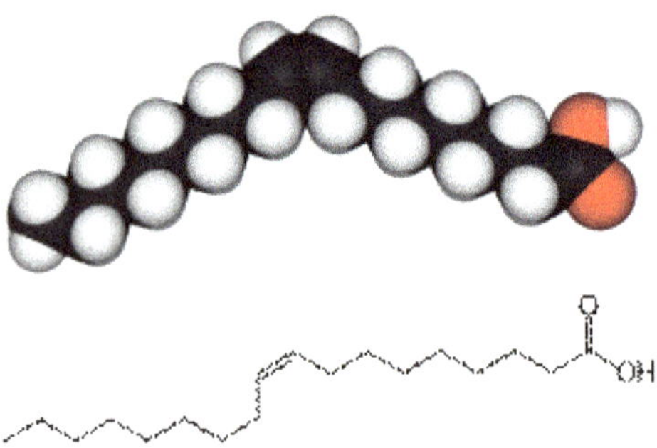

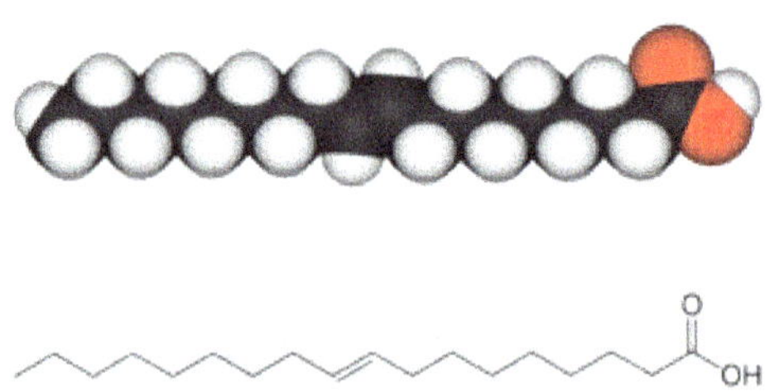

Technically speaking, the conversion from *cis* to *trans* configuration is a catalytic reaction, meaning that another atom is temporarily bonded into the fat during the conversion process and then released. The other elements used (the catalysts) are finely divided nickel, palladium, platinum or cobalt.

The amount of *trans* fatty acid in the product is dependent on reaction conditions. Increasing the pressure at which oil is hydrogenated reduces *trans* fat formation.

Researchers at the United States Department of Agriculture applied 1400 kPa (200 psi) of pressure to soybean oil in a 2-litre vessel while heating it to between 140°C and 170°C. The standard 140 kPa (20 psi) process of hydrogenation produces a product of about 40 per cent *trans* fat by weight, compared to about 17 per cent using the high pressure method. Blended with pure soybean oil, the high pressure processed oil produced margarine containing 5 to 6 per cent *trans* fat which could qualify for a label of zero grams of *trans* fat.

Trans fats are formed from a process described as partial hydrogenation because the reaction is not allowed to go to completion; if it were there would be no *trans* fatty acids left, but the resulting material would be too solid for practical use.

Sources

Trans fats occur naturally in the milk and body fat of ruminants (such as cows and sheep) at a level of 2-5 per cent of total fat. They originate in the rumens of these animals. Animal-based fats were once the only *trans* fats that were consumed but by far the largest amount of *trans* fats consumed today are plant-based *trans* fats (made from partially hydrogenated vegetable oil). These have displaced natural solid fats and liquid oils in many areas, notably in the fast food, snack food, fried food and baked good industries. Vegetable shortenings are primarily *trans* fats packaged for home use, and some margarines contain a large proportion of them. Foods containing artificial *trans* fats formed by partially hydrogenating plant fats may contain up to 45 per cent *trans* fat compared to their total fat.

Benefits of hydrogenating plant-based fats for food manufacturers include an increased product shelf life and decreased refrigeration requirement. Partial hydrogenation raises the melting point of fat, producing a semi-solid material, which is much more desirable than liquid oils for use in baking. Plant-based hydrogenated vegetable oils are much less expensive than the animal fats traditionally favored by bakers, such as butter or lard.

Because partial hydrogenation of plant oils can replace animal fats, the resulting products can be consumed (barring other ingredient and preparation violations) by adherents to Kashrut (kosher) and Halal, as well as by adherents to vegetarianism in Buddhism, ahimsa in Jainism and Hinduism, veganism, and other forms of vegetarianism.

It has been established that *trans* fats in human milk fluctuate with maternal consumption of *trans* fat, and that the amount of *trans* fats in the bloodstream of breastfed infants fluctuates with the amounts found in their milk. Reported percentages of *trans* fat (compared to total fats) in breast milk range from 1 per cent in Spain, 2 per cent in France and 4 per cent in Germany to 7 per cent in Canada.

Consumption of *Trans* Fat

The issue of TFA arose in the West, when it was propagated that consumption of margarine is a good substitute for hydrogenated fat. But margarine contains high amounts of TFAs, which have adverse effects on health. During the course of last century, the production of partially hydrogenated vegetable oils increased steadily because of their low cost, long shelf life, and suitability for commercial frying. By about 1910, the per capita production of margarine and vegetable shortening in the United States was already > 4 kg/y. Various forms of partially hydrogenated vegetable oils have replaced beef tallow, butter, and lard in homes and in many commercial applications, largely for economic and perceived (but undocumented) health benefits. Despite the continuing displacement of animal fats by partially hydrogenated fats in the United States, per capita consumption of *trans* fatty acids from vegetable sources declined slightly from a peak of ≈ 2.2 per cent of energy in the 1960s to ≈ 2.1 per cent in the mid-1980s. This resulted largely from a reduction in the degree of hydrogenation to retain more of the original polyunsaturated fats. Thus, consumption of *trans* fatty acids in other countries are sparse. In the United Kingdom, consumption was ≈ 6 per cent of total fat (≈ 2.3 per cent of energy) in the 1980s, and similar values have been reported from Sweden and Germany. Consumption of *trans* fatty acids has increased in the Indian subcontinent, where partially hydrogenated vegetable oils (vanaspathi) are replacing the traditional ghee (clarified butter). It is likely that production and consumption of these products are increasing widely throughout the developing world as populations move from relying on subsistence agriculture to being urban societies dependent on a commercial food supply.

Nutritional Guidelines

The recommendations of National Academy of Sciences (NAS) regarding *trans* fats are based on two key facts. First, "*trans* fatty acids are not essential and provide no known benefit to human health". Second, while both saturated and *trans* fats increase levels of LDL cholesterol (so-called "bad" cholesterol), *trans* fats also lower levels of HDL cholesterol (so-called "good" cholesterol); this increases the risk of coronary heart disease (CHD). The NAS is concerned "that dietary *trans* fatty acids are more deleterious with respect to CHD than saturated fatty acids".

Because of these facts and concerns, the NAS has concluded there is no safe level of *trans* fat consumption. There is no adequate level, recommended daily amount or tolerable upper limit for *trans* fats. This is because any incremental increase in *trans* fatty acid intake increases the risk of coronary heart disease.

Despite this concern, the NAS dietary recommendations have not recommended the elimination of *trans* fat from the diet. This is because *trans* fat is naturally present in many animal foods, and therefore, in most non-vegan diets; its removal from ordinary diets might introduce undesirable side effects and nutritional imbalances if proper nutritional planning is not undertaken. The NAS has therefore "recommended that *trans* fatty acid consumption be as low as possible while consuming a nutritionally adequate diet". Like the NAS, the World Health Organization has tried to balance public health goals with a practical level of *trans* fat consumption, recommending in 2003 that *trans* fats be limited to less than 1 per cent of overall energy intake.

The US National Dairy Council has asserted that the *trans* fats present in animal foods are of a different type than those in partially hydrogenated oils, and do not appear to exhibit the same negative effects.

Although the NAS has based its analysis on cardiovascular concerns, there are other deleterious effects of *trans* fat consumption too which have been reported.

Health Effects

Although synthetically created *trans* fatty acids have been a significant part of the human diet for just over 100 years, the biochemistry of *trans* fatty acids is poorly understood. Little is known about how *trans* fatty acids are incorporated into the developing fetal brain tissue, cell membranes, and arterial plaque. Some clinical studies suggest a possible association of *trans* fatty acids with cancer, coronary heart disease, obesity, metabolic syndrome and diabetes. *Trans* fats increase total and LDL (Low density lipoprotein) cholesterol in blood and decrease HDL (High density lipoprotein) cholesterol, thus adversely affecting LDL/HDL ratio. *Trans* fat consumption increases lipoprotein Lp (a) and is positively associated with CVD risk in all population-based studies. Indeed, TFA has more adverse effects than SFA vis-à-vis blood lipids, CVD risk etc. Lauric and myristic acids as SFAs are as bad as TFA in their effects on blood lipids and CVD (Cardiovascular disease) risk, while other saturated fatty acids like stearic and palmitic acids are better. It is unclear whether the naturally present *trans* fatty acids in beef, mutton and dairy products (created through fermentation processes in the stomach of ruminant animals) pose the same risks.

Trans fats are associated with an increased prostate cancer risk with researchers noting that "blood levels of *trans* fatty acids, in particular *trans* fats resulting from the hydrogenation of vegetable oils, are associated with an increased prostate cancer risk". There is preliminary evidence that other cancers may also be related to *trans* fat intake.

Human metabolism requires essential fatty acids which are destroyed by the hydrogenation process by which *trans* fat is produced. The destruction of some of the essential fatty acids is one of the intended goals of hydrogenation, since reducing the proportion of unsaturated fatty acids which are at risk of oxidation creates shortening that is less likely to undergo rancidification. For example, a typical candy bar might have a shelf life of 30 days without use of hydrogenated oils, while the same product with hydrogenated oils can last up to 18 months. For this reason, many believe that *trans* fat should be classified as a preservative.

Trans fat behaves like saturated fat by raising the level of low-density lipoprotein in the blood (LDL or "bad cholesterol") which increases the risk of coronary heart disease (CHD). It has the additional effect of decreasing levels of HDL, the "good" lipoprotein which helps remove cholesterol from arteries. The net increase in LDL/HDL ratio with *trans* fat is approximately double than due to saturated fat (Higher ratios are more deleterious).

A study of over 700 nurses showed that those in the highest quartile of *trans* fat consumption had blood levels of C-reactive protein (CRP, a pro-inflammatory cytokine which is a cardiovascular disease risk factor) 73 per cent higher than those in the lowest quartile. Although one group of researchers indicated that CRP may only be a moderate risk factor for cardiovascular disease, others have shown that CRP can exacerbate ischemic necrosis in a complement-dependent fashion and that CRP inhibition can be a safe and effective therapy for myocardial and cerebral infarcts.

The majority of clinical research reports have suggested that *trans* fats may be worse for the body than saturated fats; in fact, the 2002 summary statement by the Institute of Medicine on *trans* fatty acids concluded that there was no safe level of *trans* fatty acids in the human diet.

A confounding issue may arise from the cooking process itself, in that *trans*-fats are often associated with high temperature cooking processes which also favor the formation of Advanced glycation endproduct (AGEs) and oxidation products. It appears some of the studies have not controlled for these AGEs and oxidation products. It has been suggested that, "given the prominence of this type of food in the human diet, the deleterious effects of high-fat foods may be in part due to the high content in glycotoxins, above and beyond those due to oxidized fatty acid derivatives." The glycotoxins, as he called them, are more commonly called AGEs.

Trans fats are metabolized differently by the liver than other fats and interfere with delta 6 desaturase. Delta 6 desaturase is an enzyme involved in converting essential fatty acids to arachidonic acid and prostaglandins, both of which are important to the functioning of cells. *Trans* fats which cannot be metabolized normally end up in the liver for biotransformation. If they simply can never be metabolized, they are returned in the blood to fat cells for storage, possibly posing a risk of permanent obesity.

Research with monkeys indicates that *trans* fat may also increase weight gain and abdominal fat, despite a similar caloric intake. A 6-year experiment revealed that monkeys fed a *trans*-fat diet gained 7.2 per cent of their body weight, as compared to 1.8 per cent for monkeys on the mono-unsaturated fat diet. Monkeys eating *trans* fats also had 30 per cent more abdominal fat. Abdominal fat is associated with diabetes mellitus type 2 and heart disease.

Metabolic Effects

Although it seems likely that the effects on blood cholesterol fractions are not the same for all the *trans* isomers, there are no data on the relative potency of individual compounds. In two of the above experiments, the *trans* diet contained a mixture of *cis* and *trans* isomers similar to that of commercially available margarine; in the others, claidic acid, (the *trans* isomer of oleic acid) contributed most of the total *trans* fatty acids.

Epidemiological Studies

The prediction based on the metabolic studies, that intake of partially hydrogenated fats increases the risk of coronary disease has been supported by several epidemiologic investigations. Intake of partially hydrogenated fats has paralleled the rise in CAD mortality in the United States and other countries. Also, among the seven countries studied, average intake of *trans* fatty acids, addressed by analysis of replicate food sample, was strongly associated with regional incidence of CAD. More detailed investigations that allow for the control of individual risk factors are desirable because many other variables besides dietary fat composition differ among countries and may account for at least some of the difference in CAD incidence.

Direct associations have been reported between concentrations of *trans* isomers in adipose tissue and risk of death from myocardial infarction and between plasma concentrations of *trans* fatty acids and the presence of atherosclerosis. In the above investigations, however, other dietary factors that may affect the risk of CAD were not considered. This limitation was addressed in the Nurses' Health Study, a longitudinal study of ≈ 90000 US women. In that investigation, women in the highest quintile of intake of *trans* fatty acids from partially hydrogenated vegetable fats at baseline (median intake = 3.2 per cent of total energy) had a 35 per cent higher risk of coronary disease than women in the lowest quintile (median = 1.3 per cent of total energy), after standard cardiovascular risk factors were adjusted for. The association remained significant after further adjustment for intake of other types of fat, cholesterol, vitamins, and fibre. The positive association was limited to *trans* fatty acids from partially hydrogenated vegetable fat. The association was stronger when women who had changed their consumption of margarine during the past 10 y were excluded, suggesting that the association was not due simply to a switch to margarine by women with a suspicion of preclinical coronary disease. Also, the positive association with intake of *trans* fatty acids was due to high consumption of cookies and white bread, as well as a higher intake of margarine, indicating that the association was not simply the result of healthier behaviour by women with a perceived higher risk of CAD. A positive association between intake of *trans* fatty acids and risk of myocardial infarction was also observed in case-control study among men and women; the dose-response findings suggested a possible J-shaped relation, but a formal statistical test indicated that the data did not depart significantly from linearity. In both studies, the risk was quantitatively higher than predicted by the effect of *trans* fatty acids on blood LDL and HDL concentrations, which is compatible with the suggestion that *trans* fatty acids may have other adverse physiologic effects perhaps mediated by lipoprotein(s) or a prothrombotic mechanism.

Public Response and Regulation

The lengthy political process of balancing the public health versus private profit from the public sale of processed foods containing artificially hydrogenated oils and fats continues today. Some countries are considering a complete ban against artificial hydrogenation products in food.

Canada

Canada is one of the largest consumers of *trans* fats in the world. The food regulator, Health Canada requires the listing of the amount of *trans* fats in the food described.

In November 2004, an opposition day motion seeking a ban similar to Denmark's was introduced by Jack Layton of the New Democratic Party, and passed through the Canadian House of Commons by an overwhelming 193-73 vote.

In June 2006, a task force co-chaired by Health Canada and the Heart and Stroke Foundation of Canada recommended a limit of 5 per cent *trans* fat (to total fat) ratio in all products sold to consumers in Canada (2 per cent for tub margarines and spreads). The amount was selected such that "most of the industrially produced *trans* fats would be removed from the Canadian diet, and about half of the remaining *trans* fat intake would be of naturally occurring *trans* fats". This recommendation has been endorsed by the Canadian Restaurant and Foodservices Association and the Food and Consumer Products of Canada has congratulated the task force on the report.

Denmark

Denmark became the first country to introduce laws strictly regulating the sale of many foods containing *trans* fats in March 2003, a move which effectively bans partially hydrogenated oils. Naturally present trace amounts of *trans* fatty acids in dairy and meat products are unaffected by these bills.

European Union

The European Food Safety Authority was asked to produce a scientific opinion on *trans* fats.

United Kingdom

In October 2004, the Food Standards Agency (FSA) has asked for better labelling in the UK. In the 29 July 2006 edition of the British Medical Journal, an editorial also called for better labelling.

Some companies such as Marks and Spencer and Waitrose have voluntarily removed or reduced *trans* fats from their products. Two major supermarkets had decided to withdraw *trans* fats from their own-brand products: Sainsbury's from January 2007 and and Tesco by the end of 2006.

United States

In May 2003, Ban*Trans*Fats.com Inc., a U.S. non-profit corporation, filed a lawsuit against the food manufacturer Kraft Foods in an attempt to force Kraft to remove *trans* fats from the Oreo cookie. The lawsuit was withdrawn when Kraft agreed to work on ways to find a substitute for the *trans* fat in the Oreo. This suit was very effective at bringing the *trans* fat controversy to public attention.

Before 2006, consumers in the United States could not easily determine the presence (or quantity) of *trans* fats in food products. This information could only be inferred by reading the ingredient list on the food label. If the ingredients included the words "shortening," "partially hydrogenated vegetable oil," or "hydrogenated vegetable oil," the food probably contained *trans* fat. Because ingredients are listed in descending order of predominance, smaller amounts are present when the ingredient is close to the end of the list.

Some consumer advocates wanted a ban on *trans* fats in the US, but the United States Food and Drug Administration (FDA) responded with a labelling requirement instead. On July 9, 2003, the FDA issued a regulation (21 CFR 101.9 (c)(2)(ii)) requiring manufacturers to list *trans* fatty acids, or *trans* fat, on the Nutrition Facts panel of foods and some dietary supplements. This new information must appear below the listing of saturated fat content, which was already required. The regulation allows *trans* fat levels of less than 0.5 grams per serving to be labeled as 0 grams per serving, or *trans* fat free. (In this case, manufacturers may use the synonyms "free", "without," "no" and "zero" in their packaging claims.). However, it should be noted that small amounts may be significant, depending on how many servings are consumed. The FDA defines *trans* fatty acids as containing one or more *trans* linkages that are not in a conjugated system.

The new labeling rule took effect on January 1, 2006. The FDA created a process where companies may petition for an extension that will be reviewed on a case-by-case basis. Extensions will be granted until January 1, 2008. The FDA estimates that by 2009, *trans* fat labeling will have prevented from 600 to 1,200 cases of coronary heart disease and 250 to 500 deaths each year. This benefit is expected to result from consumers choosing alternative foods lower in *trans* fatty acids as well as manufacturers reducing the amount of *trans* fatty acids in their products.

While the FDA regulation was strictly a labeling directive, many food manufacturers used the 2006 deadline as a target date to reduce or eliminate *trans* fats from their products. This required some experimentation with alternative oils in an attempt to preserve the flavor and "mouth feel" of the food while maximizing shelf life. The solution for some products was a return to the saturated fats and tropical oils abandoned 20 years earlier, when saturated fats were a high-profile health concern. Another solution was the use of new soybean varieties and processing methods, which produce oils with many of the desirable characteristics of hydrogenated oils without requiring hydrogenation.

Trans fat: Bans Across the World

- ☆ Growing concern and action against trans fats
- ☆ Denmark bans hydrogenated oil; limits trans fats at 2 per cent
- ☆ January 2008, US Food and Drug Administration decides only to label trans fats in oils; but states protest
- ☆ In 2005, all restaurants in California go trans fats free voluntarily; In 2008, government makes it mandatory
- ☆ In 2006, New York bans trans fats in restaurants
- ☆ Mc Donald fails to limit trans fats, in 2003, agrees to pay US$ 7 million to American Heart Association
- ☆ In 2007, case filed against KFC and Burger King.

The movement away from *trans* fat has been seen in restaurant chains as well. In June 2006, the fast food chain Wendys announced that they would switch to non-hydrogenated cooking oil to reduce *trans* fat. In June 2006, Panera's food chain had removed *trans* fats from all breads and bagels, and most of their other baked goods.

Some cities are making an effort to reduce *trans* fat consumption. New York City has asked all its restaurants to eliminate *trans* fat from their offerings, on a voluntary basis. In May 2005, Tiburon, California became the first city where all restaurants voluntarily cook with *trans* fat-free oils. Chicago is considering banning oils containing *trans* fats from large chain restaurants; the ordinance would make Chicago the first city to ban *trans* fat-containing oils outright.

On 16th June 2006, research found that KFC uses *trans* fat when frying. The Center for Science in the Public Interest has sued KFC and will try to bring down the use of *trans* fat in KFC. KFC's reply was that it is looking into new methods of cooking but to use any other fat would jeopardise their unique flavour, availability and cost.

Table 6.1: Dietary Recommendations for *Trans* Fatty Acids

Organization/Authority	*Trans Fatty Acids*
US	
American Heart Association	<1 per cent energy (population)
Adult Treatment Panel III of the National Cholesterol Education Programme	Keep intake low
Health and Human Services/US Department of Agriculture	As low as possible
Institute of Medicine of the National Academy of Sciences	As low as possible
Non-US	
Health Council of the Netherlands	low as possible
Health Canada	Upper limit 1 per cent energy
Ministries of Agriculture of Austria, Germany, Switzerland and Japan	<2 per cent energy
WHO/Food and Agriculture Organization of the UN	<1 per cent energy

Adapted from Hunter (2008).

Developing Nations

Dr. Kalyanasundaram, Scientist of PORIM (Palm Oil Research Institute of Malaysia), Malaysia while presenting his paper on "Health effects of the Trans Fatty Acids – implications for the oils and fats industry" pointed out that increase in the intake of trans fatty acids (TFAs) is a global phenomenon. While Western and European countries have made attempts to reduce its intake, hardly any such efforts have been made in developing countries like India and Pakistan.

India

In India, PHVO (*vanaspati, dalda*, margarine etc) is the source of TFA and no limit has been fixed for TFA content (A.19 of PFA Act 1954 and rules 1955). Indian *vanaspati* contains 45-55 per cent of total fatty acids as TFA. It is used as a substitute for ghee and in the preparation of commercially fried/processed/ready to eat and bakery foods. In 1980s estimates of TFA intake were reported to be between 2-11g/p/d (4 per cent energy). However, in recent years due to changes in life styles, the intake of PHVO has increased in the urban population. The current annual production of PHVO constitutes 4 5 per cent of total edible oil consumption (4 5 out of 4 110 lakh tons).

In one of the studies carried out in India, the following samples of fats and oils were analyzed. Test methodology included internationally used methodology of AOAC for fatty acids using GC-FID (CSE Report, 2009).

1. *Vanaspati* – 7 brands
2. Vegetable oils: 21 brands– Soybean (4 brands), Sunflower (4), Safflower (1), Groundnut (1), Mustard (4), Coconut (1), Olive (1), Sesame oil (1), Rice bran (1) and Palm oil (2), blended oil (1 brand)
3. Desi ghee (1)
4. Butter (1)

Vanaspati is a hydrogenated vegetable fat. About 55 per cent of *vanaspati* manufactured in India is consumed in the Northern States. Trans fatty acid content of *vanaspati* ranges from 10-40 per cent, with variation observed in the trans fatty acid content due to use of several different oils. The extent of trans fatty acids formed during hydrogenation process also depends on the type of source oil used. The higher the PUFA content of the oil, the greater the formation of trans fatty acids. The following companies manufacture *vanaspati* in India:

- *Rath*: Agro Tech Foods Ltd affiliated to US ConAgra Foods
- *Dalda*: Bunge Limited, a mega-food giant US multinational
- *Gemini*: Cargill Inc, another US based company
- *Raag*: Adani group and Singapore's Wilmar International
- *Jindal*: Jindal group, a steel major
- *Gagan*: Amrit Banaspati Company,
- *Panghat*: Mawana Sugars Limited
- *Amul butter*: Gujarat Co-op. Milk Marketing Federation Ltd
- *Milk Food Desi Ghee*: Milk Food Ltd

Most of these are not small companies, they are global companies, meeting global standards for *trans* fats, but not in India. There is a growing health concern in the world about trans fats which are regulated in developed world. For example, in Denmark, the limit for trans fats in cooking oil is set at 2 per cent. WHO recommends that the energy intake from trans fats should not be more than 1 per cent.

Trans fatty acids in fat samples collected from above mentioned various *vanaspati* manufacturing companies ranged from 9-24 per cent as mentioned in Figure 6.1. These values are 5-12 times the standards set for TFAs in Denmark. CSE analysis found that Rath *vanaspati* had 16 per cent trans fats–eight times above the Denmark standard. Can we have this high level of *trans* fat? Are we not supposed to take any regulatory measures?

Indian regulations allow companies to mix – "permissible vegetable oils: cottonseed, *kardi*, *mahua*, maize, palm, soybean, mustard/rapeseed, vegetable oils imported for edible purpose". *Trans* fats will depend on the oil used in *vanaspati*. So, if soybean oil is used, it will be higher in *trans* fats. Is this why companies are reluctant

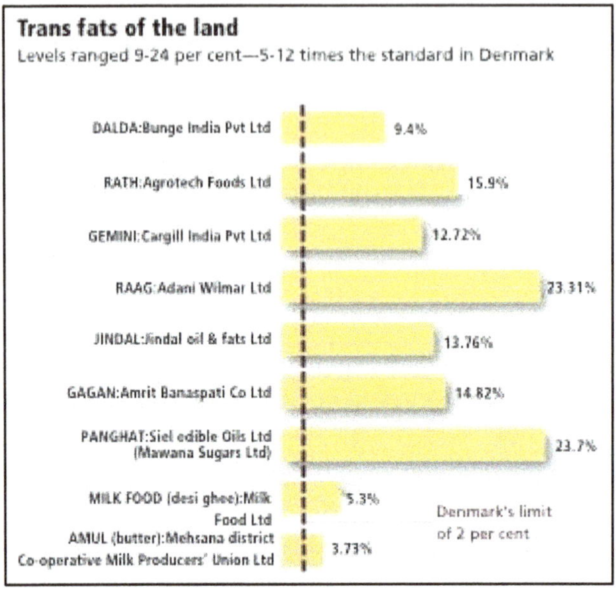

Figure 6.1: ***Trans*** **Fatty Acids in Various Indian Fats and Oils Samples**
Source**: CSE Report, 2009.**

to take on standards. Take case of *Dalda* – says 15-55 per cent *trans* fat, CSE analysis found 9.4 per cent. So, could it be higher in other times when the composition changes?

CSE's Pollution Monitoring Lab

- Set up in 2000, with state-of-the-art equipment to test for toxins, pesticides, heavy metals, other contaminants and health matters.
- ISO 9001:2000 certified by SWISO, Switzerland
- www.cseindia.org

The progress and present status of regulation on *trans* fat in India is as under:

Late 2004

Oils and Fats sub-committee of CCFS accepts that *trans* fats are health hazards. Agrees to set standards

August 25, 2006

Chair of sub-committee submits proposal for standard. Data is asked for. Industry says it will give.

April 16, 2007

Sub-committee recommends to Central Committee for Food Standards (CCFS) to set a limit of 15 per cent trans fats content. CCFS asks committee to consider the matter again and come back.

January 7, 2008

Sub-committee discusses that the issue is urgent, "in the light of growing presence of multinationals in the fast food business that have taken steps to limit trans-fat in their products in western countries, but will take advantage of the lax regulatory control in the country". A 3- phase-wise introduction of standards is recommended.

February 18, 2008

The CCFS endorses this recommendation. Wants standards to be set urgently. But asks for data from industry groups.

August 2008

CCFS meets again. Still awaiting data.

January 2009

Data is still awaited. Our health is at risk. In September 2008, government notifies food labeling. It says companies that make nutrition and health related claims must include the quantity of trans fats on their package; says food which uses hydrogenated vegetable fats, must declare on the label: "contains trans fats". If a company says it is "trans fats free", it would mean that the product contains less than 0.2 g of trans fats per serving of food. But there is no standard. So companies decide to label and get away.

To reduce trans fatty acids in food supply, the Indian vegetable oil and the food industry has the following challenges:

1. Improve hydrogenation technology and /use vegetable oil (s) with lower saturation for hydrogenation.
2. Examine regulatory issues regarding the range and upper limit for TFA in Indian *vanaspati*, shortenings and margarines, labeling TFA and SFA contents in foods. The current food label reads as 'contains PHVO', this is misleading.
3. Encourage substitution of vegetable fats soft at room temperature for hard fats.
4. Invest in adopting enzymatic inter-esterification technologies in place of hydrogenation to produce zero trans fats without increasing SFA.

Public Health Approach to Reducing Intake of *Trans* Fatty Acids

Without greater availability of information on the *trans* fatty acid content of foods, health-conscious consumers are likely to be particularly misled by claims of "low saturated fat" and "cooked in vegetable oil," as those products may contain up to 35 per cent *trans* fatty acids. Prudent dietary advice should aim to reduce specifically the amount of both saturated and *trans* fatty acids. This can be achieved by using vegetable oils in their natural, unhydrogenated form for frying, baking and at the table and avoiding animal fats and commercial products baked or fried in hydrogenated fats, which include most fried fast foods, brands of potato and tortilla chips, donuts, crackers, cookies, and other bakery items. It is difficult to argue that consumers should not be allowed to make informed choices, which would require that food labels indicate the amount of *trans* fatty acids and that special labels be created for fast foods and other products with very high *trans* fatty acid contents and that are presently exempt from labeling requirements.

Chapter 7

Role of Cholesterol in Human Health

Cholesterol an unusual waxy and fat-like substance is essential to life. It is a sterol (a combination of steroid and alcohol) and lipid (a type of fat). It's found in foods such as eggs and dairy products and is also manufactured in the body, especially the liver.

It is essential for many of the body's metabolic processes. It helps make hormones like oestrogen, testosterone and adrenaline (the name originates from the Greek 'chole' meaning bile and stereos meaning solid).

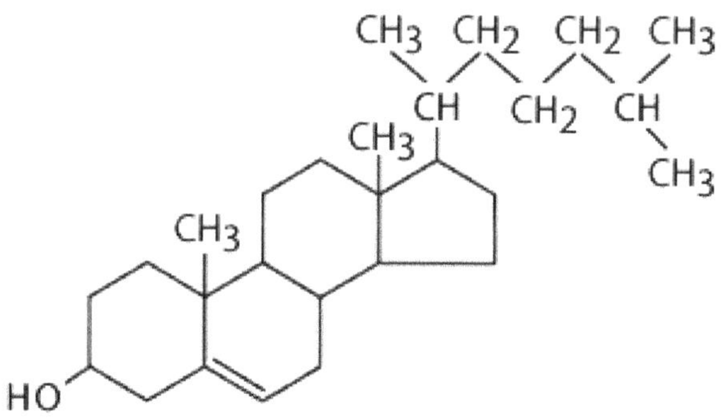

Role of Cholesterol

☆ Cholesterol helps to lubricate the skin and hair, keeping them from drying out.

- It helps in the digestion of food fats. Our digestive system relies heavily on bile salts to help emulsify and digest fats. The liver makes about a quart of these a day (just under a liter) with cholesterol as a major ingredient, storing a concentrated version in the gall bladder for controlled release as foods (especially fatty ones) enter the small intestine.
- It's present in all of our cell walls, providing watertight integrity and structural support, and is especially essential to electrically conductive nerve and brain cells- we can't have moisture and wayward ions seeping in and short-circuiting things. This might explain why the nervous system is such a large repository of cholesterol, and why a diet that includes adequate amounts of it is a must for infants and small children with growing brains. Luckily, both human and bovine (cow's) milk contain plenty of it for just this purpose.
- Mood and behaviour are also apparently linked to proper blood cholesterol levels. Studies have shown a decrease in the number of serotonin receptors as cholesterol levels lower. Serotonin is a key neurotransmitter which figures heavily in depression, among other things.
- Forming the backbone for numerous steroid hormones manufactured in the ovaries, testicles and adrenal glands, cholesterol plays a critical role in controlling the body's stress response, defense system, sexual development, and numerous other metabolic functions.
- It is used to form vitamin D. It's a major component of cholecalciferol (also known as vitamin D_3, made in skin exposed to sunlight), which assures proper absorption of calcium and phosphorus, maintains normal muscle tone and takes part in several immune and reproductive processes.

Without cholesterol, none of these functions would take place, and without these functions, human beings wouldn't exist. The liver produces all the cholesterol we need but too much cholesterol can cause serious problems.

Sources of Cholesterol

Cholesterol is nevertheless a very important molecule, because it is found in animal fats and oils, in bile, blood, brain tissue, milk, the yolk of egg, and the myelin sheaths of nerve fibers, as well as in the liver, kidneys, and adrenal glands. In fact, cholesterol is a constituent of all living animal cells.

Cholesterol comes mainly from two sources:

- *De novo* synthesis in the body
- Diet

The body manufactures roughly 80 per cent of the cholesterol present in the body. Some cholesterol, and the rest 20 per cent comes from the animal products such as meats, eggs, butter, cheese and whole milk which we take in the diet. The body produces enough cholesterol to meet its needs, so monitoring the diet is very important.

Biosynthesis of Cholesterol

About every cell in the body is potentially capable of *de novo* cholesterol synthesis, and sufficient is synthesized every day to meet body requirements.

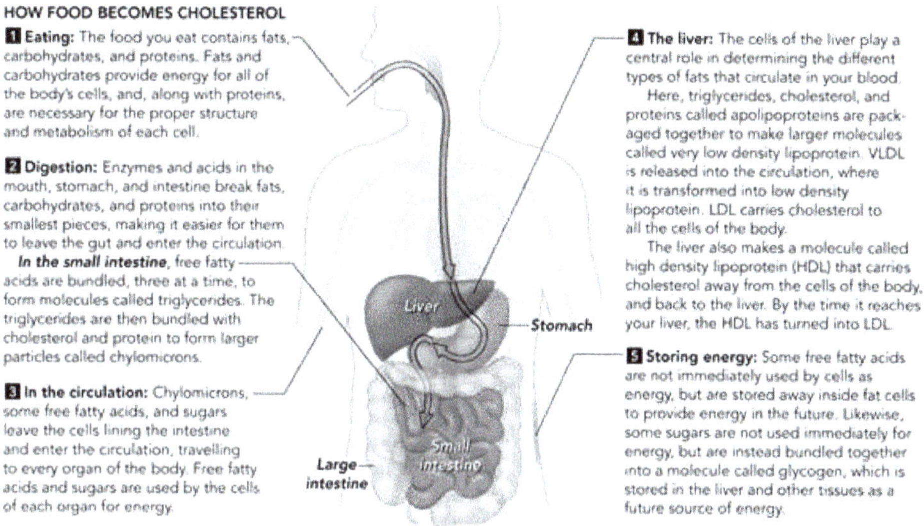

Figure 7.1: How Food Becomes Cholesterol

Synthesis is balanced, and to a certain extent regulated by the absorption of cholesterol from the diet, and under normal circumstances cholesterol homeostasis is maintained within fairly narrow limits.

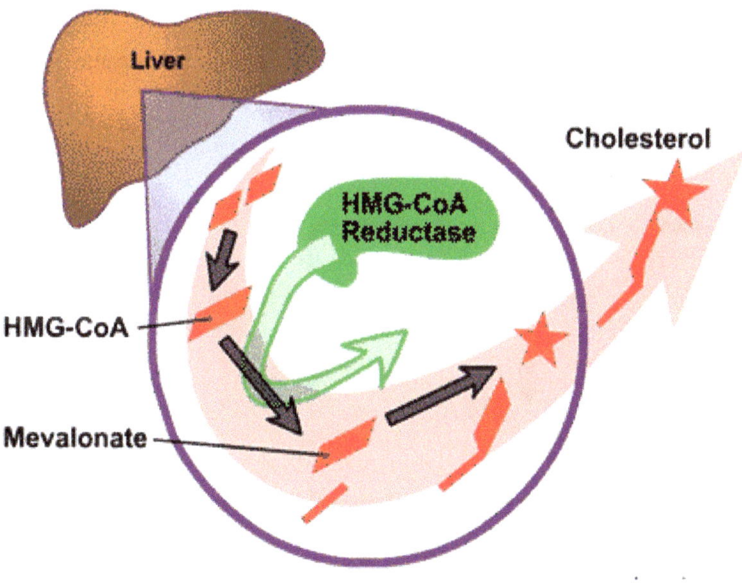

Figure 7.2: Understanding the Synthesis of Cholesterol

Cellular cholesterol content is closely controlled by several mechanisms. The circulating plasma cholesterol levels correlate more with saturated fat intake than with dietary cholesterol–meaning that the cholesterol that causes the atherosclerotic complications in the vasculature does not enter the body as cholesterol; rather, it is actually synthesized by the body in the liver from other chemicals.

The major sites for biosynthesis of cholesterol are the liver and intestines, the liver probably being responsible for the majority of production. The precursor of cholesterol is acetate, a small, ubiquitous molecule produced during the metabolism of protein, carbohydrate and fat. This undergoes a stepwise conversion involving twenty-five enzymes into squalene and, then, to cholesterol.

The first stage in the conversion is a series of reactions by which acetyl-CoA is built up into mevalonic acid. The series is catalysed by microsomal enzymes of which the most important is 3-hydroxy3-methylglutaryl-CoA reductase (HMG-CoA reductase), which is the rate-limiting enzyme of cholesterol biosynthesis and, therefore, a target for intervention. Recently, pharmacological agents which inhibit the action of HMG-CoA reductase have become available for the treatment of hypercholesterolaemia.

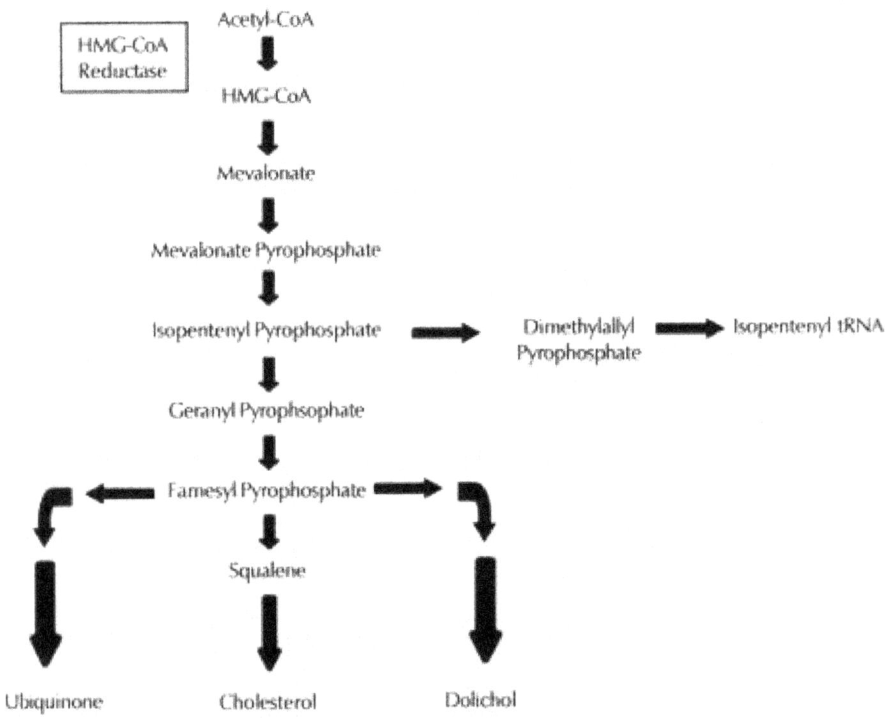

Figure 7.3: The Overall Synthesis of Cholesterol

Four Stages of Cholesterol Synthesis

1. First Stage

Three acetate molecules condense to form a 6 carbon intermediate, mevalonate. 2 acetyl-CoA molecules condense to form acetoacetyl-CoA.

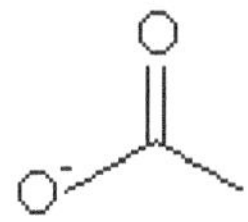

Acetate

- A 3rd acetyl-CoA is added and condenses to form a 6 carbon compound. HMG-CoA. These two reactions are reversible and do not commit the cell to the synthesis of cholesterol or other isoprenoid compounds.
- The committed step: Reduction of HMG-CoA to mevalonate.

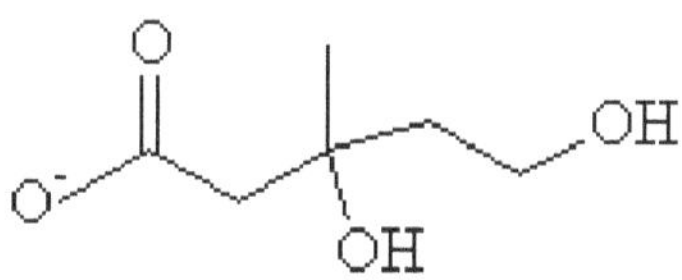

Mevalonate

2. Second Stage

The conversion of mevalonate into activated isoprene units.

- Two Activated isoprenes from mevalonate
- ATP (Adenine triphosphate) can be simply regarded as a phosphate donor.
- Three phosphate groups are added to the mevalonate. Two are added to the terminal hydroxyl end and one is added to the C-3 hydroxyl.
- The phosphate on C-3 and the nearby carboxyl group leave creating a double bond within a 5 carbon intermediate. This is the first of the isoprene units, isopentenyl pyrophosphate.

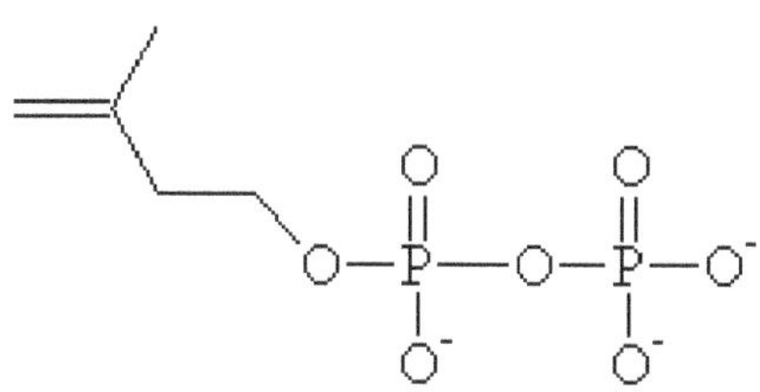

Activated isoprene. (An isoprene unit with 2 phosphate groups attached.)

- A [1, 3] hydrogen shift readily occurs to give dimethylallyl pyrophosphate, but this is reversible.

- ☆ This isomerisation of isopentylpyrophosphate yields the second isoprene unit.

3. Third Stage

The polymerisation of six 5 carbon isoprene molecules results into a 30 carbon linear squalene molecule. Formation of squalene involves the following steps:

- ☆ Squalene is formed by the condensation of 6 activated isoprene units.
- ☆ Head to tail condensation of isopentyl pyrophosphate and dimethylallyl pyrophosphate. A 10 carbon chain is formed. Elimination of 1 pyrophosphate gives geranyl pyrophosphate
- ☆ Head to tail condensation of geranyl pyrophosphate with isopentenyl pyrophosphate gives a 15 carbon intermediate farnesyl pyrophosphate.
- ☆ Head to head joining of two molecules of farnesyl pyrophosphate and elimination of 2 pyrophosphate groups gives a 30 carbon chain squalene.

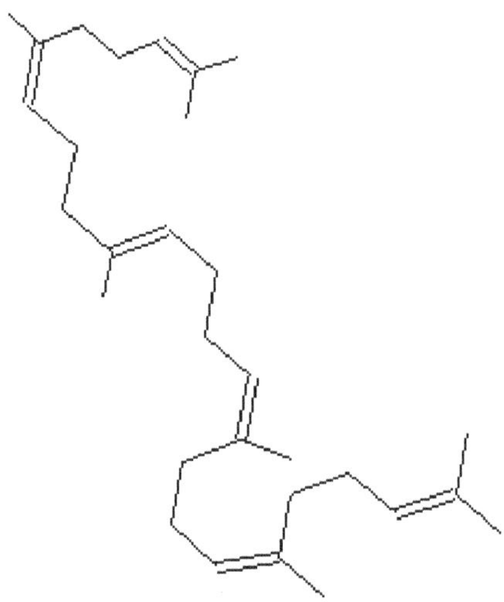

Squalene

4. Fourth Stage

Cyclisation of squalene and further reactions to yield cholesterol.

- ☆ All sterols consist of 4 fused rings, and are alcohols, with the hydroxyl group at C-3.
- ☆ It can be seen quite easily that the linear squalene molecule can be converted into the 4 fused ring structure of sterols.
- ☆ Squalene monooxygenase adds 1 oxygen atom to the end of the squalene chain, forming an epoxide.
- ☆ NADPH is an electron donor and this reduces the other oxygen of the oxygen molecule to water.

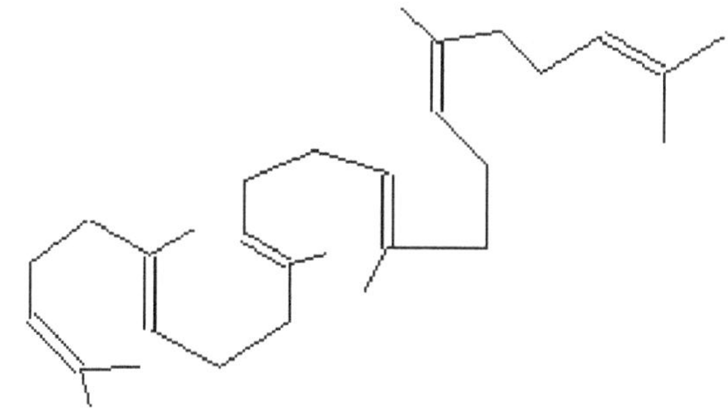

Squalene in position to cyclise

- The double bonds of squalene 2,3-epoxide are positioned such that a concerted reaction can occur, which converts the linear squalene into a cyclic structure, called lanosterol.
- Lanosterol is then converted to cholesterol.

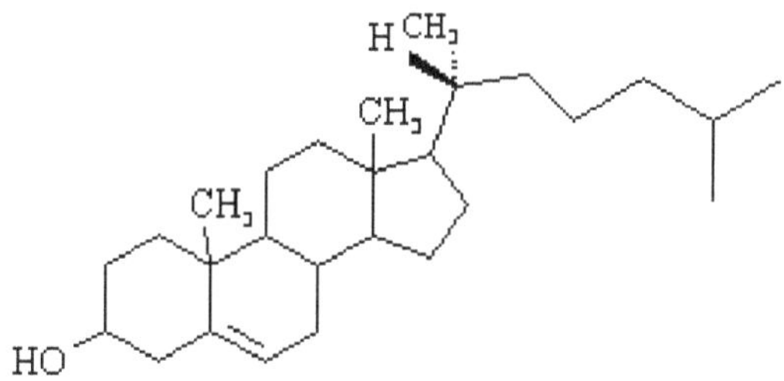

Cholesterol

Diet

Cholesterol intake through the diet should not exceed 300 milligrams a day. Animal foods like beef liver, egg yolk, chicken, whole milk and skim milk contain cholesterol. Eggs are probably the best-known source, containing 213 milligrams of cholesterol per yolk (more than two-thirds of the recommended daily allowance of cholesterol). One cup of whole milk contains 33 mg whereas one cup of skim milk provides 4mg of cholesterol. Food from plants like fruits, vegetables and cereals do not have cholesterol.

Absorption of Cholesterol

The diet and the bile are the major sources of intestinal cholesterol, thus the cholesterol absorbed from the intestine is a mixture of exogenous and endogenous cholesterol. In fact, dietary cholesterol represents only about one-third of total intestinal cholesterol pool, while endogenous sources, the bile and to some extent intestinal mucosal cholesterol account for the remaining two-thirds. An average of 400-500 mg cholesterol enters the intestines daily from the non-vegetarian human diet, mainly from animal products. In addition 800-1200 mg biliary cholesterol/d is presented to the gut.

Only free cholesterol appears to be absorbed. Lipolytic pancreatic enzymes and solubilizing properties of bile salts are needed before dietary fat is absorbed. In order to be absorbed, cholesterol is solubilized by incorporation into the hydrophobic centre of micelles comprising bile acids, fatty acids, monoacylglycerols and lysolecithin. Transport of cholesterol across the mucosal membrane occurs by simple, passive diffusion. This seems to be the rate-limiting step for cholesterol absorption and is another point at which intervention may take place.

Once absorbed into the mucosal cell, the cholesterol undergoes esterification with long-chain fatty acids. The esters thus formed combine with free cholesterol and small amounts of specific apoproteins to form chylomicrons within enterocytes and transported via the lymph to the circulation which are released into the lymphatics.

Significant inter-individual variation has been observed in cholesterol absorption, the values ranging from 15 per cent to 80 per cent. In men, dietary cholesterol absorption has been found to correlate positively with plasma total and LDL cholesterol concentration, but among subjects consuming a low-cholesterol low-fat diet the efficiency of intestinal cholesterol absorption and the amount of dietary cholesterol absorbed were not related to plasma cholesterol and LDL cholesterol. In addition, individual variation in responses to the amount and the quality of dietary fat has been observed both in animal and human studies, suggesting genetic control of cholesterol absorption. Agents inhibiting cholesterol absorption include among others dietary fiber such as guar gum and plant sterols (β -sitosterol and sitostanol) and ezetimibe, a new selective inhibitor of intestinal cholesterol absorption. Cholesterol homeostasis is partly balanced by dietary cholesterol absorption, while dietary cholesterol modifies other regulatory mechanisms inducing down-regulation of hepatic cholesterol synthesis and LDL receptors.

Transport of Cholesterol

Cholesterol needs to be transported through the watery medium of the blood to various tissues and organs. Blood is watery, and cholesterol is fatty. Just like oil and water, the two do not mix. To travel in the bloodstream, cholesterol is carried in small packages called lipoproteins. Lipoproteins are the vehicles used to transport cholesterol and triaclyglycerols in the bloodstream. They are made of fat (lipid) on the inside and proteins on the outside. The major cholesterol carrying particle is LDL, but HDL also plays an important role in cholesterol flux.

Classification of Lipoproteins

Cholesterol and TG are transported through lipoproteins. Each lipoprotein has a core of lipids and a shell of specific associated apolipoproteins. They are classified according to their density:

Chylomicron	**Chylomicron remnants**
Lipids: dietary triacylglycerols	Lipids: dietary cholesterol esters
Apoproteins: B-48, C, E	Apoproteins: B-48, E

VLDL (very low density lipoprotein)	IDL (Intermediate density lipoprotein)
Lipids: endogenous cholesterol esters	Lipids: endogenous cholesterol esters
Apoproteins: B-100, C, E	Apoproteins: B-100, E
LDL (low density lipoprotein)	**HDL (high density lipoprotein)**
Lipids: endogenous cholesterol esters	Lipids: endogenous cholesterol esters
Apoproteins: B-100	Apoproteins: A

Low-density lipoprotein (LDL) cholesterol is sometimes called bad cholesterol. High LDL cholesterol leads to a build up of cholesterol in arteries. The higher the LDL level in the blood, the greater chance of getting heart disease.

LDL is the major transporter of cholesterol from the liver to peripheral tissues. Approximately 50 per cent of LDL mass is cholesterol, which is mainly esterified, the rest being phospholipid, triacylglycerol and protein. The protein component of human LDL is almost entirely apo B_{100}. LDL particles are formed by conversion of hepatically secreted small VLDL via IDL intermediates but to some extent also by hepatic secretion. The actual mechanism for the conversion of IDL to LDL is not known, but it may involve as the hepatic LDL receptor to which IDL binds avidly.

In normal humans, all LDL is derived from VLDL by intravascular conversion. Triglyceride-rich VLDL particles are synthesized in the liver and they transport triglycerides to adipose tissue and muscle. When VLDL is hydrolyzed by lipoprotein lipase, smaller VLDL remnants, IDL particles are generated and surface lipids and apolipoproteins are transferred to HDL as in hydrolysis of chylomicrons. Remnant particles are partially removed by the liver via receptor-mediated pathway, or IDL is further converted to LDL by hepatic lipase.

Apo B is the major apolipoprotein of LDL and has a central role in LDL cholesterol metabolism. Apo B is produced by the liver and secreted in VLDL. Availability of lipids regulates whether apo B is secreted or degraded. Moreover, production of apo B is correlated with LDL cholesterol level.

The clearance of LDL cholesterol from plasma is primarily mediated by LDL receptors. In addition, some of LDL may be removed by scavenger receptors, which are responsible for the clearance of modified LDL, or by non-receptor-mediated pathways. LDL delivers its cholesterol to cells by way of a specific LDL receptor which is present in the cell membrane. The LDL receptor is a single-chain transmembrane glycoprotein that specifically binds two proteins, apo B and apo E. LDL receptors are mainly expressed in the liver, but they are also present on the surface of nearly all normal cells where the uptake of plasma LDL provides cholesterol for membrane synthesis and other requirements of these cells. Recognition of LDL by the receptor is by the apo B_{100} component. Most tissues in the body are able to express the LDL receptor, but it is thought that many cells satisfy their cholesterol needs by endogenous synthesis. The liver clears at least two-thirds of the LDL in plasma, mostly via the hepatic LDL receptor.

Binding of LDL to the receptor results in internalization of the particle by endocytosis. LDL dissociates from the receptor, which returns to the cell surface and is again able to bind lipoproteins. Within lysosomes, cholesterol esters of LDL are converted to free cholesterol by acid lipase and apolipoproteins are degraded to amino acids. Free cholesterol is delivered to the cytoplasm. Inverse correlation has been observed between LDL cholesterol and fractional catabolic rate (FCR) for LDL apo B that reflects receptor-mediated clearance of LDL with consequent suppression of further receptor expression and down-regulation of cholesterol synthesis.

High-density lipoprotein (HDL) cholesterol is sometimes called good cholesterol. HDL carries cholesterol from other parts of the body back to the liver. The liver removes the cholesterol from the body. The higher the HDL cholesterol level, the lower the chance of getting heart disease.

HDL is small, dense particle, consisting mainly of protein, but containing small amounts of phospholipid, free cholesterol, triacylglycerol and cholesteryl ester. The characteristic apoproteins of HDL are apo AI (70 per cent) and apo AII (20 per cent). The HDL fraction typically contains two sub fractions HDL_2 and HDL_3. HDL_2 has a lower density than HDL_3 and contains more cholesteryl esters which are derived from the lipolysis of CM and VLDL, from the surface coat of intact lipoproteins or from cell membranes. HDL cholesterol, mainly HDL_2 subfraction, is an antiatherogenic lipoprotein. Thus, it is responsible for the reverse transport of cholesterol from peripheral tissues to circulation and to the liver for degradation.

Nearly all the variation in plasma HDL concentration may be explained by variation in the HDL_2 sub fraction. This, in turn, is strongly related to the activity of lipoprotein lipase and, hence, to rates of triacylglycerol transport. Thus, certain dietary perturbations which increase the production or turnover of CM and VLDL will also raise HDL_2 levels.

The best known hypothetical role of HDL is in 'reverse cholesterol transport', that is, the net efflux of free cholesterol from cells. Most tissues appear to possess binding sites for HDL, and it has been demonstrated to act as an effective acceptor or cholesterol from cells. Having accepted the cholesterol, it may redistribute it to other peripheral cells, transfer it to other lipoprotein carriers or deliver it to the liver.

Intracellular Cholesterol Transport

LDL (yellow circles) carrying cholesterol and cholesterol esters bound to LDL receptors (light blue Y-shape) is internalized and transported to sorting endosomes and to late endosomes and lysosomes from which cholesterol can efflux to cellular compartments including the plasma membrane or the endoplasmic reticulum (ER). The LDL receptor recycles to the plamsa membrane via the endocytic recycling compartment (ERC). Efflux from late endosomes and lysosomes is poorly characterized as indicated by the dashed lines. Cholesterol can move from the plasma membrane to the ERC by a non-vesicular, ATP-independent process. Recycling of cholesterol back to the plasma membrane occurs by non-vesicular transport and in membrane-recycling vesicles carrying other recycling membrane components. Newly synthesized cholesterol in the ER is mostly transported from the ER directly to the plasma membrane, bypassing the Golgi, but some follows the biosynthetic secretory

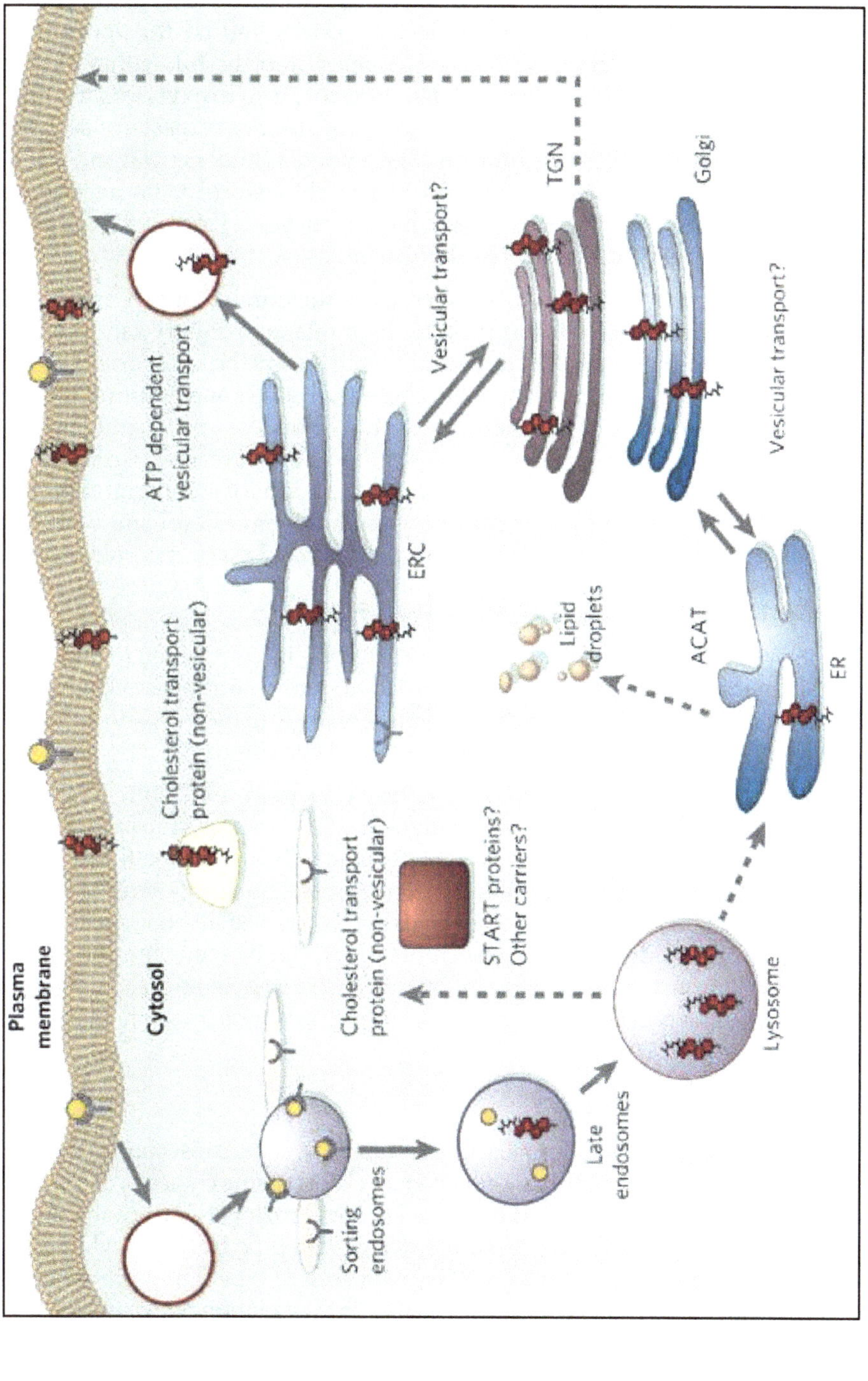

Figure 7.4: Intracellular Cholesterol Transport
Source: **Nature 438, 612-621 (1 December 2005).**

pathway from the ER to the Golgi. Excess cholesterol in the ER becomes esterified by ACAT and stored in cytoplasmic lipid droplets (Maxfield and Tabas, 2005).

In the liver, cholesterol is re-esterified by acyl coenzyme A:cholesterol acyltransferase (ACAT) and stored as cholesteryl esters, reused for lipoprotein synthesis and resecreted into the plasma or excreted into the bile either as free cholesterol or after conversion to bile acids. Cholesterol 7α-hydroxylase is the rate-limiting enzyme in bile acid synthesis. After secretion, biliary cholesterol and bile acids are either reabsorbed from the intestine or excreted as fecal neutral and acidic sterols. Finally, hepatic cells may also synthesize cholesterol from acetate by microsomal 3-hydroxy-3-methylglutaryl coenzyme A reductase (HMG CoA reductase), the rate-limiting enzyme of cholesterol biosynthesis.

The cholesterol content of hepatocytes regulates the number of LDL receptors. Excess of cellular cholesterol, for example after high intake of dietary saturated fat and cholesterol, down-regulates LDL receptors, which lowers the uptake of LDL and consequently results in elevated plasma LDL cholesterol levels and accumulation of cholesterol in peripheral cells. Cholesterol excess also induces suppression of HMG CoA reductase and cellular cholesterol biosynthesis is decreased. Conversely, cholesterol-lowering treatments with bile acid-binding resins or statins, inhibitors of HMG CoA reductase, and other causes of low cellular cholesterol stimulate the expression of hepatic LDL receptors and decrease plasma LDL cholesterol levels.

Degradation and Excretion of Cholesterol

The major pathway for the removal of cholesterol is its conversion to bile acids and excretion in the faeces. It may also be converted to steroid hormones and excreted from the skin surface. Bile acid synthesis takes place entirely in the liver and accounts for approximately one-third of the daily production of cholesterol.

The two primary bile acids formed directly in man are cholic acid and chenodeoxycholic acid. These acids are conjugated with either glycine or taurine to yield four primary bile salts which are secreted into the bile and pass through the biliary tract into the duodenum. The bile acid pool is small (2-3 g) but there is efficient hepatic recycling whereby 98 per cent of bile acids are reabsorbed in the small intestine and returned directly to the liver for resecretion. Binding, or sequestration of bile acids within the intestine by dietary components or pharmacological agents, may interrupt the recycling process, forcing new bile acids to be made from cholesterol to replete the pool.

Hypercholesterolaemia

Hypercholesterolaemia or Type II hyperlipidaemia, is the most common of the lipid disorders and is characterized by elevated levels of plasma cholesterol, most of which is found in the LDL fraction. If the raised cholesterol levels are accompanied by raised triacylglycerol levels, the disease is designated type IIb; if triacylglycerol levels are normal, the disease is type IIa. The prevalence of type II hyperlipidaemia within the population, and the relative strength of the association between elevated LDL levels and atherosclerosis compared with that of triacylglycerols, makes this hyperlipidaemia by far the most important in terms of risk from heart disease.

The existence of three divisions of hypercholesterolaemia is dependent on the degree of genetic influence. These are 'dietary hypercholesterolaemia' which is represented by cholesterol levels within the range 5.2-6.2 mmol/l, 'primary hypercholesterolaemia' which constitutes cholesterol levels above 6.2 mmol/l, and 'familiar hypercholesterolaemia' (FH) which is a specific, genetically determined form of primary hypercholesterolaemia. Genes encoding various proteins involved in cholesterol metabolism such as apolipoproteins, lipoprotein receptors, lipid transfer proteins and enzymes modify plasma LDL cholesterol levels. FH arises out of a genetic deficiency of LDL receptors. Subjects homozygous for FH have no LDL receptors, whilst heterozygous subjects have about half the normal number.

The major cause of cholesterol levels within the range 5.2-6.2 mmol/l is a diet rich in saturated fat and cholesterol. The extent to which cholesterol levels are raised depends on the responsiveness of the recipient. Dietary treatment is usually sufficient to reduce plasma cholesterol levels within this range.

What Causes High Blood Cholesterol?

A variety of factors can affect the blood cholesterol levels. Some of these can be controlled while others cannot be.

One Can Control

- *Diet*: Certain type of foods having more amounts of saturated fat, trans fatty acid and cholesterol can raise the blood cholesterol levels. Saturated fats, which contribute to high cholesterol significantly, are found mostly in meat and dairy products as well as some oils, nuts, coconut, and cocoa.
- *Body weight*: Being overweight tends to increase the LDL level, lower the high-density lipoprotein (HDL) level, and increase the total cholesterol level.
- *Physical activity*: Lack of regular exercise can lead to weight gain, which could raise the LDL cholesterol level. Regular exercise can help to lose weight and lower the LDL level. It can also help to raise the HDL level.
- *Stress*: Studies have not shown stress to be directly linked to cholesterol levels. But experts say that because people sometimes eat fatty foods to console themselves when under stress, this can cause higher blood cholesterol. On the other hand, some studies have reported that chronic stress is associated with a range of problems, including heart attacks, the common cold and even a shorter life expectancy. Steptoe's study, published in *Health Psychology*, looked at nearly 200 middle-aged men and women to see if stressful events triggered higher cholesterol three years later. After having their cholesterol levels measured, the participants were put through a series of mild, nerve-rattling tests, such as picking the correct names of various colors that were rapidly flashing on a computer screen. They were tracked for changes in heart rate and other signs to see how they handled the pressure.

  Three years later, the researchers measured cholesterol levels again. As to be expected, all showed higher levels than before, a common occurrence with growing older. But those who had the highest stress response to the test also had the highest cholesterol levels three years later. Compared to participants who seemed to take the tests in stride, the most stressed-out group was three times more likely to have dangerously high LDL, or bad cholesterol, down the road. This spike in cholesterol was independent of the usual culprits, like being overweight or smoking. Steptoe suggests that stress may produce more nervous energy in the form of harmful fatty acids and sugar, or it may even interfere with the body's ability to get rid of cholesterol. The rise in cholesterol was relatively modest, Steptoe added, at least in comparison to a poor diet or other causes (Sabo, E. 2005, Medicine: Stress now, cholesterol later. Health Centers Online Inc. Review).

One Cannot Control

- ☆ *Heredity*: High blood cholesterol can run in families. An inherited genetic condition (familial hypercholesterolemia) results in very high LDL cholesterol levels because cholesterol isn't properly cleared by the liver and builds up in the blood. These people have a high risk of arterial disease, heart attack and stroke–and at an early age. It's a dominant genetic disorder; a person inherits it from one parent, and has a one in two chance of passing it on. It affects about one person in 500.
- ☆ *Age and sex*: Some risk factors cannot be controlled. These include age (45 years or older for men and 55 years or older for women) and family history of early heart disease (father or brother stricken before age 55; mother or sister stricken before age 65).

  Starting at puberty, men have lower levels of HDL than women. As women and men get older, their LDL cholesterol levels rise. Younger women have lower LDL cholesterol levels than men, but after age 55, women have higher levels than men. Menopause is often associated with increases in LDL cholesterol in women.

Signs and Symptoms of High Blood Cholesterol

There are usually no signs or symptoms of high blood cholesterol. Many people don't know that their cholesterol level is too high. One should get the blood sample analyzed for lipid profile in the pathology laboratory to know whether blood cholesterol is high or not.

Cholesterol Test

A simple blood cholesterol test can assess the risk for heart disease.

Typically, a cholesterol test is part of a routine physical at the doctor's office. Physician can take a blood sample and send it to a pathology laboratory for analysis. To achieve the most accurate results, one should fast for 9-12 hours prior to having the blood drawn.

All adults age 20 years or older should have their cholesterol checked every five years. This check-up should measure total cholesterol, LDL cholesterol, HDL cholesterol and triglycerides. The National Heart Foundation recommends that a man over 45 or a woman over 55 should get this test done more frequently. People younger than 45 who are at higher risk of coronary heart disease – for example, those who have a family history of hypercholesterolaemia, heart disease, high blood pressure and/or diabetes, should also have a regular cholesterol test.

The National Institute of Health (NIH) now recommends that adults should strive for total cholesterol below 200 mg/dl (or LDL cholesterol less than 130 mg/dl). A blood cholesterol level of 200-239 would be considered borderline high risk and 240 or greater (or LDL over 160) would be considered high risk and may require drug therapy. An HDL cholesterol level of over 40 mg/dl is acceptable.

Table 7.1: Total Cholesterol Level (mg/100ml)

Desirable	*Borderline*	*High*
Below 200	200-239	Above 240

Table 7.2: LDL (or bad) Cholesterol Level (mg/100ml)

Optimal	*Near Optimal*	*Borderline High*	*High*	*Very High*
Below 100	100-129	130-159	160-189	Above 190

Table 7.3: Triglyceride Level (mg/100ml)

Normal	*Bordline High*	*High*	*Very High*
Below 150	150-199	200-499	Above 500

Table 7.4: HDL (or good) Cholesterol Level (mg/100ml)

Optimal	*Desirable*	*Undesirable*
Above 60	40-60	Below 40

The American Diabetes Association (ADA) and the U.S. National Institutes of Health (NIH) recommend the following cholesterol and triglyceride target levels for people with diabetes:

- ☆ LDL cholesterol: Lower than 100 mg/dL for men and women
- ☆ HDL cholesterol: Greater than 40 mg/dL for men and 50 mg/dL for women.
- ☆ Triglycerides: Lower than 150 mg/dL for men and women

Some material published by the ADA call for minimum HDL levels of 45 in diabetic men and 55 in diabetic women. Individuals should consult their physician about their cholesterol targets.

Chemcard™ Cholesterol Test

The Chemcard™ Cholesterol test is a complete, disposable, 3 minute test intended for use for early detection of elevated blood cholesterol levels associated with increased risk of coronary artery disease. The Chemcard™ uses a single drop of whole blood from a fingerstick to provide a semi-quantitative estimate of total cholesterol concentration without the use of an instrument, centrifuge or sample measurement. Results are interpreted after 3 minutes by matching color with one of the six color blocks calibrated in 25 mg/dL increments. The Chemcard™ is the simplest, most cost effective cholesterol screening device available.

New Approach to Lipid Valuation

Although the initial public focus of the National Cholesterol Education Program (NCEP) was on high cholesterol. ATP III recommends a fasting lipoprotein panel for initial assessment. This is performed after a 9-to 12-hour fast. The patient is asked to come hungry, not thirsty, as water and pills are allowed.

> Clinical Tip: If the screening opportunity is a non-fasting one (as in an evening or afternoon clinic), nonfasting total cholesterol and high-density lipoprotein cholesterol (HDL-c) should be obtained. A true fasting lipoprotein panel should be obtained if the nonfasting total cholesterol exceeds 20 mg dL or HDL-c is <40 mg/dL.

In case of persons with lipid abnormalities, low-density lipoprotein cholesterol (LDL-c) is calculated by the Friedewald formula:

LDL-c =Total cholesterol-HDL-c – (Triglycerides/ 5)

For example, if total cholesterol is 300 mg/dL, triglycerides (TGs) are 250 mg/dL, and HDL-c is 50 mg/dL, the formula determines LDL-c as:

LDL-c = 300 – 50 – (250/5);

LDL-c – 200 mg/dL by calculation

There are caveats. If used for nonfasting samples, the formula will underestimate LDL-c levels. The formula should not be used when TGs are >400 mg/dL or the cholesterol-rich, very low-density lipoproteins VLDLs) seen in familial dysbetalipoproteinemia are present. Fortunately, this condition is rare.

Calculation of non-HDL-c is particularly useful in those with elevated fasting TG levels. Simply put, non-HDL-c is:

Non-HDL-c = Total cholesterol –HDL-c

This calculation is easily done and represents the spectrum of apolipoprotein B (apo B)–carrying lipoproteins. These are considered atherogenic and include VLDL, chylomicron remnants, VLDL remnants, inter-mediate-density lipoprotein (IDL), lipoprotein (a) (Lp[a]), and low-density lipoprotein (LDL). In aggregate then, the non-HDL-c represents the sum of atherogenic particles in the circulation. Moreover, non-HDL-c measurement correlates well with total apo B measurements (Abate *et al.*, 1993).

Sniderman and associates contend that we should measure apo B directly to help determine coronary risk and as a target of therapy, particularly in those with normal cholesterol and TGs and low LDL-c (Sniderman *et al.,* 2001). An analysis of the Air Force/Texas Coronary Atherosclerosis Prevention Study (AFCAPS/TexCAPS) data supports this contention (Gotto, 2000). In a cross-sectional study of women undergoing their first angiography, apo B predicts extent of coronary disease better than other lipid markers (Westerveld *et al.,* 1998). Although the apo B measurement is standardized, its availability is limited. In addition, replacing LDL-c with apo B in treatment algorithms would require a major educational program as noted in Prevention Conference V of the American Heart Association (Grundy *et al.,* 2000). As pointed out earlier, non-HDL-c can be calculated from data already available and appears to be a useful surrogate for apo B. Indeed, in an examination of the data from the Lipid Research Clinics Prevalence data, Cui and colleagues showed that perhaps not unexpectedly, non-HDL-c predicted coronary heart disease (CHD) risk even better than LDL-c. Grundy put this in perspective in an accompanying editorial. He pondered the role for non-HDL in cholesterol management vis-a-vis LDL-c and noted that LDL-c, unlike non-HDL-c, is not confounded by other lipid markers. He suggests that a logical first step is to use non-HDL-c when hypertriglyceridemia is present. This redues the underestimation of risk in such individuals that occurs if only LDL-c is considered.

Clinical Tip: Some clinicians consider it bother-some to stop and calculate non-HDL-c. They wish to use TGs instead as a target. One advantage of using non-HDL-c instead of TGs is the reduced variability seen. Actually, once non-HDL-c is put into the flow sheet, it becomes second nature to bring LDL-c to goal and then, when TGs exceed 200 mg/dL, to bring non-HDL-c to goal (defined as 340 mg/dL more than the LDL-c goal).

Blood Cholesterol Levels of Special Population

I. Children and Adolescents

No long-term studies have been conducted showing the relationship of blood cholesterol levels measured in childhood to coronary heart disease in later life. However that relationship can be inferred based on these facts:

- Autopsy studies demonstrate that early coronary atherosclerosis often begins in childhood and is related to high cholesterol.
- Children and adolescents with elevated serum cholesterol levels, particularly LDL-cholesterol levels, often come from families with elevated values and in which there is a high incidence of coronary heart disease.

Routine testing of children starts during teens. For identifying children and adolescents who are likely to be at increased risk for coronary heart disease (CHD), their universal screening is not recommended. However, selective screening is preferred to screening all children. Children and adolescents who are recommended for selective screening in the context of regular health care are:

- Children and adolescents whose parents or grandparents (<55 years of age in males and <65 years of age in females) were found to have coronary atherosclerosis, or had a documented myocardial infarction, cerebrovascular disease, or sudden cardiac death. Such children should be screened with fasting lipoprotein profile.
- The offspring of a parent with an elevated blood cholesterol level (240 mg/dL or higher). Such children should be screened with a non-fasting blood cholesterol levels.
- Children and adolescents whom the physician may feel have a higher chance of having an elevated cholesterol. For example, adolescents who smoke, consume excessive amounts of saturated fats and cholesterol, or are overweight may also be tested at the discretion of their physician.

Cut Points for Screening

Screening of children for dyslipidemia has traditionally been focused on those with a positive family history of premature cardiovascular disease (CVD) and those whose parents have CVD or dyslipidemia (primarily hypercholesterolemia). Unfortunately, screening by family history of CVD or hypercholesterolemia fails to detect 17 per cent to 90 per cent of those with significant dyslipidemia (Haney *et al.*, 2007). Although 50 per cent of offspring of parents with premature CVD will have dyslipidemia, such parents are usually in their 40s, delaying the detection of dyslipidemia in their children. Conversely, considerable data indicate that lipid and lipoprotein concentrations track from childhood into adulthood, especially total cholesterol (TC), LDL-C, non–HDL-C (the estimated cholesterol concentration of all the apolipoprotein B–containing lipoproteins, *i.e.*, TC minus HDL-C) (Haney *et al.*, 2007). Given all of the above results, the alternative approach of universal screening is receiving greater attention.

Screening requires the use of cut points to identify individuals with dyslipidemia. Cut points in adults are primarily based on their association with CVD in middle age. Such CVD-based data are not available in children and adolescents, and cut points are primarily based on percentile values, derived from defined populations, and set at thresholds that increase the likelihood of detecting those dyslipidemic youth who will become dyslipidemic adults.

The selection of cut points is often empirically derived and arbitrarily chosen. There is no perfect paradigm. For example, as one increases the cut points for TC or LDL-C, sensitivity (the ability to detect those who are affected) decreases, but the specificity (the ability to detect those who are not affected) and the predictive value of a positive test (ability of a test results to identify an affected person) increases. Decreasing the cut point (*e.g.*, from the 95th percentile to the 75th) increases sensitivity but decreases specificity and the predictive power of a positive test.

The National Cholesterol Education Program (NCEP) Expert Panel on Blood Cholesterol Levels in Children (NCEP, 1992) recommended a single set of cut points to define paediatric dyslipidemia, primarily but not exclusively focused on LDL-C. The use of multiple cut points specific for these variables may be indicated because lipid and lipoprotein concentrations may vary with age, sex, ethnicity, and during periods of rapid growth and development, such as adolescence.

As suggested by NCEP, Table 7.5 describes the classification of acceptable, borderline, and high values for total cholesterol and low-density lipoprotein cholesterol (LDL-c).

Table 7.5: Classification of Total Cholesterol and LDL-c

Category	*Blood Cholesterol*	*LDL-c*
Acceptable	170 mg/dL	110 mg/dL
Borderline	170-199 g/dL	110-129 mg/dL
High	≥200 mg/dL	≥130 mg/dL

Abbreviation: LDL-c, low-density lipoprotein cholesterol

Report of the Expert Panel on Blood Cholesterol Levels in Children and Adolescents. NIH Publication No. 91-2732, September, 1991.

The "normal" value of cholesterol, LDL, and HDL is based on population studies and the incidences of vascular disease. It would appear that the lower the cholesterol, the lower the LDL, and the higher the HDL, there is less rate of disease. Any improvement in the child's blood values will increase their health and life span.

The report by Magnussen and colleagues (2008) examined the use of multiple cut points in part by comparing the usefulness of lipid and lipoprotein concentration measurements in adolescence, classified according to the NCEP Paediatric Panel (1992) and the National Health and Nutrition Education Survey (NHANES) cut points (Jolliffe *et al.*, 2006), to predict abnormal concentrations in adulthood. Adolescent and adult concentrations of TC, LDL-C, HDL-C, and triglycerides were measured in 365 Australian, 1185 Finnish, and 273 US individuals who participated in 3 population-based prospective cohort studies. According to diagnostic performance statistics, the NCEP cut points, compared with NHANES, were more strongly predictive of adult high TC, LDL-C, and triglycerides than NHANES, but less predictive of HDL-C.

The pooled data indicated that the risk of developing an abnormal condition in adulthood was significantly higher in those adolescents with borderline- and high-risk concentrations compared with those with normal concentrations for all lipoprotein variables. Moreover, a graded increase in the risk of developing abnormal concentrations in adulthood was observed when moving from the normal, to borderline-risk, to high-risk groups.

Magnussen *et al.* (2008) evaluated different screening strategies to identify adolescents more likely to develop dyslipidemia as adults. The best-performing high-risk cut points from the initial analyses were used in conjunction with universal screening and selective screening using:

(*a*) Positive family history of CVD

(*b*) Overweight or obesity

(*c*) Positive family history of either CVD or obesity.

For total cholesterol (TC) and LDL-C, the addition of family history or obesity to the cut points from screening only marginally improved the results of universal screening. Universal screening alone identified a much larger number of affected adults than selective screening. Universal screening identified 75 per cent of participants with high LDL-C at follow-up in adulthood, but at the expense of a high false-positive rate (66 per cent). HDL-C and TG from universal screening of adolescents was a poor predictor of low HDL-C and high TG in adulthood. The addition of obesity improved the yield of low HDL-C and high TG at follow-up from 10.8 per cent to 29.0 per cent and from 12.5 per cent to 29.2 per cent, respectively. This result highlights the important relationship of obesity in adolescence with low HDL-C and high TG later in life, and most likely reflects the proclivity of such youth to show effects of the metabolic syndrome, including insulin resistance. Although the LDL-C concentration may not be increased in such patients, they often have an increased number of small, dense LDL particles, an important part of the dyslipidemic triad in obese adolescents with multiple CVD risk factors (Kwiterovich, 2008).

According to Kwiterovich (2008) adolescence is not the only time amenable to screening. The age of 10 years precedes the changes in lipids and lipoproteins that occur during adolescence. A set of cut points might be adjusted for adolescence, but it is not clear that using cut points adjusted for each year and for sex improves the result of screening. In fact, the report by Magnussen *et al.* (2008) suggests otherwise. Therefore paediatricians, family practitioners, and other healthcare providers may not have to scrutinize screening results in such detail. The implications of multiple cut points for the clinical chemist may be problematic as well.

Thus, a clear need exists to address CVD risk factors in children and to update the NCEP Paediatric Panel's recommendations. Guidelines based on a systematic evidence review for the screening, diagnosis, and management of dyslipidemia, as well as obesity, hypertension and other risk factors in paediatric patients, are currently being developed by the National Heart, Lung and Blood Institute Paediatric Cardiovascular Risk Reduction Initiative.

Goals of Treatment

The goals of treatment are given in Table 7.6. Cholesterol and fat restriction is not intended for infants from birth to 2 years, whose fast growth requires a higher percentage of calories from fat. But for dealing with the problem of high blood cholesterol in children above 2 years and adolescents, the National Cholesterol Education Program (NCEP) Report of the Expert Panel on Blood Cholesterol Levels in Children and Adolescents suggested that all healthy children and adolescents over the age of 2 years should take a nutritious, balanced Step I diet (a therapeutic diet with 10 per cent saturated fat and 300 mg/day dietary cholesterol) with adequate energy (calories) to support growth and development.

Table 7.6: Goals of Therapy in Children and Adolescents

Category	Treatment Goals
If borderline LDL-c	Lower to 110 mg/dL
If high LDL-c	Lower to 130 mg/dL as a minimal goal, ideally ≤110 mg/dL

Abbreviation: LDL-c, low-density lipoprotein cholesterol.

Report of the Expert Panel on Blood Cholesterol Levels in Children and Adolescents. NIH Publication No. 91-2732, September, 1991.

The effort to lower the cholesterol should be mainly through diet and medications. Exercise is also important. Proper diet and exercise learned at a young age will carry over into a healthier teenager and adult. Now the panel has recommended the therapeutic lifestyle change [TLC] and diet is a component of Therapeutic Lifestyle Change.

Drug therapy is usually considered for children >10 years of age after an adequate trial of diet therapy for 6 to 12 months. Children between 5 and 10 yr old may be treated if their cholesterol is extreme *i.e.* >300 mg/dL. There are several recommended medications for the treatment of hypercholesterolemia and high LDL levels in children and adults. These newer medications are safe and do not affect the child's growth and development.

II. Elderly Persons

Cardiovascular disease is the leading cause of death and a major cause of disability in older men and women. Several studies suggest that lipid-lowering therapy may prove useful in selected older men and women.

In the Pravastatin in Elderly Individuals at Risk of Vascular Disease (PROSPER) trial and the Heart Protection Study (HPS), elderly subjects with CHD benefited from statin therapy as compared with placebo and did not show a significant increase in liver or muscle side effects. The new ATP III update paper (Grundy *et al.*, 2004) felt that "there was a strong justification for intensive LDL-c lowering in the elderly with CHD.

The potential for benefit is greatly increased in the elderly due to what is called "attributable risk". Attributable risk is the excess risk, derived by subtracting the risk of those in the lowest percentile for cholesterol from those in the highest percentile for cholesterol. A closely related statistical attribute called "relative risk" is derived by dividing the risk of those in the highest percentile of cholesterol by those in the lowest percentile of cholesterol. For example, younger hypercholesterolemic persons have a high relative risk of CHD. Their attributable risk is low because of the low prevalence of CHD in the younger age range. In the elderly, relative risk for hypercholesterolemia is small (presumably because those with the highest cholesterol values have died). On the other hand, attributable or excess risk is high because so many events of CHD occur in the older age groups.

Total cholesterol levels lose predictive power in older age groups, may be due to other serious, comorbid states associated with low cholesterol levels. In the PROSPER trial, risk reduction on pravastatin treatment risk reduction therapy exhibited a significant interaction with HDL-c. Indeed, subjects in the lowest two quintiles for HDL-c (<45 mg/dL) had a risk reduction of 33 per cent, P <0/001, whereas those with higher HDL-c had no benefit from statin therapy. They also found that the change in the LDL-c/HDL-c ratio on statin therapy appeared to account for the therapeutic benefit (Packard *et al.*, 2005). Other useful markers such as abnormal renal function (although not end-stage), metabolic syndrome, abnormal ankle-brachial index, carotid intimal-medial thickness (cIMT), or high-risk coronary calcium scores may also indicate those who would most likely benefit from lipid-lowering therapy (Eimer and Stone, 2004).

Benefit from statins in the elderly is also seen in studies of high-risk subjects without CHD. However, in elderly persons, many factors must be considered before statin therapy should be prescribed to those without CHD. These include comorbidity, cost, and tolerability as well as patient preferences. Older patients may be more prone to side effects with statins and older, frail, smaller women are especially prone to side effects such as myositis (Pasternak *et al.*, 2003). Thus, elderly patients should be carefully screened before starting with statin therapy.

Finally, high cholesterol in the elderly should always prompt a search for common secondary causes, such as hypothyroidism (TSH), nephritic syndrome (serum albumin, urine analysis), diabetes (FBS), liver disease (liver panel), and kidney disease (BUN/creatinine). Since the elderly may be more prone to muscle complaints, a baseline creatine kinase (CK) is worth obtaining before starting statin therapy.

Treating high cholesterol should never be done in isolation. In the elderly at increased risk for CHD, therapeutic lifestyle change with smoking cessation, increased regular physical exercise, and loss of excess weight are strongly advised. Treatment of systolic hypertension is also an important consideration in reducing CV events.

Risks of High Blood Cholesterol

When there is too much LDL or "bad" cholesterol in the blood, it builds up in the walls of arteries. This build up of cholesterol is called plaque. Over time, plaque can cause narrowing of the arteries. This is called atherosclerosis, or hardening of the arteries. These arteries become narrowed and blood flow to the heart is slowed down or blocked. The blood carries oxygen to the heart, and if enough blood and oxygen cannot reach the heart, it becomes weakened and one may suffer chest pain. If the blood supply to a portion of the heart is completely cut off by a blockage, the result is a heart attack. Likewise, decreased blood flow to the brain can cause a stroke.

Figure 7.5 shows a normal artery with normal blood flow (Figure A) and an artery containing plaque build up (Figure B). Special arteries, called coronary arteries, bring blood to the heart. Narrowing of the coronary arteries due to plaque can stop or slow down the flow of blood to heart. When the arteries narrow, the amount of oxygen-rich blood is decreased. This is called coronary artery disease (CAD). Large plaque areas can lead to chest pain called angina. Angina happens when the heart does not receive enough oxygen-rich blood. Angina is a common symptom of CAD.

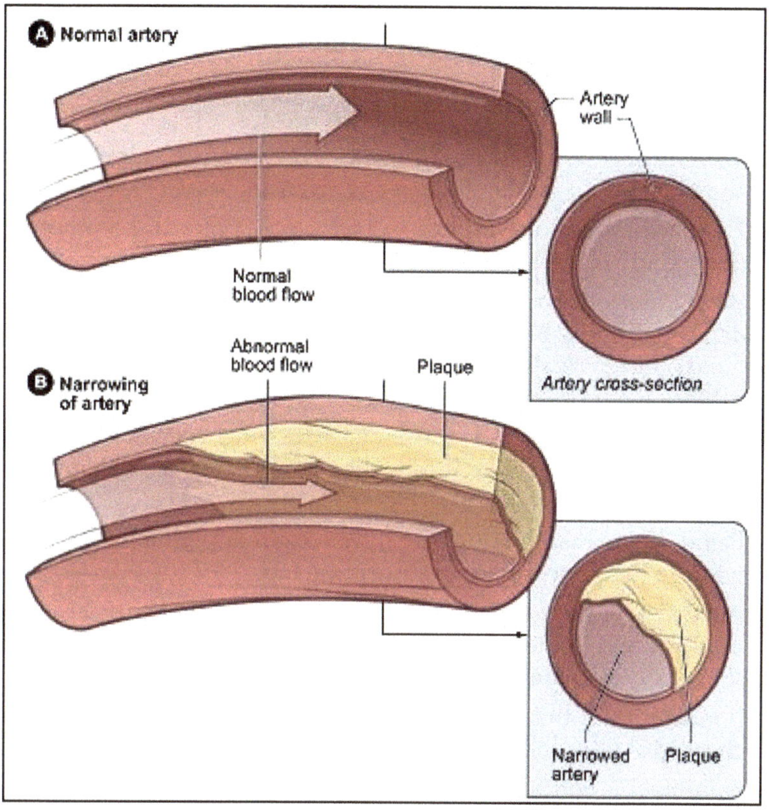

Figure 7.5: Plaque Build Up in Artery

Some plaques have a thin covering and burst (rupture), releasing fat and cholesterol into the bloodstream. The release of fat and cholesterol may cause blood to clot. A clot can block the flow of blood. This blockage can cause angina or a heart attack. Lowering cholesterol level decreases the chance for having a plaque burst and cause a heart attack. Lowering cholesterol may also slow down, reduce, or even stop plaque from building up. Plaque and resulting health problems can also occur in arteries elsewhere in the body.

The blood cholesterol level has a lot to do with the chances of getting heart disease. In fact, the higher the blood cholesterol level, the greater the risk for developing heart disease or having a heart attack. If total cholesterol is less than 200 mg/dL, the heart attack risk is relatively low, unless the person has other risk factors. In general, people who have a total cholesterol level of 240 mg/dL have twice the risk of heart attack as people who have a cholesterol level of 200 mg/dL.

How to Lower Cholesterol

Pathobiological studies have confirmed that fatty streaks appear as early as in the second trimester of pregnancy and progresses through childhood, adolescence, youth and adulthood. A strong correlation exists between the maternal cholesterol

Facts about Cholesterol

- ☆ Eating too much saturated fat and cholesterol raises the level of cholesterol in blood.
- ☆ Lowering cholesterol is important for everyone-young, middle-aged, and older adults, and both men and women.
- ☆ There are no signs or symptoms of high blood cholesterol. Many people don't know that their cholesterol level is too high.
- ☆ When there is too much cholesterol in the blood, excess cholesterol is deposited in the blood vessels. Too much cholesterol in blood can build up in the walls of arteries. This is called plaque which can lead to blockages in the arteries.
- ☆ Reducing saturated fats and increasing fruit, vegetables, fish and wholegrain foods as part of a healthy lifestyle will assist in reducing cholesterol absorption.
- ☆ Being active, maintaining a healthy weight and giving up smoking will help reduce cholesterol absorption too.
- ☆ A blood test called a lipoprotein profile measures the cholesterol levels in blood and is the recommended test. The total blood cholesterol should be less than 200 mg/dl.
- ☆ It is important that everyone age 20 and older get their cholesterol checked at least once every 5 years.
- ☆ Some people will need to take medicines prescribed by their doctor to lower their cholesterol in addition to eating a low saturated fat and low cholesterol diet, exercising, and losing weight if needed.

levels and rate of progression of plaque in the offspring. Starts in the womb and ends in the tomb! Prevention should, therefore start very early and continue throughout the life.

It's worth taking steps to lower cholesterol because lowering cholesterol by 10 per cent reduces the risk of heart attack by 20 per cent.

Type of Fat

Eating a lot of saturated fat tends to elevate the levels of LDL in the blood, so these kinds of fats are often called 'bad fats' contained in foods such as full fat dairy products, processed meats like salami and sausages, snack foods like chips, takeaway foods (especially deep fried foods), cakes, biscuits and pastries, coconut oil and palm oil should be avoided. One should choose lean meats, trim-off visible fats, eat chicken after removing skin, switch to low fat or fat free dairy products.

Eating monounsaturated or polyunsaturated fats, on the other hand, tends to increase the levels of HDL. HDL reduces cholesterol in the blood, so these fats are called 'good fats'. Eating these will reduce the risk of artery disease. Foods high in monounsaturated fats include olive oil, canola oil, avocados and most nuts. Foods high in polyunsaturated fats include oils of seeds and grains, such as sunflower, safflower, corn, soybeans and walnuts.

Table 7.7

Eat Less of	*Eat Moderate Amounts of*	*Eat More of*
Cold cuts, sausage, regular hot dogs, fried meats, organ meats (*e.g.* liver), eggs	Steak, ham, roasts, chicken or turkey hot dogs	Fish, other seafood, skinless poultry
Whole milk, canned milk, cream, sour cream, ice cream, butter, hard cheese, cream cheese	Low fat milk, frozen yogurt, low-fat cheese, ice milk, margarine	Skim milk, low fat yogurt, cheese with less then 5% fat
Cakes, cookies, pies, candy, chips	Peanut butter, unsalted peanuts, almonds, walnuts, pecans	Fresh fruits, fresh veggies, unbuttered popcorn
Regular salad dressings, gravies, sauces, and spreads	Low fat	

Fibre

Most of the cholesterol is synthesized in our body. Dietary fibre binds with the bile acid and cholesterol and helps it remove as faeces, before it is reabsorbed in the system. There are two types of fibre; soluble and insoluble fibre. Soluble fibre helps to lower blood cholesterol levels in most individuals when added to the diet. Though oat bran is the most common type of fibre next to barley, whole wheat, millet, peas, figs, apples, cherries, berries along with many vegetables and most fruits also contain soluble fibre. All citrus fruits are high in soluble fibre. Animal products have very little fibre no matter how lean they are.

Not only can a diet rich in fibre and low saturated foods reduce cholesterol it may also prevent heart disease. One should eat cracked wheat porridge, oats for breakfast, *roti* from whole grain flour, whole pulses, brown or paddy rice. One should avoid eating refined foods.

Nuts

If one is looking for a way to keep the heart healthy and still satisfy his or her snacking mood, pistachios and sunflower seeds may be the powerful cholesterol-fighting tool the body needs.

A new study, published in the *Journal of Agricultural and Food Chemistry*, shows that these nuts and seeds rank at the top of the list for containing cholesterol-lowering compounds, phytosterols. While many nuts contain this helpful compound, the study is the first to determine which of these little treats have the largest amount of this cholesterol-clobbering ingredient (Barrow, 2006).

Phytosterols are found only in plant-based foods and very closely resemble the molecular structure of cholesterol. But unlike cholesterol, phytosterols are not easily absorbed by the body. Scientists believe that because of this, the compound can partially block cholesterol from being absorbed, thereby lowering overall cholesterol levels naturally. Philips and her colleagues recognized that nuts and seeds tend to be high in phytosterols, but no study had adequately compared the amounts of the compound found in all of the varieties, which range in size from poppy seeds to walnuts. While wheat germ and sesame seeds are also found to contain the highest amount of phytosterols but most people do not eat these foods by themselves. So, the third and forth place finishers, sunflower seeds and pistachios, were considered by Philips to be the most practical nutty snack for people looking to lower their cholesterol. Even if one doesn't consider sunflower seeds or pistachios a desirable treat, any of the nuts and seeds tested were found to contain at least a small amount of phytosterols.

Exercise

Exercise lowers body weight, blood sugar, blood pressure, bad cholesterol (LDL), and triglycerides, improves insulin sensitivity, increases good cholesterol (HDL) and releases lipoprotein lipase, an enzyme that mobilizes fat from skeletal muscle. Regular exercise for example, at least 30 minutes of brisk walking daily increases HDL levels and reduces LDL levels in the body at no costs.

Medication

Some people can achieve target levels with diet and exercise. However, many require cholesterol reducing medications to keep their levels within a healthy range and reduce the risk of cardiovascular disease. People with familial hypercholesterolemia usually need medications.

Cholesterol reducing drugs are medications that lower the levels of lipids in the blood. There are five main categories of cholesterol reducers: statins, bile acid resins, nicotinic acid, fibrates and cholesterol absorption inhibitors. Most medications are available only by prescription, except for nicotinic acid, a form of vitamin B_3 (niacin), which is available over the counter. However, niacin still needs to be taken under the care of a physician to monitor possible side effects.

The different types of cholesterol reducing drugs which can be taken alone or in combination are discussed as under:

- *Statins*: Statins, also known as HMG CoA reductase inhibitors, block an enzyme (HMG CoA reductase) used in the production of cholesterol. They also accelerate turnover of cholesterol by the liver. Common statins are atorvastatin (brand name Lipitor), fluvastatin (Lescol or Vastin), pravastatin (Pravachol), and simvastatin (Lipex or Zocor). They can drop blood LDL levels by anywhere between 20 and 50 per cent, and increase HDL by 5 to 15 per cent. Side effects include stomach upset and headache.
- *Cholestyramine and colestipol*: These are older medications, also known as bile-acid-binding resins. They bind to bile acids in the intestine, preventing them from being absorbed into the body. The liver needs bile acids to make cholesterol – so less bile acids means less cholesterol. Examples include cholestyramine and colestipol. They both come in sachets of powder which

need to be mixed with water, juice or other fluid and can be taken with or without food. Constipation is a common side effect.

- *Gemfibrozil and fenofibrate*: These drugs are used when the others don't work, or when levels of triglycerides are high though they also increase the amount of HDL in the blood. Fenofibrate also lowers total cholesterol.
- *Nicotinic acid*: It can lower LDL cholesterol and triglycerides, and increase HDL cholesterol. It also can lower triglycerides. It can cause flushing of the face and neck. Because the dose needed for treatment is about 100 times more than the Recommended Daily Allowance for niacin and thus, can potentially be toxic, the drug must be taken under a doctor's care.
- *Ezetimibe*: It is a new drug in a class called the cholesterol absorption inhibitors. It works by reducing the absorption of cholesterol from the intestine into the bloodstream. It reduces total cholesterol and LDL, and increases HDL cholesterol.

Some cholesterol reducers can cause liver inflammation, which tends to resolve on its own after patients stop taking the medication. To monitor this and other complications, patients should undergo regular liver function tests and possibly other blood tests.

Some cholesterol drugs can affect the kidneys. Because kidney damage is a common consequence of diabetes, patients are advised to ask their physician about whether their medication can impair their kidney function and whether they should have regular monitoring such as microalbuminuria testing.

Women taking cholesterol reducing drugs should inform their physician at once if they are or plan to become pregnant. Although it has been found that statins do not have a negative effect on female reproductive hormone levels yet cholesterol is an important contributor to the development of the foetus. In addition, some cholesterol reducers are excreted in breast milk. Nursing mothers, therefore, should consult with their physician before taking or discontinuing these drugs.

Patients are advised not to abruptly stop taking their medications without first consulting their physician. It is also important that patients notify all physicians (including dentists) that they are taking statins before undergoing any surgical procedure. Patients should inform their physician immediately of any side effects or concerns.

Diet Recommended for Lowering Blood Cholesterol

A cholesterol lowering diet should be low in total fat, especially saturated fat, as well as cholesterol, and high in fiber.

Earlier, the Step I and Step II diets created by the National Heart, Lung, and Blood Association's National Cholesterol Education Program (NCEP) were also endorsed by the American Heart Association. Both diets were designed to reduce risk of cardiovascular disease by reducing high blood cholesterol levels.

The Step I diet restricted total fat to no more than 30 percent of total calories, saturated fat to no more than 10 percent of total calories, and cholesterol to less than 300 mg/day. It was intended as the starting point for patients who had high cholesterol levels.

The Step II diet goals were lower for saturated fat (less than 7 percent) and cholesterol (less than 200 mg/day). They were intended for people already at the Step I goals or for patients with a high-risk cholesterol level (240 mg/dL or higher) or who had a heart attack.

Now, the American Heart Association no longer uses the terms "Step I" and "Step II" in reference to heart -healthy diets. These terms, however, still appear in some older materials and journal articles. In June, 2006, AHA released new Dietary Recommendations (TLC diet) which have been described in Chapter 11. Their revised dietary guidelines have been built upon the Step I diet and emphasize the importance of a diet low in saturated and *trans*-fat, and rich in fruits, vegetables, whole grains, fat-free and low-fat dairy products, and lean meat, fish and poultry.

In the diet one should take at least five servings (cups) each of fresh fruits and vegetables a day. Whole grains, legumes, lentils, variety of nuts (almonds, walnuts, pecans), low fat milk products, soy milk, and tofu provide the body with soluble and insoluble fibre, vitamins, antioxidants, isoflavins, good fats, vegetable protein and low glycemic index sugars and help lower the homocysteine levels, prevent heart disease, diabetes and certain forms of cancer. One should take minimum amount of fried foods. Stop re-heating the edible oils for cooking. Balance the intake of omega 6 and omega-3 fatty acids in the diet. Avoid foods rich in *trans*-fats such as crispy and crunchy, fried and fast foods/desserts, cookies, cakes, pastries etc.

Other Ways to Lower Total Cholesterol and Increase HDL-Cholesterol Naturally

Natural remedies are abundantly available. With a few changes in eating habits and lifestyle, one can easily lower cholesterol naturally. A few of them as reported by various researchers are given as under:

- Vitamin E may help reduce fatty formations on arteries.
- Chromium is a proven method of maintaining correct blood sugar levels, which will help to control cholesterol.
- Red wine consumed in reasonable quantity gives a positive result. It contains antioxidants that slow down oxidation of HDL and LDL cholesterol. By drinking wine, HDL levels do not shoot up, but contain higher level of various types of blood fats, thus making it useful for the body.
- Drinking orange juice every day increases HDL level by nearly 21 per cent. This is possible due to the presence of flavonoids.
- Kidney and red beans are another source to increase HDL level. They contain low-glycemic carbohydrates which do not create insulin spikes during digestion.
- Taking flaxseed several times a week is very useful in increasing HDL level as it contains omega-3 fatty acids.

- ☆ Olive oil contains the highest number of monounsaturated fats. Having 1-2 teaspoons in the daily diet would help tremendously.
- ☆ Half raw onion per day increases HDL level by 30 per cent.
- ☆ Soy products increase HDL levels thereby decreasing LDL. Eating soy protein each day can be a healthy way to lower LDL-cholesterol and reduce the risk of CVD, which increases in women as they reach menopause.
- ☆ Eat more of soluble fiber present in barley, oat and other whole millets to reduce LDL cholesterol. Studies have shown that 2 ounces of oat bran per day helps in reducing 16 per cent LDL and 15 per cent increase in HDL.
- ☆ Green tea lowers LDL levels by increasing HDL levels.
- ☆ A multitude of medical studies confirm that garlic in several forms can reduce cholesterol. In the most recent study, using garlic pills and a placebo, researchers at Oxford University noted a 12 per cent reduction in total cholesterol.

Ratio of Total Cholesterol/HDL-Cholesterol and Essential Fatty Acids

According to some research studies, not only total cholesterol, but HDL cholesterol is also an important predictor of coronary heart disease. Total: HDL cholesterol is more sensitive and specific than is total cholesterol as a risk predictor. The ratio of TC/HDLC in blood is one of the best factors for predicting the risk that a person will develop heart disease. It is one of the standards used to guide medical treatment. In the Framingham Study, the total cholesterol/HDL cholesterol ratio gave the best prediction for the coronary heart disease risk. Persons having total cholesterol: HDL cholesterol ratio less than 6 have lower risk of CHD.

It has been reported by researchers that essential fatty acids (EFAs) are excellent predictors of the total cholesterol (TC)/ high density lipoprotein cholesterol (HDLC) ratio. Lipoproteins, such as LDL, carry cholesterol, EFAs, and other nutrients to the body's cells. Dr. Siguel proposed that TC/HDLC reflects EFA status in the body because the particles (lipoproteins) that carry cholesterol are also the main carriers of EFAs. When levels of EFAs in LDL particles decline, the amount of LDL increases so that cells can get enough EFAs. According to Dr. Siguel and his colleague Robert Lerman, a deficiency of EFAs is the missing link relating nutrition to CAD (Metabolism, 1994) and widely reported in the news media.

According to Dr. Siguel, people should be concerned primarily with total calories (achieving ideal weight) and calories from PUFA to achieve ideal w3/w6 ratios. The amount of PUFAs to eat per day depends on the number of cells in the body. In contrast to AHA recommendations, Dr. Siguel states that people should not reduce their EFA intakes when they eat fewer calories. Eating the appropriate amount and mixture of EFA-rich foods will correct EFA abnormalities and usually decrease TC/HDLC.

Researchers identify EFAs as key nutrients that regulate TC/HDLC and recommend drastic changes in nutrition policy to prevent and treat cardiovascular disease

Dr. Siguel recommends that people eat fewer calories from SFAs, MUFAs, and carbohydrates, until they achieve ideal weight. Individuals who consistently replace most fat with carbohydrates or those on low-calorie diets who strictly follow the USDA Food Pyramid may become deficient in EFAs. Although very low-fat diets may be safely prescribed to overweight individuals who have large reserves of EFAs in their bodies, Drs. Siguel and Lerman have stated that very low-fat diets, deprived of EFAs, may be counterproductive for many patients, particularly those who are not losing weight. For people who do not eat sufficient neither EFAs, nor have enough stored in their bodies, the government's dietary recommendations are ineffective (Am. J. of Clinical Nutrition, December, 1994 letter by Drs. Siguel and Lerman pertaining to the USDA Food Pyramid).

The results reported by Dr. Siguel indicated that drastic changes should be made to current recommendations for the correction of abnormal cholesterol ratios. Instead of avoiding fat, people should eat foods rich in EFAs but low in calories. Using a nutritional blood test, doctors can determine what needs to be changed in the diet to reduce the TC/HDLC ratio by as much as 50 per cent. Such drastic changes are not possible with existing dietary or drug therapy. Current strategies to lower cholesterol frequently fail and vast sums of money are spent on nutritional programs and diets which may be ineffective (New York Times, 4/25/95, p. C13).

This research is based on the analyses of more than 500 subjects from the Framingham Heart Study. The relationship between EFAs and cholesterol had not been found previously, because the technology needed to accurately measure EFAs in human blood is highly complex and was only developed recently. The researchers used a method patented by Dr. Siguel, and described as "state-of-the-art" by NIH reviewers, to report as follows:

- ☆ Levels of EFAs in the blood are highly correlated with TC/HDLC. The relationship is similar for men and women, suggesting that PUFA or EFA metabolism is a key mechanism that mediates sex differences in TC/HDLC plasma levels (PUFA = EFA + EFA derivatives = w3 + w6 fatty acids).
- ☆ In individuals with low PUFA levels or biochemical evidence of EFA insufficiency, treatment with diets consisting of different fatty acid mixtures or oil supplements are indicated. Bringing the fatty acid profiles of patients with high TC/HDLC closer to those of healthy people should precede any decisions for drug therapy. The risks of such treatment are minimal and the potential benefits highly significant.

On average, subjects with low levels of EFAs had high levels of TC/HDLC, and subjects with high levels of EFAs had low levels of TC/HDLC. Furthermore, when subjects with high TC/HDLC eat more EFAs, TC/HDLC declines (ISSFAL, 1995).

According to Edward Siguel, the principal author of this research, blood levels of EFAs are a major nutritional factor regulating blood levels of TC/HDLC. EFA abnormalities are a cause of acquired (not genetic) atherosclerotic disease through their effects on membrane function.

Dr. Siguel's research leads to a new treatment for abnormal cholesterol ratios, a treatment that is substantially different from the one proposed by the AHA and NIH. The NIH recommends that people decrease their intake of SFAs, and increase their intake of both carbohydrates and MUFAs. Dr. Siguel proposed that people achieve ideal weight by reducing caloric intake from all sources. He also suggested that people eat EFAs as needed to bring their EFA blood profile closer to that of healthy subjects. Because EFAs are essential, Dr. Siguel emphasizes that patients with low blood levels of EFAs should not follow very low-fat diets devoid of EFAs. Instead, they should eat diets to correct their fatty acid abnormalities. The changes recommended by Dr. Siguel should lead to substantial revisions in the way abnormal cholesterol ratios are treated today. They offer a practical alternative to save billions of dollars in health care costs while improving quality of life and life expectancy.

Chapter 8
Cardiovascular Disease and Risk Factors

It is time to make cardiac health a top priority. If the heart is not working, nothing else works. Life to some extent can remain even without a fully functioning brain, but one cannot survive without a heart. Heart is a leading cause of death and is one of the most preventable too. Cardiovascular disease claim 17 million lives worldwide annually. It is the single greatest killer and takes more lives than the next seven leading causes of death put together. Heart diseases or disorders are surprisingly high in new borns and then it usually strikes when we have spent two thirds of our lives. However, heart disease often begins in childhood.

What Is 'Heart Disease', or 'Coronary Heart Disease'?

Heart disease refers to more than 30 cardiovascular conditions. The heart muscle is living and needs food and oxygen to survive. There are arteries within the heart muscle which supply the food and oxygen to the heart muscle. These arteries are known as coronary arteries. When one or more of these arteries in the heart get narrowed, or partially blocked, then it leads to Coronary Artery Disease. When one or more of these arteries get blocked then some part of the heart muscle does not get food and oxygen. This condition is called a heart attack or infarction. The term, coronary artery disease is used for problems which include angina, heart attack, and heart failure. Among cardiovascular diseases, those resulting from thromboembolic complications such as coronary occlusion, infarction, and stroke are the main cause of death and disability.

Atherosclerosis

The root cause of most cases of coronary artery disease or cardiovascular disease is atherosclerosis *i.e.* a buildup of atheroma–a fatty deposit within the inside lining of arteries. A blockage caused by the development of complex atheromatous plaques, composed of inflamed tissues and fatty deposits on the inner surface of the artery. These plaques develop slowly over time and may cause chronic restriction of blood flow leading to pain on exertion (angina) or it may lead to as acute blockage. This most often occurs when the irregular, inflamed surface of the plaque leads to the formation of a blood clot. When this occurs, a region of heart muscle is suddenly deprived of blood and gets damaged. This is what is known as a heart attack. If the damage is relatively limited the heart can recover but major damage can lead to death. Similar degeneration of arteries in the brain leads to loss of blood supply and stroke or death.

Formation of Atheroma

Three distinct layers make up arterial walls. The intima, or innermost layer bordering the lumen, consists of flattened endothelial cells. A fenestrated membrane composed largely of elastin separates the intima from the middle layer. This is formed of concentric wrappings of smooth muscle cells, elastin, and fibrous material supported in a matrix of glycoproteins, proteoglycans, and glucosaminoglycans. The adventitia, or outermost layer, contains fibroblasts and smooth muscle cells loosely arranged among bundles of collagen fibres. The outer half of the arterial wall is supplied by the capillary network of the vasa vasorum while the inner half relies on diffusion from the lumen for its nutriment.

Injury to the endothelial cells of the arterial wall increases their permeability and initiates atherosclerosis. This allows the entry of cholesterol from circulating lipoproteins into the deeper layers of the arterial wall. Lipoproteins, which are macromolecular complexes synthesized by the liver for the transport of cholesterol and triglycerides, are also composed of phospholipids and specific proteins termed apoproteins. The various classes of lipoproteins, which include very low density (VLDL), low density (LDL), and high density (HDL) lipoproteins, differ in size and relative proportion of constituent components (triglycerides, cholesterol, phospholipids). The source of cholesterol in atherosclerotic lesions is believed to be the low density lipoproteins (LDLs). Lipid droplets are deposited and can form a dense coating on elastin and collagen fibres. Fat-filled cells derived from smooth muscle cells or circulating monocytes also appear.

Localized thickenings or plaques of fatty and fibrous material on arterial walls cause narrowing of the vessel lumen. Clumps of aggregated platelets called thrombi may form at the sites of atherosclerotic lesions, and impaired circulation and ischemia occur when atherosclerotic lesions and thrombi obstruct the flow of blood.

Various Theories Regarding Atherosclerosis

The exact molecular sequence of events in atherosclerosis is still debated. Three different theories (not mutually exclusive) include the following (Boren *et al.*, 2000).

- Response-to-injury hypothesis, emphasizing injury to endothelium and smooth muscle cells by:
  - Oxidized low-density lipoprotein (LDL)
  - Cigarette smoking
  - Hypertension
- Oxidation hypothesis, emphasizing oxidative modification of LDL-c and its involvement in the recruitment of macrophages and other inflammatory cells to lesions.
- Response-to-retention hypothesis, emphasizing that the initial event in cholesterol-induced atherosclerosis is the retention and accumulation of LDL and other atherogenic (apolipoprotein [apo] B-containing) lipoproteins in the arteries.

The latter theory holds that subendothelial retention of apo B-100-containing lipoproteins is the initiating event in atherogenesis. The events described above lead to a series of biologic responses that promote growth of the atherosclerotic plaque and lead to the formation of "vulnerable" plaques.

Thus emerging risk factors, such as ultrasensitive C-reactive protein, carotid ultrasound, ankle-brachial index, or calcium quantification by computed tomography (CT) scan, might prove useful in certain situations to indicate those who need more intensive therapy. However, it remains to be proven whether any of these novel risk factors provide clinically useful information beyond that provided by the well-established risk factors, including:

- Age
- Gender
- High LDL-c
- Low HDL-c
- Cigarette use
- Diabetes mellitus
- Hypertension

Burke looked at CHD risk factors and plaque anatomy and found the following significant correlations:

- Cigarette smoking and plaque erosion
- Glycosylated hemoglobin with stable plaque and healed infarct.
- Hypertension with stable plaque with healed infarct
- Women >50 years of age and plaque rupture.

The focus of therapy then is to prevent the plaque from rupturing and to decrease the thrombogenicity of the plaque.

Atherosclerosis, Lipids, and Acute Coronary Syndromes

Coronary atherosclerosis begins in youth and develops over a lifetime. Progression of atherosclerosis varies according to:

- ☆ Heredity
- ☆ Gender
- ☆ Well-defined coronary heart disease (CHD) risk factors

Complications of atheroma in advanced stages may occur suddenly, but not necessarily expectedly, as acute events are more likely to occur during:

- ☆ Early morning hours (6 to 11 AM) due to circadian variation and a host of physiologic variables
- ☆ Winter months
- ☆ Heavy physical exertion
- ☆ Emotional stress
- ☆ Sexual activity

Yet the most concerning and frustrating manifestation of CHD is acute, out of-hospital sudden death (Tarven *et al.*, 1995). This emphasizes of the need to find susceptible but asymptomatic persons in the population and bring them to treatment before sudden death can occur. Since this chapter is on lipids and CHD, the focus will be on how cholesterol lowering favorably alters both:

- ☆ The chronic process that begins in youth and develops over a lifetime.
- ☆ The acute process in which a sudden plaque rupture in a region of underlying atherosclerosis gives way to dynamic changes in the coronary circulation that can lead to myocardial infarction (MI) and death.

The chronic process of atherosclerosis begins in youth. The American Heart Association has developed a grading system to standardize terminology. Table 8.1 shows the summary provided by the Pathobiological Determinants of Atherosclerosis in Youth (PDAY) study. This study was a multi center collaborative effort that examined relationships between cardiovascular (CV) risk factors and atherosclerosis in young (15 to 34-year-old) black and white men and women who were presented for autopsy after a traumatic death (Strong *et al.*, 1999). As expected from autopsy studies of US military personnel from the Korean War and the Vietnam conflict, intimal lesions were found in the youngest age group (15 to 19 years of age) and increased in prevalence and extent up to the oldest group (30 to 34 years of age).

McGill *et al.* (2000) evaluated 760 subjects from the PADY study and noted that grade 4 or 5 lesions in the proximal left anterior descending (LAD) coronary artery were present in 2.4 per cent of 15- to 19-yer-old men and 20.3 per cent of 30- to 34-year old men. Although no such lesions were found in 15- to 19-year-old women, they were found in 7 per cent to 8 per cent of 30- to34-year-old women. Importantly, by age 30 to 34, 19 per cent of men and 8 per cent of women had atherosclerotic narrowing >40 per cent. This end point was chosen due to Glagov's findings that plaque

Table 8.1: American Heart Association Criteria for Pathologic Coronary Arterial Lesions

Grade	Criteria			Comments/Corresponding Gross Classification
	Macrophage Foam Cells	Extracellular Lipid	Adaptive Intimal Thickening	
0	None	None	With or without	Normal tissue
1	Isolated	None	Variable	Initial atherosclerotic lesion, sometimes visible grossly with lipid staining.
2	Numerous, often in layers	No distinct pools	Variable	Fatty streak, visible grossly with lipid staining
3	Numerous, often in layers	One or more pools	Variable	Fatty plaque, raised fatty streak, intermediate lesion
4	Numerous often in layers	Well-defined core		Luminal surface covered by relatively normal initima, atheroma, fibrous plaque, or raised lesion
5	Numerous	Well-defined or multiple cores	–	Reactive fibrotic cap, vascularization, or calcium, fibroatheroma, fibrous plaque, or raised lesion.
6	All of the above plus surface defect, hematoma, hemorrhage, or thrombosis			Complicated lesion

Adapted from: McGill HC, *et al.*, Circulation 2000; 102: 374-379.

accumulation does not encroach on the coronary lumen with lesions <40 per cent (Glagov *et al.*, 1987). This is because of compensatory remodeling with arterial dilation that occurs until the external elastic membrane by approximately 40 per cent.

This important study gave evidence that significant early atherosclerosis was related to CHD risk factor. Only 22 per cent of adolescents and young adults had no risk factors, whereas 43 per cent had one and 35 per cent had two or more risk factors. Of note in this sample with a high prevalence of metabolic syndrome risk factors, high non-high-density lipoprotein cholesterol (HDL-c) was associated with greater odds of grade 2 or 3 lesions, grade 4 to 5 lesions, and stenosis with about 60 per cent higher prevalence of grade 4 or 5 lesions (Table 8.2).

In a meta-analysis consisting of three studies with long-term follow-up, Stamler provided a summary of epidemiologic evidence supporting the importance of cholesterol control at an early age (Stamler *et al.*, 2000) (Table 8.3). In all three studies, the relative risk (RR) of CHD death was particularly high for those with the highest levels of cholesterol as contrasted with those with low levels. This supports the concept that hypercholesterolemia, even when it is present in early life, contributes to the risk of developing CHD. Thus, there is a need to work at improving life-habit risk factors such as:

- Atherogenic diet
- Sedentary lifestyle
- Weight gain, leading to overweight and obesity

Table 8.2: Metabolic Risk Factors in Pathobiologic Determinants Atherosclerosis in Youth Study

Risk Factors	Classification	Prevalence (per cent)
High Non-HDL-Cholesterol	≥160mg.dL or ≥4.14 mmol/L	28
Low HDL- Cholesterol	<35mg/dL or<0.91 mmol/L	18.7
Smoking	≥90mg/L (thiocyanate level)	44
Hypertension	Renal artery algorithm110 mm Hg	15.5
Obesity	Body mass index ≥30kg/m^2	14.3
Impaired glucose tolerance	Glycohemoglobin ≥8 per cent	4.3

Adapted from: McGill HC, *et al.*, Circulation 2000; 102:374-379

Clinical Tip. Non-HDL-c is now a secondary target of treatment for those with triglycerides (TGs) >200 mg/dL after the low density lipoprotein cholesterol (LDL-c goal has been achieved. The goal for non-HDL-c is 130 mg/dL more than the LDL-c goal.

Table 8.3: Meta Analysis of Risk for Coronary Heart Disease Death Overtime in Younger Men with High Cholesterol*

Criteria of Trials	MRFIT	Chicago Heart Association Detection Project	Peoples Gas Company
Number of male subjects	69.205	11.017	1.266
Age ranges at onset of study (Years) Follow up (years)	37 to 53 16	30 to 55 25	32 to 66 34
Absolute risk (per 1000) TC≥240mg/dl	15.5	54.2	154.0
Absolute excess risk (per 1000) TC≥240mg/dl	12.1	43.6	81.4
Relative risk T≥280 mg/dl	8.1	11.9	8.1

Abbreviations. MRFIT-Multiple Risk Factor Intervention Trial; TC- total cholesterol

· All members are rounded off to one decimal place

· Difference in risk of those with TC 240 mg/dl. as compared with TC 200mg/dl.

· Risk of those with TC 180 mg/dl. divided by risk of those with TC 160 mg/ dl.

Adapted from. Stamler J. *et al.*, JAMA 2000;284:311-318

Obesity and CHD

The increased risk of mortality associated with excess weight extends over the entire range from very thin to very heavy. This increase in risk is seen over the entire spectrum of ages studied, but it is of greater magnitude among younger individuals (Stevens *et al.*, 1998). In the Nurses' Health Study, this was shown for women; slightly more than 115,000 women were enrolled in this study. The 12-year risk of dying was 2.2 times higher for women with a body mass index (BMI) of 32.0 (equivalent to 175 lbs and 62 inches tall) than for women with a BMI <19.0 (equivalent to 104 lbs and 62 inches tall). The risk gradient for death due to CHD was much steeper, those with a BMI ≥ 32.0 were at 5.8 times the risk of those with a BMI <19. Similar results are seen in other data involving men.

In accord with these data on mortality from CHD, the National Health and Nutrition Evaluation Survey (NHANES) III has demonstrated that obesity is associated with an increased prevalence of CHD both in men and in women (Must *et al.*, 1999). Furthermore, the Pathobiologic Determinants of Atherosclerosis in Youth (PDAY) study showed that obesity is associated with a >2-fold increase in raised coronary lesions in 25- to 34-year-old individuals who died of external causes (homicide, suicide, or accidents) (McGill *et al.*, 2000).

It is now well-known that there has been a substantial reduction in CHD rates over the past 3 decades. Data from the Nurses' Health Study showed a 31 per cent decline in CHD rates between the 2-year period 1980 to 1982 and the 2-year period 1992 to 1994. However, analysis of data from that study showed that were it not for increased rates of obesity, the improvement in CHD incidence would have been 8 per cent better (Hus *et al.*, 2000). Some previous analyses had identified a U-shaped relationship between mortality and measures of obesity, with a major increase in risk for the thinnest members of the population. However, the conclusion that being thin causes increased risk is erroneous. This erroneous conclusion stems from:

- Failure to control for cigarette smoking (smokers tend to be thinner)
- Inappropriate control for biologic effects of obesity, such as hypertension, diabetes, and hyperlipidemia
- Failure to account for weight loss that has been caused by serious disease (Manson *et al.*, 1987)

The increased risk associated with obesity appears to be due not only to changes in lipoprotein metabolism. Weight gain is associated with a clustering of risk factors termed "the metabolic syndrom." These risk factors include the following (Wilson *et al.*, 1999; Grundy, 1999):

- Abdominal obesity
- Hypertriglyceridemia
- Low HDL-chosterol
- Hypertension
- Glucose intolerance
- Small, dense LDL
- Hypercoagulable state
- Insulin resistance.

Overweight appears to confer coronary risk independent of its association with hypertension, hypercholesterolemia, and glucose intolerance, as demonstrated in the 26-year follow-up in the Framingham Study. Additionally, gaining weight after early adulthood appears to contribute independently to CHD risk.

Distribution of Body Fat and CHD Risk

A growing body of evidence indicates that the impact of obesity on health is determined to a great extent by the location of excess body fat. In the Nurses' Health Study, for example, waist-to-hip ratio (ratio of body circumference at waist to that at the hip) was used as an index of visceral fat deposition. This measurement was a better predictor of CHD risk than BMI. The 12-year risk of developing CHD for those in the highest quintile of waist-to-hip ratio was 8.7 times that for those in the lowest quintile. Most other studies have similarly shown that abdominal obesity is a better predictor of risk.

Lipoprotein Disorders Associated with Obesity

Much of the adverse impact of obesity on risk of CHD can be accounted for by the effects of obesity on lipoprotein metabolism. Obesity is associated with undesirable changes in VLDL, LDL, and HDL (Table 8.4).

Obesity may have a striking impact on serum levels of VLDL and, therefore, on fasting TGs. Marked hypertriglyceridemia in an obese individual can often be effectively treated by loss of weight. Furthermore, body weight is a major factor in the expression of type III hyperlipoproteinemia (dysbetalipoproteinemia).

Table 8.4: Effects of Obesity on Plasma Lipoprotein Levels

- ☆ Very low-density lipoprotein (fasting triglyceride) increased
- ☆ Low-density lipoprotein (LDL) cholesterol increased
- ☆ High-density lipoprotein cholesterol reduced
- ☆ Atherogenic pattern of small, dense LDL fostered

In the Lipid Research Clinics Prevalence Study, BMI was significantly correlated with high TG levels, high LDL levels, and low HDL levels. From 2692 adult males in this study, BMI accounted for 20 per cent to 27 per cent of the population variance in HDL-c after adjustment was made for covariation of BMI with age, cigarette use, exogenous sex hormone use, and alcohol consumption. Among the 2413 adult females, BMI accounted for 17 per cent to 27 per cent of the variation in HDL-c levels after accounting for the impact of the same covariates. The univariate correlation coefficient for BMI with log of TG was approximately 0.3 for both men and women. Similar result are seen in the NHAANES II with data obtained 1976 to 1980 (Denke *et al.*, 1993 and 1994). In this study, the inverse relationship of BMI with HDL was strong in all age groups and in both genders; the relationship with LDL was the strongest in young men and in young and middle-aged women. Among overweight young men (BMI >25.0), total serum cholesterol level averaged 19 mg/dL, greater than in those with a BMI of 25.0. Stamler calculated that for this group, the elevated cholesterol level associated with overweight would result in a 15 per cent increase in CHD events. He further concluded that "with prevention of overweight and overweight-related higher cholesterol, CHD mortality over the next 15 or more years for the whole cohort of younger men would be lowered by 14 per cent." Recent analyses have shown a frightening 1.5-fold increase in the prevalence of obesity during the past decade (Mokdad *et al.*, 1999; Flegal *et al.*, 2002). In the United States, the age-adjusted prevalence of obesity (BMI ≥30 kg/m^2) among adults in 1999-2000 was 30.5 per cent. There were also substantial increases in the prevalence of overweight (BMI ≥25 kg/m$^{2)}$ (from 55.9 per cent to 64.5 per cent) and in the prevalence of severe obesity (BMI ≥40 kg/m$^{2)}$ (from 2.9 per cent to 4.7 per cent) during the decade ending 1999-2000. Thus, the benefits resulting from prevention of obesity should be considerably greater than the 14 per cent reduction in CHD mortality calculated by Stamler using older data. Furthermore, there has been speculation that a continuing increase in the prevalence of obesity will soon lead to a decline in life expectancy in the United States (Olshansky *et al.*, 2005).

The adverse impact of obesity on LDL-c and HDL-c levels was confirmed in the Framingham Offspring Study. These findings were extended with the observation that increasing BMI led to an increased prevalence of the atherogenic LDL pattern B (predominance of small, dense LDL).

The mechanisms producing the lipoprotein abnormalities seen with obesity are complex. Obesity leads to increased production of inflammatory cytokines, which produce insulin resistance (Dandona *et al.*, 2005; Neels and Olefsky, 2006). Insulin resistance leads to increased hepatic secretion of VLDL, and this is manifested by elevated fasting TG levels. Furthermore, obesity is associated with reduced lipoprotein lipase activity and, thereby, with reduced clearance of VLDL from plasma. Weight loss increases both lipoprotein lipase activity and LDL receptor activity (Patalay *et al.*, 2005).

Since LDL is a metabolic product of VLDL, one might expect obesity to be associated with some elevation of LDL levels. Additionally, the hypertriglyceridemia occurring in obesity will reduce HDL levels by mechanisms involving cholesterol ester transfer protein.

Excess body weight attenuates the impact of dietary cholesterol (but not of saturated fats) on serum cholesterol levels. Thus reduction of dietary cholesterol will lead to greater reduction of serum cholesterol in overweight individuals after reduction of weight.

A number of observations suggest the particular importance of visceral adipose tissue in influencing lipoprotein physiology (Table 8.5). Visceral adipocytes seem to be especially sensitive to stimulation of lipolysis and to have reduced sensitivity to the antilipolytic effects of insulin. Additionally, lipolysis in visceral adipocytes deposits free fatty acids (FFAs) directly into the portal blood stream and, therefore, increases hepatic exposure to FFAs. This, in turn, increases the hepatic secretion of VLDL. The foregoing indicates mechanisms by which visceral obesity may increase the secretion of TG-rich lipoproteins. Additionally, visceral obesity retards the clearance of postprandial TG-rich lipoproteins (Taira *et al.*, 1999; Mekki *et al.*, 1999), this prolonging the residence in plasma of atherogenic particles. Visceral obesity is associated with increased levels of hepatic TG lipase and this speeds the catabolism of HDL, reducing HDL levels.

Table 8.5: Impact of Visceral Obesity on Lipoprotein Physiology

- ✰ Increased sensitivity of visceral adipocytes to lipolytic stimul
- ✰ Reduced sensitivity of visceral adipocytes to antilipolytic effects of insulin
- ✰ Increased hepatic exposure to free fatty acids with lipolysis in visceral location
- ✰ Increased hepatic triglyceride lipase activity

Insulin Resistance, Dyslipidemia, and Coronary Heart Disease

Hyperinsulinemia and insulin resistance have been reported to be associated with CHD and with other metabolic disorders that themselves predispose to development of CHD.

Association of Insulin Resistance with Coronary Risk

The reports of association of insulin resistance with CHD have not been consistent (Wingard *et al.*, 1995). In virtually all of these studies, measurement of elevated insulin levels was used as a surrogate for insulin resistance. Most of the studies that reported an absence of association between hyperinsulinism and CHD were hampered by a small number of CHD events, this limited their power to detect a relationship. Two recent reports of large studies do indicate that hyperinsulinism is associated with increased CHD risk and that this risk is independent of associations with established CHD risk factors (Despres *et al.*, 1996; Perry *et al.*, 1996). However, a nested case control study from the very large population of the Multiple Risk Factor Intervention Trial (MRFIT) did not show any relationship between fasting serum insulin levels and CHD risk (Orchard *et al.*, 1994). The question of whether hyperinsulinism (fasting or after a glucose load) is an independent risk factor for CHD thus, remains controversial.

When insulin sensitivity was measured directly in a large epidemiologic study, insulin resistance was associated with increased carotid atherosclerosis in Hispanics and in non-Hispanic whites, but not in blacks (Howard *et al.*, 1996).

Association of Hyperinsulinism with Coronary Risk Factors

In addition to any independent effect on CHD risk, it is clear that hyperinsulinism is associated with other abnormalities, which themselves increase risk of CHD (Table 8.6). Hyperinsulinism is associated with increased prevalence of established risk factors, including reduced HDL-c, hypertension, and obesity. Insulin resistance and hyperinsulinism are felt to be central to the metabolic syndrome, in which there is a clustering of several risk factors (Grundy *et al.*, 1999; Eckel *et al.*, 2005). In addition to these very well-established independent risk factors for CHD, hyperinsulinism is also associated with a predominance of small, dsnse LDL particles, elevated TG levels, impaired hemostasis, and a heightened inflammatory state. It is not clear whether insulin resistance has an impact on LDL-c levels; reports in the literature have not been consistent.

Table 8.6: Coronary Heart Disease Risk Factors Associated with Hyperinsulinism

- ✰ Low high-density lipoprotein cholesterol concentrations
- ✰ High low-density lipoprotein (LDL) cholesterol concentrations
- ✰ Small, dense LDL particles
- ✰ Hypertension
- ✰ Hyperglyceridemia
- ✰ Abdominal obesity

Mechanisms by which Insulin Resistance Influence Lipoproteins

Insulin resistance can influence lipoprotein metabolism in a variety of ways (Table 8.7). Insulin stimulates the expression of the gene for apoA-1, the major protein of HDL (Murao *et al.*, 1998). Thus insulin resistance may limit the production of apoA-1. Furthermore, free unsaturated fatty acids are increased by insulin resistance; they reduce the expression of ATP cassette transporter A1 (ABCA1) in hepatocytes. They do this by preventing oxysterols from binding to liver X receptor α, a key nuclear transcription factor (Ou *et al.*, 2001; Uchara *et al.*, 2002).

Table 8.7: Influences of Insulin Resistance on Lipoprotein Metabolism

Primary Effect	*Impact on Lipoproteins*
VLDL Metabolism	
↑ Flux of FFA to liver	↑ Secretion of TG and increased VLDL apo B-100 secretion
↓ Adipose tissue LPL activity	↓ Clearance of VLDL from circulation
LDL Metabolism	
↑ Secretion of VLDL apo B-100	↑ LDL synthesis (because of increased precursor)
↓ Adipose tissue LPL activity	↓ Conversion of VLDL to LDL
↓ LDL receptor activity	↓ Clearance of LDL from plasma
HDL Metabolism	
↑ Hypertriglyceridemia	↑ HDL catabolism by mechanisms involving CETP
↑ Hepatic TGL activity	↑ Catabolism of HDL, TG, and PPL
↓ LPL activity	↓ HDL synthesis due to reduced production of "surface remnants" of VLDL and CM

Abbreviations: apo, apolipoprotein; CETP, cholesteryl ester transfer protein; CM, chylomicron; FFA,free fatty acid; HDL, high-density lipoprotein; LDL, low-density lipoprotein; LPL, lipoprotein lipase; PPL, phospholipid, TG, triglyceride; TGL, triglyceride lipase; VLDL, very low-density lipoprotein.

In a transgenic mouse model, insulin resistance in skeletal muscle resulted in increased body fat and increased plasma levels of FFAs and of TGs (Moller *et al.*, 1996). Thus, insulin resistance per se can influence lipoprotein physiology.

Although we speak of insulin resistance, much of the impact of insulin on lipoprotein physiology is mediated by hyperinsulinism and an increased insulin effect. In obesity and other insulin-resistant states, resistance develops to the glucose-regulatory effects of insulin, which are mediated via IRS-2, a component of the glucose-regulatory system in the liver. However, resistance does not develop to most of the lipid-regulatory effects of insulin, which are mediated via sterol regulatory element binding proteins (Shimomura *et al.*, 2000).

Insulin resistance affects the metabolism of TG-rich lipoproteins (VLDL and chylomicrons). Crucial events are effects on hormone-sensitive lipase (HSL), the enzyme responsible for hydrolysis of TG stores in adipose tissue, and LPL, the enzyme responsible for hydrolysis of TG in circulating VLDL and chylomicrons. HSL is suppressed by insulin. Thus in insulin-resistant states, lipolysis in adipose tissue is stimulated, and there is an increased flux of FFA to the liver. This provides substrate for synthesis of TG and leads to the secretion of increased amounts of VLDL, TG and apoB-100 by the liver.

Furthermore, LPL activity is stimulated by insulin, therefore, in insulin-resistant states, adipose tissue activity of LPL is reduced, and the clearance of VLDL and chylomicrons from the circulation is retarded.

Some metabolic effects of insulin resistance increase LDL levels, while other effects of insulin resistance reduce LDL levels:

- ✰ Enhanced secretion of apo B-100 in VLDL provides increased precursor for the production of LDL.
- ✰ Reduced LPL activity slows the conversion of VLDL to LDFL and may result in reduced production of LDL.
- ✰ Reduced activity of LDL receptors leads to retarded clearance of LDFL from plasma and increases LDL levels (insulin stimulates LDL receptor activity).

Insulin resistance can reduce HDL levels by several mechanisms. As detailed above, insulin resistance and the consequent increase in plasma concentrations of FFAs will reduce HDL levels by reducing the synthesis of apoA-1 and by reducing the expression of ABCA1. Increased plasma levels of TG-rich lipoproteins (generated as indicated above) will reduce HDL levels by mechanisms involving the cholesteryl ester transfer. Additionally, insulin-resistant states are associated with elevated activity of hepatic TG lipase, and this may speed the catabolism of HDL in plasma. The reduced activity of adipose tissue LPL seen with insulin resistance may lead to reduced synthesis of HDL. A portion of the synthesis of HDL is attributed to the production of "surface remnants" of TG-rich lipoproteins by the action of LPL.

Diabetes Mellitus and Coronary Risk

Diabetes carries with it a great burden of atherosclerotic risk. In 1974, the 16-year follow-up experience of the Framingham Study was reported, the risk of CHD death among diabetics was 3.2 times that of nondiabetics. The increased risk persists after adjustment is made for other known risk factors, and the impact of diabetes on relative risk of CHD is greater for women than for men. Diabetes eliminates the female advantage in CHD rates. The increased relative risk imposed by diabetes in women appears to be due at least in part to increased risk in women with low HDL-c ($\leq$50 mg/dL) and/or high VLDL-c ($\geq$20 mg/dL) levels (Goldschmid *et al.*, 1994).

In the Nurses' Health Study (Manson *et al.*, 1991), of 116,117 women who were followed prospectively for 8 years, the risk of nonfatal MI and CHD death among diabetics was 6.7 times that for nondiabetics. Risk of nonfatal MI for those treated with oral hypoglycemic agents (relative risk {RR} 8.7) was similar to that for those treated with insulin (RR 8.2), it was somewhat lower for those treated with diet alone (RR 5.7), probably reflecting reduced severity of disease.

Coronary heart disease mortality in diabetics has been reported to be markedly elevated, being 50 per cent to 100 per cent of that seen in patients with a prior MI (Lotufo *et al.*, 2001; Whiteley *et al.*, 2005). This provides some of the rationale for particularly energetic management of risk factors in diabetics.

Even mild, asymptomatic hyperglycemia leads to increased coronary risk. When serum glucose repeatedly exceeds 200 mg/dL in individuals without previously known diabetes within 1 hour after a 50-g oral glucose challenge, the 19-year risk of CHD death increases 2.4-fold compared with those with lower serum glucose levels (Vaccaro *et al.*, 1992).

Atherogenic disorders of plasma lipoproteins have been associated with asymptomatic hyperglycemia, diagnosed type 1 diabetes, and type 2 diabetes. The major lipoprotein abnormalities of type 2 diabetes are low HDL concentrations, high TG concentrations, and prevalence of small, dense LDL (Table 8.8). These abnormalities and their pathophysiology are very similar to what is seen in nondiabetics with insulin-resistant states.

Table 8.8: Lipoprotein Abnormalities Characteristic of Type 2 Diabetes

- ✰ Hypertriglyceridemia (high very low-density lipoprotein)
- ✰ Low high-density lipoprotein cholesterol concentration
- ✰ Small, dense low-density lipoprotein (LDL)
- ✰ Glycosylated LDL

Additionally, glycosylation of lipoproteins in diabetics may enhance the atherogenicity of lipoproteins. Data from NHANES II clearly show a tendency to lower HDL cholesterol levels and higher fasting TG levels in patients with type 2 diabetes. This is seen in both men and women, and in blacks and whites.

Type 2 diabetes is strongly associated with a predominance of atherogenic small, dense LDL particles (LDL subclass phenotype B). This association is at least partially a result of hypertriglyceridemia in type 2 diabetes, in men, but not in women, the association of type 2 diabetes with small, dense LDL could be entirely accounted for on the basis of hypertriglyceridemia (Austin and Edwards, 1996).

A different pattern is apparent for type I diabetes in the recent data from the Diabetes Control and Complications. Trial (DCCT) in an analysis involving over 1500 patients, the lipid and lipoprotein levels in people with type 1 diabetes were found to be similar to those in the general population (DCCT Research Group, 1992). Previous studies, however, have shown increased LDL levels, low HDL levels, and high TG levels in association with poorly controlled type 1 diabetes (Howard, 1987). The better lipoprotein profiles seen in the more current DCCT data may be caused by:

- ☆ A secular trend toward improved glycemic control
- ☆ Altered dietary recommendations for diabetics with a current emphasis on restriction of cholesterol and saturated fats
- ☆ Increased use of lipid-lowering medication

In untreated type 1 diabetes, a deficiency of LPL causes reduced clearance of VLDL and chylomicrons, thus plasma levels of these TG-rich lipoproteins are markedly increased. FFA levels in plasma are high because of increased activity of hormone-sensitive lipase, the enzyme responsible for hydrolysis of stores of TG in adipose tissue; this enzyme is suppressed by insulin. When insulin is present in the small amount sufficient to allow hepatic lipogenesis and protein synthesis, the increased FFA flux to the liver provides substrate for production of VLDL, and VLDL secretion is increased.

Hyperglycemia, whether due to type 1 or type 2 diabetes, leads to glycosylation of LDL, and this may be atherogenic (Table 8.9). Recognition of glycosylated LDL by the LDL receptor is impaired. Thus glycosylated LDL is cleared more slowly from plasma than is native LDL and clearance by atherogenic, non-LDL receptor pathways is greater for glycosylated LDL. Macrophages internalize glycosylated LDL at an enhanced rate; thus the glycosylation of LDL fosters the formation of foam cells. Glycosylated LDL is immunogenic, and diabetics have been shown to have circulating complexes of immunoglobulins with glycosylated LDL. These immune complexes are internalized by macrophages in unregulated fashion favoring the formation of foam cells. Additionally, glycosylated LDL has been shown to foster platelet aggregation.

Table 8.9: Glycosylation of LDL Potential Atherogenic Effects

- ☆ Impaired recognition by low-density lipoprotein (LDL) receptor
- ☆ Enhanced uptake by macrophages
- ☆ Stimulation of platelet aggregation
- ☆ Glycosylated LDL is immunogenic

Women, Lipids, and CHD

Approximately 50 per cent of all deaths from CHD occur in women. The onset of CHD in women occurs, on average, about 10 years later than in men. As women age, however, the rates of CHD increase; in the postmenopausal woman, the risk from CHD and stroke far exceeds that from cancer. Risk factors in women are similar to those seen in men, although there are some important differences.

HDL-c is a major risk factor in women, and low HDL-c levels are important predictors of CHD mortality in older women. Lp(a) levels in some, but not all, studies are a risk factor for premature CHD. Certainly Lp(a) levels rise after the menopause.

Estrogen status must be strongly considered because of the important effects of estrogen not only on the lipid profile, but also on the vessel wall and other risk factors. After menarche, women have higher HDL-c levels than men of similar ages. When women enter the menopause, they often have a rise in weight, higher levels of LDL-c, and lower levels of HDL-c. Oral estrogen therapy improves LDL-c and HDL-c. One study showed that oral therapy with 2 mg of micronized estradiol or 0.625 mf of conjugated estrogens lowered LDL-and raised HDL-c by 14 per cent to 16 per cent (Walsh *et al.*, 1993). The decrease in LDL particles results from accelerated catabolism. TGs rise even more with oral estrogens therapy; this seems to reflect the production of large TG-rich particles of very low-density lipoprotein (VLDL).

Progestins and estrogen have essentially opposite actions as far as the lipid profile is concerned (although if given alone, some progestins can lower HDL-c and LDL-c together). In addition, those progestins with more androgenic activity lower HDL-c more. In the Postmenopausal Estrogen/Progestin Intervention (PEPI) trial, however, micromized progesterone actually improved HDL-c. Finally, there is great concern about the negative effects of progestin on the arterial wall and the oxidation of LDL.

Oral contraceptives have evolved to offer reduced doses of estrogen and progestin. It appears that the relative risk of CV disease is not increased by past use. Yet, oral contraceptives may affect the lipid profile adversely. Obese women with a familial lipid disorder might develop severely elevated TG levels. Women with multiple risk factors for CHD who take a formulation whose progestin has high androgenic activity can have their HDL-c values lowered.

To look at this aspect, it is useful to divide women into three categories based on coronary risk.

- ☆ Those who are healthy and at low risk (most premenopausal women)
- ☆ Those who have ≥2 risk factors (many of these have the metabolic syndrome)
- ☆ Those with known CHD or "CHD risk equivalents".

A recent evidence-based guideline for coronary disease prevention in women converts this into four categories (Table 8.10).

Table 8.10: Evidence-Based Guidelines for Disease Prevention in Women

Risk Group	*Framingham Global Risk*	*Clinical Examples*
High risk	>20 per cent	CAD, noncoronary forms of atherosclerosis, chronic kidney disease
Intermediate risk	10-20 per cent	Coronary calcification, metabolic syndrome, multiple risk factors, markedly elevated levels of a single risk factor, first-degree relatives with premature CHD (age <55 in men and <65 in women)
Lower risk	<10 per cent	May include women with multiple risk factors, metabolic syndrome, or ≤1 risk factor
Optimal risk	<10 per cent	Optimal levels of risk factors and heart-healthy lifestyles

Abbreviations: CAD- coronary artery disease; CHD -congestive heart disease.

Modified from Mosca L. *et al.*, 2004. J. Am. Coll. Cardiol. 43: 900-921.

In the lower-risk categories, careful review of primary prevention trials shows no compelling evidence that treatment of high cholesterols reduces total mortality. Within this essentially low-risk group, however, may reside women with FH. For middle-aged women with FH and one risk factor, aggressive treatment of the hypercholesterolemia is actually cost-effective (Goldman *et al.*, 1993). Moreover, weight gain after 18 years of age leads to increased risk of CHD, for women in this group, therapeutic lifestyle change (TLC), regular exercise, and smoking cessation would seem to be prudent (Manson *et al.*, 1995).

The above advice is also important for those women with two or more risk factors for CHD but no evidence of overt CHD. This group includes women with the metabolic syndrome with its characteristic clustering of metabolic risk factors. Framingham investigators showed that clusters of three or more risk factors occurred at twice the rate as predicted by chance (Wilson *et al.*, 1999). Moreover, a 5-lb (2.25-kg) weight increase over the 16 year observation period was associated with a marked increase in risk factor sum as well as CHD risk (Table 8.11).

Table 8.11: Multiple Risk Factors in Framingham, Experience in Men and Women Aged 18 to 74 Years

	Men (per cent) (n=2406)	*Women (per cent) (n=2569)*
Weight increase 5 lb (2.25 kg)		
Risk-factor sum	20*	37†
Clusters of ≥3 risk factors	2.39†	5.9†

*$P = 0.002$; † $P < 0.001$.

Source: Wilson FW, *et al.*, 1999. Arch Intern Med. 159:1104-1109.

Use of Framinghan Tables for Assessment of Major Risk Factors Causing CHD

In the ATP III, diabetics (both types 1 and 2) are regarded as having a CHD risk equivalent and so no longer appear in the tally of risk factors that determine LDL-c goals.

Table 8.12: Major Risk Factors

- ☆ Cigarette smoking (in the past month)
- ☆ Hypertension (BP ≥140/90 mm Hg or taking antihypertensive medication)
- ☆ Low HDL-c (<40 mg/dL)*
- ☆ Family history of premature CHD (CHD in male, first-degree relative <55 years or in female, first-degree relative < 65 years)
- ☆ Age (men ≥45 years, women ≥55 years)

Abbreviations BP- blood pressure; CHD- coronary heart disease; HDL-c -high-density lipoprotein cholesterol.

* HDL-c >60 mg/dL, counts as a "negativ≥ risk factor, its presence reduces the tally of risk factors by one.

i) How to Assess 10-Year CHD Risk

If two or more major risk factors are present, special Framinghan tables designed for use by the ATP III (Tables 8.13 and 8.14) can be used to assess 10-year (near-term) "hard" CHD risk. There are three levels of risk:

- ☆ Highest risk: >20 per cent CHD risk equivalent
- ☆ Intermediate: 10 per cent to 20 per cent
- ☆ Low risk: <10 per cent

ATP III has a web site that allows downloading of an Excel-based spreadsheet to calculate risk as a continuous function. Also there is a Palm application that allows calculation on a handheld device using this software: (http: www.nhlbi.nih/gov).

> **Clinical Tip:** The 10-year "hard" CHD risk determined by the Framingham table cannot be as accurate as the continuous function that calculates risk when you use the spreadsheet calculator or the Palm application. This become apparent when you use values close to the end points.

Table 8.13: Farmingham Point Scores Estimate of 1-Year Risk for Men

Age (Years)	*Points*
20-34	–9
35-39	–4
40-44	0
45-49	3
50-54	6
55-59	8
60-64	10
65-69	11
70-74	12
75-79	13

Points by Age (years)

TC (mg/dL)	*20-39*	*40-49*	*50-59*	*60-69*	*70-79*
<160	0	0	0	0	0
160-199	4	3	2	1	0
200-239	7	5	3	1	0
240-279	9	6	4	2	1
≥280	11	8	5	3	1
Nonsmoker	0	0	0	0	0
Smoker	8	5	3	1	1

Contd...

Table 8.13–*Contd...*

HDL (mg/dL)	Points
≥60	–1
50-59	0
40-49	1
<40	2

Systolic BP (mm Hg)	Points	
	Untreated	Treated
<120	0	0
120-129	0	1
130-139	1	2
140-159	1	2
≥160	2	3

Point Total	10-Year Risk (per cent)
<0	<1
0	1
1	1
2	1
3	1
4	1
5	2
6	2
7	3
8	4
9	5
10	6
11	8
12	10
13	12
14	16
15	20
16	25
≥17	≥30

Abbreviations: BP, blood pressure, HDL, high-density lipoprotein; TC, total cholesterol

Source: Executive Summary of the Third Report of the NCEP Expert Panel on Detection, Evaluation, and Treatment of High Blood Cholesterol in Adults (ATP III). JAMA 2001; 285: 2486-2497.

Table 8.14: Farmingham Point Scores Estimate of 10-Year Risk for Women

Age (Years)	*Points*
20-34	–7
35-39	–3
40-44	0
45-49	3
50-54	6
55-59	8
60-64	10
65-69	12
70-74	14
75-79	16

Points by Age (years)

TC (mg/dL)	*20-39*	*40-49*	*50-59*	*60-69*	*70-79*
<160	0	0	0	0	0
160-199	4	3	2	1	1
200-239	8	6	4	2	1
240-279	11	8	5	3	2
≥280	13	10	–	4	2
Nonsmoker	0	0	0	0	0
Smoker	9	7	4	2	1

HDL (mg/dL)	*Points*
≥60	–1
50-59	0
40-49	1
<40	2

Systolic BP (mm Hg)	*Points*	
	Untreated	*Treated*
<120	0	0
120-129	1	3
130-139	2	4
140-159	3	5
≥160	4	6

Contd...

Table 8.14–*Contd...*

Point Total	*10-Year Risk (per cent)*
<9	<1
9	1
10	1
11	1
12	1
13	2
14	2
15	3
16	4
17	5
18	6
19	8
20	11
21	14
22	17
23	22
24	27
≥25	≥30

Abbreviations: BP- blood pressure; HDL- high-density lipoprotein; TC- total cholesterol

Source: Executive Summary of the Third Report of the NCEP Expert Panel on Detection, Evaluation, and Treatment of High Blood Cholesterol in Adults (ATP III). JAMA 2001;285:2486-2497.

ii) Risk Category

Determine risk category and hence goals and LDL-c levels at which therapeutic lifestyle change is initiated (Table 8.15). The goals for the categories are similar to ATP II with a few important differences:

Highest Risk (Those with CHD and Coronary Artery Disease (CAD) Risk Equivalents)

The primary goal is an LDL-c <100 mg/dL: If this is attained, and TGs are ≥200 mg/dL, then a secondary goal of a non-HDL-c <130 should be sought.

The guidelines were updated in July 2004 (Grundy *et al.*, 2004) to indicate that certain patients felt to be very high risk could have an LDL-c goal of <70 mg/dL. This is optional because complete data is not at hand; several ongoing clinical trials will soon provide further information to guide decisions.

Patients to be considered for an LDL-c goal <70 mg/dL include those with established cardiovascular disease (CVD) and

- ☆ Acute coronary syndrome

Table 8.15: LDL Cholesterol Goals and End Points for Therapeutic Lifestyle Changes and Drug Therapy in Different Risk Categories*

Risk Category	*LDL-c Goal*	*Initiate TLC*	*Consider Drug Therapy*
High Risk			
CHD* or CHD risk equivalents‡ (10-year risk 20 per cent)	<100 mg/dL, (optional goal: 70 mg/dL) ¶	≥ 100 mg/dL§	≥100 mg/dL¶ (100 mg/dL consider drug options)†
Moderately High Risk			
2 risk factors(10-year risk 10 per cent-20 per cent)	130 mg/dL**	≥130 mg/dL §	≥130 mg/dL (100-129 mg/dL, consider drug options) ‡‡
Moderate Risk			
2 risk factors(10-year risk 10 per cent)	130 mg/dL	≥130 mg/dL	≥160mg/dL
Lower Risk			
0-1 risk factors §§	160mg/dL	≥160mg/dL	≥190mg/dL (160-189 mg/dL, # -lowering drug optional)

Abbreviations: BP- blood pressure; CHD- congestive heart disease; HDL- high-density lipoprotein; HDL-c- HDL cholesterol; LDL- low-density lipoprotein; LDL-c- LDL, cholesterol; TLC- therapeutic lifestyle changes

* CHD includes history of myocardial infarcation, unstable angina, stable angina, coronary artery procedures (angioplasty or bypass surgery) or evidence of clinically significant myocardial ischemia

† When LDL-lowering drug therapy is employed, it is advised that intensity of therapy be sufficient to achieve at least a 30 per cent to 40 per cent reduction in LDL-c levels.

‡ CHD risk equivalents include clinical manifestations of noncoronary forms of atherosclerotic disease (peripheral arterial disease; abdominal aortic aneurysm, and carotid artery disease [transient ischemic attacks or stroke of carotid origin or >50 per cent obstruction of a carotid artery D, diabetes, and 2 risk factors with 10-year risk for hard CHD 20 per cent.

§ Any person at high risk or moderately high risk who has lifestyle-related risk factors (*e.g.* Obesity, physical inactivity, elevated triglyceride, low HDL-c, or metabolic syndrome) is a candidate for TLC to modify these risk factors regardless of LDL-c level.

|| If baseline LDL-c is <100 mg/dL, institution of an LDL-lowering drug is a therapeutic option on the basis of available clinical trial results if a high-risk person has high triglycerides or low HDL-c, combining a fibrate or nicotinic acid with an LDL-lowering drug can be considered.

¶ Very high risk favors the optional LDL-c goal of 70 mg/dL, and in patients with high triglycerides, non HDL-c 100 mg/dL.

\# Risk factors include cigarette smoking, hypertension (BP ≥140/90mm Hg or on antihypertensive medication), low HDL cholesterol (<40 mg/dL), family history of premature CHD (CHD in male first-degree relative <55 years of age: CHD in female first-degree relative <65 years of age), and age (men ≥45 years; women ≥55 years)

** Optional LDL-c goal <100 mg/dL.

†† Electronic 10-year risk calculators are available at www.nhlbi.nih.gov/guidelines/cholesterol.

‡‡ For moderately high-risk persons, when LDL-c level is 100 to 129 mg/dL, at baseline or on lifestyle therapy, initiation of an LDL- lowering drug to achieve an LDL-c level <100 mg/dL is a therapeutic option on the basis of available clinical trial results.

§§ Almost all people with zero or 1 risk factor have a 10-year risk <10 per cent, and 10-year risk assessment in people with zero or 1 risk factor is thus not necessary

Source: Grundy SM, *et al.*, Circulation, 2004:110:227-239

- ☆ Multiple metabolic risk factors, such as diabetes
- ☆ Metabolic syndrome
- ☆ Severe or uncorrected risk factors, such as cigarette smoking

Moderately High Risk (Two or More Risk Factors and 10-Year CHD Risk of 10 per cent to 20 per cent)

The primary goal is an LDL-c <130 mg/dL as before but certain factors may suggest a lower goal of <100 mg/dL; these include:

- ☆ Continued cigarette smoking
- ☆ Strongly positive family history of premature atherosclerotic CVD
- ☆ High TG >200 mg/dL plus non-HDL-c >160 mg/dL
- ☆ Low HDL-c <40 mg/dL
- ☆ Metabolic syndrome
- ☆ Emerging risk factors, such as:
- ☆ High-sensitivity C-reactive protein (CRP) >3 mg/L
- ☆ Coronary calcium ≥75th age and gender percentile

Moderate Risk (Two or More Risk Factors and 10-Year CHD Risk of <10 per cent)

The LDL-c goal is still <130 mg/dL.

Lower Risk (Zero to one Risk Factors and 10-Year CHD Risk Almost Always < 10 per cent)

The LDL-c goal is < 160 mg/dL and Framingham risk assessment is usually not required. Drug therapy can be considered for those with LDL-c >190 mg/dL after secondary causes have been ruled out and a trial of therapeutic lifestyle change considered. In this category are young patients with heterozygous familial hypercholesterolemia.

> Clinical Tip: The increase in CHD risk with age presents an opportunity for tests of subclinical atherosclerosis (ankle-brachila index, computed to-mography [CT] of the coronaries for calcium) to help the clinician decide whether the expected increased coronary atherosclerosis based on the Framingham risk score with age is truly present in certain cases.

Although this approach is rational and quite useful, there are situations in which additional data are available or considered worth obtaining in order to justify more aggressive efforts at therapy. ATP III recognizes emerging factors (Table 8.16) that affect risk to varying degrees and may be considered after the ATP III algorithm has been used to help guide intensity of risk-reduction therapy.

Initiate Therapeutic Lifestyle Change

ATP III does define as life-habit risk factors the following:

- Atherogenic diet (high in saturated fats, cholesterol, extra calories)
- Physical inactivity
- Overweight and obesity

For those not at the very highest level of risk (CHD and CHD risk equivalents), undertaking Therapeutic Lifestyle Change (TLC) for 3 months and then rechecking LDL-c is recommended.

Table 8.16: Emerging Risk Factors: Lack of Definite Evidence of an Independent Contribution

- Lp(a)
- Homocysteine
- Prothrombotic risk factors (plasminogen-activator inhibitor-1 [PAI-1], fibrinogen)
- Inflammatory markers
- Impaired fasting glucose
- Subclinical atherosclerosis (noninvasive assessment)
  - Carotid imaging with intimal-medial thickness
  - Computed tomography (CT) scan of coronary arteries for calcium
  - Ankle-brachial index

Source: Smith SC, *et al.*, Circulation, 2000: 101:111-116.

Drug Therapy

Consider adding drug therapy if LDL-c exceeds levels shown in Table 8.6. This means considering drug therapy simultaneously with TLC for CHD and CHD risk equivalents if LDL-c is >130 mg/dL or after 3 months for other risk categories.

Metabolic Syndrome

Identify the metabolic syndrome, if present (Table 8.17). One of the new features of ATP III is the emphasis on those with multiple (>2) risk factors. These individuals may have 10-year rates of hard CHD exceeding those with known CHD, and they deserve to have similar goals of therapy and end points for initiation of TLC and drug therapy. In Framingham, atherogenic risk-factor clustering was common and associated with a striking increase of CHD risk for those with ≥3 risk factors. Looking at age-specific quintiles for total cholesterol, TGs, HDL-c, body mass index, glucose, and systolic blood pressure:

- Males: relative risk (RR) 2.39 (confidence interval [CI] 1.6-3.4)
- Females: RR 5.9 (CI 2.5-13.7)

Table 18.17: Clinical Identification of the Metabolic Syndrome*

Risk Factor	*Defining Level*
Abdominal obesity †‡	Men ≥102 cm (≥40 in)
Women ≥88 cm (≥35 in)	
Triglycerides §	≥150 mg/dL
HDL-c §	Men <40 mg/dL
Women <50 mg/dL	
Blood pressure §	≥130 or ≥85 mm Hg
Fasting glucose	≥100 mg/dL

* Any three of the five risk factors constitutes a diagnosis of the metabolic syndrome

† Measure waist circumference on the right at the top of the iliac crest perpendicular to the floor at the end of a nominal expiration; tape should be snug, but not compress the skin.

‡ Some US adults of non-Asian origin (*e.g.* White, Black, Hispanic) with marginally increased waist circumference (*e.g.* 94-101 cm [37-39 inches] in men and 80-87 cm [31-34 inches] in women) may have strong genetic contribution to insulin resistance and should benefit from changes in lifestyle habits, similar to men with categorical increases in waist circumference. Lower waist circumference cutpoint (*e.g.* ≥90 cm [35 inches] in men and ≥80 cm [31 inches] in women) appears to be appropriate for Asian Americans.

§ Having risk factor or on therapy for this abnormality

Source: Adapted from: Grundy S.M. *et al.*, Circulation, 2005; 112:2735-2752

After adjustment for age and obesity level, a 2.25 kg (5-lb) weight increase over 16 years in this cohort was associated with a highly significant increased tally of risk factors in men (+20 per cent) and women (+37 per cent). Not surprisingly, a 2.25 kg (5-lb) weight loss was associated with a decreased risk factor tally in men (-48 per cent) and women (-40 per cent) as well (Wilson *et al.*, 1999). Thus, identification of those with multiple metabolic risk factors culls out, so to speak, a very high-risk group for subsequent CHD.

ATP III recognizes that there is a constellation of major risk factors (low HDL-c, hypertension), life-habit risk factors (atherogenic diet, physical inactivity, overweight and obesity), and emerging risk factors [impaired fasting glucose, plasminogen-activator inhibitor-1 (PAI-1), ultrasensitive C-reactive protein (CRP)] that is overrepresented among populations with CHD. A clue to this high-risk clinical syndrome is a distinctive body type with increased abdominal circumference, suggesting increased visceral fat.

Thinking of an aggregation of several risk factors as a 'metabolic syndrome' is useful clinically, because it is very difficult to accurately assess the independent contributions of all of the elements that comprise this diagnosis in an individual (Grundy, 1997). Although insulin resistance is at the core of the factors that comprise this syndrome, there probably is a multifactorial etiology resulting from:

- Abdominal (visceral) obesity
- Physical inactivity

- ☆ High intakes of calories and cholesterol-raising nutrients
- ☆ Aging
- ☆ Genetic factors

Small amounts of weight loss, preferably through intensified weight management and increased physical activity, can improve this high-risk state. Treatment, however, should extend to the nonlipid risk factors associated with this syndrome as well (Figure 8.1). These include:

- ☆ Treatment of hypertension (angiotensin-converting enzyme inhibitors [ACEs] or, if not tolerated, angiotensin receptor blockers [ARBs] may be particularly useful).
- ☆ Aspirin to reduce prothrombotic state
- ☆ Treatment of elevated TGs and/or low HDL-c

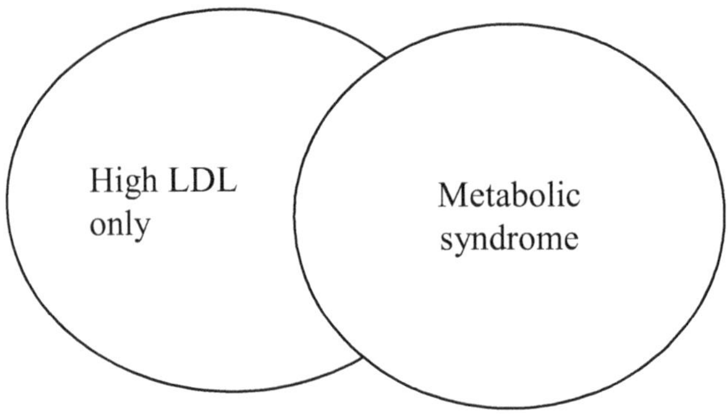

Figure 8.1: Extending Treatment to Those at Risk of a Metabolic Syndrome

Triglyceride Therapy

Treat the person if TGs are high (≥150 mg/dL), then consider low HDL-c. TGs have great variability and one should note any recent changes that can affect TG levels, such as:

- ☆ Weight change
- ☆ Change in diet, especially regarding consumption of carbohydrates
- ☆ Significant change in exercise status

If this is not a stable time, it may be prudent to have the individual return for a repeat fasting lipid panel in 4 weeks. Nonetheless, the ATP III has changed the end points for TGs to place a greater emphasis on hypertriglyceridemia (Table 8.18).

Treating a person with very high TGs can be a medical urgency. Health professionals should note that individuals with very high TGs are at risk for acute pancreatitis. This can come on suddenly in a person with TGs >500 mg/dL, typically occurring with one of the following scenarios:

Clinical Tip: Remember that accurate measurement of TGs requires the person to be fasting for 9 to 12 hours. Alcohol is preferably omitted for the 24 hours prior to the blood draw as well TG values are highly variable and a second blood draw is very helpful in getting a good baseline if the TGs are high. Severe elevations can be suspected when the plasma is creamy on blood draw or when there is a substantial creamy cap (supernatant) overlying the clear (infranatant) in blood that has been spun down and chilled in an upright test tube at 4°C. A very light topping of a creamy layer calls into question whether the patient was truly fasting!

- ☆ A spree of alcoholic and dietary excess
- ☆ A state of gradual insulin lack with increased intake of fat calories to compensate for glucose urinary losses
- ☆ A postmenopausal woman in whom unopposed estrogen (and rarely tamoxifen) is given (often after hysterectomy) in the setting of very high TGs.
- ☆ The third trimester of pregnancy in a woman who started the pregnancy with a very high TG level due to a previously unsuspected lipid disorder.

Table 8.18: The Adult Treatment Panel III Classification of Serum Triglycerides

Category	*Level of Fasting Triglycerides*	*Clinical Decisions*
Normal	<150 mg/dL	Encourage continued good diet and exercise
Borderline high	150-199 mg/dL	Improved diet and regular exercise can result in a small weight loss that can improve these values to <150 mg/dL
High	200-499 mg/dL	Once LDL-c goal has been reached, triglycerides at this level trigger non HDL-c as a secondary target
Very high	≥500 mg/dL	Patient is at risk for acute pancreatitis as well

Abbreviations: HDL-c, high-density lipoprotein cholesterol; LDL-c, low-density lipoprotein cholesterol

Source: Adapted from: Executive Summary of the Third Report of the NCEP Expert Panel on Detection, Evaluation, and Treatment of High Blood Cholesterol in Adults (ATP III). JAMA 2001; 285: 2486-2497

Clinical Tip: One of the few times that a nonfasting TG value is important is in the person with acute abdominal pain and the suspicion of acute pancreatitis. A tube of blood spun down and put in the refrigerator may show a creamy appearance indicative of chylomicron excess and the substrate for acute pancreatitis. This is important because often the amylase is artifactually low in hyperlipidemic pancreatitis.

Measures employed to reduce very high TGs include:

- ☆ Reduce intake of fat calories in marked fashion (<15 per cent of calories ingested should be from fat sources)
- ☆ Weight management and physical activity
- ☆ Consideration of a fibrate or nicotinic acid and possibly fish oil (≥3 grams)
- ☆ LDL-lowering therapy when TG levels are >500 mg/dL.

Treating the patient with high TGs is a secondary goal after the LDL-c goal is reached in ATP III. If TGs are in the 200-to 499-mg/dL range after the LDL-c goal is reached, consider adding drug therapy to reach the non-HDL goal (set 30 mg/dL above the LDL-c goal) (Table 8.19).

Table 8.19: Comparison of LDL-c and Non-HDL-c Goals for Three Risk Categories in Persons with Hypertriglyceridemia*

Risk Category	*LDL-c Goal (mg/dL)*	*Non-HDL-c Goal (mg/dL)*
CHD and CHD risk equivalent; 10-year risk for CHD > 20 per cent	<100	<130
Multiple (2+) risk factors and 10-year risk <20 per cent	<130	<160
Zero to one risk factor	<160	<190

* Triglycerides ≥ 200 mg/dL

To lower non-HDL-c to goal, there are two major pharmacologic options:

- ☆ Intensify therapy to reduce LDL-c
- ☆ Add nicotinic aid or fibrate to further lower VLDL

Caveat: Bile acid-binding resins should not be given if TGs exceed 250 mg/dL as they can elevate TGs

Borderline high TGs (150 to 199 mg/dL often respond to:

- ☆ Intensified weight management
- ☆ Increased emphasis on regular physical activity

Treating Low HDL

Treatment of persons with low HDL cholesterol (<40mg/dL) should be considered. Clinicians should remember that for most patients, behavioral strategies that lower TGs raise HDL-c. In individuals with isolated low HDL-c, particularly <25 mg/dL, the usual increase in HDL-c seen with weight loss, regular physical activity, smoking cessation, and lower carbohydrate intake may not occur. Nonethless, ATP III recommends the following sequence if low HDL-c is present:

- ✰ First reach LDL goal (potentially markedly effective in lowering CHD events in the setting of low HDL-c) (Table 8.15).
- ✰ Intensify weight management and increase physical activity.
- ✰ If TGs are 200 to 499 mg/dL, achieve non-HDL goal (30 mg/dL more than LDL-c goal) (Table 8.13); then consider nicotinic acid or fibrate if HDL-c remains low.
- ✰ If TGs are <200 mg/dL (isolated low HDL-c) in the presence of CHD or CHD equivalent, the clinician should consider nicotinic acid or fibrate.

Some have questioned whether HDL-c should be the primary target of therapy. Potent arguments in support of including HDL-c as a target of therapy (Boden, 2000) include:

- ✰ An inverse marker of risk for CHD in major epidemiologic studies
- ✰ The most potent lipid predictor in men and women >49 years of age (Framingham)
- ✰ For every 1 per cent increase in HDL-c with fibrate therapy, there was a 3 per cent reduction in all-cause mortality and MI (Veterans Affairs High-Density Lipoprotein Cholesterol Intervention Trial [VA HIT]
- ✰ HDL-c identifies those who benefit from statin therapy (in the AFCAPS/TexCAPS, a striking benefit from treatment was noted in 45 per cent of the participants if HDL-c ≤ 35 mg/dL at baseline)
- ✰ HDL-c serves as marker for identifying metabolic syndrome.

These arguments certainly justify HDL-c as a major, independent CHD risk factor. Those who do not include it as a target of therapy contend:

- ✰ All persons at risk for CHD deserve the behavioral changes that benefit HDL-c, such as:
  - Weight loss
  - Cessation of cigarette smoking
  - Regular physical activity
- ✰ Confusing epidemiologic data where some prospective studies show that the highest quintiles of HDL-c do not have the lowest risk for CHD
- ✰ Confusing relationship to CHD in genetic syndromes where low HDL-c is associated with reduced CHD risk (*e.g.* Apo A-1 Milano) or where higher values for HDL-c are associated with increased CHD (certain Japanese kindreds with cholesteryl ester transfer protein [CETP] deficiency).
- ✰ Confusing clinical trial data in which the VA HIT, utilizing gemfibrozil, showed a reduction in CHD with increased HDL-c, while the Bezafibrate Infarction Program (BIP), utilizing bezafibrate, did not, and HDL-c was increased significantly more in the latter trial.
- ✰ Difficulty with drug therapy in which HDL-c increases are not easily obtained. Niacin can raise HDL-c about 30 per cent, but statins and fibrates raise it less.

Chapter 9

Role of Polyunsaturated Fat in Cardiovascular Disease

Cardiovascular disease is often termed as 'lifestyle illness'. Several risk factors have been implicated in the etiology of atherosclerosis and ischemic heart disease. As explained in the previous chapter, these factors include the levels of various plasma constituents, especially lipoproteins, and the lifestyle patterns, personality traits, and genetic background of individuals. Some of these factors are modifiable, meaning that they can be changed, and include things like diet, exercise, obesity, smoking and stress. Other factors are non-modifiable and cannot be controlled, such as age, gender, race, ethnicity, family history etc. These aspects cannot be changed but knowing about them helps in the health assessment.

Indians have a higher rate of serious heart disease at a younger age. And, the major risk factors include-less physical activities, less consumption of fruits and vegetables, more consumption of deep fried foods which also lead to quite a bit of obesity and heart disease. Indians also have some different kinds of lipid abnormalities, which are more harmful. It is not sure whether it is genetic or it is because of the diet or life style. So, Indians have a bunch of these risk factors that put them at higher risks. In fact, currently one out of ten (10 per cent) of those between 45-60 years of age (males) in India have established heart diseases.

Among the dietary factors, intake of fats and oil matters a lot. It has been observed that total plasma cholesterol and VLDL and LDL concentrations have positive associations with subsequent incidence of heart disease, whereas HDL concentrations are negatively associated with risk. Risk is heightened by an increase in the ratio of total to HDL cholesterol.

Plasma Lipid Changes Associated With Diets Rich in Cholesterol and Saturated Fat

It is known from human feeding trials that an increase in dietary cholesterol is usually accompanied by an increase in the amount absorbed by the body. Increased absorption leads to higher levels of cholesterol in plasma and body pools. Generally, greater amounts of cholesterol in the diet raise the concentration of LDLs, although the mechanism remains unclear. The influx of excess dietary cholesterol to the liver may increase the production of LDLs. Although most data suggest that these lipoproteins arise largely from the degradation of VLDLs, it has been proposed that the liver may also secrete LDLs or lipoproteins that are quickly converted to LDLs directly in the plasma. It also has been suggested that increased dietary cholesterol augments the formation of abnormally large LDLs with an extra content of cholesterol. Both mechanisms may facilitate the increased deposition of cholesterol in arterial walls.

Plasma Lipid Changes Associated With Diets Rich in Polyunsaturated Fats

In feeding trials, the replacement of saturated fats and cholesterol in the diet by polyunsaturated fats from vegetable sources caused changes that are associated with a decreased risk of cardiovascular disease. Diets rich in saturated fat caused increases in plasma cholesterol; the consumption of polyunsaturated fats had the opposite effect. The cholesterol lowering effect of polyunsaturated fats is related to the magnitude of the difference between P/S ratios (polyunsaturated to saturated fatty acids) of the saturated and polyunsaturated fat diets and to the presence of cholesterol. With larger differences in P/S ratios, a greater drop in cholesterol concentration can be expected. When cholesterol is absent from diets, plasma cholesterol levels are less responsive to changes in the dietary P/S ratios.

Table 9.1: Common Biological Saturated Fatty Acids

Symbol	*Common Name*	*Systematic Name*	*Structure*	*mp(°C)*
12:0	Lauric acid	Dodecanoic acid	$CH_3(CH_2)_{10}COOH$	44.2
14:0	Myristic acid	Tetradecanoic acid	$CH_3(CH_2)_{12}COOH$	52
16:0	Palmitic acid	Hexadecanoic acid	$CH_3(CH_2)_{14}COOH$	63.1
18:0	Stearic acid	Octadecanoic acid	$CH_3(CH_2)_{16}COOH$	69.6
20:0	Arachidic aicd	Eicosanoic acid	$CH_3(CH_2)_{18}COOH$	75.4

The consumption of polyunsaturated fats reduce plasma cholesterol concentrations are still poorly understood. An increased faecal excretion of cholesterol and its derivatives often accompanies a fall in plasma cholesterol, perhaps representing the enhanced elimination of the cholesterol lost from the plasma compartment. A number of other potential mechanisms have also been suggested *i.e.*

a decrease in cholesterol absorption in the gut; a reduction in its synthesis by the body; a shift in its content from the plasma to other body components; changes in the rates of synthesis or catabolism of individual lipoproteins; depressed hepatic synthesis of fatty acids and triglycerides for LDLs; or an increase in the polyunsaturated fatty acid content of LDLs, which alters their structure so they only can accommodate a smaller quantity of cholesterol.

Dietary Polyunsaturated Fatty Acids

Recognition of a correlation between dietary fat and cardiovascular disease has led to dietary recommendations that advocate replacing dietary saturated fats and cholesterol with polyunsaturated fatty acids (PUFAs).

Table 9.2: Common Biological Unsaturated Fatty Acids

Symbol	*Common Name*	*Systematic Name*	*Structure*
16:1	Palmitoleic acid	Hexadecenoic acid	$CH_3(CH_2)_5CH{=}CH\text{-}(CH_2)_7COOH$
18:1	Oleic acid	9-Octadecenoic acid	$CH_3(CH_2)_7CH{=}CH\text{-}(CH_2)_7COOH$
18:2	Linoleic acid	9,12 -Octadecadienoic acid	$CH_3(CH_2)_4(CH{=}CHCH_2)_2$ $(CH_2)_6COOH$
18:3	Linolenic acid	9,12,15 -Octadecatrienoic acid	$CH_3CH_2(CH{=}CHCH_2)_3$ $(CH_2)_6COOH$
20:4 [5,8,11,14]	arachidonic acid	5,8,11,14- Eicosatetraenoic acid	$CH_3(CH_2)_4(CH{=}CHCH_2)_4$ $(CH_2)_2COOH$
20:5 [5,8,11,14,17]	EPA	5,8,11,14,17-Eicosapen-taenoic- acid	$CH_3CH_2(CH{=}CHCH_2)_5$ $(CH_2)_2COOH$
22:6 [4,7,10,13,16,19]	DHA	Docosohexaenoic acid	22:6w3

There are four families of polyunsaturated fatty acids derived from the parent fatty acids; linoleic acid (C_{18}:2n-6), α-linolenic acid (C_{18}:3n-3), oleic acid (C_{18}:1n-9), and palmitoleic acid (C_{16}:1n-7). The principal families of polyunsaturated fatty acids of major interest are the n-6 and n-3 families, characterized by the position of the first double bond (at the sixth and third carbon atom, respectively, counting from the methyl end of the carbon chain).

PUFAs and n-6 PUFAs are applied to omega-3 and omega-6 fatty acids, respectively. These fatty acids use the Greek alphabet (α,β,γ,.,ù) to identify the location of the double bonds. The "alpha" carbon is the carbon closest to the carboxyl group (carbon number 2), and the "omega" is the last carbon of the chain because omega is the last letter of the Greek alphabet. Linoleic acid is an omega-6 fatty acid because it has a double bond six carbons away from the "omega" carbon. Linoleic acid plays an important role in lowering cholesterol levels. Alpha-linolenic acid is an omega-3 fatty acid because it has a double bond three carbons away from the "omega" carbon. By subtracting the highest double-bond located in the scientific name from the number of carbons in the fatty acid we can obtain its classification. For arachidonic acid, we subtract 14 from 20 to obtain 6; therefore, it is an omega-6 fatty acid. This type of terminology is sometimes applied to oleic acid which is an omega-9 fatty acid. The two families derived from the n-6 and n-3 (ω3) polyunsaturated fatty acids, linoleic and α-linolenic acids (ω6), are known as the essential fatty acids. They cannot be synthesized by the human body and must be obtained from the diet. These two families of essential fatty acids have distinct nutritional and metabolic effects and they should be differentiated.

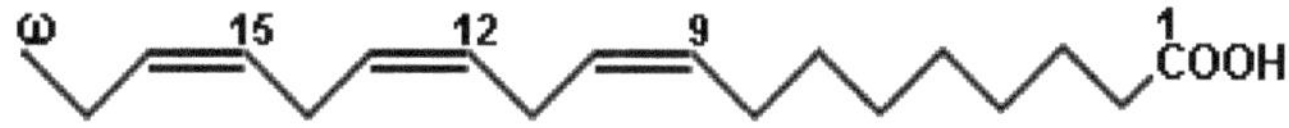

Alpha-Linolenic Acid (omega-3)

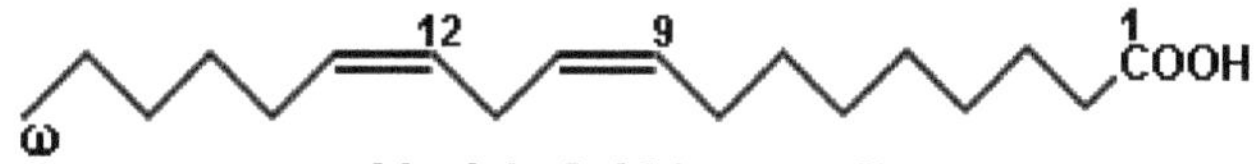

Linoleic Acid (omega-6)

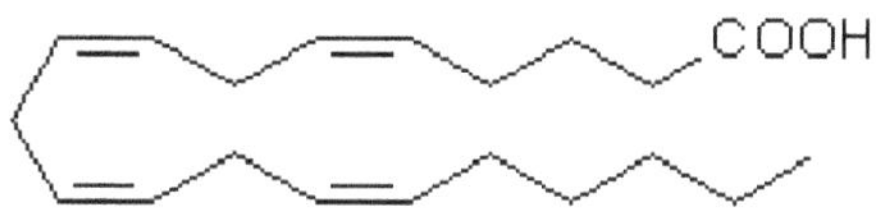

arachidonic acid

Linoleic and α-linolenic acids are furthermore the parent fatty acids for the directed precursors of the various classes of eicosanoids, dihomo-linolenic, arachidonic, and eicosapentaenoic acids. The other two families derived from palmitoleic and oleic acids are considered to be non-essential fatty acids, because humans can synthesize them from saturated fatty acid precursors. Interconversion among these four families of unsaturated fatty acids does not occur in humans. However, the enzymes for the desaturation and elongation reactions by which the parent fatty acids are converted to their derivative fatty acids are shared by all four families. The rates of desaturation and elongation differ among the families, and the rank of the families by order of decreasing rates is n-3 > n-6 > n-9 fatty acids. Evidence for this sequence *in vivo* in humans has been found. Thus, the amounts of fatty acids in our diet determine the competition among substrates and the relative rates of the desaturation-elongation reactions and finally influence cellular lipid metabolism.

Table 9.3: Major Classes of Fatty Acids and their Sources

Family	*Fatty Acids*	*Formula*	*Source*
Omega-9	Oleic acid	C16: 1	Olive oil, other vegetable oils, animal fats
Omega-6	Linoleic acid	C18: 2	Vegetable oils
Arachidonic acid		C20: 4	Poultry, meats
Omega-3	α-linolenic acid	C18:3	Marine and land plants
EPA		C20: 5	Marine oils and fish
DHA		C22: 6	Marine oils and fish
Saturated fats	Palmitic acid	C16: 0	Animal and vegetable fats
Stearic acid		C18: 0	Butter, lard, palm oil, palm kernel oil, coconut oil

Source: Messerli FH, 1996. Cardiovascular Drug Therapy, Second Edition, p. 1608.

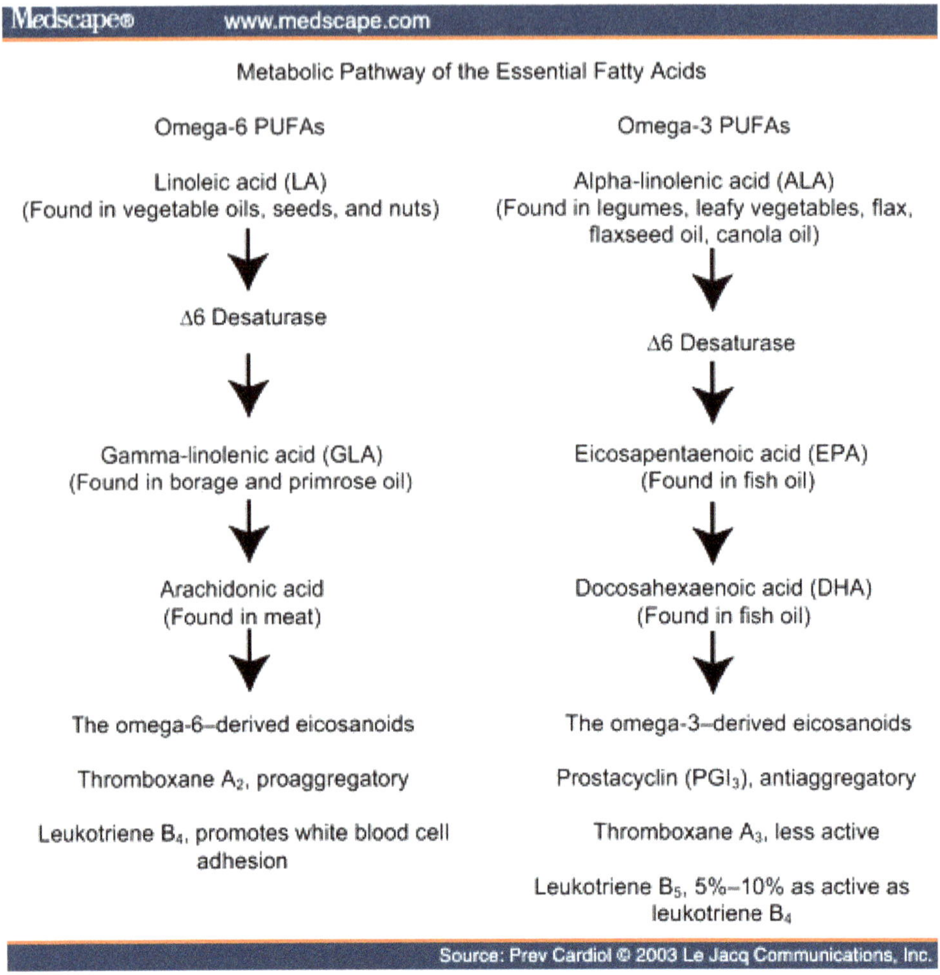

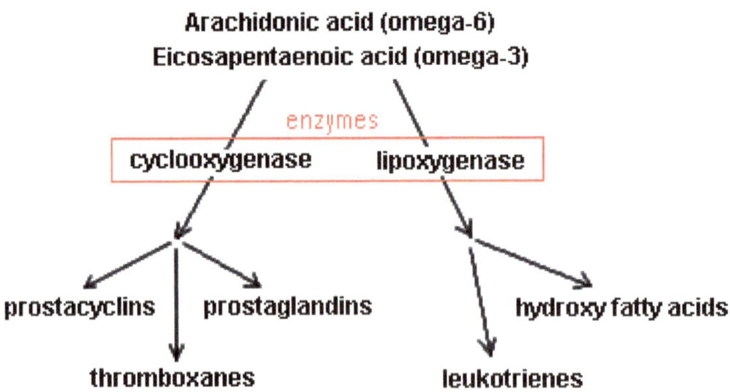

EPA and DHA also are derived from linolenic acid. Although linoleic acid competes with linolenic acid for the same enzymes in the desaturation and elongation reactions, the formation of arachidonic acid from linoleic acid is favoured.

Under normal conditions humans may generate about 1 mg of prostanoids per day, mainly from arachidonic acid, as estimated by urinary metabolites. Thus, all eicosanoids formed in the tissues of humans are generated from polyunsaturated fatty acids that must be derived from the diet.

Structure and Functions of EPA and DHA

The most common long chain Omega-3 PUFA fatty acids are known as EPA (eicosapentaenoic acid) and DHA (docosahexanoic acid). Eicosapentaenoic acid (EPA) is a member of the Omega-3 fatty acid family. EPA is required for the production of a special group of substances in the body called prostaglandins, which control blood clotting and other arterial functions.

EPA also provides a natural approach in lowering blood cholesterol and triglycerides. Thus, EPA is a direct source of an important substance called prostaglandin E_3. Prostaglandin E_3 is directly responsible for making blood platelets less sticky thus, leading to an easier flow of blood throughout our bodies. This means that EPA is intimately involved in bodily process that inhibit blood clots, particularly in the small capillaries of the heart.

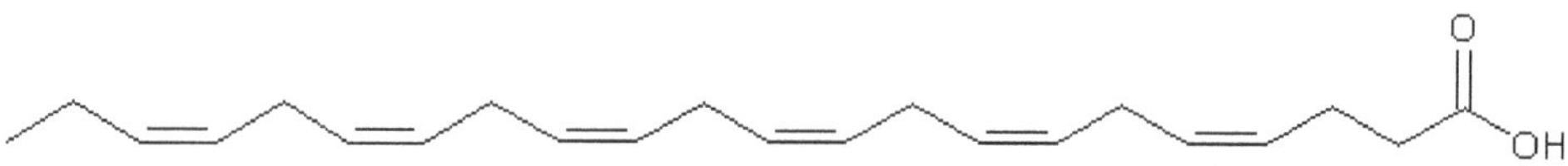

Docosahexaenoic Acid (DHA) (22:6 n-3)

Figure by RMB

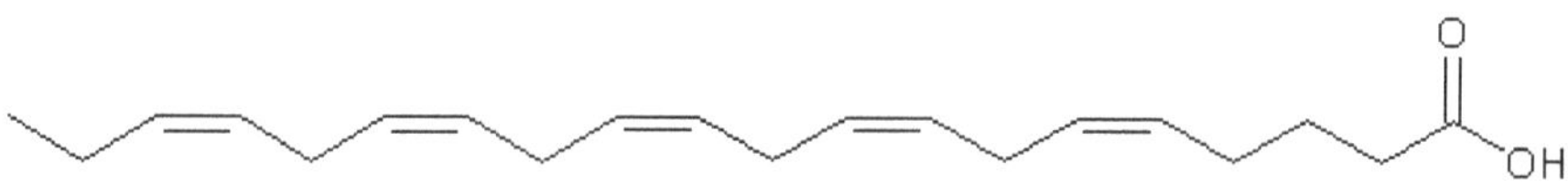

Eicosapentaenoic Acid (EPA) (20:5 n-3)

Figure by RMB

Structure of DHA and EPA

Due to the body's inability to synthesize EPA and DHA, it has to depend on external source. In early infancy and old age the body is not capable of producing adequate amounts of EPA and is true of people suffering from cardiovascular disorders, diabetes and peroxisomal disorders. As these fatty acids offer nutritional as well as medical benefits, it is recommended that the intake should be on regular basis.

DHA (Docosahexaenoic Acid)

Of almost equal importance, but not as widely researched is Docosahexaenoic acid (DHA). It comprises of a significant amount of the tissue, which makes up our brains as well as a large part of retina of eye.

Omega-3 Fatty Acids and Atherosclerosis

Mortality caused by atherosclerosis-related diseases accounts for more than 50 per cent of all morality in developed countries. The most prone diseases are

Effects of EPA

EPA is known to:

- ✰ Lower lipids – decrease TG, increase HDL
- ✰ Have an anti-thrombotic – decrease blood clotting effect
- ✰ Have an anti-arrhythmic effect
- ✰ Have an anti-inflammatory- via eicosanoids, weakens the effect of pro-inflammatory hormones

Effects of DHA

DHA is known to:

- ✰ Lower lipids – decreases TG, increases HDL
- ✰ Have anti-hypertensive effect – lowers blood pressure
- ✰ Have an anti-inflammatory effect- attacks early phase of effect inflammation, anti-chemotaxis
- ✰ Facilitate the normal growth – incorporated into membrane, development and function of the lipids of brain, nerves and eyes
- ✰ Improve the clinical symptoms – corrects abnormalities of depression and schizophrenia membrane PL-A_2, which is an essential component of the nervous system
- ✰ The importance of DHA and AA in infant nutrition is well established, and both substances are routinely added to infant formulas.

cardiovascular diseases like coronary heart disease and cerebral stork. Atherosclerosis is usually caused by life style related factors such as smoking, elevated blood lipids and hypertension, whereas hereditary factor is the most common cause.

The first traces of atherosclerosis formation may be found in children; it consists of fatty streaks beneath the endothelial layer of arteries containing lipid-filled macrophages. A high intake of Omega-3 fatty acids seems to prevent atherosclerosis. This has been documented in epidemiological studies and by intervention. Omega-3 fatty acids induce beneficial effects through several of the mechanisms that play a role in the development of the disease.

Omega-3 fatty acids have multiple effects which are very relevant for the prevention and treatment of atherosclerosis. The most potent effect is related to triglyceride reduction which will induce a shift from small, dense LDL-particle to normal LDL. This may offer a way of reducing oxidized LDL and reduce the inflammatory stimuli in the arterial wall.

Omega-3 also reduces the amount of adhesion molecules measured as soluble ICAM-1 and E-selectin. This is attributed to a reduction of the presentation of these molecules at the transcription level. A reduction of leukotriene B_4 which is regularly induced by Omega-3 could add to this effect. A reduction of oxidized LDL could also indirectly down-regulate the production of adhesion molecules.

Furthermore, Omega-3 increases the concentration of HDL which is responsible for the transportation of surplus cholesterol from the periphery back to the liver. A low level of HDL-C regularly coincides with hypertriglyceride and is related to increased coronary heart disease risk. Regarding the build-up of atherosclerotic thrombic Omega-3 fatty acids interfere with the aggregation phase of early thrombus formation preventing arterial occlusion with aspirin-like mechanisms. Omega-3 with multiple effects on causes and features relevant to atherosclerosis is an anti-atherosclerotic drug more than only a triglyceride-lowering drug.

Omega-3 fatty acids – Bare facts

- ☆ Polyunsaturated fatty acids (PUFAs) play a critical role in maintaining good health and ensuring normal development.
- ☆ PUFAs are made up of chains of fatty acids that differ in length and the number and position of double bonds. These differences determine PUFAs biological properties.
- ☆ Molecules with the first double bond between the third and fourth carbon atom from the methyl end are called Omega-3 or n-3 fatty acids. Those with a double bond between the sixth and seventh carbon atoms are known as Omega-6 or n-6 fatty acids.
- ☆ The most common long chain Omega-3 PUFA fatty acids are known as Eicosapentaenoic acid and DHA (Docosahexaenoic acid).
- ☆ We need to obtain two key PUFAs – Linoleic acid and alpha-linolenic acid – from our diets. These are the 'essential' fatty acids that the body converts into other PUFAs.
- ☆ Eating 200 to 300 g of oily fish weekly fulfills the dietary requirements. Some patients may need to increase their intake through supplements.
- ☆ Babies, pre-term infants and pregnant women need PUFAs to ensure normal development of the brain and other nerve tissues.
- ☆ People with a personal or family history of heart disease or circulatory problems may also benefit from a higher Omega-3 PUFA intake.
- ☆ People suffering from rheumatoid arthritis often find increasing consumption of Omega-3 PUFA reduces pain and stiffness.
- ☆ Omega-3 PUFAs may alleviate infantile seborrhoeic dermatitis and diaper dermatitis, also protect smokers from chronic obstructive pulmonary disease and reduce the likelihood of relapse in Crohn's disease.
- ☆ Still to be confirmed roles for PUFAs include treating pre-menstrual syndrome, diabetes, multiple sclerosis, migraine, depression and cancer.

By the same mechanism, Omega-3 also reduces the concentration of thromboxane thereby counteracting the vasoconstriction related to the formation of acute-thromboses. Lastly Omega-3 has antihypertensive effects in patients with arterial hypertension.

Omega-3 reduces morbidity and mortality associated with cardiovascular disorders, as numerous studies show that increased long-term intake of marine oils, rich in EPA and DHA reduces the morbidity and mortality associated with cardiovascular disorders in middle-aged men. It is generally agreed that Omega-3 fatty acids reduce the triglyceride levels in the blood by a reduced-synthesis and secretion of VLDL particles.

The influence of Omega-3 fatty acids on platelet aggregability at rather low doses, whereas significant effects on blood lipids and blood pressure can be achieved at higher doses. Recent data show that DHA produce a 30-40 per cent greater reduction in triglyceride levels in plasma than a corresponding amount of EPA. DHA also seems to have a more marked effect on increasing HDL-cholesterol, whereas EPA was found to slightly decrease both total cholesterol and APO-1 in normal subjects. Moreover, it is reported that DHA-rich oils are less active than EPA-rich oils on both fasting and post-prandial triglyceride levels. Positive correlation has been observed between supplementation with EPA and DHA and improvements in blood pressure and heart rates in subjects suffering from milk hypertension.

Even short time supplementation with large amounts or a combination of EPA and DHA has shown to have long-lasting effects on the human platelet aggregation, an effect suggested by inhibition of TXA_2/PGH_2 receptor by EPA and or DHA-sensitive mechanisms.

Recent data also show that DHA has more pronounced inhibitory effect on the expression of cytokines in endothelial cells, which clearly down regulate the inflammatory process and may inhibit the progression of atherosclerosis.

Omega-A Boon for Cardiac Patients

- ☆ Omega-3 are polyunsaturated fatty acids found almost exclusively in fish and shell fish. They have become a "hot topic" because they can reduce chance of heart attack in patients with heart disease.
- ☆ Omega-3 reduces the chances of having heart attack, even if we already have heart disease.
- ☆ It is reported that Omega-3 are vital from childhood to age old adults.
- ☆ The protective effects of Omega-3 were discovered by observing Eskimos who eat large amount of these polyunsaturated fatty acids in their foods.
- ☆ The Eskimos almost never developed heart disease. Thus, researchers looked for the link and found Omega-3 in fish oils.
- ☆ Omega-3 makes cardiac patients risk-free due to presence of EPA and DHA.

Epidemiological and clinical researches have shown that Omega-3 fatty acids intervene in the atherosclerotic process at all steps, and that there probably are synergistic effects of EPA and DHA at many levels.

Omega-3 PUFAs and Plasma Lipids

Dietary PUFAs depress serum VLDL and LDL lipids and cholesterol and, in this respect, different families of PUFAs show varying efficacies. The PUFAs of vegetable oils, containing mostly linoleic acid (LA), are effective in counteracting the effects of dietary saturated fatty acids but the n-3 PUFAs of fish oils may be equally or more hypolipidemic.

Earlier trials indicated that even though they contained cholesterol, fish oils were effective in reducing plasma lipids. More recent epidemiological observations, which showed low plasma lipids in populations consuming seafood and fish, indicated the effectiveness of dietary fish oils in reducing plasma lipids, especially TGs, and their association with a decreased incidence of atherosclerosis, thrombosis, and coronary infarction. The relationship between seafood consumption and the reduced incidence of cardiovascular disorders has been observed with Eskimos and Japanese fishermen. Eskimos consume a marine food diet (500 g/d), supplying ~ 40-45 per cent of calories from fat (< 10 g EPA) and 700 mg cholesterol, and have significantly lower plasma LDLs and VLDL than do Eskimos living in Denmark and consuming a Western-type diet. The fatty acid composition of the plasma and platelet lipids reflected the dietary fatty acids with regard to the relative concentrations of n-6 and n-3 PUFAs (Table 9.4).

The lower incidence of atherosclerosis and ischemic heart disease in Japan has been attributed to the lower plasma cholesterol and LDL values resulting from (among other factors) the higher consumption of fish, *i.e.* ~ 90 and 250 g/d by Japanese farmers and by fishermen and women, respectively, compared with < 20 g fish/d in the United States. Japanese fishermen have lower blood pressures and lower incidences of heart disease than do farmers, and the Japanese population has a sixfold lower incidence of atherosclerosis and heart disease than do Americans. In both Eskimos and Japanese, the EPA and DHA contents of plasma and platelet and tissue phospholipids (PLs) are significantly increased whereas the relative concentration of arachidonic acid (AA) is decreased (Tables 9.4 and 9.5). The overall effects of dietary seafood lipids in reducing the incidence of CADs, when consumed over a long time period, may reflect the effects of the n-3 PUFA components on several metabolic indices. Thus, n-3 PUFAs may reduce plasma lipids, depress tissue AA synthesis, alter the composition of cell and tissue PUFAs, improve vascular tone, and modify cell-to-cell interactions by altering eicosanoid balance.

Effects of N-3 PUFAS on Lipoproteins

Dietary n-3 PUFAs can modify plasma lipids and lipoprotein metabolism. Most clinical trials with human subjects consistently showed a decrease in VLDL TGs and some observed decreased plasma cholesterol. The preferential depression of serum TGs and a slight decrease in the plasma cholesterol of normolipidemic subjects after consumption of salmon oil compared with vegetable oils. Dietary fish oil attenuated

Table 9.4: Composition of Dietary Fat in Eskimo and Danish Diets and Relative Amounts of n-6 and n-3 PUFAs in plasma and blood platelets

	Eskimos	Danes
Total calories from fat (per cent)	39	49
n-3 PUFAs (g/d)	14	3
n-6 PUFAs (g/d)	5	10
Cholesterol (g/d)	0.7	0.42
Fatty acids (dietary fat) (per cent)		
Saturated	23	53
Monounsaturated	58	34
Polyunsaturated	19	13
Plasma PLs (fatty acid) (per cent)		
18:2n-6	6.6	22.3
20:4n-6	0.8	8.4
20:5n-3	7.1	1.8
22:6n-3	3.9	2.2
Cholesterol esters (per cent)		
18:2n-6	20.3	51.0
20:4n-6	1.0	5.8
20:5n-3	15.8	0.9
22:6n-3	1.0	0.4
Platelet lipids (per cent)		
18:2n-6	3.9	8.2
20:4n-6	8.5	22.1
20:5n-3	8.0	0.5
22:6n-3	5.8	1.5
Bleeding time (min)	8.1	4.7

Table 9.5: Differences in Fatty Acid Composition of Serum PLs in American Subjects and in Japanese Living in Farming and Fishing Villages

Fatty Acids (per cent)	*Japanese*		*Unites States (Nashville)*
	Mountain Farm	*Fishing Village*	
18:1	16	16	22
18:2 (n-6)	16	14	20
20:4 (n-6)	7	7	7
20:5 (n-3)	3	3	0.1
22:6 (n-3)	8	10	0.1

the expected increase in plasma cholesterol. Twenty g fish oil + EPA/d (~ 5 g n-3 PUFAs/d) significantly reduced plasma TGs in humans whereas cholesterol reduction was observed only in those subjects with high initial plasma cholesterol concentrations. A significant decrease in serum VLDLs, an insignificant drop in LDLs, and an increase in HDLs occurred. An increased removal of VLDL particles and increased excretion of bile were observed after fish-oil consumption. Postprandial reduction of VLDL remnants may be beneficial.

Dietary n-3 PUFAs are more hypotriglyceridemic than are equivalent amounts of n-6 PUFAs. Fish oil supplements (15-20 mL/d providing 4.5 g n-3 PUFAs) caused a decrease in plasma TG and cholesterol concentrations but increased LDL apoprotein B concentrations. This may be partly explained by the decreased size and increased density of the LDL particles formed after fish-oil ingestion. These changes may reduce the atherogenicity of these lipoprotein particles.

In some studies, doses of < 5 g fish oil/d (1 g EPA) had negligible effects on plasma lipoproteins. Maximum TG lowering was observed at doses of ~ 4.5 g n-3 PUFA/d in normal human subjects. The response, however, may be affected by the amount and composition of other dietary fat components. Increasing the dosage of fish oils (*e.g.* up to 30-50 g/d) resulted in significant decreases in serum TGs, VLDLs, and, frequently, LDLs; occasionally fish oils depressed cholesterol concentrations, particularly in patients with elevated plasma cholesterol, and caused slight increases in HDLs. Generally, reduction of serum lipids and lipoproteins has been observed in both normal and hyperlipidemic patients, with the effects being greater in hyperlipidemic patients.

The effect of n-3 PUFAs from fish oils on plasma TGs is sustained with continued feeding, is dose responsive, and is reversible. Fish oils depress plasma lipids when the oils are being ingested, and this effect is reversed after removal of the fish oils (*i.e.* there is negligible residual effect on plasma lipids beyond 2-4 d).

Fish oil may be effective in the treatment of hyperlipidemic patients. Salmon oil at 30 g/d decreased plasma TG concentrations 32 ± 7.5 per cent in hyperlipidemic patients. The decrease in TG concentrations was dose dependent, with a 41 per cent and 52 per cent decrease in total plasma TGs in subjects given 6 and 9 g salmon oil/d, respectively. Fish oil + EPA reduced plasma TG concentrations (28 per cent) in patients with type II hyperlipidemia. Salmon oil or fish oil + EPA supplementation caused a 64 per cent decrease in the plasma TG concentrations of type IIb-hyperlipidemic subjects.

A significant reduction was observed in cholesterol, LDL cholesterol, and total apoprotein B in subjects consuming n-3 or n-6 PUFAs in place of saturated fatty acids. When salmon oil was administered to subjects with familial combined hyperlipidemia (FCH) there was a marked reduction in TGs, however, LDL cholesterol and apoprotein B concentrations tended to increase. This may reflect a change in size of LDL lipoprotein particles. Diets containing 24 or 200 mg cholesterol /1000 kcal and 22 g fish oil /1000 kcal reduced lipoprotein cholesterol in patients with familial hypercholesterolemia. LDL concentrations were decreased from 6.57 ± 1.16 to 5.59 ± 1.16 mmol/L in patients on the high-cholesterol diet and to 5.36 ± 1.06 mmol/L in patients on the low-cholesterol diet. The observation that fish oils suppress VLDL synthesis suggests that they may be useful in treating persons with FCH, who are at an increased risk of coronary heart disease. Fish oils could be useful in reducing LDL and hyperchylomicronemia by facilitating clearance of chylomicrons and via reduced competition from fewer LDL particles.

In addition to the effects on TGs, fish oils may also alter the concentrations of cholesterol associated with lipoprotein, especially HDLs. Greenland Eskimos consuming a seafood diet had consumed much less n-3 PUFAs. Clinical trials with normolipidemic and hyperlipidemic patients revealed that dietary fish oil increased HDL cholesterol concentrations. Fish oil + EPA increased HDL cholesterol concentrations from 1.19 ± 0.027 to 1.31 ± 0.037 mmol/L in both normal and hyperlipidemic human subjects, while VLDL and LDL cholesterol removal from extra hepatic tissues. These findings were consistent in both types of patients after 6 mo-2y of fish-oil + EPA administration. Fish oil concentrate given to hypercholesterolemic patients caused a 40 per cent increase in the HDL_2 sub fraction and an increase in the ratio of HDL_2 to HDL_3 from 0.17 to 0.25. Increased HDL_2 may improve cholesterol transport in hypercholesterolemic patients. Fish oil + EPA also increased the HDL_2 cholesterol concentrations of male insulin-dependent diabetic patients. Fish oil may increase HDL cholesterol in a dose-dependent manner (*e.g.* a 4-g dose did not significantly alter HDL cholesterol concentrations in hypercholesterolemic patients but 7.5 g increased HDL cholesterol concentrations from 0.83 ± 0.05 to 0.98 ± 0.05 mmol/L). Dietary n-3 PUFAs increased the cholesterol content of the HDL particles without altering the number of particles.

Dietary fish oil altered the fatty acids of platelets and decreased plasma TG concentrations in non-insulin-dependent diabetics but did not change TG concentrations in insulin-dependent diabetics. In non-insulin-dependent diabetics, however, dietary fish oil reduced plasma TG concentrations by 37 per cent from 1.9 ± 0.08 to 1.2 ± 0.5 mmol/L. Insulin-stimulated glucose uptake *in vivo* was increased by 25 per cent in non-insulin-dependent diabetic patients after consumption of 3 g n-3 PUFAs/d (cod liver oil) for 8 wk. Thus, dietary n-3 PUFAs appear to improve insulin sensitivity while simultaneously reducing plasma TG concentrations. Dietary n-3 PUFAs increased erythrocyte-membrane fluidity, decreased platelet activity, and increased the LDL and HDL cholesterol concentrations in diabetic patients. n-3 PUFA supplementation caused rapid but reversible metabolic deterioration in non-insulin-dependent diabetic patients. These conflicting reports concerning the effects of n-3 PUFAs on diabetics need to be clarified.

Possible Mechanisms of the Effects of N-3 PUFAS on Serum Lipids

The hypolipidemic effects of fish oils may be mediated by several mechanisms. Dietary n-3 PUFAs can reduce TG synthesis and chylomicron secretion from intestinal cells, and suppress hepatic fatty acid synthesis and TG production, thereby limiting VLDL secretion. In rats, n-3 PUFAs reduce hepatic glucose-6-phosphate dehydrogenase, malic enzyme, and acetyl-CoA carboxylase. Dietary EPA reduces hepatic TGs inhibiting phosphatidate phosphohydrolase and acyltransferases.

Increased ketogenesis was observed in perfused livers from rats fed diets rich in EPA and DHA, accompanied by increased peroxisomal β-oxidation of these acids. Dietary fish oil decreases the VLDL TG pool by suppressing TG synthesis and possibly enhancing the clearance of VLDL TGs.

There is evidence that n-3 PUFAs also reduce apoprotein synthesis. Fish oil + EPA diminish the production of apoprotein B in humans and rats and may reduce the daily flux or transport of VLDL apoprotein B. Diets rich in LA also suppress VLDL and LDL apoprotein B concentrations but n-3 PUFAs appear to be more effective. Both EPA and DHA markedly inhibit the capacity of Hep G2 cells to incorporate glycerol and leucine into TGs and apoprotein B, indicating that n-3 PUFAs suppress hepatic VLDL TGs and apoprotein B secretion. Herring and lamprey oils suppress the expression of mRNA for apoproteins A_1 and B whereas safflower oil enhances expression of apoprotein B suggesting n-3 PUFAs may inhibit hepatic and intestinal synthesis of apoproteins A_1 and B. In miniature pigs MaxEPA increased the conversion of VLDL to LDL but decreased the LDL apoprotein B pool size.

LDL binding was decreased after incubation of Hep G2 cells with either EPA or LA, and EPA inhibited LDL binding to the hepatic B/E receptor without affecting binding to the apo E receptor. Dietary fish oil decreased hepatic LDL-receptor activity in rats by 37 per cent and this was associated with decreased cholesterol synthesis. Fish oil + EPA depressed LDL-receptor mRNA concentrations in Hep G2 cells. Fish oil + EPA reduced the receptor-mediated clearance of LDL apoprotein B from 0.029 to 0.014/h in miniature pigs whereas in rats, dietary fish oil stimulated LDL-receptor activity (200 per cent) and reduced VLDL, LDL and HDL cholesterol concentrations. Six weeks of fish-oil supplementation did not significantly alter LDL surface binding, internalization, or degradation by isolated human skin fibroblasts. Fish-oil ingestion increased hepatic HDL-receptor activity by 71 per cent rats.

Dietary n-3 PUFAs may promote lipoprotein metabolism by altering the activity of certain lipolytic and transfer enzymes functioning in the plasma. n-3 PUFAs facilitate the transfer of fatty acids from VLDLs to HDLs. Fish oil increased plasma lecithin:cholesterol acyltransferase (LCAT) concentrations by 45 per cent in rats. Administration of fish oil to 14 cardiac patients for 6 wk increased serum LCAT activity by 25 per cent whereas it was significantly decreased in normolipidemic humans on a mackerel-steak diet. The decreased LCAT activity would reduce the cholesterol ester (CE) content and the size of LDL particles. Fish-oil consumption reduces CEs and the size of LDLs in monkeys. This was attributed to a change in LCAT concentrations and the altered composition of substrate plasma PLs of animals ingesting fish oil. Thus, position sn-2 of the PL was enriched fourfold in n-3 PUFAs, and LCAT was 10 times less active towards these than when linoleic acid was present. Thus, PLs enriched in n-3 PUFAs are apparently poor substrates for LCAT; consequently, less CE is formed and LDL particles are smaller and conceivably less atherogenic.

The effects of dietary n-3 PUFAs on lipoprotein lipase (LPL), which catalyzes the degradation of VLDLs and chylomicrons in extrahepatic tissues, is unclear. In one study LPL concentrations in rats fed fish oil or corn oil were unchanged whereas another reported that fish oil decreased LPL activity by 50 per cent in male rats.

Intracellular acyl-coenzyme A-cholesterol acyltransferase (ACAT), which regulates the intracellular catabolism of CE, was higher whereas hydroxy methylglutaryl (HMG)-CoA reductase activities were lower in intestine and liver of rabbits fed menhaden oil than in those fed cocoa butter. The aortas from rhesus monkeys fed a mixture of coconut menhaden oil (1:1) had less ACAT, acid lipase, and cholesteryl esterase activity than did those of monkeys fed coconut oil.

These reports indicate that the n-3 PUFAs of dietary fish can affect plasma lipids and lipoprotein metabolism at several loci, which may partly account for the metabolic effects of n-3 PUFAs. However, data from many studies of the effects of dietary n-3 PUFAs are inconsistent because of differences in dosages and composition of the fish oils; differences in age and health status of subjects, plasma lipid concentrations, and duration of study; and limited control of other dietary factors, especially saturated fatty acids and n-6 PUFAs. Generally, although fish oils tend to reduce serum TGs, especially in hypertriglyceridemic patients, they rarely reduce cholesterol and may actually increase LDL cholesterol.

The data indicate that the collective actions of dietary n-3 PUFAs involve more than alteration of plasma lipids and lipoproteins, and the growing evidence suggests that n-3 PUFAs of fish oils may exert several beneficial effects via modulation of eicosanoid synthesis and functions of various cells associated with the cardiovascular system.

Intake of Fish Oils

Although many of the clinical trials are flawed, the available evidences indicate that the n-3 PUFA components of seafoods are effective in lowering plasma TGs and reducing eicosanoid-mediated reactions. Thus, fish oils may be useful for diabetics and subjects with familial hypertriglyceridemia. Consumption of seafoods as a regular dietary practice would appear to be prudent for prophylactic effects, whereas, for therapeutic purposes, ingestion of fish oil enriched with n-3 PUFAs on a frequent basis may be beneficial.

Table 9.6: Approximate Amount (in mg) of Omega-3 (n-3) Fatty Acids in Raw 100 g Portion of some Fish

Fish	*EPA*	*DHA*	*Total*
Mackerel, Atlantic	900	1600	2500
Herring, Atlantic	700	900	1600
Bluefish	400	800	1200
Salmoan, Atlantic	300	900	1200
Tuna	100	400	500
Cod, Atlantic	100	200	300
Shrimp	200	100	300
Flounder	100	100	200
Haddock	100	100	200
Swordfish	100	100	200

Source: Clinical Dietetics and Nutrition, F.P. Antia and Philip Abraham, Fourth Edition, Pg. 401, 1997

The effective dosage of n-3 PUFAs has not been established. It may vary depending on the subject's age and health, the desired effect (specific ailment, disease status,. remission, prophylaxis), the duration of administration, the type of seafood or fish oil being used, and the amount of other fatty acids, especially n-3 PUFAs, being concomitantly consumed in the diet. Eskimos consume ≤ 10 g n-3 PUFAs/d whereas the Japanese ingest ~ 1 g/d with low-fat diets. Most of the clinical trials to date have used fish oils providing very high concentrations of n-3 PUFAs (3-10 g/d). These concentrations are not typical for long-germ ingestion. However, consistent ingestion of lower amounts (2-3 g/d) may exert effective prophylactic actions. Consumption of 30 g fish/d appeared to have beneficial effects whereas Japanese data indicate that 200-250 g fish/d in a low-fat diet (20 per cent calories as fat), may be efficacious.

Consumption of sufficient fish to provide an average of 2-3 g n-3 PUFAs three to four times per week, combined with a prudent diet, might be feasible by consuming high-fat fish (*e.g.* salmon).

Sources and Intake of Polyunsaturated Fatty Acids

w-6 polyunsaturated fatty acids occur most commonly in plant oils. Linoleic acid (18:2n-6), the major dietary source of the w-6 PUFAs, is abundant in vegetable oils (soybean, corn, and safflower) and is the precursor of arachidonic acid (20:4n-6). The n-3 family occurs in small amounts in most foods except fish. Linoleic acid (18:3n-3) is present in low concentrations in leafy plant tissues and soybean oil. Eicosapentaenoic acid (EPA) (20:5n-3) and docosahexaenoic acid (DHA) (22:6n-3) originate in unicellular phytoplankton and seaweeds, and once incorporated into the lipids of fish and other marine animals that consume the algae, they are passed on through the food chain to other species. Persons consuming a normal diet have low tissue levels of EPA and DHA, but persons who regularly consume fish have increased tissue levels.

Linoleic acid is by far the prevailing polyunsaturated fatty acid in the typically Western diet at 9.8 per cent of the total fatty acids. Besides linoleic acid, the most abundant polyunsaturated fatty acid is α-linolenic acid, at 1.6 per cent. Arachidonic, eicosapentaenoic, and docosapentaenoic/docosahexaenoic acids represented 0.5, 0.1, and 0.4 per cent of the total fatty acids, respectively. Compared to the Western diet, the Eskimo diet contains less fat and its saturated fatty acids represent a lower percentage of the total fatty acids. Furthermore, Eskimos consume a greater percentage of polyunsaturated fatty acids, and the ingested polyunsaturated fatty acids are dominated by the n-3 class, in contrast to the dominance of the n-6 class in the Western world. Thus, in Europe and North America 7-15 g linoleic acid is ingested daily, making it the major polyunsaturated fatty acid, whereas Eskimos consume about 13 g/day of eicosapentaenoic and docosahexaenoic acids.

Ratio of Omega-6 and Omega-3 Fatty Acids in Diet

Excessive amounts of omega-6 polyunsaturated fatty acids and a very high omega-6/omega-3 ratio have been linked with pathogenesis of many diseases, including cardiovascular disease, cancer, and inflammatory and autoimmune diseases. The ratio of omega-6 to omega-3 in modern diets is approximately 15:1, whereas ratios of 2:1 to 4:1 have been associated with reduced mortality from cardiovascular disease, suppressed inflammation in patients with rheumatoid arthritis, and decreased risk of breast cancer.

Role of Other Dietary Constituents in Cholesterol Metabolism and CVD

Attempts to reduce coronary risk have focussed largely on the fat content and composition of diets, but some preliminary evidence indicates that other aspects of diet may warrant rigorous investigation.

Antioxidants

Free radicals, that is to say atoms or molecules that contain one or more unpaired electrons are potentially injurious to living organism, for example, by lipid peroxidation to form lipid peroxides. Antioxidants may play a role in gvolacting against such effects. Two epidemiological studies showed that the use of large doses of vit E supplements, an antioxidant vitamin, was associated with a decreased risk of coronary heart disease.

Experiments were done with Se and vit E on hyperlipidemic rats to see this effect on the plasma total and high density lipoprotein cholesterol level. Rats fed on vit E diet in the presence of Se were shown to lower the total cholesterol and plasma HDL-cholesterol.

Fibre

Cholesterol reduction has been observed in some clinical trials of isolated forms of dietary fibre but the type of fibre seems important. The soluble fibre diet from barley, beans, oat bran etc has been reported to cause a 5 per cent greater reduction in total cholesterol, while HDL-cholesterol was lowered by 3.5 per cent. In healthy subjects, the cholesterol lowering effect of dietary fibre may be indirect, through replacement of dietary saturated fat and cholesterol.

Legumes

Anti-hypocholesterolemic effect of the indigested high molecular fraction of soybean protein is known in rats, but such an effect has not been shown in man. A study was conducted with female university students who had relatively high serum cholesterol levels. These students were given two types of diet, (1) supplying 8 per cent of this total energy from casein, soybean protein isolates or high molecular fraction, (2) supplying 4 per cent of total energy from casein or HMF. Energy intake and daily activities were kept constant. A decrease in LDL-cholesterol and increase in HDL-cholesterol were observed in the HMF group as compared to the casein group.

Inclusion of purified alfalfa saponin in bengal gram diet showed no interference with food intake and food efficiency ratio. Saponin supplemented diet lowered total plasma cholesterol the effect being prominent, when cholesterol was absent in the diet. In addition, saponin appeared to be a patent anti-atherogenic when supplemented to cholesterol free and cholesterol containing bengal gram diets. The saponin supplementation did not exert any significant effect on total liver lipids. The hypercholesterolemic and antiatherogenic effect of saponin could be directly correlated with their ability to decrease intestinal cholesterol absorption and to increase the faecal excretion of bile acids.

Soybean milk, soybean milk lipid extract and defatted soybean milk cause an inhibition in the increase in the total serum cholesterol and serum triglycerides.

Fruits and Vegetables

The extract of nutmeg kernels has an effect on hyperlipidemia. The total cholesterol: HDL and LDL: HDL ratio was significantly lowered when 500 mg/kg of the extract was administered to rabbits. The total cholesterol, LDL and triglyceride level was lowered significantly but no significant decrease in HDL-cholesterol was observed.

The effect of the water soluble viscous substance of the leafy vegetables on cholesterol metabolism was studied. When powder of leaves was given, there was a fall in the total serum cholesterol and liver cholesterol concentrations. On feeding a diet containing water soluble viscous substance (1.7 per cent), about 1 per cent as dietary fibre, there was decrease on serum and liver cholesterol concentrations and increase in faecal excretion of bile acids and neutral olerols.

The effect of garlic on plasma cholesterol was examined in a meta analysis of 16 randomized controlled trials of at least 4 weeks duration, this showed a 12 per cent reduction in total cholesterol. A water soluble fraction of garlic also is reported to specifically lower LDL cholesterol. The water soluble component of garlic added to the diet at level of 0.2 per cent to 1.6 per cent lowered LDL-cholesterol level by 38 per cent.

Milk

Cultured milk has a potential for cholesterol lowering in man. The cultured milk containing *Enterococcus faecivia* and two strains of *Streptococcus thermophilus* (200 ml of cultured milk/day) were given. After 2 and 6 weeks, total cholesterol was reduced. This reduction in total cholesterol in completely ascribed to a 10 per cent fall in LDL-cholesterol since HDL-cholesterol and triglyceride were unchanged.

Microorganisms

Recently, a unique bacterium, *Eubacterium coprostanoligenes*, that reduces cholesterol to coprostanol was isolated. Because coprostanol is absorbed poorly it was hypothesised that oral administration of *E. coprostanoligenes* might decrease the absorption of endogenous and dietary cholesterol by conversion to coprostanol.

Total serum cholesterol concentration in rats fed on the mixture of organisms (*Bacillus, Lactobacillus, Streptococcus, Clostridium, Saccharomyces* and *Candida*) was decreased by 15-33 per cent. Hepatic cholesterol concentration was also decreased.

Mushrooms

A hypocholesterolemic effect of different varieties of mushrooms has also been observed. The oyster mushrooms lowered the serum cholesterol and cholesterol in VLDL. A fall in serum and liver cholesterol values was observed as 32 and 55 per cent, respectively. Mushroom extract grifalin also had a hypocholesterolemic action. But farm mushrooms (*Agaricus compestris*) do not have plasma cholesterol lowering properties.

Chapter 10
Role of Omega-3 Fatty Acids in Health and Disease

An adequate n-3 (omega-3) polyunsaturated fatty acid (n-3 PUFA) status is important for the maintenance of health and could reduce the risk of chronic and inflammatory diseases, such as coronary artery disease and, potentially, dementia, diabetes, and asthma, although the evidence is weaker. Dietary n-3 PUFAs are either plant-derived [e.g, short-chain α-linolenic acid (ALA)] or marine-derived [e.g, longer-chain eicosapentaenoic acid (EPA) and docosahexaenoic acids (DHA)].

Plant Sources

ALA is the major plant-based n-3 PUFA and its dietary sources include flaxseeds and flaxseed oil, walnuts and walnut oil, soybeans and soybean oil, pumpkin seeds, rapeseed (canola) oil, and olive oil. In addition to providing ALA, these foods are good sources of a variety of nutrients, such as fiber, monounsaturated fatty acids, vitamins, and minerals. The intake of various oils needed to meet current recommendations of ALA for women and men varies from 2.2–3.2 mL/d (0.15–0.22 tablespoons/d) of flaxseed oil to 158–229 mL/d (10.7–15.5 tablespoons/d) of olive oil. The intake of various nuts and seeds needed to meet current recommendations of ALA for women and men varies from 12.2–17.6 g/d (0.43–0.62 oz/d) of English walnuts to 4.8–7.0 g/d (0.17–0.25 oz/d) of flaxseeds to 612–890 g/d (21.6–31.4 oz/d) of pumpkin seeds. The intake of food sources lower in ALA, such as olive oil or pumpkin seeds, alone to meet current recommendations is impractical because of the calories associated with the amounts needed to meet current recommendations. Therefore, a combination of oils, nuts, seeds, and other foods rich in ALA, such as leafy greens (*i.e.*, 1 cup of kale contains 0.121 g ALA, H≈25 per cent of total fat from

ALA), is optimal (Gebauer *et al.*, 2006). ALA content of selected oils, seeds, and nuts and the amount of each needed to reach the AI levels for men and women are shown in Table 10.1.

Table 10.1: Linolenic Acid (ALA) Content of Selected Oils, Seeds, and Nuts and amounts Needed to meet Adequate Intakes *1*

Source of ALA	*ALA (g/tbsp.)*	*Amount Needed by Men to Meet Recommendation (1.6g ALA/d)*	*Amount Needed by Women to Meet Recommendation (1.1g ALA/d)*
Pumpkin seeds	0.051	31.4	21.6
Olive oil	0.103	15.5	10.7
Walnuts, black	0.156	10.3	7.05
Soybean oil	1.231	1.3	0.89
Rapeseed oil	1.302	1.2	0.84
Walnut oil	1.414	1.1	0.78
Flaxseeds	2.350	0.68	0.47
Walnuts, English	2.574	0.62	0.43
Flaxseed oil	7.249	0.22	0.15

1: 1 tbsp oil = 13.6 g; 1 tbsp seeds or nuts= 28.35 g.

Source: Gebauer *et al.* (2006)

Marine Sources

Fish is a very good source of long chain n-3 fatty acids. In addition to being an excellent source of the marine-derived n–3 fatty acids, fish is a good source of protein, B vitamins, and minerals, such as potassium, phosphorous, and selenium too. All fish contain EPA and DHA; however, the quantities vary among species and within a species according to environmental variables such as diet and whether fish are wild or farm-raised. Farm-raised catfish tend to have less EPA and DHA than do wild catfish, whereas farm-raised salmon and trout contain similar amounts versus their wild counterparts.

EPA and DHA range from as low as 0.134 g/85 g for cod (3-oz serving) to as much as 1.825 g/85 g for salmon (3-oz serving). The total EPA and DHA content of the most commonly eaten fish and shellfish in the United States is shown in Table 10.2.

Intake of Omega-3 Fatty Acids

The intake of total omega-3 fatty acids in the United States is ≈1.6 g/d (≈0.7 per cent of energy intake) (Kris-Etherton *et al.*, 2000). Of this, α-linolenic acid accounts for ≈1.4 g/d, and only 0.1 to 0.2 g/d comes from EPA and DHA. The major food sources of α-linolenic acid are vegetable oils, principally canola and soybean oils in US diets. Other food sources that are rich in α-linolenic acid include flaxseed (23 g/100 g) and English walnuts (7 g/100 g). Although some α-linolenic acid is converted to the longer-chain omega-3 fatty acids, the extent of this conversion is modest and controversial. For example, Emken *et al.* (1994) reported a 15 per cent conversion, whereas Pawlosky *et al.* (2001) found 0.2 per cent; both reported that the conversion to DHA was much less than that to EPA.

Table 10.2: Top Finfish and Shellfish Consumed in the United States and Eicosapentaenoic Acid (EPA) and Docosahexaenoic Acid (DHA) Content [1]

Fish	*EPA DHA*	*Amount Needed to get 500 mg EPA DHA/d[2]*	*Amount Needed to get 500 mg EPA DHA/d[2]*	*Mean mercury Concentration*
	mg/serving	*serving*	*servings/wk*	*ppm*
Cod	134	3.7	25.9	0.11
Catfish	151	3.3	23.1	0.05
Haddock	203	2.5	17.5	0.03
Clams	241	2.1	14.7	ND
Shrimp	267	1.9	13.3	ND
Flounder	426	1.2	8.4	0.05
Pollock	460	1.1	7.7	0.06
Flatfish	498	1	7	0.05
Tuna, canned	733	0.68	4.8	0.12 (light); 0.35 (Albacore)
Salmon	1825	0.27	1.9	0.01

1: ND, mercury concentration below the level of detection (0.01 ppm).

2: 1 serving 85 g (3 oz) cooked portions.

Source: Gebauer *et al.* (2006).

Studies on Role of Omega-3 Fatty Acids in Health and Disease

As conversion from ALA to EPA and DHA is limited, fish, particularly fatty fish, is a source of the long-chain omega-3 polyunsaturated fatty acids (PUFAs) eicosapentaenoic acid and docosahexaenoic acid. Therefore, individuals who do not eat fish or fish oils (e.g, vegans and non-fish-eating vegetarians and meat-eaters) could be at risk of low or inadequate n-3 PUFA status.

Various aspects of omega-3 fatty acids through consumption of fish or fish oil and their therapeutic effects have been discussed as under.

I. Cardiovascular Disease (CVD)

Since the first cross-cultural epidemiologic studies conducted in the 1970s, evidence has been accumulating regarding the role of n–3 polyunsaturated fatty acids in fish (EPA and DHA) in the prevention and management of cardiovascular disease (CVD). α-Linolenic acid (ALA), a plant-derived n–3 fatty acid and a precursor to EPA and DHA (found in walnuts and certain vegetable oils such as flaxseed, canola and soybean), is also of interest for CVD prevention. The AHA Scientific Statement reported by Kris-Etherton *et al*. (2002) had addressed distinctions between plant-derived (α-linolenic acid, C18:3n-3) and marine-derived (eicosapentaenoic acid, C20:5n-3 [EPA] and docosahexaenoic acid, C22:6n-3 [DHA]) omega-3 fatty acids.

Evidence from prospective cohort studies in generally healthy populations and randomized controlled trials (RCTs) in patients with known coronary heart disease suggest that the n–3 polyunsaturated fatty acids in fish are likely to prevent sudden cardiac death, manifested as fatal ischemic heart disease or arrhythmic death (Lemaitre *et al.*, 2003; Siscovick *et al.*, 1993; Albert *et al.*, 1998; Mozaffarian and Rimm, 2006) and possibly as ischemic stroke (Mozaffarian *et al.*, 2005). However, the effects of modest fish consumption (*e.g.*, 1–2 servings/wk) on other CVD events, such as nonfatal myocardial infarction or nonischemic strokes, have been less consistent (He *et al.*, 2004a; He *et al.*, 2004b). In aggregate, available RCTs show a beneficial effect of dietary and supplemental omega-3 fatty acids, including EPA+DHA and α-linolenic acid, on CHD. This has been summarized in a recent meta-analysis of 11 RCTs with 7951 patients in the intervention groups (Bucher *et al.*, 2002). In this meta-analysis, the risk ratio of nonfatal MI was 0.8, for fatal MI it was 0.7, and for sudden death (in 5 trials) it was 0.7.

Major studies showing a cardioprotective effect of EPA and DHA and fish intake on CVD risk in healthy subjects include the Nurses' Health Study (Hu *et al.*, 2002), the Physicians' Health Study (Albert *et al.*, 1998), the Cardiovascular Health Study (Lemaitre *et al.*, 2003), the Chicago Western Electric Study (Daviglus *et al.*, 1997; Orencia *et al.*, 1996), an ecologic study by Zhang *et al.* (1999), and, most recently, the Japan Public Health Center-Based Study Cohort I (Iso *et al.*, 2006).

A systematic review of the literature on the effects of n–3 FAs (consumed as fish or fish oils rich in EPA and DHA or as α-linolenic acid) on cardiovascular disease outcomes and adverse events was conducted by Wang *et al.* (2006). Studies from MEDLINE and other sources that were of ≥1 y in duration and that reported estimates of fish or n–3 FA intakes and cardiovascular disease outcomes were included in this review. They screened 8039 abstracts and evaluated 842 full text articles for potentially relevant data. They identified 46 unique eligible studies on CVD outcomes, including 14 RCTs, 25 prospective cohort studies, and 7 case-control studies. They also reviewed 395 clinical studies for potentially relevant human data on adverse events associated with n–3 FA consumption. Secondary prevention was addressed in 14 randomized controlled trials (RCTs) of fish-oil supplements or of diets high in n–3 FAs and in 1 prospective cohort study. According to them studies on the relation between dietary n–3 fatty acids (FAs) and cardiovascular disease varied in quality, and the results were inconsistent. No significant effect on overall deaths was reported in 3 RCTs that evaluated the effects of fish oil in patients with implantable cardioverter defibrillators. Most trials reported that fish oil significantly reduced all-cause mortality, myocardial infarction, cardiac and sudden death, or stroke. Primary prevention of cardiovascular disease was reported in 1 RCT, in 25 prospective cohort studies, and in 7 case-control studies.

Most cohort studies have reported that fish consumption was associated with lower rates of all-cause mortality and adverse cardiac outcomes. Three large prospective cohort studies that comprised >53 000 participants from China, Japan, and the United States (Nagata *et al.*, 2002; Yuan *et al.*, 2001; Dolecek, 2001) provided data on fish-oil intake and reported significant reductions in all-cause mortality. In a cohort study conducted by Folsom *et al.* (2004) of 41 836 US women initially free of heart disease, the estimated marine n–3 FA intake was not associated with total mortality. However, the authors reported in a secondary analysis that ALA intake was modestly inversely associated with total mortality after multivariate adjustment.

One prospective cohort study from Finland followed 415 patients with coronary artery disease for 5 y and compared those who consumed fish with those who consumed no fish. The study reported a significant decrease in all-cause mortality (RR = 0.37) in patients who consumed >57 g fish/d (Erkkila *et al.*, 2003). Most of the large cohort studies reviewed, which involved >340 000 participants in total, reported significant reductions after multivariate adjustment in one or more of the CVD outcomes of interest (Iso *et al.*, 2001; Ascherio *et al.*, 1995; Folsom *et al.*, 2004; Nagata *et al.*, 2002;. Morris *et al.*, 1995; Yuan *et al.*, 2001; Dolecek, 1992; Egeland *et al.*, 2001; Sauvaget *et al.*, 2003;. Rodriguez *et al.*, 1996; Oomen *et al.*, 2000; Orencia *et al.*, 1996).

Two prospective cohort studies (Pietinen *et al.*, 1997; Dolecek, 1992) reported data on n–3 FA consumption and cardiac death. A 6-y cohort study from Finland by Pietinen *et al.* (1997) of 21 930 middle-aged men who smoked found no association of cardiac death with either ALA or EPA+DHA intake. Cardiac death was defined in the Finnish study as International Classification of Disease (revision 9) codes 410-414, which specifies coronary heart disease (CHD) as the underlying cause of death. The Multiple Risk Factor Intervention Trial (MRFIT), which followed 12 866 middle-aged men at high risk of CHD for 10.5 y, found no association between ALA intake and risk of cardiac death, whereas the highest quintile of EPA+DHA intake was associated with a 40 per cent lower risk (Dloecek, 1992). In MRFIT, cardiac death is defined as deaths due to MI within 30 d of symptoms or hospitalization, sudden death, congestive heart failure due to CHD, or death during hospitalization for surgery for CHD or from attendant complications (Multiple Risk Factor Interventional Trial, 1982).

There were 15 cohort studies that reported data on fish consumption and cardiac death, 4 of which showed a statistically significant reduction in fatal and total coronary heart disease with higher fish consumption. Eight cohort studies showed some protective benefit, and 4 showed none. The Cardiovascular Health Study by Mozaffarian and Rimm (2006), which followed 3910 older subjects for 9.3 y, found that a statistically significant lower risk of total ischemic heart disease associated specifically with higher intakes of oily fish (*i.e.*, tuna and other nonfried fish). Of note, in this study, trends for increased cardiac events were observed with increasing consumption of fried fish or fish sandwiches.

Two prospective cohort studies and 1 case-control study reported data on sudden death (Morris *et al.*, 1995; Siscovick *et al.*, 1995; Daviglus *et al.*, 1997). The Physicians' Health Study followed 20 551 men for 11 y and reported an H"50 per cent lower relative risk even in participants who ate fish only once a month (>0.3 g/mo n–3 FA) (Morris *et al.*, 1995). The case-control study of 827 subjects conducted in the United States by Siscovick *et al.* (1995) reported a significant decrease in sudden death with increasing fish intake and fish-oil consumption (*i.e.*, 5.5 g of omega-3 fatty acids per month, equivalent to two fatty fish meals per week, was associated with a 50 per cent reduced risk of primary cardiac arrest). Another prospective cohort study, the Chicago Western Electric Study, followed 1822 men for 30 y and provided data on fish consumption and also found an association between higher fish consumption and lower rates of sudden death (Daviglus *et al.*, 1997).

Five cohort studies and 1 case-control study reported data on both fatal and non-fatal MI. Three of these large cohort studies–the Nurses' Health Study (Hu *et al.*, 2002), the Health Professionals Follow-Up Study (Ascherio *et al.*, 1995)–and a study from China by Yuan *et al.* (Yuan *et al.*, 2001)–as well as 1 case-control study by Tavani *et al.*, of 148 802 participants from Italy (Tavani *et al.*, 2001) showed benefits of FA intake. Among 84 688 female nurses, higher EPA+DHA intakes were associated with a lower risk of nonfatal MI, *i.e.*, a 31 per cent lower risk in the highest compared with the lowest quintile of intake. On the other hand, neither the Physicians' Health Study nor the Zutphen Elderly Study (which followed 667 Dutch elderly men free of coronary artery disease for 10 y) reported reductions in the risk of MI with increasing intakes of EPA+DHA or fish (Morris *et al.*, 1995; Oomen *et al.*, 2001).

Nine prospective cohort studies and 4 case-control studies reported data on fish consumption and MI. Four of the 9 cohort studies (Hu *et al.*, 2002; Ascherio *et al.*, 1995; Yuan *et al.*, 2001; Daviglus *et al.*, 1997) and 1 case-control study (Tavani *et al.*, 2001) showed a statistically significant reduction in CHD, whereas 3 cohort studies (Folsom *et al.*, 2004; Albert *et al.*, 1998; Fraser *et al.*, 1992) and 1 case-control study (Gramenzi *et al.*, 1990) found no such reduction in risk.

Evidence suggested that increased consumption of n–3 FAs from fish or fish-oil supplements, but not of α-linolenic acid, reduced the rates of all-cause mortality, cardiac and sudden death, and possibly stroke. The single primary-prevention RCT of n–3 FA supplementation by Natvig *et al.* (1968) included 13 578 subjects between 50 and 59 y of age who were randomly assigned to receive 10 ml flaxseed oil (5.5 g ALA/d) or sunflower seed oil (0.14 g ALA/d) for 1 y. This trial was conducted in Norway >30 y ago and reported a very-low CVD event rate (<1 per cent) in the control group and no significant cardiovascular benefit of ALA supplementation. Background fish and fish-oil intake was already quite high in this population, which possibly limited any potential benefit of additional ALA.

Overall, the data from the secondary- and primary-prevention studies support the hypothesis that consumption of very-long-chain n–3 FAs from fish and fish-oil supplements reduces all-cause mortality, cardiac and sudden death, and stroke. This conclusion agrees with 2 recent meta-analyses by He *et al.* (2004a and 2004b), which were more limited in scope than the current review, and with the results of a 1999 ecologic study by Zhang *et al.* (1999). The latter showed a significant association between fish consumption and total mortality across 36 countries on the basis of data from the Food and Agriculture Organization and the World Health Organization.

However, this conclusion is not applicable to the population of patients with an ICD, in whom 3 recent RCTs found inconsistent antiarrhythmic effects and no significant overall effect on mortality.

The evidence appears strong for a beneficial effect of very-long-chain n–3 FA intakes on CVD risk in secondary, but not in primary, prevention because data from RCTs are available for the former, but less evidence exists to support a beneficial effect on MI. There is no high-quality evidence to support a beneficial effect of ALA.

Combined Effect of Fish-Oil Supplements with Regular Aerobic Exercise on Cardiovascular Disease Risk Factors

Regular exercise and consuming long-chain n–3 fatty acids (FAs) from fish or fish oil can independently improve cardiovascular and metabolic health, but combining these lifestyle modifications are more effective than either treatment alone (Hill *et al.*, 2000). They examined the individual and combined effects of n–3 FA supplements and regular exercise on body composition and cardiovascular health.

Overweight volunteers [body mass index (BMI; in kg/m^2): >25] with high blood pressure, cholesterol, or triacylglycerols were randomly assigned to one of the following interventions: fish oil (FO), FO and exercise (FOX), sunflower oil (SO; control), or SO and exercise (SOX). Subjects consumed 6 g tuna FO/d (H"1.9 g n–3 FA) or 6 g SO/d. The exercise groups walked 3 d/wk for 45 min at 75 per cent age-predicted maximal heart rate. FO supplementation lowered triacylglycerols, increased HDL cholesterol, and improved endothelium-dependent arterial vasodilation ($P < 0.05$). Exercise improved arterial compliance ($P < 0.05$). Both fish oil and exercise independently reduced body fat ($P < 0.05$) (Hill *et al.*, 2000). They concluded that FO supplements and regular exercise both reduce body fat and improve cardiovascular and metabolic health. Increasing intake of n–3 FAs could be a useful adjunct to exercise programs aimed at improving body composition and decreasing cardiovascular disease risk.

Mechanism of Action Proposed

New information about how omega-3 fatty acids affect cardiac function (including antiarrhythmic effects), hemodynamics (cardiac mechanics), and arterial endothelial function have helped clarify potential mechanisms of action. In previous studies, the postulated biological mechanisms underlying the relation between n–3 FAs and the prevention of CVD included decreased arrhythmias, lower triacylglycerol concentrations (Adkins and Kelley, 2010; Breslow, 2006), lower blood pressure, improved vascular reactivity and decreased platelet aggregation (Kris-Etherton *et al.*, 2002; Appel *et al.*, 1993; Kristensen *et al.*, 2001).

Thrombosis and Hemostasis

Omega-3 fatty acids decrease platelet aggregation, resulting in a modest prolongation of bleeding times. Some evidence indicates that fish oil supplementation may enhance fibrinolysis. Although omega-3 fatty acid intake has been negatively associated with levels of fibrinogen, Factor VIII, and von Willebrand factor (Shahar *et al.*, 1993), more recent evidence from the Coronary Artery Risk Development in young

Adults (CARDIA) study found no significant associations between customary intakes of fish (4 to 39 g/d) and omega-3 fatty acids (0.9 to 4.1 g/d) and these coagulation factors (Archer *et al.*, 1998). Marckmann *et al.* (1997) also found no effect of omega-3 fatty acids (0.9 g/d) on levels of Factor VII, fibrinogen, endogenous fibrinolysis, ß-thromboglobulin, and von Willebrand factor. In contrast, a recent study reported that coronary patients taking 5.1 g/d of omega-3 fatty acids for 6 months experienced a reduction in von Willebrand factor (128 per cent versus 147 per cent for controls) and thrombomodulin (25 versus 33 ng/mL) (Johansen *et al.*, 1999). Although it seems clear that omega-3 fatty acids beneficially influence collagen-induced platelet aggregation (thereby affecting hemostasis), their effects on thrombosis remain unclear. There is little evidence to suggest that an intake <3 g/d of omega-3 fatty acids would cause clinically significant bleeding.

Arrhythmias

The possibility that omega-3 fatty acids (including α-linolenic acid) may reduce risk for sudden cardiac death is based on evidence from a prospective cohort study (Albert *et al.*, 1998), a case-control study (Siscovick *et al.*, 1995), and four prospective dietary intervention trials (deLorgeril *et al.*, 1999; Burr *et al.*, 1989; Singh *et al.*, 1997). Proposed mechanisms to explain these observations center not on lipid or blood pressure lowering or on antithrombotic effects, but on a novel stabilizing effect of omega-3 fatty acids on the myocardium itself. Evidence for a direct effect of these fatty acids on the heart has come from several observations. First, increased heart rate variability in survivors of MI was associated with the consumption of one fish meal per week (Christensen *et al.*, 1997) or fish oil supplements (4.3 g/d of omega-3 fatty acids (Christensen *et al.*, 1996). Increases in this parameter predict a lower risk of mortality due to arrhythmic events in post-MI patients. EPA and DHA also have been shown to reduce resting heart rate and increase left ventricular filling capacity (Grimsgaard *et al.*, 1998). Animal experiments and cell culture studies have shown that fish oil has potent antiarrhythmic effects. For example, studies with rats (Pepe *et al.*, 1996) and dogs (Kinoshita *et al.*, 1994; Billman *et al.*, 1997) have shown that pretreatment with omega-3 fatty acids reduced damage to cardiac tissue and forestalled the development of ventricular dysrhythmias when heart attacks were induced. Similar observations were made in fish oil–fed cats that were protected from cerebral damage after stroke induction (Black *et al.*, 1979). *In vitro* induction of tachyarrhythmias in cultured neonatal rat ventricular myocytes by various pharmacological agents (such as ouabain) can be prevented or abolished by the addition of omega-3 fatty acids to the culture medium (reviewed by Kang and Leaf, 1996). This seems to be due to the ability of omega-3 fatty acids to prevent calcium overload by maintaining the activity of L-type calcium channels during periods of stress (Hallaq *et al.*, 1992), and to increase the activity of cardiac microsomal Ca^{2+}/Mg^{2+}-ATPase (Grimsgaard *et al.*, 1998). In addition, omega-3 fatty acids (including α-linolenic acid) are potent inhibitors of voltage-gated sodium channels in cultured neonatal cardiac myocytes, which may contribute to the reduction in arrhythmia (Kang and Leaf, 1996).

Blood Pressure

Omega-3 fatty acids seem to have a small, dose-dependent, hypotensive effect, the extent of which seems to be dependent on the degree of hypertension (Howe *et al.*,

1997). In a meta-analysis, Morris *et al.* (1993) found a significant reduction in blood pressure of -3.4/-2.0 mm Hg in studies with hypertensive subjects who consumed 5.6 g/d of omega-3 fatty acids. Likewise, Appel *et al.* (1993) found that blood pressure was decreased -5.5/-3.5 mm Hg in trials of untreated hypertensives given >3 g/d of omega-3 fatty acids. DHA seems to be more effective than EPA in lowering blood pressure. (Mori *et al.,* 2000). Still, in view of the high dose required to lower blood pressure and the proven efficacy of other nutritional factors and of antihypertensive medications, an increased intake of omega-3 fatty acids has a limited role in the management of hypertension.

Hypertriglyceridemia

Fish oil can have a therapeutic role in the treatment of marked hypertriglyceridemia (>750 mg/dL). Effective doses of omega-3 fatty acids range from 3 to 5 g/d, which can only be obtained consistently by supplementation. At present, it seems that both EPA and DHA have triglyceride-lowering properties (Grimsgaard *et al.,* 1997). Patients taking >3 g of EPA+DHA from supplements should do so only under a physician's care because the FDA has noted that an intake in excess of this level could result in excessive bleeding in some individuals (CFS and AN, 2002). In contrast, cardioprotective intakes seem to be considerably lower (≈1 g/d), have almost no potential for adverse effects, and can be achieved by diet.

Other Biological Effects

Goode *et al.* (1997) showed that acetylcholine-stimulated relaxation of small arteries taken from hypercholesterolemic patients was significantly improved after three months of supplementation with 3 g/d of EPA+DHA. Fish oil feeding has also been shown to improve endothelial function (reviewed by Chin and Dart, 1995) and to increase arterial compliance (McVeigh *et al.,* 1994). These effects may be secondary to fish oil's ability to enhance nitric oxide production (Harris *et al.,* 1997) and may be the mechanism by which fish oil elicits a small hypotensive effect.

Mechanisms to explain the antiatherogenic (inhibition of new plaque development) effect of omega-3 fatty acids have recently been proposed (Eritsland *et al.,* 1996). For example, EPA and DHA seem to alter the metabolism of adhesion molecules such as vascular cell adhesion molecule-1 (VCAM-1), E-selectin, and intercellular adhesion molecule-1 (ICAM-1). Abe *et al.* (1998) reported a 9 per cent reduction in soluble ICAM-1 and a 16 per cent reduction in soluble E-selectin but not in soluble VCAM-1 in hypertriglyceridemic subjects receiving 3.4 g/d of highly purified omega-3 fatty acid ethyl esters for 7 to 12 months. There is also *in vitro* evidence that DHA reduces endothelial expression of VCAM-1 and the expression of E-selectin, ICAM-1, interleukin (IL)-6, and IL-8 in stimulated cell (DeCaterina *et al.,* 1996; DeCaterina *et al.,* 2000). On the other hand, a study in male smokers with hyperlipidemia showed that six weeks of omega-3 fatty acid supplementation (4.8 g/d) increased soluble forms of E-selectin and VCAM-1 (Seljeflot *et al.,* 1998). A subsequent study in coronary patients given supplemental omega-3 fatty acids (5.1 g/d for 6 months) found similar results (Johansen *et al.,* 1999).

Fish oil also affects the metabolism of inflammatory mediators like the interleukins and tumor necrosis factor-α, (Endres *et al.*, 1996) molecules also believed to play a role in atherogenesis and plaque stability (Lee and Libby, 1997).

Another potential antiatherogenic mechanism of omega-3 fatty acids is their interference with the arachidonic acid cascade that generates a wide variety of eicosanoids (reviewed by Uauy *et al.*, 1999). EPA not only can replace arachidonic acid in phospholipid bilayers, but it is also a competitive inhibitor of cyclooxygenase, reducing the production of the 2-series prostaglandins, thromboxanes, and prostacyclins and the 4-series leukotrienes. The 3- and 5-series (respectively) produced from EPA are generally less biologically active. DHA, although not a direct inhibitor of arachidonic acid metabolism, nevertheless can inhibit platelet aggregation by reducing the affinity of platelet TxA_2/PGH_2 receptor for its ligand (Bayon *et al.*, 1995). The net effects of omega-3 fatty acids are thus to reduce inflammatory processes, vasoconstriction, and platelet aggregation, all known to be antiatherogenic.

Influence of Fish Oils on Lipid Metabolism

i) Triacylglycerol-Rich Lipoproteins

The concentrations of endogenously derived triacylglycerol-rich lipoproteins, VLDLs, and intermediate-density lipoproteins have been almost uniformly reported to be lowered with fish oil. Fish oils have been effective in normal subjects and in patients with common phenotypes of hyperlipidemia in which VLDL concentrations are raised. The minimum effective dose of n–3 fatty acids appears to be slightly more than 1 g/d. At intakes >2 g/d, VLDLs decreased an average of 25 per cent in normal subjects and even more in hypertriglyceridemic subjects (≈50 per cent in those with the type 4 or 5 phenotype and ≈40 per cent in those with combined hyperlipoproteinemia) (Harris, 1989). Furthermore, this response is maintained. What of chylomicrons and chylomicron remnants? In more severe forms of hypertriglyceridemia, such as type 5 hyperlipoproteinemia, in which both VLDLs and chylomicrons (or remnants) are present, excess n–3 fatty acids can be highly effective. Whether this result reflects enhanced removal of chylomicrons is uncertain. Catabolized VLDLs and chylomicrons compete for similar removal mechanisms; diminished chylomicron removal may therefore occur whenever VLDL overproduction increases the need for VLDL removal, as in type 5 hyperlipoproteinemia. Chylomicronemia after a fatty meal is diminished when fish oil is eaten over 2 wk (Weintraub *et al.*, 1988) but not after a single meal. Remnants in type 3 hyperlipoproteinemia are partly cleared with fish-oil treatment (Dallongeville *et al.*, 1991).

Dietary fish oils also modify the type of hypertriglyceridemia that is normally inducible by carbohydrates (Harris *et al.*, 1984). This modification might be expected from the known effects of these 2 nutrients on triacylglycerols: carbohydrates stimulate and fish oils inhibit VLDL production. This is seen strikingly in hepatocytes from obese hyperlipidemic rats in which the usual overproduction of lipid is suppressed with DHA (Wong *et al.*, 1985).

In summary, fish oils affect VLDL metabolism by *1*) reducing VLDL triacylglycerol secretion, as clearly shown in kinetic studies in humans, animal liver perfusions, and isolated hepatocytes (Nestel, 1990); *2*) generally, but not always, increasing VLDL apoliprotein B secretion (Nestel *et al.*, 1984) [at least in rat liver, this may be related to increased apolipoprotein B degradation (Wang *et al.*, 1993), thus assembly of VLDL is impaired]; *3*) reducing triacylglycerol transport, resulting in smaller VLDLs, which are largely converted to LDLs; and *4*) less certainly, increasing VLDL clearance. The key enzyme lipoprotein lipase has mostly been found to be unaffected by fish oil in humans (Harris *et al.*, 1988).

ii) Chylomicron Metabolism

Although there is agreement that chylomicron assembly and secretion are reduced in isolated intestinal cells incubated with EPA, the interpretations of results differ. The mechanisms appear to include the reduction of apolipoprotion B formation and the diversion of EPA from triacylglycerols to phospholipids (Murthy *et al.*, 1988).

iii) Hepatic Triacylglycerol Metabolism

Reduced triacylglycerol formation is ascribed largely to reduced fatty acid availability. Studies have confirmed that *1*) fish oil increases oxidation of fatty acids by peroxisomal as well as mitochondrial routes, which may be mediated by peroxisome proliferator in the liver; *2*) fish oil reduces fatty acid synthesis (owing to suppression of key enzymes); *3*) fish oil diverts fatty acids to phospholipids; *4*) although fish oil reduces plasma fatty acids, this may be due to increased hepatic uptake through a transporter protein; *5*) within the liver, triacylglycerol assembly is impaired through down-regulation of esterifying enzymes (Nestel, 2000).

iv) Cholesterol Metabolism

Fish oil reduces cholesterol absorption in humans and in monkeys. Cholesterol synthesis in the liver is reduced and cholesterol secretion within VLDLs is lowered (Nestel, 2000).

v) LDL Metabolism and Oxidation

The effects of fish oil on LDL metabolism represent the more controversial aspects of the n–3 fatty acid effects. Some studies have shown that omega-3 fatty acids may increase the susceptibility of LDL to oxidation (Hau *et al.*, 1996; Sorensen *et al.*, 1998) whereas others have not (Brude *et al.*, 1997; Higdon *et al.*,2001).

Why does fish oil cause LDL-cholesterol concentrations to sometimes rise, at least in humans, when all the evidences suggest it should not? Fish oil depresses cholesterol synthesis and may reduce cholesterol absorption (Nestel, 1990). This focuses attention on LDL removal and particularly on the LDL (apolipoprotein B/E) receptor. There is evidence that fish oil down-regulates the receptor in hepatic cells. Abnormal LDL binding to the receptor in human monocytes and to skin fibroblasts has been ascribed to abnormalities in the LDL itself. Reduced LDL synthesis has been reported with large amounts of fish oil (Nestel, 2000).

The n–3 enrichment renders LDLs susceptible to oxidation, as has been shown in several reported studies, with some exceptions. The obvious relevance is to atherogenesis, which is favored by oxidized lipoproteins. The evidence includes increases in *in vitro* copper-oxidized and macrophage-modified changes in LDL that lead to their increased uptake by macrophages. These findings define a potential atherogenic property of dietary fish oil, although it must be emphasized that these are *in vitro* observations and that the sum of the metabolic outcomes of marine n–3 fatty acids appears to be antiatherogenic in life. Nevertheless, findings of Nestel (2000) indicate a need for increased antioxidant action, such as that provided by α-tocopherol, if large amounts of fish oil are to be consumed. It has in fact been shown that, at least *in vitro*, the addition of vitamins E and C to n–3 fatty acid–enriched macrophages inhibits their capacity to oxidize LDLs (Suzukawa *et al.*, 1996). In a study in pigs fed atherogenic diets, however, atherosclerosis was not increased in animals fed fish oil, despite evidence of raised in vitro LDL oxidizability (Whitman *et al.*, 1994).

It therefore remains to be established whether LDL oxidative status in vivo is affected by omega-3 fatty acids and, if so, whether this has any adverse clinical implications in humans. Current inability to identify and quantify *in vivo* oxidative damage and to relate it to clinical outcomes makes it difficult to draw firm conclusions about the impact of omega-3 fatty acids on these processes in humans.

vi) HDL Metabolism

Most reports indicate a favorable effect of fish oil on HDLs. The number of larger cholesterol-rich HDLs (in the HDL_2 range) increases at the expense of HDL_3. However, very high intake of fish oil may lower HDL concentrations.

The major effect of fish oil on HDL metabolism is mediated by a reduction in activity of cholesterol ester transfer protein (Abbey *et al.*, 1990), which transfers cholesterol esters from HDLs to VLDLs and LDLs, largely in exchange for VLDL triacylglycerols. Because triacylglycerol concentrations are also reduced, exchange is further diminished, favoring large cholesterol-rich HDL (and LDL) particles over the formation of triacylglycerol-enriched HDLs (and LDLs), which are more susceptible to catabolism.

Limitations of Studies done on Omega-3 Fatty Acids and CVD

In many of the studies that examined the above mentioned mechanisms, the n–3 FA intakes were high, and the effects were small and limited to subsets of the population or were not consistently observed. It is unresolved whether all forms of n–3 FAs have similar biological activity *in vivo* and similar effects on CVD risk. Notably, most studies suggest that humans convert <5 per cent of ALA to EPA or DHA.

The totality of the data available on the effect of n–3 FAs on CVD outcomes suffered from many limitations that make drawing firm conclusions difficult. The evidence to support cardiovascular benefits from n–3 FA intakes in the secondary-prevention population came mostly from one large RCT. All the evidence for beneficial effects in the general population is derived from cohort studies. Data in women are limited, but the results are similar to those in men. Also, the studies analyzed were heterogeneous with regard to the methods of estimating fish or n–3 FA intakes, background diets, background risks for heart disease, settings, and the methods of reporting results. Different species of fish contain different amounts of EPA and DHA, and it is difficult to derive an accurate assessment of n–3 FA intakes from food frequency questionnaires. The method of food preparation, often not specified, may affect the n–3 FA content or add saturated and *trans* fatty acids, which can affect the outcome variables.

Data on the effects of ALA on CVD outcomes are limited and typically of poor quality. Only one comparative trial of ALA and fish oil was identified, and serious concerns were recently raised about the validity of these data. Dose-response effects of n–3 FAs on CVD outcomes are inconsistent: no direct comparisons of doses in fish-oil- or ALA-supplement trials have been attempted. Only 2 cohort studies reported outcome data using the ratio of n–6 to n–3 FAs, but these data were presented in inconsistent formats and with different degrees of quality, which makes the interpretation difficult. In addition, such a ratio may provide little useful information without knowledge of the absolute intakes of linoleic acid, ALA, EPA, and DHA. Finally, data on the effects and associations of n–3 FAs with CVD outcomes in different subpopulations are limited. Future research needs to address all of these lingering issues. Well-designed large RCTs that assess the effects of EPA and DHA on CVD outcomes with long follow-up periods are needed, especially in the general population. Future trials should not only attempt to confirm the findings of the GISSI trial in countries with different background dietary habits and risk but should also explore the various underlying mechanisms. Such studies should adequately assess background diet and fish consumption, particularly the species of fish and the methods of fish cooking and preparation. Attempts should also be made to determine the effect of higher fish intakes on the displacement of other foods from the diet, specifically meat and cheese, which are high in saturated fat (Wang *et al.*, 2007).

II. Stroke

Fish, the major source of long-chain omega-3 PUFAs may potentially reduce risk of stroke through several mechanisms. First, randomized clinical trials have shown that fish-oil supplementation decreases systolic and diastolic blood pressure, especially in older and hypertensive persons (Geleijnse *et al.*, 2002). Second, increasing evidence indicates that omega-3 PUFAs reduce blood triglyceride concentrations. A meta-analysis of 47 placebo-controlled randomized trials found that supplementation with fish oil produced a clinically significant reduction of fasting blood triglycerides (Eslick *et al.*, 2009). Third, limited and inconsistent evidence indicated that fish oil may have beneficial effects on inflammation and endothelial function. Intervention studies conducted in persons at high risk of cardiovascular diseases or patients with clinical cardiovascular disease have shown that fish-oil supplementation significantly decreased the concentration of soluble intercellular cell adhesion molecule-1 (Hjerkinn *et al.*, 2005) or interleukin-6 (Seierstad *et al.*, 2005) but had no effect or an adverse effect on inflammatory markers (Johansen *et al.*, 1999). Other potential mechanisms by which long-chain omega-3 PUFAs may reduce risk of stroke include antiatherogenic, neuroprotective, and antiplatelet effects (Massaro *et al.*, 2008, Dyall and Michael-Titus, 2008). Fatty fish is a major determinant of serum 25-hydroxyvitamin D concentrations in the Swedish population during winter at a latitude of 60°. Prospective studies reported an inverse association between blood concentrations of 25-hydroxyvitamin D and incident hypertension.

Fish is also an important source of selenium, which might have a protective role against stroke by acting as an antioxidant and preventing methyl mercury toxicity (Ralston and Raymond, 2010). However, randomized controlled trials in China and the United States have not shown a protective effect of selenium supplementation on stroke risk. Fish is a good source of protein and low in saturated fat. The amino acid taurine is concentrated in fish and has been shown to decrease blood pressure and triglyceride concentrations in animals and humans (Zhang *et al.*, 2004). Lean fish consumption has been shown to reduce systolic and diastolic blood pressure in subjects with ischemic heart disease (Erkkila *et al.*, 2008). Moreover, a randomized trial in patients with ischemic heart disease showed that circulating soluble intercellular cell adhesion molecule-1 concentrations significantly decreased in the group assigned to consume lean fish but not in the group assigned to consume fatty fish (de Mello *et al.*, 2009).

Many studies of fish consumption in relation to stroke incidence or mortality have produced conflicting results. Methodologic differences among studies may have been responsible for some of the inconsistency. Importantly, fish was not a major constituent of the diet of some of the populations studied (Keli *et al.*, 1994; Gillum *et al.*, 1996), and for populations, the type of fish typically consumed may not have been particularly healthful (*e.g.*, salted, smoked, or deep-fried fish). The method by which the fish was usually prepared (*e.g.*, deep frying) may have negated any health benefits. Some studies were too small to allow for separation of stroke or fish subtypes. The failure to accomplish such separation could have hid beneficial associations because fatty fish contain higher concentrations of omega-3 PUFAs than do lean fish, and fish consumption may not affect all stroke subtypes equally.

Previous studies have shown that the effects of fish oil on stroke were inconsistent. Five prospective cohort studies and 1 case-control study provided data on estimates of n–3 FA intake and stroke. These studies included the large US cohorts of the Nurses' Health Study (Iso *et al.*, 2001) and of the Health Professionals Follow-Up Study (He *et al.*, 2004b). Only the latter study, which followed 43 671 men free of CVD for 12 y, reported a significant reduction in ischemic strokes at all fish-oil intakes above the lowest quintile. The Nurses' Health Study found a nonsignificant trend of decreased strokes with increasing fish-oil intake (Iso *et al.*, 2001).

Twelve prospective cohort studies and 1 case-control study provided data on fish consumption and stroke. Three large cohort studies (He *et al.*, 2002; Sauvaget *et al.*, 2003; Mozaffarian *et al.*, 2005) showed a statistically significant reduction in stroke, particularly ischemic stroke. The Health Professionals Follow-Up Study reported a significant reduction in ischemic strokes with any level of fish consumption (He *et al.*, 2002). The Hiroshima/Nagasaki Life Span Study, which followed 30 827 male and female survivors of the atomic bomb in Japan, found that those in the highest tertile of fish consumption had a lower risk of death from stroke than did those in the lowest tertile (Sauvaget *et al.*, 2003a). In the Cardiovascular Health Study by Mozaffarian *et al.* (2005), increased consumption of tuna or other nonfried fish was associated with a decrease in total stroke and ischemic stroke. In contrast, increased consumption of fried fish and fish sandwiches was associated with an increased risk of stroke. There was no association with hemorrhagic stroke in either of the latter 2 studies. Three cohort studies and 1 case-control study (Oomen *et al.*, 2001; Gillum *et al.*, 1996; Keli *et al.*, 1994) found a nonsignificant trend of decreased strokes with increasing fish consumption. An additional 5 cohort studies provided no evidence to support the hypothesis that fish consumption reduces the risk of stroke.

In the prospective cohort of Swedish women, Larsson *et al.* (2011) observed an inverse association between the consumption of fish, especially lean fish, and stroke incidence. Women who consumed ≥3 servings of lean fish/wk had a 33 per cent lower risk of total stroke compared with the risk for women who never consumed lean fish. Other types of fish, including salmon, whitefish, and char and herring and mackerel were not significantly associated with risk of stroke.

Their findings for total fish consumption and incidence of stroke were similar to results of a meta-analysis that combined data from 8 prospective studies (with a total of 3491 stroke events) published through October 2003 (He *et al.*, 2004). Results from that meta-analysis showed that, compared with individuals who never consumed fish, subjects who consumed fish 2-4 times/wk had an 18 per cent lower risk of stroke, and subjects who consumed fish ≥5 times/wk had a 31 per cent lower risk of stroke (He *et al.*, 2004b). On the basis of data from 3 studies that provided results for cerebral infarction (ischemic stroke) and hemorrhagic stroke, the association was stronger for cerebral infarction; the pooled RRs for the highest compared with the lowest category of fish consumption were 0.65 (95 per cent CI: 0.46, 0.93) for cerebral infarction (1138 cases) and 0.80 (95 per cent CI: 0.44, 1.47) for hemorrhagic stroke (548 cases). Larsson *et al.* (2011) observed a stronger inverse association for hemorrhagic stroke, but the number of hemorrhagic stroke cases was relatively small (233 cases) and the results were not significant. In a cohort of 4775 US women and men, the high consumption of tuna or other broiled or baked fish was associated with lower risk of total stroke and ischemic stroke, whereas consumption of fried fish or fish sandwiches was associated with increased risk (Mozaffarian *et al.*, 2005). Results from a British cohort study showed no association between total fish consumption and stroke incidence; however, fatty fish consumption was significantly inversely associated with risk of stroke in women (Myint *et al.*, 2006). In contrast, a nested case-control study in northern Sweden showed a significant positive association between fish consumption and stroke incidence in men but no association in women (Wennberg *et al.*, 2007). Four other cohort studies observed no association between fish consumption and stroke incidence (Montonen *et al.*, 2009) or mortality (Yamagishi *et al.*, 2008).

According to Larsson *et al.* (2011), their findings from the prospective cohort of women suggested that a high consumption of fish, especially of lean fish, may reduce risk of stroke. The association between the consumption of specific types of fish and stroke subtypes merits further investigation.

III. Cancer

Fish consumption may also have various effects on cancer risk (Maclean *et al.*, 2006). For example, in prospective cohort and case-control studies, men with higher EPA+DHA intakes had a lower incidence of prostate cancer and longer survival after prostate cancer diagnosis (Leitzmann *et al.*, 2004: Chavarro *et al.*, 2007), but neither fish nor EPA+DHA intake were associated with colon cancer or bladder cancer (Holick *et al.*, 2006). Additionally, concern has been raised that contaminants in some fish may lead to increases in total cancer risk because of organochlorine contaminants (Huang *et al.*, 2006).

IV. Chronic Diseases

To elucidate the sum of effects on chronic disease endpoints, Virtanen *et al.* (2008) investigated the relations of fish and dietary EPA+DHA consumption, assessed with serial food-frequency questionnaires (FFQs), with total major chronic disease, including total CVD, cancer, and death due to other diseases. Given the hypotheses that n–6 fatty acids compete with or counteract potential benefits of fish or n–3 fatty acid intake, they also investigated whether n–6 fatty acid intake modified associations between fish or EPA+DHA consumption and risk of major chronic disease. They assessed lifestyle and other risk factors every 2 y and diet every 4 y in 40,230 US male health professionals aged 40–75 y and free of major chronic disease at baseline in 1986. During 18 y of follow-up, 9715 major chronic disease events occurred, including 3639 cardiovascular disease events, 4690 cancers, and 1386 deaths from other causes. After multivariable adjustment, neither fish nor dietary n–3 fatty acid consumption was significantly associated with risk of total major chronic disease. Compared with fish consumption of <1 serving/mo, consumption of 1 serving/wk and of 2–4 servings/wk was associated with a lower risk of total cardiovascular disease of ≈15 per cent. No significant associations were seen with cancer risk. Higher or lower n–6 fatty acid intake did not significantly modify the results. They concluded that modest fish consumption was associated with a lower risk of total cardiovascular disease, consistent with cardiac mortality benefits but not with total cancer or overall major chronic disease; n–6 fatty acid consumption did not influence these relations.

V. Dementia Risk

Long-chain omega-3 (n-3) polyunsaturated fatty acids, specifically EPA and DHA present in fish are critical for brain structure and function (Salem *et al.*, 2001). Experimental evidence indicates that a DHA-enriched diet can reduce neurodegenerative pathology (*e.g.* β-amyloid accumulation and oxidative stress) and improve learning ability in aged rats (Lim and Suzuki, 2000; Gamoh *et al.*, 2001) and rodent models of Alzheimer disease (AD) (Calon *et al.*, 2004; Hashimoto *et al.*, 2002). Furthermore, DHA treatment of human neuronal cells can decrease β-amyloid secretion and counteract the proinflammatory and proapoptotic effects of β-amyloid (Lukiw *et al.*, 2005).

Some (Morris *et al.*, 2003: Kalmijn *et al.*, 1997; Barberger-Gateau *et al.*, 2007; Larrieu *et al.*, 2004), but not all (Schaefer *et al.*, 2006; Engelhart *et al.*, 2002; Huang *et al.*, 2005), epidemiologic studies suggest that higher intakes of fish and omega-3 PUFAs from dietary sources are related to reduced dementia risk.

In 2 separate publications from the Rotterdam Study, researchers found that fish consumption was associated with a lower risk of dementia over 2 y of follow-up (Kalmijn *et al.*, 1997), but total omega-3 PUFA consumption was not related to dementia risk over 6 y (Engelhart *et al.*, 2004). In addition to overall inconsistent results, few studies have explored the longer-term effects of these dietary factors on dementia risk. However, because dementia develops over many years, earlier exposures may influence dementia risk in later life (Launer *et al.*, 2005). To address this issue, Devore *et al.* (2009) examined the dietary consumption of fish and omega-3 PUFAs in relation to long-term dementia risk over an average follow-up of 10 y in the Rotterdam Study, thus taking advantage of longer follow-up and substantially more dementia cases than were available in previous analyses. The population for analysis consisted of 5395 participants who were free of dementia and provided valid dietary information at baseline. They found no relation of total fish intake with long-term risk of dementia and Alzheimer disease (AD) in either age-and sex- adjusted or multivariate-adjusted models. Specifically, in multivariable models, those with a higher fish intake had a risk of dementia similar to participants who typically ate no fish. Likewise, when examined intake according to fish type, they found no difference in dementia risk comparing participants who ate fatty fish to those who did not typically eat fish. Results were very similar when AD was evaluated as the outcome, as might be expected because most dementia cases (78 per cent) were attributable to AD in this cohort. In this cohort of Dutch older adults, no evidence was found that higher intakes of fish and omega-3 PUFAs from food sources were associated with long-term risk of dementia over an average 10 y of follow-up.

V. Cognitive Performance among the Elderly

Modern studies of the role of nutrition in cognition among the elderly began in the 1980s and were reviewed by Rosenberg and Miller (1992). In 1997, Grant highlighted the possible role of diet in the development of Alzheimer disease (AD). After the initiation of large-scale observational epidemiologic studies in the Netherlands in the 1990s, it was suggested that the intake of fish might protect the elderly from developing cognitive impairment or dementia (Kalmijn *et al.*, 1997a, 1997b). This idea has been supported by several independent studies (Grant, 1997, Kalmijn *et al.*, 2004; Morris *et al.*, 2005) that have led to a debate about whether modification of the diet might be one way to prevent cognitive decline and dementia in the elderly (Friedland, 2003; Luchsinger and Mayeux, 2004). It is clearly important to resolve the question of whether such a relatively simple change in lifestyle as eating more fish can reduce the burden on the individual and on society of cognitive decline and dementia in the elderly. Although intervention studies ultimately will be required to answer this question, it is possible to test some hypotheses by additional observational studies. The purpose of the cross-sectional study carried out by Nurk *et al.* (2007) on community-dwelling elderly people was to seek answers to the following questions: *1*) Is the intake of fish and fish products associated with better cognitive performance? *2*) Is dietary intake of seafood associated with the performance of all, or only some, cognitive abilities? *3*) Is there any relation between the type of seafood product consumed and cognitive test results? and *4*) Is there any relation between the amount of fish consumed and cognitive test results? The subjects (n = 2031 subjects; 55 per cent women), aged 70–74 y, were recruited from the general population in Western Norway who underwent cognitive testing in this study. They reported that the subjects whose mean daily intake of fish and fish products was ≥10 g/d (n = 1951) had significantly better mean test scores and a lower prevalence of poor cognitive performance than did those whose intake was <10 g/d (n = 80). The associations between total intake of seafood and cognition were strongly dose-dependent; the maximum effect was observed at an intake of ≈75 g/d. Most cognitive functions were influenced by fish intake. The effect was more pronounced for nonprocessed lean fish and fatty fish. They concluded that in the elderly, a diet high in fish and fish products is associated with better cognitive performance in a dose-dependent manner.

VI. Role in Age-Related Hearing Loss

Age-related hearing loss (HL) (presbycusis) is a common and under recognized health problem in the older subpopulation. The cochlea of the inner ear is the site at which most of the HL in older adults is believed to arise. The cochlea is highly vascularized and is supported by a single artery. Apart from biological degeneration that results from the aging process itself, genetic risk factors, exposure to noise, and the occurrence of certain diseases may predispose individuals to presbycusis. Although many of these factors cause disruption to the hair cells of the cochlea, per se, it is assumed that disruptions to cochlear blood flow can also cause significant permanent HL. Gates *et al.* (1993) examined the association between cardiovascular disease events and risk factors and hearing status in the Framingham cohort of 1662 older adults. A moderate association between cardiovascular disease events (i.e, ischemic heart disease, myocardial infarction, and stroke) and HL was shown (Gates *et al.*, 1993). With the assumption of the hypothesis that atherosclerosis is common to the pathogenesis of age-related HL and cardiovascular disease, clinical evidence has shown that diets high in unsaturated fats reduce cardiovascular events. The polyunsaturated group of fats, particularly long-chain omega-3 polyunsaturated fatty acids, has been shown to be protective against cardiovascular disease (Wijendran and Hayes, 2004; Hooper *et al.*, 2006). As fish contain n-3 PUFAs (particularly EPA and DHA) which have been shown to be cardioprotective (Connor, 2000), it was plausible to think the role of n-3 PUFAs and fish in vascular function may also be important for the auditory system. Gopinath *et al.* (2010) determined the association between dietary intakes of omega-3 (n-3) PUFAs and fish and the risk of presbycusis. This Blue Mountains Hearing Study conducted by them was a population-based survey of age-related hearing loss (1997–1999 to 2002–2004). They collected dietary data by using a semiquantitative food-frequency questionnaire and calculated PUFA and fish intakes. In 2956 participants (aged ≥50 y), they measured presbycusis, which they defined as the pure-tone average of frequencies 0.5, 1.0, 2.0, and 4.0 kHz >25 decibels of hearing loss. They found an inverse association between total n-3 PUFA intake and prevalent hearing loss. There was an inverse association between long-chain n-3 PUFAs and incident hearing loss. Participants who had ≥2 servings of fish/wk compared with participants who had <1 serving of fish/wk had a significantly reduced risk (42 per cent) of developing presbycusis at follow-up. There was an association between consumption of ≥1 to <2 servings/wk of fish and a reduced risk of a progression of hearing loss. Their findings may have important public health implications, given that regular consumption (≥1 but <2 servings/wk) of fish in the diet was shown to slow the progression of an existing HL and, thus, could provide a rare opportunity to preserve residual hearing function. However, it needs to be highlighted that fish consumption >2 servings/wk did not protect against the progression of HL. This could indicate a threshold effect at 1–2 servings of fish/wk, with no increased protection at increased amounts of intake (Gopinath *et al.*, 2010). They concluded that as there was an inverse association between higher intakes of long-chain n-3 PUFAs and regular weekly consumption of fish and hearing loss, dietary intervention with n-3 PUFAs could prevent or delay the development of age-related hearing loss by having direct beneficial effects on hearing function by preserving the cochlear microcirculatory flow or by other mechanisms not yet defined (Liew *et al.*, 2007).

VII. Diabetes

Omega-3 fatty acids from seafood sources, alter the expression of peroxisome proliferator–activator receptor genes, which are involved in signaling nutrition status, and of the production of inflammatory cytokines, which are associated with T2DM. These findings suggested that omega-3 fatty acids could lower the risk of T2DM.

In epidemiologic studies, intake of long-chain omega-3 fatty acids was associated with better glucose tolerance in some studies but not in others. Some intervention studies have found that omega-3 intake resulted in an increase in glycated hemoglobin (Hb A_{1C}) (Woodman *et al.*, 2002; Sirtori *et al.*, 1998) and in fasting blood glucose (range: 2-25 mg/dL) (Toft *et al.*, 1995; Sirtori *et al.*, 1998). According to Vessby *et al.* (1994), eating long chain omega-3 polyunsaturated fats from fish does not protect against diabetes, even though there is much evidence that these marine omega 3 fats help prevent heart disease. If one is already diabetic, eating fish can help protect against a heart attack or dying from heart disease (Yokoyama *et al.*, 2007).

Epidemiologic studies of the relation of long-chain fatty acid intake with T2DM have reported conflicting results (Nkondjock and Receveur, 2003; Salmeron *et al.*, 2001; Meyer *et al.*, 2001; Wang *et al.*, 2003). This could be related to background differences in intake of α-linolenic acid (ALA), an omega-3 fatty acid from plant sources. Therefore, Kaushik *et al.* (2009) also investigated the interplay between long-chain omega-3 fatty acids and ALA in relation to T2DM risk in 3 large cohorts of women and men: the Nurses' Health Study (NHS), the Nurses' Health Study 2 (NHS2), and the Health Professionals Follow-Up Study (HPFS). Following 195,204 US adults (152,700 women and 42,504 women) for 14 to18 years, researchers found that the more fish or omega-3 fatty acids participants consumed, the higher their risk of developing diabetes. The risk increase was modest for occasional fish eaters, but rose to a 22 percent increased risk for women consuming five or more fish servings per week (Kaushik *et al.*, 2009).

Keeping in view the limited and inconsistent data regarding the effects of omega-3 fatty acids on glucose metabolism and insulin sensitivity, Djousse *et al.* (2011) also carried out a prospective study on 36,328 women (mean age 54.6 y) and followed them from 1992 to 2008 to find out the relationship between dietary omega-3 fatty acids, fish consumption and risk of T2D. They have also reported an increased risk of T2D with the intake of long-chain omega-3 fatty acids, especially with higher intakes (0.20 g omega-3/d or 2 servings of fish/d). During the follow up, 2370 women developed T2D. Marine but not plant-based omega-3 fatty acids were positively associated with incident T2D. The relation between marine omega-3 fatty acids and T2D was observed in hypertensive and nonhypertensive subjects and in women who reported infrequent fish consumption.

According to recent Dr. Bernard's blog on PCRM (Physicians Committee for Responsible Medicine), prior studies have also suggested that fat accumulation within muscle cells can lead to insulin resistance which, in turn, contributes to diabetes. People who eat no animal products have less fat in their cells and much less risk of developing diabetes. A low-fat vegan diet is required to improve type 2 diabetes. However, according to Kaushik *et al.* (2009), it is unclear whether such increases in glucose concentrations are associated with changes in insulin resistance. Previous studies have shown that omega-3 fatty acids may contribute to higher glucose concentrations through other mechanisms. Long-chain omega-3 can lower glucose utilization and increase glucagon-stimulated C-peptide (Mostad *et al.*, 2006) or could increase hepatic gluconeogenesis (Woodman *et al.*, 2002) by increasing uptake and oxidation of free fatty acids in liver (Puhakainen *et al.*, 1995) and lowering triacylglycerols (Carpentier *et al.*, 2006). Thus, omega-3 fatty acid and fish consumption may increase the diagnosis of T2DM by increasing circulating concentrations of glucose, but without causing other adverse metabolic abnormalities (insulin resistance, high triglycerides, and low HDL cholesterol). Recent studies have also reported that toxins such as dioxins and methyl mercury may interrupt insulin signaling pathways. This suggests that the findings for omega-3 fatty acids (Kaushik *et al.*, 2009) could be related to confounding by other factors in fish, but evidence to support this hypothesis is limited and requires further investigation. Furthermore, because studies have suggested that environmental contaminants such as dioxins (Lee *et al.*, 1999), found in fish, might raise the risk of T2DM, the risks and benefits of fish intake remain controversial.

Dietary Recommendations for Omega-3 Fatty Acids

General Population

A number of countries (Canada, Sweden, United Kingdom, Australia, Japan) as well as the World Health Organization and North Atlantic Treaty Organisation have made formal population-based dietary recommendations for omega-3 fatty acids. Typical recommendations are 0.3 to 0.5 g/d of EPA+DHA and 0.8 to 1.1 g/d of α-linolenic acid. In 2002, the Food and Nutrition Board, Institute of Medicine, and The National Academies, in collaboration with Health Canada, released the Dietary Reference Intakes for Energy and Macronutrients (IOM, 2002). The Acceptable Macronutrient Distribution Range (AMDR) for α-linolenic acid is estimated to be 0.6

per cent to 1.2 per cent of energy, or 1.3 to 2.7 g/d on the basis of a 2000-calorie diet. This is ≈10 times the current intake of EPA+DHA. The lower boundary of the range is based on an Adequate Intake set for α-linolenic acid, which represents median intake levels that prevent an essential fatty acid deficiency. The upper boundary corresponds to the highest α-linolenic acid intakes from foods consumed by individuals in the United States and Canada. Thus, the intent of the AMDR range for omega-3 fatty acids is to provide guidance for healthy people, not to prevent chronic disease. These recommendations can easily be met by following the AHA Dietary Guidelines to consume two fish meals per week, with an emphasis on fatty fish (ie, salmon, herring, and mackerel), and by using liquid vegetable oils containing α-linolenic acid. Commercially prepared fried fish (e.g, from restaurants and fast food establishments, as well as many frozen, convenience-type fried fish products) should be avoided because they are low in omega-3 and high in trans-fatty acids.

Prevention and Treatment of CVD

Dietary recommendations have been made for n–3 fatty acids, including α-linolenic acid (ALA), eicosapentaenoic acid (EPA), and docosahexaenoic acid (DHA) to achieve nutrient adequacy and to prevent and treat cardiovascular disease. Several health agencies worldwide recognize the importance of increasing EPA and DHA intake from fish to decrease the risk of CVD and therefore, many national, international, and professional organizations have made recommendations for fish or EPA and DHA consumption (Table 10.3).

A greater intake of the long-chain n–3 fatty acids (FAs) eicosapentaenoic acid (EPA) and docosahexaenoic acid (DHA) has been recommended by a variety of scientific and regulatory bodies to reduce population risk for coronary artery disease (CAD) (Harris, 2011). The evidence base supports a dietary recommendation of ≈500 mg/d of EPA and DHA for cardiovascular disease risk reduction. For treatment of existing cardiovascular disease, 1 g/d is recommended. These recommendations have been embraced by many health agencies worldwide. A dietary strategy for achieving the 500-mg/d recommendation is to consume 2 fish meals per week (preferably fatty fish). Although 1g/d intake of EPA and DHA potentially can be attained through fish consumption, the requisite amount of fish intake may be difficult to achieve and sustain over the long term. For those individuals who do not eat fish, have limited access to a variety of fish, or cannot afford to purchase fish, a fish oil supplement may be considered (Gebauer *et al.*, 2006). Depending on the preparation, up to three 1-g fish oil capsules per day will be necessary to provide ≈1 g/d of omega-3 fatty acids. The most common fish oil capsules in the United States today provide 180 mg of EPA and 120 mg DHA per capsule. It is important that consumers read the nutrition label to determine EPA and DHA levels in the fish oil capsule.

The American Heart Association has divided its recommendations into 3 categories: persons without known CAD, those with CAD, and those with elevated serum triacylglycerol concentrations (Kris-Etherton *et al.*, 2002). The intakes suggested for persons in those categories are, respectively, ≥2 fish meals/wk (preferably oily fish), ≈1 g EPA+DHA/d (from oily fish or from capsules), and 2–4 g EPA+DHA/d from capsules. A presumption of an equivalence between oily fish and fish-oil capsules is inherent in these recommendations, and yet few studies have examined whether n–3 FAs are equally bioavailable from these 2 very different matrixes.

Table 10.3: International Recommendations for Long-Chain n-3 Fatty Acids[1]

Source	Date	Total n-3	ALA	EPA DHA	n-6 : n-3
		% of Energy	g	mg	
NATO workshop	1989	–	3	800	4:1
UK Committee on Medical Aspects of Food Policy	1994	0.2	–	100–200	–
ISSFAL workshop	1999	1	2.2	650	–
ANC (France)	2001	0.8–1	1.8	450 (DHA, 110–120)	5:1
Eurodiet	2000	–	2	200	–
Health Council of the Netherlands	2001	1	–	200	7.5:1
American Heart Association (51)	2002	–	–	1 g/d (2° prev CHD)	–
US National Academics of Science, Institute of Medicine	2002	–	1.4	140	–
European Society of Cardiology	2003	–	–	1 g/d (2° prev CHD)	–
WHO FAO	2003	1–2	–	400–1000 (1–2 fish meals/wk)	–
ISSFAL	2004	–	1.6	500	
UK Scientific Advisory Committee on Nutrition	2004	–	–	Minimum 2 portions fish/wk (1 oily); assumes 450 mg	

1: ALA, -linolenic acid; ANC, Apports Nutritionnels Conseilles; DHA, docosahexaenoic acid; EPA, eicosapentaenoic acid; FAO, Food and Agriculture Organization; ISSFAL, International Society for the Study of Fatty Acids and Lipids; NATO, North Atlantic Treaty Organization; WHO, World Health Organization.

Source: Gebauer *et al.*, 2006.

GI symptoms associated with fish-oil or ALA supplementation are the most commonly reported adverse events. Most GI symptoms were reported at dosages >3 g/d for EPA+DHA. Because current recommendations do not exceed 1 g/d for secondary prevention of CVD risk (AHA, 2001), it is unlikely that GI symptoms are a limiting factor for the implementation of this intervention. Overall, adverse events related to the consumption of fish-oil or ALA supplements appear to be minor and bothersome but not clinically relevant.

Challenges in Meeting the Recommendations

One of the main considerations when trying to meet current recommendations for n–3 fatty acids is that current intake of PUFAs consists primarily of n–6 fatty acids. The competition for desaturases and elongases in n–3 and n–6 PUFA metabolism results in inverse affects on tissue concentrations of these fatty acids (Cunnane, 2003). Therefore, this would be a concern for those consuming a diet, which is characterized by foods high in refined carbohydrates, saturated and *trans* fatty acids, and vegetable oils high in n–6 fatty acids that contain little n–3 fatty acids (Simopoulos, 2003). This is of even greater concern in vegetarians and vegans, who have relatively high intakes of LA combined with low intakes of EPA and DHA (Davis *et al.*, 2003). Cross-sectional data collected in this population indicate that plasma DHA concentrations are lower but stable compared with those in nonvegetarians and are inversely correlated with plasma LA. This illustrates the inverse relation between n–3 and n–6 fatty acids and the particular concern for vegetarians and vegans in attaining n–3 fatty acid recommendations (Rosell *et al.*, 2005).

Fish or Fish Oil?

The underlying support for fish oil in the management of cardiovascular risk is the apparent protection that eating fish provides. Several large studies have documented such protection from relatively small amounts of fish eaten regularly The current consensus is that eating fish is beneficial at surprisingly modest intakes, and the benefit probably depends on the fatty acid profile of the fish consumed.

In a pilot study including 4–8 volunteers who had consumed either salmon or fish-oil supplements, Visioli *et al.* (2003) found similar increases in serum phospholipid EPA (per mg EPA consumed) from either source, but a 3 times greater increase in serum DHA concentrations when the DHA came from salmon than when it came from fish-oil capsules. This study was small and retrospective; moreover, the EPA and DHA intakes from these 2 sources were not matched, and the study was not randomized. A larger study compared the effects of eating salmon and taking cod liver oil on serum n–3 FAs; it found that the former was a more efficient vehicle (Elvevoll *et al.*, 2006). However, in neither of these studies were EPA and DHA intakes prospectively matched. Harris *et al.* (2007) compared the effects of equivalent, nutritionally relevant intakes of marine n–3 FAs (i.e, ≈500 mg/d that are currently recommended by several health organizations and agencies) from oily fish given 2 times/wk and of daily 1000 mg fish-oil capsule supplementation on the EPA and DHA content of blood cell membranes [(i.e, red blood cells, RBCs, or the omega-3 index, a proposed risk marker for cardiovascular mortality and of the plasma phospholipid (PPL) fraction]. They also compared the tolerability of each approach. Their study showed that, regardless of whether n–3 FAs were consumed from oil-rich fish or fish-oil capsules, there was, after 16 wk of treatment, no difference in the effect on the major long-chain n–6 or n–3 FAs, whether measured in RBCs or in PPL. Over that period, the consumption of ≈485 mg EPA+DHA/d from fish or capsules produced a 40–50 per cent rise in RBC EPA+DHA and a 60–80 per cent rise in PPL EPA+DHA. They found that EPA+DHA concentrations rose more quickly in PPL than in RBCs; the former stabilized by 4 wk and the latter continued to rise over the span of the 4-mo test period. Fish consumption was associated with fewer episodes of a fishy aftertaste than was capsule consumption, which suggests increased tolerability of the former. Fish also provides high-quality protein and trace minerals (especially selenium and iodine) that are not provided by supplements. In contrast, capsules are more convenient to consume, and they provide none of the mercury or chemical contaminants (Foran *et al.*, 2003) that can be found in fish. However, a recent risk-benefit analysis indicated that the cardiovascular benefits of consuming fish (ie, salmon) far outweigh (≈400:1) any risks due to the potential presence of these contaminants (Mozaffarian and Rimm, 2006).

Overall, this study concluded that the EPA+DHA content of RBCs or PPLs did not differ significantly when equivalent doses of n–3 FAs were provided twice a week from fish or daily 1000-mg from fish oil capsules for 4 mo. Accordingly, either source could be used to bolster tissue n–3 concentrations, and evidence from past randomized trials suggests that both would be expected to result in a lower risk of CAD events (Harris *et al.*, 2007).

Whether one decides to get omega-3 fatty acids from fish or from supplements, heed precautions about potential exposure to environmental contaminants, including mercury. Pregnant women and children should avoid fish that has the highest likelihood of being contaminated with mercury such as tilefish, swordfish and king mackerel. One should eat a variety of other fish and seafoods to reduce risk of contamination even further.

n–3 Fatty Acid–Rich Foods of the Future

The extensive evidence of the health benefits of n–3 fatty acids has prompted the development of food products enriched in these fatty acids. Genetic modification has been used to develop a new generation of plants (*e.g.*, corn and soybeans) that produce seeds that have a modified fatty acid profile. Strategies are available to increase or decrease specific fatty acids in the target plant. Research is ongoing to increase the n–3 fatty acid content of animal products, such as eggs, milk, and cuts of meat by altering the composition of animal feed. The n–3 fatty acid content of animal feed is increased with the addition of fishmeal, flax, and n–3 fatty acids. New n–3 fatty acid–enriched products include oils, bakery products, eggs, mayonnaise, margarines, salad dressings, pasta, milk, meat, and poultry. Consequently, the evolving marketplace will help individuals meet fatty acid recommendations in a way that could not be envisioned 25 y ago. Thus, it will be far easier for individuals to meet the contemporary recommendations for n–3 fatty acids than in the past (Gebauer *et al.*, 2006).

Another consideration for meeting recommendations for marine-derived n–3 fatty acids is that some populations do not consume fish because of concerns about environmental toxins, taste preferences, or ethical reasons. Studies have shown that certain fish contain high levels of environmental toxins, such as mercury and polychlorinated biphenyls (PCBs) (Guallar *et al.*, 2002; Yamaguchi *et al.*, 2003). Therefore, one challenge faced when increasing dietary fish intake is methylmercury, a heavy metal toxin found in varying amounts in different types of fish. Of particular importance is the neurologic damage to developing fetuses and young children caused by toxic levels of methylmercury. In response to these concerns, the Food and Drug Administration and the Environmental Protection Agency issued a joint advisory in March 2004 for women who are pregnant or might become pregnant, nursing mothers, and young children (FDA, 2004). Three recommendations made in the advisory, such that these women and young children can benefit from n–3 fatty acid intake while minimizing their exposure to mercury are

1. Do not eat shark, swordfish, king mackerel, or tilefish because they contain high levels of mercury.
2. Eat up to 340 g/wk (2 average meals) of a variety of fish and shellfish that are lower in mercury, such as shrimp, canned light tuna, salmon, pollock, and catfish. Furthermore, albacore (white) tuna has more mercury than canned light tuna. So, when choosing 2 meals of fish and shellfish, one may eat up to 170 g /wk (1 average meal) of albacore tuna.
3. Check local advisories about the safety of fish caught by family and friends in local lakes, rivers, and coastal areas. If no advice is available, eat up to 170 g/wk (one average meal) of fish you catch from local waters, but do not consume any other fish during that week.

In addition to mercury, PCBs, which were reported to be higher in farm-raised than in wild salmon, are another concern for persons who consume fish. Hites *et al.* (2004) found median PCB concentrations of 42 ppb in farmed and 3 ppb in wild salmon (including the skin in the analysis). To put these amounts in context, the FDA limit for PCBs in foods is 2000 ppb; thus, neither presents a significant risk. Preparation methods, such as cooking the fish and removing its skin, reduces the amount of environmental toxins in the fish. New research is focusing on assessing amounts of PCBs in other species of fish besides salmon, determining ways to minimize contaminants in farm-raised fish, and establishing consistent methods for consumption advice. Because of the varying amounts of mercury and PCBs in fish, consumption of a variety of fish species, both wild and farmed, is recommended to minimize exposure to environmental toxins while maximizing health benefits.

Another challenge in meeting n–3 fatty acid recommendations is that some persons do not enjoy the taste of fish; whereas some vegetarians, such as vegans, do not consume any animal products, including fish. Because only a small amount of ALA can be converted to DHA and a minimal amount is converted to EPA, other options need to be utilized by vegetarians and persons who do not eat fish. One dietary option for increasing dietary intake of EPA is seaweed, which is incorporated into dishes growing in popularity, such as sushi. Kelp, laver, and wakame are types of seaweed that range in EPA content from 0.004 to 0.186 g per 100-g portion.

Another option for increasing the intake of EPA and DHA for persons who do not consume fish is DHA-rich microalgae supplementation or fish oil supplementation. DHA-rich microalgae, which is available in supplement form, provides 10–40 per cent DHA by dry weight. When supplementing with DHA-rich microalgae capsules, a direct DHA source, 100–300 mg/d is suggested. Fish oil capsules vary widely in amounts of EPA and DHA, with the most common fish oil capsules currently in the US providing 180 mg EPA and 120 mg DHA per capsule. A recent review suggests that an EPA-to-DHA ratio in fish oil capsules between 2:1 and 1:2 appears optimal. The reasons for this recommendation are the apparent synergistic relation of EPA and DHA and that substantial evidence to suggest that either one is the principal bioactive fatty acid is currently lacking. Studies have also shown that several over-the-counter brands of fish oil supplements contain negligible amounts of mercury; whereas PCBs are below the limit of detection. Thus, persons concerned with environmental toxins from fish may also opt for fish oil supplementation.

Chapter 11

Dietary Component of Therapeutic Lifestyle Change in CVD

Diet is the hallmark of therapy for hyperlipidemia, hypercholesterolemia and cardiovascular diseaseses. Its usefulness extends beyond simply providing additional low-density lipoprotein cholesterol (LDL-c) lowering for those with hypercholesterolemia. It also can help improve the abnormal high-density lipoprotein cholesterol (HDL-c) and triglyceride (TG) values seen in combined hyperlipidemia. In fact, patients with combined hyperlipidemia are often quite sensitive to weight reduction and exercise. Diet may play an important role in those with low HDL-c and premature coronary heart disease (CHD). Knowledge of the effects of dietary fat, kind of dietary fat, effect of dietary carbohydrate and effect of alcohol may prove useful in the overall care of such individuals. In those with severe hypertriglyceridemia who are prone to pancreatitis, reduction of all dietary fats and cessation of alcohol is crucial to avoiding exacerbations that could lead to the chylomicronemia syndrome and acute pancreatitis. Also, dietary antioxidants may reduce risk of CHD through mechanisms independent of lipid effects. Finally, antithrombotic and antiarrhythmic effects of diet may prove useful.

Nutritionist and clinicians need to know and understand the changes in dietary composition that affect LDL-c, HDL-c and TGs. Denke has shown that the higher the initial serum cholesterol value, the greater the response to diet. Also, excess body weight is a factor that must be considered. It is a strong contributor to elevated cholesterol levels in men. Weight gain in adult life can lead not only to abnormal lipid values, but to increased risks for diabetes mellitus and CHD also. Genetic influences on dietary responsiveness are considerable. Those persons with familial hypercholesterolemia cannot usually hope to achieve goal LDL-c values with diet alone.

Those with apo E-IV phenotype absorb more dietary cholesterol than those with apo E-II. This may become clinically useful since some patients who do not respond well to statins are thought to have increased absorption and hence decreased synthesis of LDL. On the other hand, those with familial combined hyperlipidemia or metabolic syndrome (often a strong genetic component) may improve markedly with diet, weight loss, and exercise. A genetically influenced atherogenic lipoprotein phenotype characterized by a predominance of small, dense LDL-particles giving an undesirable Pattern B phenotype can be induced by low-fat diets (that are high in carbohydrates) in healthy subjects with large LDL particles and the desirable Pattern A (Dreon *et al.*, 2000).

Previously, the two diets recommended by the National Cholesterol Education Program (NCEP) Adult Treatment Panel (ATP) II were the Step I and Step II Diets. The Step I diet was really the "population" diet and the Step II diet was the high-risk patient diet. Yet diet alone may not be effective unless advice on regular physical activity and a program of weight control is added. ATP III offers a therapeutic diet (Tables 11.1 and 11.2) and combined lifestyle advice on diet, exercise, and weight loss in an intensified program called Therapeutic Lifestyle Change (TLC).

Therapeutic Lifestyle Changes (TLC) Diet and its Recommendations

For people at high risk or who have known cardiovascular disease, they should adopt the Therapeutic Lifestyle Changes (TLC) diet. This is the "next generation" of the Step II diet recommended in May 2001. That's when the NCEP released new guidelines for cholesterol management in its Third Report of the Expert Panel on Detection, Evaluation, and Treatment of High Blood Cholesterol in Adults (Adult Treatment Panel III [ATP III]). ATP III continues to recommend the Step I diet for the general public. The American Heart Association accepted and endorsed new guidelines given in the above mentioned Third Report (ATP III). ATP III recommends that therapy for elevated cholesterol begins with more intensive life-habit intervention to lower cholesterol and reduce the risk for developing heart disease and having a heart attack. This approach is referred to as the "Therapeutic Lifestyle Changes (TLC)" diet.

For people at higher risk, the new (TLC) dietary goals offer dietary therapy for subgroups of people with specific medical conditions and risk factors such as these:

- ☆ High LDL cholesterol or other lipid disorders
- ☆ Coronary heart disease or other cardiovascular disease
- ☆ Diabetes mellitus, insulin resistance or metabolic syndrome

TLC diet is targeted to people whose LDL cholesterol is above the goal level for their category of risk for heart disease. The TLC diet contains recommendations on the daily intake of fats, carbohydrates, and proteins. Additionally, the diet also includes recommendations on fiber-containing products. This regimen basically focuses on the consumption of a balanced diet, emphasizing the difference between "good" fats and "bad" fats as well as the difference between "good" and "bad" carbohydrates.

The essential components of TLC diet are:

Table 11.1: Essential Components of TLC Diet

Component	*Recommendation*
LDL Raising nutrients	
Saturated fats*	Less than 7 per cent of total calories
Dietary Cholesterol	Less than 200mg/day
Therapeutic options for LDL-lowering	
Plant stanois/sterols	2g/day
Increased viscous (soluble) fibre	10-25g/day
Total calories(energy)	Adjust total calorie intake to maintain desirable body weight/prevent weight gain
Physical activity	Include enough moderate exercise to expend at least 200 kcal per day

*Trans fatty acids also raise LDL and should be kept at a low intake.

TLC Diet and Fat Recommendations

Total and Saturated Fat

In ATP II, the recommended intake for saturated fat was low. Total fat should be 30 per cent of calories for most. ATP III offers a range of 25 per cent to 35 per cent , allowing an increased intake of unsaturated fat in place of carbohydrates in those with metabolic-syndrome and diabetes. ATP III does not advise dietary fat intake 25 per cent due to concerns of decreased compliance with such a diet and an unwanted increase in TGs and decrease in HDL that is often seen when fat intake is so lowered.

In view of the fact that only saturated fats and trans fatty acids increase LDL cholesterol levels, serum levels of LDL cholesterol are unrelated to total fat intake per se. For that reason, the ATP III suggests it is not crucial to limit total fat intake for the specific goal of reducing LDL cholesterol levels, provided saturated fats are decreased to goal levels.

People who have high cholesterol because they eat too many fatty foods may be able to lower their cholesterol 10 per cent to 20 per cent with diet changes alone, while others may only achieve a 5 per cent to 8 per cent reduction. Those who are most successful using diet changes to lower their cholesterol are those who lose excess weight. Diet changes are usually the first step in lowering cholesterol before medicines are added.

Table 11.2: TLC Diet Guidelines – One Should Eat

Nutrient	*Recommended Intake as Percent of Total Calories*
Total Fat[1]	25-35 per cent
Saturated fat	Less than 7 per cent
Polyunsaturated fat	Up to 10 per cent
Monounsaturated fat	Up to 20 per cent
Carbohydrate[2]	50-60 per cent of total calories
Protein	Approx. 15 per cent
Cholesterol[3]	Less than 200mg/day
Total calories	Balance energy intake and expenditure to maintain desirable body weight and prevent weight gain

1. The 25–35 per cent fat recommendation allows for increased intake of unsaturated fat in place of carbohydrates in people with the metabolic syndrome or diabetes.
2. When saturated fats are replaced with carbohydrates, LDL cholesterol levels are reduced. On the other hand, very high intakes of CHOs (60 per cent total energy intake) are associated with a reduction in HDL cholesterol and an increase in serum TG. Increasing soluble fibre intake can sometime reduce these responses. On an average, increasing soluble fibre to 5-10g/day is accompanied by an approx. 5 per cent reduction in cholesterol.
3. Carbohydrate should come mainly from foods rich in complex carbohydrates. These include grains (especially whole grains), fruits and vegetables.
4. Options include adding 10–25 grams of viscous (soluble) fiber; 2 g/day of plant-derived sterols or stanols. Soy protein may be used as a replacement for some animal products.
5. Daily energy expenditure should include at least moderate physical activity (contributing about 200 Kcal a day).

Source: NCEP resources page. Third report of the National Cholesterol Education Program (NCEP) Expert Panel on Detection. Evaluation, and Treatment of High Blood Cholesterol in Adults (Adult Treatment Panel III). Executive Summary Available at http:// www.nhlbi.nih.gov/guidelines/ cholesterol/atp3xsum.pdf.

The main focus of Therapeutic Lifestyle Changes (TLC) diet is to reduce the amount of saturated fat we eat because it elevates the blood cholesterol. One can reduce the saturated fat in the diet by limiting the amount of meat and milk products. Choose low-fat products from those food groups instead. Replace most of the animal fat in the diet with unsaturated fat, especially monounsaturated oils, such as olive, canola, or peanut. Monounsaturated fat lowers LDL ("bad") cholesterol if it is substituted for saturated fat and keeps HDL ("good") cholesterol up.

MUFA

The TLC diet recommends the substitution of MUFA fat for saturated fats at an intake level of up to 20 per cent of total energy intake because MUFA fats lower LDL cholesterol levels relative to saturated fats without decreasing HDL cholesterol or TG levels. It is recommended that plant oils and nuts be used because they are the best sources of MUFA fats.

PUFA Fats

PUFA fats, in particular linoleic acid, reduce LDL cholesterol levels when used instead of saturated fats. However, they can also bring about small reductions in HDL cholesterol when compared side by side with MUFA fats. The TLC Diet recommends liquid vegetable oils, semi liquid margarines, and other margarines low in trans fatty acids be used because they are the best sources of PUFA fats, intakes can range up to 10 per cent of total energy intake.

Other Recommendations

The TLC diet also includes recommendations on soluble fiber and phytosterol, both of which are known to lower cholesterol levels. Soluble, or viscous fiber includes oatmeal, psyllium, pectin, and bran. Phytosterols, also known for their ability to lower cholesterol. Current recommendations for soluble fiber consumption are 10 to 25 grams each day, whereas two grams a day of phytosterol intake is recommended. Additionally, the TLC diet recommends that salt intake be limited to 2400 milligrams a day.

The TLC diet might seem complicated because of the many guidelines given for each main nutrient. However, it basically encourages eating a heart-healthy, balanced diet and lowering cholesterol through decreased fat intake and increased consumption of fiber. An example of TLC diet is given in Table 11.3.

Table 11.3: An Example of TLC Diet

Food Group	*Number of Servings*	*Serving Size*
Lean meat, poultry, fish, dry beans, and dry peas	No more than 5 ounces total per day	☆ 5 ounces maximum per day of lean meat, poultry, or fish ☆ Substitute ¼ cup dry beans or peas for 1 ounce of meat.
Eggs	No more than 2 yolks per week	1 whole egg. Egg whites or substitutes are not limited.
Low-fat milk and milk products	2 to 3 per day	☆ 1 cup nonfat or 1 per cent milk ☆ 1 cup nonfat or low-fat yogurt ☆ 1 ounce fat-free or low-fat cheese (3 grams of fat or less per ounce)
Fruits	2 to 4 per day	☆ 1 piece fruit, such as apple, orange, or ½ a banana ☆ ½ cup canned fruit ☆ 1 cup berries or melon ☆ ¾ cup fruit juice
Vegetables	3 to 5 per day	☆ 1 cup raw leafy greens ☆ ½ cup cooked or raw vegetables ☆ ¾ cup vegetable juice
Bread, cereals, pasta, rice, and other grains	6 to 11 per day	☆ 1 slice of bread ☆ ½ hot dog or hamburger bun, bagel, or English muffin ☆ 1 ounce cold cereal ☆ ½ cup cooked pasta, rice, noodles, or other grains

Contd...

Table 11.3–*Contd...*

Food Group	*Number of Servings*	*Serving Size*
Fat and oils	6 to 8 per day	☆ 1 teaspoon monounsaturated oil, such as canola, olive, or peanut ☆ 1 teaspoon polyunsaturated oil, such as corn or safflower ☆ 1 teaspoon soft margarine (one that does not contain hydrogenated oils) ☆ 1 tablespoon salad dressing ☆ 1 teaspoon mayonnaise ☆ 2 tablespoons nuts or seeds
Sweets and snacks	Within calorie limit	Choose snacks that are low in fat or are made with unsaturated fat.

Source: Grundy SM, et al. (2001). Executive summary of the third report of the National Cholesterol Education Program (NCEP) Expert Panel on Detection, Evaluation, and Treatment of High Blood Cholesterol in Adults (Adult Treatment Panel III). JAMA, 285(19): 2486–2497.

Dietary Influence on Lipids and Lipoproteins

The classic equation of Keys and Hegstedt established the important role of saturated fat and dietary cholesterol in determining change in blood cholesterol when changes were made in the metabolic ward setting. Their classic experiments showed that dietary saturated fat is twice as potent in raising blood cholesterol values as polyunsaturated fats are in lowering them. Dietary cholesterol is also important but quantitatively has less effect (Hegstedt et al., 1995).

Dietary Cholesterol

Sources of dietary cholesterol include:

- ☆ Animal meat
- ☆ Egg yolk
- ☆ Milk or dairy fat

Dietary cholesterol affects LDL-c by suppression of cholesterol production in the liver. While the effects of dietary cholesterol on some animal species are striking, with massive hypercholesterolemia seen, the effects in humans are highly variable. Hyper- and hypo- responders are seen. There are gender differences as well, with women increasing their HDL-c more than men with cholesterol feeding. Nonwhites appear to be particularly responsive to cholesterol feeding as compared with whites, in whom LDL-c increases more strikingly in response to saturated fat intake (Fielding et al., 1995). Two large prospective studies found little effect on blood cholesterol of one egg per day except in diabetics (Hu et al., 1999).

Saturated Fats

Sources of saturated fat in the diet include:

- ☆ Fatty meats

- ✰ High-fat dairy products
- ✰ Vegetables sources, such as coconut and palm kernel oil (Table 11.4).

Table 11.4: Sources of Fatty Acids in the Diet

Name	*Structure**	*Common Sources*
Saturated		
Lauric	C12.0	Coconut oil, palm kernel oil
Myristic	C14.0	Coconut oil
Palmitic	C16.0	Palm oil, beef
Stearic	C18.0	Cocoa butter, beef
Monounsaturated (n-9) †-oleic	C18.1	Olive oil, canola oil, beef, peanut oil, avocado
Polyunsaturated (n-6) † - linoleic	C18.2	Corn, cottonseed, safflower, sunflower, soybean oils
Polyunsaturated (n-3) † - linolenic	C18.3	Flaxseed oil, canola oil, soybean oil, nuts (English walnuts)
Eicosapentaenoic	C20.5	Fatty fish such as mackerel, sardines, salmon, and bluefish
Docosahexaenoic	C22.6	Fatty fish such as mackerel, sardines, salmon, and bluefish

* Carbon chain length; double bonds.

† By convention, named for the location of the first double bond from the methyl position on the carbon chain.

Saturated fats appear to raise blood cholesterol and LDL-c through their influence on the LDL receptor. Among saturated fats, lauric, myristic, and palmitic are the most cholesterol raising (Table 11.5). Stearic acid has not been found to be cholesterol raising and may, in some circumstances, lower blood cholesterol. Nonetheless, in the St. Thomas Atherosclerosis Regression Study (STARS), progression of coronary disease was directly, strongly, and independently associated with intake of saturated fatty acids from lauric through stearic. This fact was not fully explained by the effects of these fatty acids on cholesterol. Certainly, at the population level, dietary saturated fatty acids are strongly associated with CHD; this was best seen in the 16 cohorts from 14 countries followed in the landmark, Seven Countries study. In that study, there were also significant associations with dietary cholesterol and trans fatty acids, but independent effects could not be shown due to high correlations between those dietary components. An informative study from eastern Finland with the excessive CHD mortality noted that cohorts from the past 20 years who had decreased their intake of high-fat liquid dairy products and spreadable fats had lower rates of CHD (Kromhout *et al.*, 1995). Thus, in the TLC program, saturated fat intake should be 7 per cent of total calories.

Table 11.5: Dietary Factors that Affect Lipids/Lipoproteins

	Lower LDL-c	*Raise HDL-c*	*Lower Triglycerides*
Fats			
Saturated	No, raises LDL-c	Yes	No
Monounsaturated	Yes*	No	Yes, if substitute for CHO
Polyunsaturated (n-6)	Yes	No	Yes, if substitute for CHO
Trans fatty acids	No, † raise LDL-c	No†	No
Dietary cholesterol	No‡	Yes‡	No
Fiber	Yes	No	No
Soy protein	Yes δ	No	No
Weight loss	Yes	Yes	Yes
Alcohol	No	Yes	No, raises triglycerides
Dietary carbohydrate	Yes*	Lowers HDL-c	No, raises triglycerides
Fish oil (n-3)	NoZ**	Variable	Yes

Abbreviations: CHO, carbohydrate, HDL-c, high-density lipoprotein cholesterol, LDL-c, low-density lipoprotein cholesterol.

* When substituted for saturated fat in the diet.

† In high amounts, raise LDL-c and lower HDL-c.

‡ Response to diet is variable, may increase LDL-c significantly in some but not in others, may increase HDL-c more in women than in men.

δ LDL-c lowering seen in hypercholesterolemia. Isoflavones appear to be most important component.

** May raise LDL-c as triglycerides are lowered in cases of combined hyperlipidemia.

Trans Fatty Acids

Trans fatty acids (TFAs) also raise cholesterol. The most common TFA is the trans isomer of oleic acid, claidic acid. Its structure is such that it is straighter than the usual cis isomer and thus, can be more tightly packed and hence solid at room temperature. Common sources include:

- ☆ Stick margarines and shortenings
- ☆ Dairy items, such as milk, butter and cheese
- ☆ Commercially processed baked goods

In terms of the potential of raising blood cholesterol, butter, which contains both dietary cholesterol and saturated fat, is the most harmful, followed closely by stick margarine with its higher content of TFAs. On the other hand, small amounts of soft tub or liquid margarine should impact the lipid profile in minimal fashion.

Fast-food restaurants partially hydrogenate vegetable oils, which increases their content of TFA. Feeding studies show that TFA in usual amounts in the American diet do not raise cholesterol as much as saturated fats. Nonetheless, in increased amounts, they raise LDL-c and lower HDL-c. The current recommendation is to keep consumption of TFAs low. Ideally, saturated fatty acids and TFA would be 10 per cent .

Polyunsaturated Fats

Polyunsaturated fats (n-6) are essential fatty acids, thus a diet completely devoid of these fats is not healthy. These fats are represented by the seed oils and often are components of soft margarines. They lower blood cholesterol and LDL-c in relation to their intake in the diet. No population has a long-term experience with high amounts of polyunsaturated oils, so their usage is initiated to 10 per cent of energy. Potential side effect from consuming excessive amounts of polyunsaturated oils include:

- Obesity (fats have 9 kcal/g)
- Gallstones
- Lower HDL-c levels

Although excess polyunsaturated fat intake is associated with tumor growth in animals, this has not been seen in the many clinical studies of humans.

Monounsaturated Fats

Monounsaturated fatty acids (MUFAs) are omega-9 fatty acids that are good choices for replacing saturated fatty acids in the diet. The chief monounsaturated fatty acid is oleic acid. Common sources include:

- Olive oil
- Canola (rapeseed) oil
- Peanut oil
- Avocados
- Almonds

Canola oil is low in saturated fatty acids and is a source of omega-3 fatty acid as well (alpha linolenic acid). This makes it a good choice for home use.

In addition to lowering blood cholesterol and LDL-c by replacing saturated fats in the diet, MUFAs appear to make LDL less susceptible to oxidation. This tendency may be particularly advantageous in those with combined hyperlipidemia and diabetes where small dense LDL particles are more likely to be present. MUFAs should not be consumed in excess.

Advocating a Mediterranean-type diet is reasonable for many patients. In this diet, the source of fats is usually olive oil, but it can be canola oil. Fatty sources of fish, poultry and red meat are eaten less frequently. Fruits and vegetables and whole grain products are abundant. This diet may be useful in the diabetic whose low HDL-c and high TGs worsen on a high-carbohydrate diet. One potential difficulty is for the patient who overdoes the use of olive oil and gains weight.

Low Fat, High-Carbohydrate Diets

Low-fat diets with high intakes of complex carbohydrate are typical of an Asian-style diet. These permit levels of fat intake as low as 10 per cent to 15 per cent of total energy. When these diets are introduced gradually, the marked carbohydrate induced hypertriglyceridemia that occurs with an abrupt shift in diet may not be seen (Ullmann et al., 1991). One of the problems with these diets is the decline in HDL-c that occurs.

Two strategies of clinical importance are weight loss and exercise. Tufts investigators compared a low-fat, high-complex-carbohydrate diet with body weight kept constant to one in which there was decreased caloric intake permitting weight loss. Only in the circumstance in which there was weight loss was the overall change in LDL-c/HDL-c favorable.

Regular aerobic exercise is a useful strategy to help raise low HDL-c. When aerobic exercise was added to a prudent weight-reducing diet, HDL-c levels in men increased by approximately 13 per cent and the expected decline in HDL-c with diet was prevented. The message is clear – it is not enough to restrict saturated fats and cholesterol. Regular physical activity and weight loss, when appropriate, are crucial as well to impact the lipid panel in the most favorable way.

Dietary Fiber

Practically speaking, there are two kinds of fiber or nondigestible carbohydrate. The first, which is insoluble, aids in bowel function. An example is wheat bran. The second is soluble fiber, now referred to as viscous fiber, which has an additional cholesterol-low-ering effect. Examples include:

- ☆ Dried beans
- ☆ Grains
- ☆ Certain fruits
- ☆ Vegetables

Psyllium is a source of soluble fiber used as a dietary supplement or in dry cereals. Psyllium can be a useful adjunct to bile acid sequestrants and augment the LDL-c lowering response.

Oat products have the most soluble fiber of any grain. A simple way to improve the diet is that oatmeal, oat bran, or any of the single or multigrain dry cereals be substituted for higher-fat breakfast items.

Vegetable Protein

A meta-analysis of clinical studies involving soy protein showed a small benefit in hypercholesterolemic subjects (total cholesterol 255 mg/dL). Recent data point to the value of soy with isoflavone for beneficial effects. This is a practical point because commercial products vary greatly in isoflavone content. The Food and Drug Administration (FDA) has indicated that a daily intake of 25 g/day can reduce cardiovascular (CV) risk.

As far as safety, soy is not new to the diet. Some Asian populations have consumed soy protein daily for centuries. Further work is needed, however, to establish the benefits and negative aspects of large amounts of soy in CHD risk reduction.

Other Dietary Factors

Coffee

Boiled coffee can raise total cholesterol and LDL-c, whereas usual amounts of filtered caffeinated coffee do not. There is disagreement as to whether decaffeinated coffee raises LDL-c. Moderate amounts of filtered coffee or decaffeinated coffee do not appear to increase the risk of CHD.

When patients ask about coffee, it is important to counsel that it is what the patient has with the coffee that is often more detrimental to their coronary risk profiles. Patients need to be told to avoid nondairy coffee creamers with cholesterol-raising ingredients, such as coconut oil or palm kernel oil, to use skim milk instead of whole milk or cream, and to avoid large amounts of sugar. It has been pointed out that cappuccino with skim-milk is even more frothy than that with whole milk.

Garlic

Although a meta-analysis suggested a small benefit of garlic on cholesterol levels, recent double-blind trials have not shown significant benefit of garlic over placebo on HDL subclasses, lipoprotein (a) L-p{a}) apolipoprotein B, postprandial TGs, or LDL subclass distribution.

Patients must consider the price of garlic supplements in the same way they consider cost of drug therapy. If significant lowering of LDL-c is required, a low dose of a statin and diet (TLC) has the advantage of proven efficacy and safety in high-risk populations and would be preferred over garlic supplements.

Excess Caloric Intake

Losing weight continues to be both difficult and controversial. It is difficult because helping obese people to lose weight and then keep it off over the long term is still a challenging problem for many. It is controversial because patients have been counseled in the past 10 years to try either a very low-fat diet or a very low-carbohydrate diet as alternatives to the recommended modified-fat diets of the American Heart Association (AHA). Two clinical trials in obese subjects (with a high proportion of metabolic syndrome/diabetes) that contrasted a low-carbohydrate, high-protein, high-fat diet compared with a modified-fat diet showed fairly consistent results (Foster et al., 2003; Stern et al., 2004), Both trials reported 1'-year follow-up data that showed the following:

- ✰ The low carbohydrate diet produced a greater weight loss during the first few months, but the differences were not significant at 1 year.
- ✰ The low-carbohydrate diet was associated with a greater improvement in TGs and HDL-c.
- ✰ Diabetics improve measures of glycemic control such as HbA_{1c} with low carbohydrate regimens.

- ☆ Weight loss interventions are characterized by high dropout rates when diet is the only intervention.

For obese persons with high TGs/low HDL-c, avoiding sugar-sweetened foods and drinks (especially sweetened fruit juices) and "white-flour" and white potatoes, can help with these lipid abnormalities as well as glycemic control. The data does not suggest that advising high animal fat or high dairy fat to achieve a very low carbohydrate diet is worth the increased risk of a high saturated fat diet over the long term.

The above experience should be contrasted with two studies that emphasized a low saturated fat, high dietary fiber program reducing calories to achieve a modest weight loss, and regular exercise in overweight/obese subjects with impaired fasting glucose tolerance (DPP, 2002; Tuomilehto et al., 2001). Subjects were followed for 3 years on average. Although weight loss was modest, the overall lifestyle changes resulted in a reduction of new-onset of diabetes of almost 60 per cent .

Dansinger and coworkers at Tufts contrasted four popular weight-loss diets: Ornish, Weight Watchers, Zone, and Atkins. They found that the greatest effects were observed in the study completers. The amount of weight loss seen in this study was associated with self-reported dietary adherence level ($r = 0.60$; $P = 0.001$), not with diet type ($r = 0.07$; $P = 0.40$). An improvement in metabolic parameters (Total/HDL-c, C-reactive protein, insulin) was significantly associated with weight loss (mean $r =$ 0.36, 0.37, and 0.39, respectively) but with no significant difference between diets ($P = 0.48$, $P = 0.57$, $P = 0.31$, respectively) (Dansinger *et al.*, 2005). The Dansinger study indicated that success goes most often to those who truly wish to change.

Alcohol

In cross-population studies, moderate intake of alcohol has been associated with reductions in CHD. Alcohol has several beneficial actions, including raising HDL-c and potentially beneficial effects on thrombotic susceptibility involving actions on plasminogen activator, fibrinogen, and platelets. The beneficial effects of alcohol were shown by a case-control study comparing those with a genetic polymorphism resulting in slow metabolism of alcohol with those who had a rapid metabolism. In both men and women, moderate drinkers with a slow metabolism of alcohol (homozygous for the slow oxidizing alcohol dehydrogenase allele) had increased HDL-c and decreased rates of CHD (Hines et al., 2001).

Although touted as more beneficial, red wine has not been shown to reduce CHD risk more than white wine in ecologic and epidemiologic studies. In patients with familial lipid disorders in which TG abnormalities are prominent, alcohol consumption can greatly increase TG values. In fact, excess alcohol intake is a common cause of secondary hyperlipidemias. A clue is the associated high rather than low HDL-c. In addition to concerns regarding alcohol and substance abuse, chronic, heavy drinking can exacerbate hypertension and lead to increased rates of:

- ☆ Stroke
- ☆ Cardiac dysrhythmia, especially atrial fibrillation

- ☆ Left ventricular hypertrophy
- ☆ Cardiomyopathy
- ☆ Liver disease
- ☆ Accidents and suicide (those who consume ≥5 drinks per occasion are nearly twice as likely to die from injuries than persons who drink less).

Thus, there can be no public health recommendation for alcohol usage to reduce CHD risk.

Small amounts of alcohol with meals on the order of 1 or 2 units or drinks daily for men and one-half to one drink daily for women are associated with lower rates of CHD and do not need to be proscribed in adults who have shown they can control their intake. A drink is defined as 3½ oz wine, 12 oz beer, or 1 oz hard liquor.

One should suspect alcohol excess exacerbating a familial lipid disorder in men who present with severe hypertriglyceridemia and acute pancreatitis. After recovery, elevated lipids remain as a clue to the underlying genetic lipid disorder that was exacerbated by the alcohol excess. Clues to increased intake of alcohol on a chronic basis include a high mean corpuscular volume, abnormal transaminase values, high serum iron, and the picture of a high TG associated with a high HDL-c. In the common metabolic syndrome, a high TG is accompanied by a low HDL-c.

Fish Oils and Fish Intake

Fish oils and fish intake are rich in the long-chain n-3 polyunsaturated fatty acids (PUFAs) known as eicosapentaenoic acid (EPA) or docosahexaenoic acid (DHA). The amount of n-3 PUFA is determined by summing up the EPA and DHA of a product. Good sources of marine n-3 PUFA include oily fish, such as:

- ☆ Salmon
- ☆ Mackerel
- ☆ Herring
- ☆ Sardines (watch out for the salt!)
- ☆ Tuna

Alpha linolenic acid (ALA) is a plant-based n-3 PUFA. Humans can synthesize some EPA and DHA from ALA. Good sources of ALA (grams of ALA/100 g of raw material) include:

- ☆ Flaxseed (20.0)
- ☆ Butternuts (dried) (8.7)
- ☆ Soybeans (raw) (3.2)
- ☆ Leeks (0.7)
- ☆ Oils high in ALA, including flaxseed, canola, and soybean oil (Harper *et al.*, 2001).

Feeding studies have documented the great efficacy of high-dose fish oil in lowering severe hypertriglyceridemia. In high doses (3 g), fish oil can elevate LDL-c in subjects with diabetes or combined hyperlipidemia. It can also elevate blood glucose levels in diabetics. High doses may lower blood pressure slightly and prolong bleeding times. Low doses (3 g g/day) are generally safe in that they do not produce the significant metabolic effects seen with higher-dose fish oil. One study of fish added to a Step-II diet noted immunologic changes of uncertain significance. Fish intake in epidemiologic studies appears to vary inversely with CHD risk, although this is not invariably the case. One large prospective study with careful dietary assessment noted a reduction in nonfatal myocardial infarction (MI), while others have suggested a reduction in sudden death. There are emerging data suggesting that a diet that includes a mild increase in n-3 PUFA may reduce sudden death (Table 11.6).

- The Diet and Reinfarction Trial (DART) noted a 29 per cent reduction in death, although not in reinfarction, in postinfarction male survivors randomized to a high-fish diet (25 per cent were given low-dose fish oil capsules if they could not eat fish).
- The Lyon Diet Heart Study compared a Mediterranean-style diet low in cholesterol and saturated fat with increased monounsaturated and n-3 PUFA compared with a control diet high in cholesterol and saturated fat in MI survivors. The experimental group increased their n-3 PUFA primarily through a canola-based margarine. Alcohol intake was the same in the two diet groups. There was a striking reduction in CHD death in the treatment group that was maintained at the 47-month follow-up.
- A Seattle case-control study measured n-3 PUFA in sudden-death victims and found that victims were characterized by lower intakes of fish. Their data suggested a small amount of fish weekly could provide significant benefits.
- The Gruppo Italiano per to Studio della opravvivenza nell'Infarton miocardico (GISSI) Prevenzione trial in over 11,000 MI survivors showed that low-dose (850 mg n-3 PUFA) fish oil capsules reduce significantly the combined primary end point of death, nonfatal MI, and nonfatal stroke compared with placebo. Vitamin E had no significant effect.
- Electrophysiologic studies in animals and possibly in humans have shown that n-3 PUFA increases the arrhythmia threshold for ischemia-induced sudden death. While the data do not yet show conclusively that low-dose fish oil capsules should be taken to reduce sudden death, they do support an increase in fish-based mealts per week (i.e., 2 per week) or an increase in vegetable-based n-3 PUFA in those with CHD.

Fish remain a good source of dietary protein that is low in saturated fat. For those without heart disease, the AHA suggests two servings of oily fish per week. For those with heart disease, the recommendation is for 1 g of long-chain n-3 PUFA (omega-3 fatty acids) per week. This is best obtained with fish oil capsules. Remember to check the label for the amount of eicosapentanoic acid (EPA) and docosohexanoic acid (DHA). The EPA and DHA summed together are the amount of omega-3 fatty acids in the capsule (Kris-Etherton et al., 2002).

Table 11.6: Trials of Fish or Fish Oils in Secondary Prevention

Intervention Trial	*Subjects and Duration of Study*	*Trial Design*	*Intervention*	*Results*
DART	2033 men post-MI 2 years	Randomized placebo controlled	Two fish meals/wk,	29% reduction in all-cause mortality in fish group, occurred early
Indian Experiment of Infarct Survival	360 subjects with suspected MI for 1 year	Randomized double blind, placebo controlled	Fish oil (EPA) 1.08 g/d and mustard oil (ALA) 2.9 g/d and placebo	Significant reduction in total cardiac events in EPA and ALA groups vs placebo, 50% reduction in sudden death in EPA group vs placebo
GISSI Prevention	11,324 men and women post-MI for 3.5 years	Randomized, open label, controlled, no external monitoring; 2 – 2 factorial design	Fish oil (875 mg/d; FPA + DHA) vs placebo vs vitamin E 300 mg/d vs combined therapy	Reduction in combined end point of death, nonfatal MI, and stroke
Lyon Diet Heart Study	605 men and women post-MI for 27 mo	Randomized; blood samples from intervention group showed increased n-3 fatty acids	Canola oil margarine enriched in ALA; intervention group with more fiber, MUFA, less saturated fat, cholesterol	Reduction in CHD death and nonfatal MI; no significant change in lipids
Study on Prevention of Coronary Athero-sclerosis by Intervention With Marine Omega-3 Fatty Acids	223 men and women with angiographically proven CHD	Randomized double blind placebo controlled trial; single center	Fish oil concentrate (55% EPA and DHA) or placebo with a fatty acid composition resembling average European diet-6 g/d for 3-mo; then 3 g for 21 mo	Fewer CV events in fish oil group but not significant P = 0.10, mild improvement angiographic and points' increase in LDL-c
Harvard Fish Oil Angiographic Study	31 men and women randomized to fish oil vs 28 controls; both with angiographically proven CHD; followed for 28 mo	Randomized, double blind, placebo controlled trial, single center	6 g fish oil vs placebo	No significant effect on atherosclerosis by quantitative angiography

Abbreviations: ALA, alpha linolenic acid; CHD, coronary heart disease; CV, cardiovascular; DART, Diet and Reinfarction Trial; DHA, docosahexaenoic acid; EPA, eicosapentaenoic acid; GISSI, Gruppo Italiano per lo Studio Della Sopravvivenza nell'Infarcto Miocardico, LDL-c. low-density lipoprotein cholesterol; MI, myocardial infarction; MUFA, monounsaturated fatty acids.

Antioxidants

There are many sources of antioxidants in the diet, including:

- ☆ Vitamin E (alpha-tocopherol)
- ☆ Vitamin C (ascorbic acid)
- ☆ β-Carotene
- ☆ Flavonoids

Vitamin E and β-carotene are lipid soluble, whereas vitamin C is water soluble. It is not easy to obtain large amounts of vitamin E from the diet. Food sources of vitamin E include:

- ☆ Seed oils
- ☆ Avocados
- ☆ Whole grain and fortified cereals
- ☆ Eggs
- ☆ Green vegetables

Food sources of β-carotene include:

- ☆ Carrots
- ☆ Red and yellow coloured fruits and vegetables
- ☆ Green leafy vegetables
- ☆ Papaya
- ☆ Pumpkin
- ☆ Broccoli

Vitamin C is widely available in fruits and vegetables, but loss of vitamin C can occur during cooking. Flavonoids are another source of dietary antioxidants that occur naturally in foods such as:

- ☆ Vegetables
- ☆ Fruits
- ☆ Beverages such as tea and wine

On a milligram-per-day basis, the intake of the antioxidant flavonoids still exceeds that of the antioxidants β-carotene and vitamin E. Thus, flavonoids represent a potentially important source of dietary antioxidants. These antioxidants may make LDL less susceptible to oxidation. Until recently, there were no randomized clinical trials of antioxidant therapy. Now there are four randomized, controlled clinical trials examining the effects of vitamin E supplementation for secondary prevention.

Larger-scale, carefully done, randomized, blinded clinical trials have not supported the contention that prescribing antioxidant vitamins for patients makes a clinical difference. A review of available clinical trials concluded that β-carotene supplementation was associated with a significant excess of all-cause mortality and

CV death, whereas vitamin E did not reduce the risk of CHD (Vivekanathan, 2003). Moreover, randomized angiographic trial of postmenopausal women with coronary artery disease showed that both hormone therapy and vitamin E (400 IU) and vitamin C (500 mg) were associated with adverse CHD outcomes (Waters, 2002). Indeed vitamins can interfere with proven CHD therapy such as niacin.

An angiographic trial of middle-aged men and women with low HDL-c demonstrated that a vitamin cocktail reduced both the beneficial effects of niacin therapy on HDL-c and apo A-1 levels as well as subsequent clinical and angiographic coronary end points (Brown et al., 2001). The current AHA Science Advisory on antioxidant supplements and CV disease concluded that routine use of antioxidant supplements for the prevention and treatment of CV disease is not justified by available evidence (Kris-Etherton *et al.*, 2004).

Increased dietary intake of carotenoids, particularly lutein and zeaxanthin, may reduce the risk of age-related macular degeneration. Increased intake of dark green leafy vegetables, such as spinach and collard greens, is associated with a substantial reduction in age-related macular degeneration. One should add fruits and vegetables to the diet on a daily basis as a good way of adding antioxidants; this may prove cheaper than supplements while greatly improving the quality of the diet.

Homocysteine, Folic Acid, B_6 and B_{12}

Homocysteine (H {e}) is a thiol-containing amino acid that requires folic acid, vitamins $B_{6,}$ and B_{12} for remethylation. By convention, the free and protein-bound forms of the amino acid and derived disulfides are called H (e). Elevated H (e) may occur due to an enzyme deficiency involving cystathionine synthase, deficiency of 5, 10-methylene tetrahydrofolate reductase, or dietary deficiencies of folic acid, $B_{12,}$ and B_6. Cross sectional analysis of H (e) levels and vitamin levels in elderly subjects in the Framingham Study showed that plasma H (e) levels exhibited a strong inverse association with plasma folate. Moreover, a 14-year follow-up of 80.082 women using a food questionnaire showed that daily intake of 400 μg folate and 3 mg vitamin B_6 was associated with the lowest risk of CHD. Fortunately, adequate folic acid intake can be obtained either through fortified cereals or a multivitamin (Rimm et al., 1998).

High H (e) levels are seen with renal insufficiency and renal failure. It seems clear that high H (e) levels have potentially deleterious effects on endothelial cells, platelets, and smooth-muscle cells, which could promote a prothrombotic, atherogenic state. Clinical studies have shown those cohorts with high levels of H (e) have increased rates of atherosclerosis involving coronary, cerebral, or peripheral arterial vessels. Among patients with hyperlipidemia, elevated levels of H (e) are independent predictors of atherosclerotic events. The predicament is that due to increasing public awareness, many patients ask for H (e) measurements and treatment regimens.

Two randomized, double-blind, controlled clinical trials of a folic acid, $B_{6'}$ B_{12} cocktail in patients either post-MI or at high risk with vascular disease or diabetes failed to show significant benefit from such a treatment strategy (Table 11.7) (Bonaa et al., 2006, HOPE 2, 2006). In the post-MI trial, there was a near-significant trend toward more MIs, as well as marginally significant trend toward fewer strokes, among

Table 11.7: Randomized Trials of Folic Acid, B_{12}, and B_6 on Clinical End Points

Trial/Duration	*Subjects/Age/Status*	*Intervention*	*Primary Outcome*
HOPE 2 Study/5 years	5522, ≥55 years of age, with vascular disease or diabetes	Folic acid 2.5 mg/d; B_6	Composite of death from cardiovascular causes, MI, and stroke
	Results: Mean plasma homocysteine levels: -2.4 intervention group; +0.8 placebo group; primary outcome events 18.8 per cent in intervention group assigned to active therapy 19.8 per cent in placebo (RR, 0.95, 95 per cent CI, 0.84 to 1.07, $P = 0.41$). No significant decrease in the risk of death from cardiovascular causes (RR, 0.96, 95 per cent CI, 0.81 to 1.13), MI (RR, 0.98, 95 per cent CI, 0.85 to 1.14), or any of the secondary outcomes as compared with placebo. Fewer patients assigned to active treatment than to placebo had a stroke (RR, 0.75, 95 per cent CI, 0.59 to 0.97). More hospitalizations for unstable angina (RR, 1.24, 95 per cent CI, 1.04 to 1.49) in intervention group vs placebo.		
NORVIT Trial 40 months	1749 men and women who had had an acute MI within 7 days before randomization	Subjects were randomly assigned in a 2-2 factorial design to receive either 1) folic acid 0.8 mg, B_{12} 0.4 mg, B_6 40 mg, 2) folic acid 0.8 mg, B_{12} 0.,4 mg, 3) B_6 40 mg, 4) placebo	Composite of recurrent MI, stroke, or sudden death from coronary artery disease
	Results: Mean total hemocysteine were lowered 27 per cent from baseline if given folic acid and B12, but no significant effect of intervention on the primary end point (RR, 1.08, 95 per cent CI, 0.93 to 1.25, $P = 0.31$). Also B_6 treatment was not associated with any significant benefit with regard to the primary end point (RR of the primary end point, 1.14, 95 per cent CI, 0.98 to 1.32, $P = 0.09$) to the folic acid, B_{12} and B_6 group, there was a trend toward an increased risk (RR, 1.22, 95 per cent CI, 1.00 to 1.50, $P = 0.05$)		

Abbreviation: CI, confidence interval, HOPE 2, Heart Outcomes Prevention Evaluation-the ongoing outc9omes, MI, myocardial infarction, NORVIT, Norway Vitamin {trial}, RR, relative risk

Bonna KH et al. HOPE 2 Investigators. *N Engl J Med* 2006; 354.

patients receiving folic acid, vitamin B_{12}, and vitamin B_6 than among those receiving placebo. In the high-risk trial, there was an increase in hospitalizations for unstable angina, although a decrease in stroke with the vitamin cocktail as compared with placebo. Alternate ways to lower homocysteine will need to be developed and tested before we can recommend routine lowering of homocysteine levels (Loscalzo, 2006).

For the general population, a recommendation for routine measurement of H(e) is unwarranted. For those with atherosclerotic vascular disease or familial premature CHD unexplained by other risk factors or those at high risk due to multiple risk factors or with diabetes, the measurement of H (e) and the recommendation of a multiple vitamin supplement containing 400 µg/d folic acid with small amounts of B_{12} and B_6 for those with elevated values may be considered. Higher doses of folic acid are required in chronic renal failure.

Folate deficiency is rarely seen due to supplementation of the food supply. Avoid folate supplementation alone in anorectic patients or the elderly as the addition of folic acid could mask the signs of B_{12} deficiency. Instead, a screen for B_{12} deficiency should be considered before empirically prescribing folic acid.

Vegetarian Diets

The use of a vegetarian diet is entirely consistent with a healthful, nutritional approach to reducing risk factors for CHD. Among vegetarians, levels of both LDL-c and HDL-c are low. An informative trial in India involved advising patients recovering from an acute MI to eat more fruit, vegetables, nuts, and grain products in addition to the usual post-MI fat-reduced diet. The improvements in weight and LDL-c levels were paralleled by improvements in rates of coronary events.

Patients who wish to adopt a true vegetarian lifestyle need nutritional counseling to be sure that they obtain adequate sources of nutrients. For example, vegans who eat no eggs or milk products need to provide for adequate protein and vitamin B_{12}. This is particularly important if they take folic acid supplements. Fortified soy milk may be useful. Fortified cereal can be a source of vitamin D. Ovolactovegetarians need to choose low-fat dairy products to keep the diet low in saturated fat.

A major problem for most physicians is finding the time to provide positive, useful message on diets. A useful exercise is to review the behaviors that affect dietary adherence. The DIET CAGE Questionnaire is brief, easily answered by the patient, and can give the health professional an idea as to dietary behaviors (Table 11.8). This or the validated MEDFICTS questionnaire allows the physician to highlight specific steps the patient can take to improve his or her nutritional patterns. For example, a person who orders high-fat food when they eat out (fast-food) should discuss healthier ways of eating out when they seek dietary counseling. For others, tips on how to make a lower-saturated-fat lifestyle more interesting in terms of food studies, preparation and involvement of ethnic cuisine should receive more attention.

Another option to physicians is to introduce a Mediterranean style diet at Visit I because these diets are naturally low in saturated fats and dietary cholesterol. Moreover, they emphasize a high intake of fruits, vegetables, whole-grain bread, unsweetened cereals, beans, nuts, seeds, and either olive or canola oil. Dairy products, fish, and poultry should be kept to low or moderate amounts. There should be little red meat and 0-4 eggs per week.

Table 11.8: The DIET CAGE Questionnaire

D.	Dietary counseling in the past? Would you like to see a dietitian?
I.	Imbibe alcohol? Regularly? Ever in excess? Ever criticized for drinking?
E.	Educated regarding labels? What is a saturated fat?
T.	Try cholesterol- lowering foods? How often?
C.	Cheese/high fat dairy products?
A.	Animal fats?
G.	Get high-fat food if eating out?
E.	Eat commercially prepared high-fat, high-sugar, and /or salt products?

When the physician is able to endorse a healthier eating style in a positive manner, patient satisfaction and compliance may improve. In addition, the physician needs to review how the patient is doing periodically. In ATP III, the following approach was suggested to help the patient achieve first the LDL-c goals and then if needed, the secondary goals of non-HDL-c and/or an underlying metabolic syndrome:

Visit 1: Emphasize Reduction in Saturated Fat and Cholesterol

- ☆ Reduce animal-high-fat dairy
- ☆ Order lower fat food if eating out
- ☆ Regular physical activity (Table 11.9)

Table 11.9: Goals of Physical Activity*

People of All Ages, Male and Female Benefit From Physical Activity
☆ Include a moderate amount of physical activity on *most*, if not all days of the week
☆ Additional health benefits can be derived from greater amounts of activity
☆ Emphasis is on amount not intensity, goal is 30 minutes
Suggestions on Activity
☆ Scheduled physical activity
☆ Walking, treadmill, jogging
☆ Swimming, biking, volley

Surgeon General's Report, 1995.

Visit 2: Evaluate LDL-c response

- ☆ Intensify LDL-c lowering with dietary adjuncts
- ☆ Plant stanols/sterols (not for pregnant women/children)
- ☆ Increase viscous fiber intake
- ☆ Consider consultation for medical nutrition therapy with a registered dietitian (actually appropriate at any stage)

Visit 3: Evaluate LDL Response

- ☆ Initiate therapy for metabolic syndrome
- ☆ Intensify weight management (Table 11.10)
- ☆ Regular physical activity
- ☆ Consider drug therapy if LDL-c goal not achieved.

Table 11.10: Goals of Weight Loss with Therapeutic Lifestyle Change*

- ☆ Reduce body weight in the short-term
- ☆ Maintain a lower body weight for the long-term
- ☆ Prevent further weight gain-minimum goal
- ☆ Rate of weight loss
  - – 10 per cent reduction in body weight in 6 months of therapy
  - – Rate is 1 to 2 lbs per week

* Clinical Guidelines on the Identification, Evaluation and Treatment of Overweight and Obesity in Adults, 1998.

Chapter 12

Hypocholesterolemic Effects of Cereal and Millet Fibers

Healthful effects of cereal grains were recognized by ancient cultures. A growing body of evidence suggests a protective effect of dietary fibre from cereal grains against atherosclerosis and other diseases common to modern society. Specific components of dietary fibre from cereals have been shown to moderate or prevent hypercholesterolemia, one of the primary factors contributing to atherosclerosis and heart disease. Although there are considerable differences in the composition of dietary fibre from oat bran, rice bran, and barley, yet hypocholesterolemic effects have been demonstrated with each of these cereal fibres.

I. Oat Bran and Components

Oat products such as oatmeal, and oat bran, have important hypocholesterolemic properties as demonstrated in both humans and animals. Oat bran supplementation (50 g/d) in the diets of 12 healthy young people for 6 weeks decreased serum cholesterol by 12 per cent (Storch *et al.*, 1984). Larger intakes of oat bran (100 g/d) lowered serum total cholesterol by 13-19 per cent and low-density-lipoprotein (LDL) cholesterol by 14-23 per cent with no significant changes in high-density-lipoprotein (HDL) cholesterol (Anderson *et al.*, 1984). Decreases in LDL cholesterol may significantly decrease the risk for coronary heart disease (CHD).

In other study, the intake of as little as (25 g oat bran/d) for 2 wk, in the form of a ready-to-eat cereal, significantly lowered serum total cholesterol by 5.4 per cent in men with high serum cholesterol values. If sustained, a 5.4 per cent reduction in serum cholesterol would have lowered estimated risk for CHD by 10.8 per cent

(Anderson *et al.*, 1990). Similar results have been documented with other sources of soluble fibre such as guar (Jenkins *et al.*, 1980), psyllium (Anderson *et al.*, 1988) and pectin (Reiser, 1987).

Supplementing the diets with defatted rolled oats or its extracted fat showed that the cholesterol-lowering effect was equally divided between the oat fat and nonfat materials. Other investigators in later studies focused on the hypocholesterolemic effects of the fibre component of oats. Studies in which cholesterol and cholic acid were either added to rat diets or not, resulted in significant plasma cholesterol reductions with oat bran. Adding fish oil to the oat diet resulted in further significant reductions in plasma cholesterol values over those found with the oat bran diet (Roach *et al.*, 1992). Plasma high-density lipoprotein (HDL) cholesterol levels were raised with oat bran diets in the studies by Chen *et al.* (1981) and Ney *et al.* (1988), but were significantly lowered in studies carried out by Mongeau and coworkers (1991). Some research workers did not observe significant plasma cholesterol reductions in rats fed oat bran diets containing cholesterol. Liver cholesterol was significantly lowered by oat bran in cholesterol-fed rats in several studies (Kahlon and Chow, 1997).

The cholesterol-lowering ability of oat bran has been reported to be lost by extracting oat bran with *n*-pentane, and it was not restored by adding back the lipid extract. A few workers observed that the cholesterol-lowering effects were related to a pentane-soluble component of oat bran but not to tocotrienols or tocopherols, since their content in the diets was similar in treatments that lowered cholesterol and in those that had no effect. Oat bran β-glucan (1.5 per cent) diets significantly lowered plasma cholesterol in cholesterol-fed rats compared with plasma cholesterol in those fed a cellulose control diet. Treating oat bran with endo-β-D-glucanase significantly elevated liver cholesterol compared with levels in rats fed untreated oat bran (Tietyen *et al.*, 1995).

Significant increases in faecal cholesterol excretion and bile acid excretion with oat bran diets have been reported. An inverse linear relationship ($r = -0.80$) was observed between plasma cholesterol concentration and bile acid excretion.

A significant reduction was reported in plasma cholesterol with oat bran diets in chickens. Significant reductions in liver cholesterol and increases in small intestine length with oat bran and oat gum diets in chickens were also found. Increased length of the small intestine may be associated with alterations in hormonal regulation of cholesterol metabolism. Tocotrienol-extracted oat bran diets resulted in significant serum cholesterol reduction, similar to those with an intact oat bran diet, compared with levels found with β-glucanase-treated oat bran. The cholesterol-lowering effect of oat bran was due to its soluble fibre rather than to tocotrienols. Significant reductions were reported in plasma total and low-density lipoprotein (LDL) cholesterol in chicks fed a 2.2 per cent soluble β-glucan (Oatrim) diet containing cholesterol. In hamster studies, with diets containing added cholesterol, it was observed that an oat bran diet showed significantly lower elevations of plasma and liver cholesterol compared with a cellulose control diet (Kahlon *et al.*, 1993).

In human studies, a significant cholesterol-lowering effect of rolled oats was observed in 21 male hypercholesterolemic volunteers (average 40 years) after three weeks of consuming 140 g/day of rolled oats incorporated in bread; cholesterol levels decreased significantly from 251 to 223 mg/dL (-11 per cent). Replacing rolled oat bread with their usual bread resulted in rise in serum cholesterol to 246 mg/dL in two weeks. Nearly 20 years later, renewed interest in cholesterol-lowering effects with oats resulted in a number of studies in which significant reductions in total and LDL cholesterol were observed in hypercholesterolemic men who consumed oat bran or oat gum. In several reports, oat bran diets resulted in a significant increase in the HDL/LDL ratio and in faecal bile acid excretion.

A study reported results of feeding 60 g/day of oat bran (10.8 g/day of total dietary fibre (TDF) consisting of 5.2 g of insoluble dietary fibre (IDF) or oat meal (4.9 g/day of TDF consisting of 2.2 g of SDF and 2.7 g of IDF) for six weeks to subjects consuming the American Heart Association's National Cholesterol Education Program (NCEP) step I diet (30 per cent of calories from fat, with a 1:1:1 ratio of saturated, monounsaturated and polyunsaturated fats, and less than 250 mg of cholesterol per day). The supplemented diet significantly lowered total plasma cholesterol (TC) in free-living moderately hypercholesterolemic (208 mg/dL) adults. The NCEP Step I diet lowered TC 5 per cent; oat bran further lowered it by 5 per cent and oat meal by 3 per cent, compared with results from the control group consuming an unsupplemented diet. Consumption of 100 g/day of oat bran for four weeks resulted in a significant reduction in total and LDL cholesterol in subjects who had initial plasma cholesterol levels of 227 mg/dL and who were following a low-fast (24.2 per cent of calories from fat), low-cholesterol (166 mg/day) diet (Kelley *et al.*, 1994). In another study, with three weeks of oat bran supplementation (106 g/day), serum total cholesterol in hypercholesterolemic men was significantly lowered by 12.8 per cent and LDL by 12.1 per cent compared with pretreatment control values. Plasma acetate, one of the short-chain fatty acids that are reported to inhibit cholesterol synthesis, was significantly increased (45 per cent) with oat bran supplementation compared with control values, which may have contributed to oat bran's cholesterol lowering effects. Evidence for cholesterol reductions with oat bran in children was reported on consumption of oat bran (1 g/kg of body weight per day for three weeks) by hypercholesterolemic (247 mg/dL) 5- to 12 year olds resulted in significant reductions also in LDL and in LDL/HDL ratios, plus significant elevations in HDL (Blumenschein *et al.*, 1991). On feeding a daily supplement of 38 g of oat bran for four weeks to school age children (mean age, 10 years) following the NCEP Step I diet, initial cholesterol levels (>185 mg/dL) were lowered by 9 mg/dL, LDL by 8 mg/dL, and HDL by 1 mg/dL, but the results were not significant compared with those of the NCEP Step I control (Gold *et al.*, 1991). A decrease in apo B in the oat bran group was significant compared with that in the low-fat control group, suggesting that oat bran may reduce risk factors for atherosclerosis in hypercholesterolemic children.

Soluble fibres of oat bran appear to exert their principal effects on cholesterol metabolism through decreases in bile acid absorption. These soluble fibres bind bile acids in the small intestine, alter micelle formation and decrease their absorption in the small intestine. Consequently, more bile acids are excreted with the faeces. Oat bran, for example, increases faecal bile acid loss more than twofold and increases loss of deoxycholic acid (DCA) by 24 per cent. Acting somewhat like bile-acid binding resins, these soluble fibres of oat bran deplete the bile salt pool and divert cholesterol synthesis from lipoprotein precursors to bile acid synthesis. Short-chain fatty acid (SCFA) effects on the liver may hamper the ability of the liver to compensate for these changes in cholesterol synthetic needs. Hence, adding oat products to the diet in moderate and realistic levels can produce significant reductions in plasma cholesterol and /or improve beneficial lipoprotein ratios to reduce the risk of heart disease in hypercholesterolemic individuals.

II. Rice Bran and Rice Bran Oil

Human consumption of rice bran has been limited, primarily because of the rapid onset of rancidity in rice bran, but methods to stabilize rice bran and to extract its oil have been developed. Interest in rice bran grew from the determination that the inclusion of oat bran in the diet lowers serum cholesterol. Studies of rice bran supplementation in humans found similar beneficial effects on lipoproteins. In a 10-wk controlled feeding trial, rice bran was as effective as oat bran in lowering blood cholesterol concentrations in men and women with moderately high blood cholesterol concentrations.

Rice bran oil (RBO) is not popular oil worldwide, but it is in steady demand as so-called "healthy oil" not only in Japan but also in Asian countries, particularly India. Approximately 80 thousand tons of RBO, corresponding to only 3.5 per cent of total vegetable oils, is consumed annually in Japan. Rice bran oil, since immemorial times, has been used by Japanese women to keep their skin smooth. Today, rice bran oil is extensively used in the cosmetics industry in products such as lips sticks, nail polish, hair conditioners and sunscreens. Apart from cosmetic applications, rice bran oil, extracted from the germ and inner husk of rice, is well-liked cooking oil in several Asian countries as India, China, Indonesia, Korea and Japan.

Appreciative nutty flavor, high smoke point of 490°F and oxidative stability are some important properties that make rice bran oil suitable for all high-temperature cooking methods as deep-frying, stir-frying and pan-frying. Additionally, rice bran oil imparts ideal color, desirable texture and longer shelf life to all types of fried foods. In recent years, interest in rice bran oil has grown significantly, mainly due to the health benefits that it offers.

Wide-ranging studies have shown that rice bran oil, when included in diet, produces hypocholesterolemic effect, that is, it reduces LDL cholesterol and triglycerides, but increases HDL cholesterol. It is believed that for every one percent decrease in cholesterol, the risk of coronary heart disease is reduced by two percent. Unlike pharmaceutical drugs, rice bran oil lowers cholesterol without generating any harmful side effects.

The hypocholesterolemic production capability of rice bran oil stems from its chemical composition. About 14g of rice bran oil contains 2.5g of saturated fat (SFA), 6g of monosaturated fat (MUFA) and 5.5g of polysaturated fat (PUFA). In addition to these, 4 percent of unsaponifiable fraction, which is rich in vitamin E complex, tocopherols, tocotrienols, gamma oryzanol, phytosterols, polyphenols and squalene, is also present. All these ingredients work together to produce hypocholesterolemic effect.

Studies have shown that the minor constituents, particularly gamma oryzanol, of rice bran oil exhibit anti-cancer and antioxidant properties. Consumption of gamma oryzanol retrieved from rice bran oil is found to help in muscle development, weight gain, enhancement of physical strength, reduction of early arteriosclerosis, inhibition of platelet aggregation and amplification of fecal bile acid excretion. Rice bran oil fulfills all the AHA and FDA/WHO recommendations and protocols. Hence, it is absolutely safe for human consumption. In fact, rice bran oil has also earned the GRAS status in the U.S. With all these benefits, it wouldn't be wrong to called rice bran oil, "The Health Oil".

A number of studies in humans and animals have shown that RBO is as effective as other vegetable oils in lowering plasma cholesterol levels (Lichtenstein *et al.*, 1994; Rukmini and Raghuram 1991). In some cases, RBO lowered plasma cholesterol more effectively than other commonly used vegetable oils rich in linoleic; this effect can be attributed to the occurrence of specific components in RBO, γ-oryzanol (and its constituents, triterpene alcohols) and perhaps tocotrienols (Nicolosi *et al.*, 1994; Rukmini and Raghuram 1991).

The amount of linoleic acid in RBO is rather moderate among the vegetable oils (~40 per cent of total fatty acids), but it is still a rich source. RBO also contains a relatively high proportion of oleic acid (40 per cent). Thus, RBO has a nonspecific fatty acid profile, but it does contain a detectable amount of α-linolenic acid, ranging from 1 to 3 per cent (mean value, 2 per cent). This amount may be enough to increase the content of (n-3) highly polyunsaturated fatty acids such as eicosapentaenoic and docosahexaenoic acids in tissue phospholipids compared with other vegetable oils such as corn oil (Edwards and Radcliff, 1994). The remaining major fatty acid in RBO is palmitic acid (17 per cent).

RBO is characterized by its relatively high content of unsaponifiable material. The content of the unsaponifiable material in refined edible RBO is regulated to be <5 per cent under the Japan Agricultural Standard; this value is considerably higher than that of other vegetable oils, <1-1.5 per cent (Sugano and Tsuji, 1997). The most characteristic component of RBO is γ-oryzanol, the ferulate esters of triterpene alcohols (Itoh *et al.*, 1973). The content of γ-oryzanol differs with the source of RBO, ranging from 115 to 780 ppm, depending on the degree and possibly the method of processing (Rogers *et al.*, 1993). Cycloartenol and 24-methylene cycloartanol are the major component terpene alcohols, followed by cycloartanol. RBO also contains campesterol and β-sitosterol at a relatively high level. Diverse effects of γ-oryzanol have been reported, including the hypolipidemic effect, growth promotion, gonadotrophic action and stimulation of the hypothalamus (Kanbara *et al.*, 1992; Nakamura, 1967; Rukmini and Raghrum 1991).

A significant reduction in serum cholesterol was reported in 15 and 30 days when 12 hypercholesterolemic subjects replaced their customary cooking oil with rice bran oil (Kahlon and Chow, 1997). A significant increase was observed in HDL cholesterol-TC ratio after four weeks of feeding 11.8 g of dietary fibre from rice bran or oat bran (total nonstarch-polysaccharides, 21 g/day) to mildly hypercholesterolemic free-living men. Consumption of stabilized rice bran (100 g/day) for two three-week periods resulted in a 4-10 per cent reduction in total cholesterol in moderately hypercholesterolemic subjects fed diets containing 37 per cent of calories as fat (Hegsted *et al.*, 1993). In normocholesterolemic men, feeding rice bran (15 or 30 g/day) for three weeks resulted in non-significant plasma cholesterol reductions (Sanders and Reddy, 1992).

Hence, rice bran has been shown to have cholesterol-lowering activity in hypercholesetrolemic animals and human subjects. This activity is apparently in the unsaponifiable matter and oil as well as in other components of rice bran. Proposed mechanisms of cholesterol-lowering by rice bran include increased faecal excretion of fat, cholesterol, and bile acids. Soluble fibre and viscosity do not appear to play a significant role in the hypocholesterolemic activity of rice bran (Kahlon *et al.*, 1999).

Rice bran contains 10–23 per cent oil and (unlike oat bran) negligible amounts of water-soluble ß-glucans and larger amounts of insoluble dietary fiber. Because of these differences, it is believed that rice bran lowers cholesterol by a mechanism different from that of oat bran. Decreases in cholesterol were found in hypercholesterolemic subjects who replaced their usual cooking oils with rice bran oil and in middle-aged and elderly subjects consuming a low-fat diet containing rice bran oil. Yet rice bran oil typically contains 20 per cent saturated fatty acids and approximately equal amounts of oleic and linoleic fatty acids. Previous research showed the deleterious effects of saturated fatty acids on total cholesterol concentrations, and the fact that rice bran oil lowers cholesterol is contrary to these findings. Research now suggests that rice bran oil's cholesterol-lowering properties are explained by its unsaponifiable components more than by its fatty acid composition. Attention has begun to focus on the components of rice bran oil, including phytosterols, triterpene alcohols, tocopherols, and tocotrienols, as possible hypocholesterolemic agents (Most *et al.*, 2005).

III. Barley Fibre and Fractions

The hypocholesterolemic effects of barley are influenced by the type of barley (hull-less or covered with an attached hull), starch content (normal or waxy) and cultivar tested, the solubility and content of the β-glucans present, and environmental conditions during growth. Processing and formulating food products with barley may alter the functionality of both the products and the barley, aspects that also must be taken into consideration when evaluating the hypocholesterolemic effects of barley.

Hypocholesterolemic effects of barley appear to be due to its soluble β-glucans, tocotrienols, and other components. Possible mechanisms for cholesterol-lowering by barley are increased feacal fat and bile acid excretion and inhibition of HMG-CoA reductase and 7α-hydroxylase, the rate-limiting enzymes for cholesterol and bile acid synthesis.

The effect of dietary fibre on cholesterol metabolism has been studied extensively. Barley and oats have a similar concentration of soluble fibres called β-glucan (3.5 per cent -5.9 per cent of the dry matter), whereas wheat and rice do not posses this

Table 12.1: Characteristics of Included Randomized Controlled Trials of Barley

Reference	*Design*	*Type of Patient*	*Double-Blinding*	*N*[a]	*Duration of Treatment (wk)*	*Preparation of Barley*	*β-Glucan Intake per Day*	*Concurrent Diet Modification*
Shimizu *et al.*, 16: 2007	Parallel	Hyper-cholesterolemic	Yes	39	12	Pearled barley	7g	Low saturated (<10 per cent) and low trans unsaturated fat diet
Keenan *et al.*, 17: 2007	Parallel	Hyper-cholesterolemic	Yes	155	6	Barley concentrate in cereal and juice	3 or 5 g of either HMW or LMW	Low saturated
Biörklund *et al.*, 18: 2005	Parallel	Hyper-cholesterolemic	No	55	5	Barley concentrate as beverage	5 or 10 g	None
Keogh *et al.*, 19: 2003	Crossover	Hyper-cholesterolemic	No	18	4	Naturally extracted barley β-glucan as a gel	9.9 g	None
Li *et al.*, 22: 2003	Crossover	Healthy	No	10	4	Barley bran in whole grain	NR	None
Lupon *et al.*, 20: 1994	Parallel	Hyper-cholesterolemic	No	79	4	Barley bran flour or oil extract in capsules	NR	Step I diet
McIntosh *et al.*, 21: 1991	Parallel	Hyper-cholesterolemic	No	21	4	Barley grain (bran and flakes)	8g	None
Newman *et al.*, 10: 1989	Parallel	Healthy	No	14	4	Barley grain flour in cereal and baked goods	4.5g	None

HMW or LMW = high or low molecular weight β-glucan; NR = not reported; step I= diet consisting total fat to ≤30 per cent of total calories, saturated fat to ≤10 per cent of total calories, and cholesterol upto 300 mg/d.

a: Number of patients evaluated.

b: Crossover trial treated as parallel trial with only the first phase of the study data taken into account.

constituent type of fibre. Unlike wheat and rice, a diet high in β-glucan has been shown to slow gastric emptying, digestion, and absorption. These effects are associated with increased excretion of bile acids and neutral sterols, increased catabolism of cholesterol, and reduced absorption of cholesterol and fat (Talati *et al.*, 2009). Talati *et al.* (2009) performed a meta-analysis of randomized controlled trials of barley to better characterize its effect on various lipid parameters (Table 12.1).

Table 12.2: Results of the Meta-analysis of Randomized Controlled Trials Evaluating Effect of Barley Cholesterol Levels

Study Type	*Total Cholesterol mg/dL (95 per cent CI)*	*LDL Cholesterol mg/dL (95 per cent CI)*	*HDL Cholesterol mg/dL (95 per cent CI)*	*Triglycerides mg/dL (95 per cent CI)*
All studies	13.38 (−18.46 to −8.31) [8 studies]	−10.02 (−14.03 to −6.00) [7 studies]	0.99 (−0.09 to 2.06) [6 studies]	−11.83 (−20.12 to −3.55) [6 studies]
Fixed–effects model	−13.38 (−18.46 to −8.31) [8 studies]	−10.02 (−14.03 to −6.00) [7 studies]	0.99 (−0.09 to 2.06) [6 studies]	−11.83 (−20.12 to −3.55) [6 studies]
Excluding cross over studies	−13.75 (−19.24 to −8.26) [6 studies]	−9.76 (−14.64 to −4.88) [5 studies]	−0.97 (−3.31 to 1.36) [4 studies]	−13.68 (−12.74. 0.39) [4 studies]
Excluding studies not double blind	−17.39 (−26.05 to −8.74) [2 studies]	−13.43 (−20.58 to −6.29) [2 studies]	0.85 (−4.71 to 6.41) [1 studies]	−22.45 (−50.65 to 5.76) [1 studies]
Excluding studies in patients without hypercholesterolemia	−12.56 (−17.89 to −7.24) [6 studies]	−9.38 (−14.13 to −4.63) [5 studies]	1.08 (−0.01 to 2.17) [4 studies]	−11.06 (−24.97 to 2.85) [4 studies]
Trim and fill	−10.49 (−15.09 to −5.89)	−8.45 (−12.21 to −4.69)	1.34 (0.31 to 2.37)	−11.83 (−20.12 to −3.55)
(+4 studies)	(+3 studies)	(+3 studies)	(0 studies)	
Studies evaluating barley with diet modification	−17.14 (−25.02 to −9.23) (2 studies)	−14.57 (−21.69 to −17.45) (2 studies)	1.53 (−2.98 to 6.05) (2 studies)	−17.36 (−40.66 to 5.94) (2 studies)
Studies evaluating barley without diet modification	−10.75 (−17.38 to −4.12) (6 studies)	−7.89 (−12.75 to −3.04) (5 studies)	−0.16 (−2.33 to 2.02) (4 studies)	−11.03 (−19.90 to −2.17) (4 studies)

CI: Confidence interval; LDL: Low density lipoprotein; HDL: High density lipoprotein; +: Analysis-imputed missing studies.

Note: All results reported as weighted mean differences.

A total of 8 randomized controlled trials (evaluating 391 participants) were included in this meta-analysis (Table 12.1). Five of the studies were conducted using a parallel study design, whereas 2 studies used a crossover design with a 4-week washout period, and 1 study used a crossover design with no washout period and was treated as a parallel trial by taking into account only the first phase of the study data. Each study enrolled relatively few participants (median sample size, 30 participants; range, 10-155 participants) and had a short duration of treatment (median duration, 4 weeks; range, 4-12 weeks). The dosage of β-glucan in reported included studies ranged from 3 to 10 g/d (median dose, 7 g/d) and was administered in various forms, including pearled barley, barley bran flour, oil extracts in capsules, barley concentrates, barley-containing beverages, and gelling agents. Only 2 studies administered barley along with some type of dietary modication. Of the 8 studies, 6 were not double-blind.

Figure 12.1: Impact of Barley on Serum Lipids

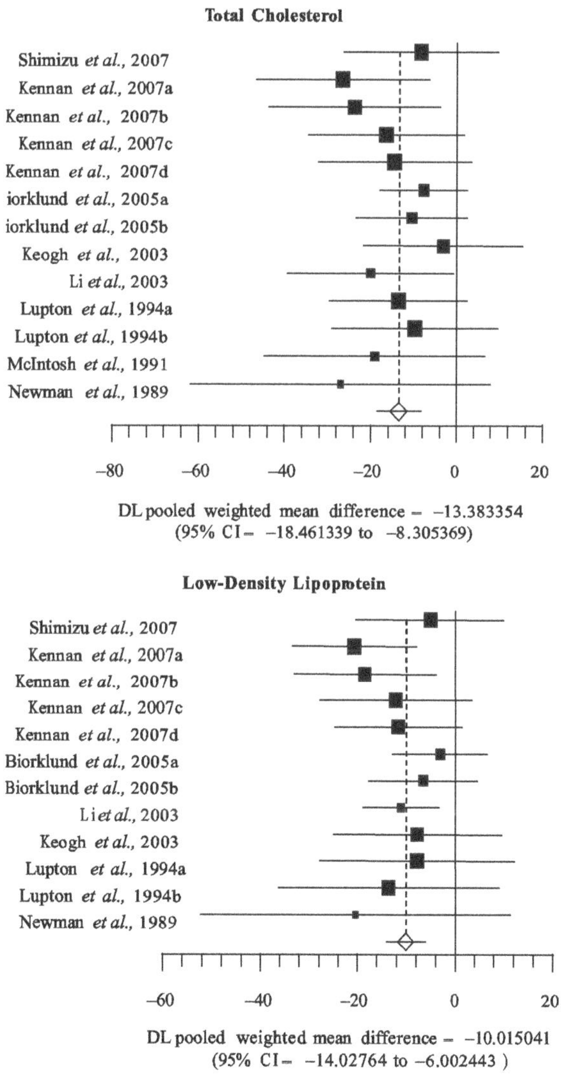

Contd...

Figure 12.1–*Contd...*

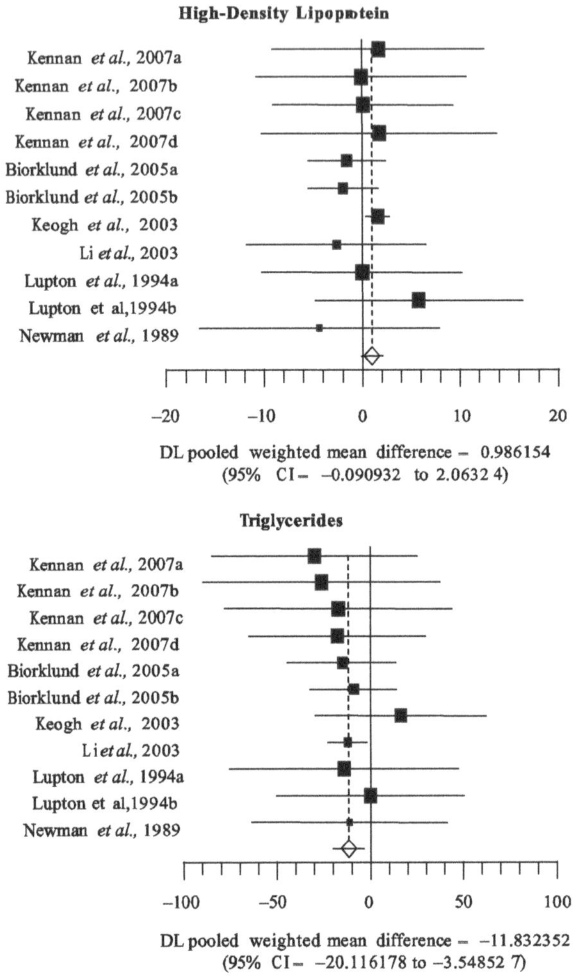

DL: DerSimonian and Laird random-effects model.

Upon meta-analysis, participants receiving barley had statistically significant reductions in total cholesterol (–13 mg/dL), LDL cholesterol (–10 mg/dL), and triglycerides (–12 mg/dL) but not HDL cholesterol compared with control participants (Table 12.2, Figure 12.1). Because studies have shown that for each milligram per deciliter reduction in a patient's LDL cholesterol level, their relative risk of having a coronary heart disease event is decreased by 1 per cent, this modest reduction in LDL cholesterol observed with barley is likely clinically significant as well.

The Food and Drug Administration (FDA) has stated that daily intakes of 3 g or more of soluble fibre (β-glucan) in whole oats or barley may reduce the risk of heart disease by its ability to lower total cholesterol and LDL cholesterol. This meta-analysis results support this FDA decision, because 3 to 10 g of β-glucan from various forms of barley lowered total cholesterol, LDL cholesterol, and triglycerides in the study participants. Furthermore, a signicant reduction in total cholesterol and LDL cholesterol was found regardless of whether a low-fat or step I diet was mandated equally in both arms of the studies. This finding is important because of the potential for a dietary substitution effect. If study participants are replacing their normal foods (*e.g.*, eggs, bacon, sausage) with barley, it may be difficult to discern whether the improvements in cholesterol resulted from the healthier diet or from barley. That signicant reductions in total cholesterol and LDL cholesterol were seen regardless of whether diet modications were mandated equally in both study groups helps guard against the issue of dietary substitution and strengthens the benecial effects of barley use.

Conclusions

Cereal fibres (oat, rice, and barley) contribute significantly to reducing TC in a variety of animal species and in hypercholesterolemic human subjects. Long-term population studies have demonstrated that, for each 1 per cent reduction in total plasma cholesterol, a two- to fourfold decrease in atherosclerosis occurs in otherwise healthy individuals. In a six-year prospective study of U.S. male health professionals free of diagnosed cardiovascular disease, cereal fibre was found to be most strongly associated with reduced risk of total myocardial infarction. Increasing the soluble fibre of diets by including barley and oat bran, in addition to other foods with high soluble fibre, proved efficacious in lowering cholesterol even further in subjects on the NCEP Step 2 diet. In normocholesterolemic subjects, although the effect of cereal dietary fibre on plasma lipids and lipoproteins is small, these changes would have a significant potential for reducing cardiovascular risk for the whole population.

Future research needs include more studies evaluating the ability of rice bran and barley to prevent hypercholesterolemia in humans; testing combinations of oat bran, rice bran, and barley for possible synergistic effects on cholesterol metabolism; development of cultivars that contain enhanced levels of the cholesterol-lowering constituents of these cereals; investigating the effects of antioxidant activity in these cereal fibres on ameliorating or preventing the development of atherosclerosis; and development of palatable food products incorporating these cereal fibres to increase the availability of healthful cereal-based foods to consumers.

Chapter 13

Hypocholesterolemic Effects of Legumes

As interest in the relationship between diet and lipid metabolism has developed, many investigations into the influence of legumes on cholesterol and triacylglycerol levels in the blood have been made. Particular interest has been shown in two legume derivatives *i.e.* guar gum and soybean protein.

Several investigators have studied the effects of leguminous diet on human subjects, but many more have utilized animal models, particularly the rat. Whilst it is necessary to use animals for certain experimental manipulations, inherent differences in the metabolism of blood lipids in different animal species may sometimes make the results of such studies difficult to interpret. A less consistent hyper- hypo-phenomenon occurs in humans consuming cholesterol-rich diet. The hyperlipidaemias observed in man may have their origin in quite different metabolic defects from those deliberately induced in animals, and it is by no means certain that the effects of dietary components will be the same in both cases.

Definition and Nutritional Characteristics of Legumes

Legumes may be defined as the dried seeds of plants from the *Leguminosae* family, the members of which are characterized by having their fruit in a pod. Many different *Leguminosae* species are grown as food or feed crops. Their seeds usually fall into one of two main classes: pulses, in which the principal storage material is a polysaccharide, usually starch, and oilseeds, in which the principal storage material is fat. Legume seeds are typically rich in protein and non-starch polysaccharides (NSP), and contain significant levels of oligosaccharides which contribute to the flatulence often experienced following their consumption. Table 13.1 shows the major components of some common pulses and oilseeds.

Table 13.1: Typical Composition of some Common Legumes (g/kg, dry matter)

Legume	*Protein*	*Fat*	*Starch*	*Sugars*	*Non-starch Polysaccharides*		
					Total	*Soluble*	*Insoluble*
Butter beans(*Phaseolus lunatus*)	241	10	530	51	178	74	104
Haricot beans(*Phaseolus vulgaris*)	219	17	525	27	183	91	112
Dried peas(*Pisum sativum*)	232	13	613	30	151	44	107
Red lentils(*Lens culinaris*)	272	18	581	29	59	18	41
Soybeans(*Glycine max*)	391	197	132	120	166	72	94
Peanuts(*Arachis hypogaea*)	254	513	57	32	66	20	46

Compiled from Paul and Sothgate, 1978; Duke, 1981; Englyst *et al.*, 1988.

The amount of protein in legume seeds ranges from 200 to 400 g/kg dry matter, one of the richest sources of legume protein being the soybean (*Glycine max*). The proteins of legumes are relatively good sources of lysine, aspartic acid, glutamic acid and leucine, but are generally deficient in the sulphur-containing amino acids methionine and cystine.

With the exception of oilseeds, legume seeds tend to contain only small amounts of lipid (g/kg), for example, lentils (*Lens culinaris*) 6, *Phaseolus beans* 10-20 and chick peas (*Cicer arietinum*) 50-60. However, the lipid component is highly unsaturated, consisting of 55-78 mol unsaturated fatty acids/100 mol, and often contains relatively high levels of other constituents such as plant sterols, isoflavones and saponins which may be physiologically active.

Legume starches are particularly rich in the unbranched moiety amylose, which is found at levels in the range 100-600 g/kg total starch. Thus, they are particularly prone to retrogradation and the development of resistant starch after heat treatment. Legume starch may also resist digestion due to entrapment within thick-walled cells. These, and possibly other aspects of legume starches, undoubtedly contribute to the exceptionally low rate at which they are digested *in vivo*, and the low blood glucose and insulin responses that follow their ingestion.

The non-starch polysaccharide (NSP) of legumes is present in both the hull and the cotyledon, but the hull tends to contain more cellulose and other insoluble NSP fractions than the cotyledon which contains more soluble NSP. Generally, legumes are considered to be rich sources of soluble NSP, which ranges from 18 g/kg dry matter in split red lentils to 91 g/kg in haricot beans (*Phaseolus vulgaris*). Also present, at varying levels, are oligosaccharides, particularly raffinose, stachyose and verbascose. The amount and type of oligosaccharide present is dependent on the species of legume.

Influence of Legumes on Lipid Metabolism

Studies using Whole Pulses

Since 1965 at least fifteen studies of the effects of whole pulses on plasma lipid levels have been carried out. Of these, eight have involved hyperlipidaemic subjects (mainly types IIa, IIb, and IV) and seven have used normolipidaemic subjects, either healthy or diabetic. Despite major differences in the protocols of the studies reviewed, all but one showed a significant reduction in the total plasma cholesterol level of the study group by the end of the study period. On average, legumes produced a fall in total cholesterol of 16 per cent of the initial level of the study group, but in individual studies reductions of from 7 to 26 per cent have been reported. The observed differences in the magnitude of cholesterol reduction between the studies are undoubtedly related to the experimental protocols followed, which have differed in such aspects as the amount of legume consumed, species eaten, background diet, initial lipid level of the group, and the time course of the study (Kingman, 1991).

Quantity

The quantity of legume seeds that must be consumed in order to achieve a significant reduction in plasma cholesterol has not been clearly defined. In the long term it may be possible to sustain a hypocholesterolaemic effect by habitual consumption of relatively small quantities of beans. The minimum quantity of mixed legumes to have an effect on plasma cholesterol levels in free-living Chinese subjects was 1 kg dry weight/month (about 33 g/d) (Bingwen *et al.*, 1981). Over 60 per cent of subjects consuming legumes at this rate experienced reductions in plasma cholesterol, compared with only 16.7 per cent of subjects consuming half this quantity per month over a period of 3 months. In shorter experiments, there seems to be a lower limit of between 60 and 100 g at which inclusion of beans in an otherwise uncontrolled diet can influence the cholesterol levels of normolipidaemic people. The consumption of one 450 g can of baked beans in tomato sauce daily (approximately 120 g dry weight of beans) significantly reduced the plasma cholesterol level of male students eating a self-selected diet over a period of 2 weeks (Shutler *et al.*, 1989). However, a subsequent experiment following a similar protocol by using one 225 g can of baked beans (approximately 60 g dry weight) daily failed to show any reduction in plasma cholesterol in normal subjects. In controlled studies using hyperlipidaemic subjects, similar quantities of beans have shown to have a hypocholesterolaemic effect.

It is not clear whether consumption of legumes in excess of about 100 g dry weight/d results in any further benefit with regard to plasma cholesterol. In an uncontrolled experiment with free-living hyperlipidaemic subjects who were already stabilized on a lipid-lowering diet, Jenkins *et al.* (1983) found that the individual changes in serum cholesterol were largely unrelated to the quantity of mixed legumes consumed, within the range 95-190 g/d. All subjects had reduced serum cholesterol levels but there was a broad spread of individual response that was not attributable to adherence to the diet. Subjects who adhered conscientiously to a long-term bean diet did experience greater cholesterol reductions than those whose compliance was only fair or poor. In this case, good compliance required the consumption of 100 g (dry weight) beans/d or an equivalent amount of oat bran (Anderson *et al.*, 1984).

Very few studies have addressed the question of a dose-response to legume seeds. Anderson *et al.* (1990) were the first to study the effects of different doses of the same legume species on cholesterol levels in a controlled situation. They compared diets containing either 120 or 162 g wet weight of *Phaseolus* beans given to hypercholesterolaemic subjects either in a single dose or at two separate meals. Although marked reductions in serum cholesterol were observed, there were no significant differences between the cholesterol levels of the groups consuming the higher and lower doses, whether these were eaten at a single meal or at two meals. However, the two doses were not very different from each other, and the quantities eaten were small compared with other studies, making a differential response difficult to detect.

Species

The level of inclusion of legumes required to have an effect on plasma cholesterol may depend upon the type of legume consumed. However, species specific differences are difficult to assess as there have been no direct comparisons of single legume species using the same study group or protocol. In majority of cases the need for variety in the diet, particularly in long-term studies, has prompted investigators to use mixtures of different legume seeds, usually varieties of *Phaseolus* beans, peas, lentils and chick peas (Jenkins *et al.*, 1983, Nervi *et al.*, 1989). However, several different types of legumes, including various cultivars of *Phaseolus vulgaris*, chick peas, roasted lucerne (*Medicago sativa*) seeds and fenugreek (*Trigonella foenum* graecum) seeds have been studied in short-term single-species experiments. Because of the unpredictability of individual responses to legumes and differences in protocols, it is difficult to compare species efficacy across studies. However, there is some evidence to suggest that some legumes are more effective than others. For example, Molgaard *et al.* (1987) observed a significant reduction in serum cholesterol of hypercholesterolaemic subjects following consumption of only 40g roasted lucerne seeds/d when other researchers have had to use more than twice this quantity of *Phaseolus* beans or fenugreek flour in order to achieve the same effect (Sharma and Raghuram, 1990). The greater apparent potency of lucerne may be related to the chemical structure of its saponins which, when isolated, bind cholesterol *in vitro* and have shown to have a hypocholesterolaemic effect in animals (Story *et al.*, 1984). Other legume saponins such as those from soybean do not interact with cholesterol *in vitro*, and are apparently ineffective at reducing plasma cholesterol *in vivo*. For legumes with a significant content of saponins, their concentration and structure may go some way to explaining species-specific differences in effectiveness. Further experiments in humans are needed to determine to what extent differences occur between other legumes. Using pigs, it has been shown that legume seeds from the species *Phaseolus vulgaris*, *Phaseolus lunatus*, *Pisum sativum*, and *Lens culinaris* reduce cholesterol levels to different extents when substituted at the same concentration into a diet based on casein and maize starch. Thus, it is likely that legumes from different sources will also have different potencies as part of a human diet.

Background Diet

In general, the background diet against which a legume diet has been studied has not been reported in detail. Whereby hyperlipidaemic subjects have been used, some investigators have chosen to use a standard lipid-lowering diet as a control situation (Jenkins *et al.*, 1983), whilst others have preferred a 'traditional' high-fat background diet (Anderson *et al.*, 1990). However, the actual sources of nutrients replaced by the beans usually remain unspecified, even in controlled studies. In an exceptional case, the carbohydrate and protein components of mixed pulses were hypocholesterolaemic when substituted isoenergetically for sucrose and soybean protein, but in a later study were unable to demonstrate a hypocholesterolaemic effect of mixed pulses or chick peas substituted isoenergetically for combinations of sucrose, wheat flour, gluten and egg white (Grand *et al.*, 1974). In a study, *chapatis* made with defatted fenugreek flour reduced cholesterol levels compared with *chapatis* made with wheat flour and groundnut protein (Sharma and Raghuram, 1990). It is interesting to note that in two of these three studies, pulses lowered cholesterol compared with products containing a legume protein and a non-legume carbohydrate source.

The fat content of the background diet against which legumes are studied appears to have a major influence on the outcome of the study. The greatest reductions in plasma cholesterol are observed when the normal diet is high in fat. For example, introduction of 100 g *Phaseolus* beans into daily regimen of hyperlipidaemic subjects consuming a controlled metabolic diet containing 37 per cent energy as fat, and reported a mean reduction in serum cholesterol of 18 per cent after 3 weeks. In contrast, on introduction of a mean of 140 g mixed legumes into the daily diet of hyperlipidaemic subjects who were already adhering to a standard lipid-lowering diet (25 per cent energy as fat) a reduction of only7 per cent in total serum cholesterol was observed (Jenkins *et al.*, 1983). It is possible that the action of legumes is particularly effective against elevations in plasma cholesterol caused by consumption of fat. Certainly, chick peas were highly effective at reducing the cholesterol levels of men in whom mild hypercholesterolaemia had been induced artificially by feeding 50 per cent of energy as butterfat (Mathur *et al.*, 1968).

It has recently been suggested that certain legumes do not reduce plasma cholesterol unless they also displace fat in the diet (Cobiac *et al.*, 1990). In uncontrolled studies, displacement of fat and reduction in energy intakes cannot be ruled out as contributory factors in the hypocholesterolaemic effect attributed to legumes. However, there is good evidence from closely controlled studies in humans (Anderson *et al.*, 1984) and in animals (Kingman *et al.*, 1992) to indicate that legume seeds do offer a benefit that is independent of changes in dietary fat or energy intake.

Initial Lipid Level

Whilst the plasma cholesterol levels of both hyperlipidaemic and normolipidaemic subjects have been reduced in response to a leguminous diet, the greatest reductions have generally been seen when starting cholesterol levels are high. Seventy seven percent of hypercholesterolaemic subjects experienced a reduction in cholesterol while consuming approximately 33 g mixed legumes daily, whereas only 48 per cent of subjects with cholesterol levels within the normal range had lower cholesterol levels as a result of the same diet (Bingwen *et al.*, 1981). Similarly, administration of 40 g lucerne seeds daily to hyperlipidaemic subjects affected the cholesterol levels of type II subjects, but not those of the type IV subjects who tended to have lower initial cholesterol levels (Molgaared *et al.,* 1987). However, Jenkins *et al.* (1983) did not find a consistent relationship between the initial lipid levels of seven subjects (three type II and four type IV) and the reduction in cholesterol seen as a result of a legume-rich diet. In fact, in this study, the greatest reduction was seen in a type IV subject with a relatively low starting cholesterol level.

Individual responses to a legume diet may be quite diverse. In uncontrolled studies it is possible that differences in response are related to compliance with the diet, but under controlled conditions they are more likely to be related to the metabolic origin of the hyperlipidaemic state exhibited by the subject.

Time-Course

Short term studies have shown that the initial phase of cholesterol reduction on commencement of a leguminous diet is very rapid, being evident within 1 week. A significant reduction was observed in the mean total cholesterol level of thirteen male students after only 3 d daily baked bean consumption (Shutler *et al.,* 1989). Subsequently a progressive decline was observed over the 14 d of the study. A similar pattern was described by Anderson *et al.* (1990) who made daily measurements of plasma cholesterol in their subjects over a period of 3 weeks on a diet of canned beans. After an initial rapid decline, levels continued to fall slowly until they reached a lowest point at between 11 and 17 d. After this they tended to rise slightly, and were higher at the end of the study than at the lowest point. Thus, studies of the cholesterol-lowering effect of legumes that last less than 3-4 weeks may overestimate the effect potentially achievable in the long term.

During sustained consumption of legume seeds a new steady-state for plasma cholesterol appears to be reached after 4-8 weeks, after which no additional benefit is observed if the diet is continued unchanged. For those subjects consuming more than 1 kg legumes/month, the significant reduction in plasma cholesterol evident after 1 month was maintained for the duration of the study (at least 3 months) (Bingwen *et al.,* 1981). Other long-term studies confirm that the reduction in plasma cholesterol caused by legumes persist as long as the diet is followed (Anderson *et al.,* 1984).

Lipoprotein Fractions

In more recent studies where the distribution of cholesterol between the lipoprotein fractions has been reported, the LDL fraction has been the most responsive to intervention with legumes, with changes in HDL being less pronounced. The LDL cholesterol is usually reduced in parallel with the reduction in total cholesterol. Of the fifteen studies reviewed, ten reported measurements of the LDL cholesterol fraction, and this was significantly reduced in all but one by a mean of 18 per cent (range 8-28 per cent). In a study, concentrations of apolipoproteins B and A-1 were measured in the plasma of hyperlipidaemic subjects consuming 40 g roasted lucerne seeds daily (Molgaard *et al.,* 1987). It was found that apo B was reduced in proportion to the reduction in LDL-cholesterol, suggesting a decrease in the number rather than the size of circulating LDL particles. Apo A-1 and its HDL counterpart were unchanged.

In the three studies where VLDL-cholesterol has been measured, no significant change in the blood concentration of this fraction has been observed. This suggests that the reduced LDL concentration is the result of either a change in the proportion of VLDL converted to LDL, or a specific increase in the catabolism of LDL particles. Since changes in LDL turnover in response to a leguminous diet have not been studied in humans, the metabolic events occurring are open to speculation. From work in pigs (Shutler, 1988), there is some evidence to suggest that the fractional catabolism of LDL is not increased by *Phaseolus vulgaris* beans, and that, by inference, it is the rate of synthesis of LDL from VLDL, that is affected. Further metabolic studies, preferably in humans, are much needed if progress is to be made in this area.

HDL-cholesterol levels are usually unchanged by a legume diet. In a few cases, significant reductions in HDL-cholesterol have contributed to the overall decline (Anderson *et al.*, 1990; Shutler, 1989), but in these cases the HDL: LDL or HDL: total cholesterol ratio has always been maintained at initial levels. HDL-cholesterol levels fell significantly while their subjects were consuming a controlled diet containing beans. However, when the same subjects were subsequently maintained on a high-fibre diet containing oat bran and beans for a further 24 weeks in a free-living environment, their HDL-cholesterol levels gradually rose to starting levels whereas LDL-cholesterol remained at a lower level. Thus, in the long term the HDL: LDL-cholesterol ratio of these subjects increased. Occasionally the HDL-cholesterol is found to be raised by legumes.

Opinions are divided as to the effects of a legume diet on plasma triacylglycerol levels. Approximately half the studies reviewed reported no significant change in triacylglycerol levels while the other half detected significant reductions, particularly in hypertriglyceridaemic subjects (type IIb and IV). It was observed that triacylglycerol levels were not affected by a high-legume diet in patients with insulin-dependent diabetes mellitus, but that they were reduced in non-insulin-dependent diabetics. Triacylglycerol levels were also significantly reduced in non-insulin-dependent diabetics in response to fenugreek *chapatis* (Sharma and Raghuram, 1990). It is possible that this effect is related to the reduced glycaemic and insulinaemic responses occurring after legume consumption.

Steroid Excretion

The extraction of steroids in faecal matter has been measured in only two studies using whole pulses. In the first study, twenty subjects consumed a very-high-fat diet containing an unspecified quantity of chick peas for a period of 55 weeks (Mathur *et al.*, 1968). During this period it was observed a significant increase in the excretion of total bile acids, but there was no change in the output of neutral sterols in comparison with the high-fat diet alone. In the second study, it was discovered that men consuming a controlled diet containing approximately 115 g dry weight of *Phaseolus* beans/d excreted significantly less bile acid in their faeces than they had while they were consuming a control diet (Anderson *et al.*, 1984). As in the chick pea study, neutral sterol excretion was unaffected. An additional observation from this study was that faecal weight and faecal dry weight were not significantly increased by eating beans. These results were in contrast to those obtained for oat bran in the same study, which increased both faecal weight and steroid output, and seemed to be in conflict with those normally obtained for diets containing rich sources of NSP. However, the results are supported by a study of the effects of four legume species on plasma cholesterol levels in cholesterol-fed pigs in which neither faecal weight nor faecal steroid excretion (neutral or acid) was increased as a result of legume consumption, compared with a control group. It is clear that further studies of the effects of legume seeds on faecal weight and composition in humans are required before any reliable conclusions can be drawn on this point.

Biliary Saturation

In epidemiological studies the consumption of large quantities of beans has been associated with increased prevalence of cholesterol gallstones, particularly in South America, suggesting that legumes somehow alter the cholesterol saturation characteristics of the bile. In a study especially designed to investigate the effect of legumes on biliary cholesterol saturation, it was revealed that, under controlled conditions, a diet containing beans, peas and lentils (120 g dry weight/d) increased biliary cholesterol and decreased biliary phospholipid in such a way that the biliary cholesterol saturation index rose from 110 to 169 per cent (Covarrubias *et al.*, 1984). At the same time plasma total and LDl-cholesterol levels were significantly reduced. Whilst an epidemiological association between cholesterol-reducing diets and the prevalence of cholesterol gallstones has also been noted, the metabolic connection between the two is unclear.

Studies using Legume Polysaccharides

The most frequently studied legume polysaccharide is guar gum, the storage polysaccharide of the Indian Cluster Bean (*Cyanopsis tetragonoloba*). Guar gum can be readily isolated in a purified power form and is principally a galactomannan. In solution guar gum is highly viscous, and it is its effect on viscosity within the small intestine that is thought to be at the heart of its physiological effects, particularly its attenuation of the rate of post-prandial glucose absorption. It has been investigated as a potentially useful therapeutic measure in both diabetes and hyperlipidaemia.

Another legume polysaccharide that has been studied for its effects on plasma lipids is locust bean gum (Zavoral *et al.*, 1983). This gum, the storage polysaccharide of the species *Ceratonia siliquya*, is almost identical to guar gum in its chemical and physical properties, but appears to be easier to incorporate into palatable food products. The only leguminous cell-wall polysaccharide that has been concentrated and fed to humans is that from the soybean (*Glycine max*). Soybean polysaccharides have been concentrated in various forms.

Guar and Locust Bean Gums

There have been numerous studies of the effects of guar gum on plasma lipids in man (Jenkins *et al.*, 1980; Aro *et al.*, 1981; Uusitupa *et al.*, 1984; Turner *et al.*, 1990). In all these studies, reductions in total and/or LDL-cholesterol have been observed, although in two studies the change was not significant. The magnitude of the reduction has been in the range 8.5-16 per cent of the total plasma cholesterol level.

Guar gum on its own is an unpalatable product and researchers have sought different ways of introducing it into the diet of volunteers. The most popular mode of administration has been to disperse the dry power in a fluid, usually soup or fruit juice, which is taken at the start of each meal. However, some investigators have used other vehicles such as crisp bread (Jenkins *et al.*, 1980; Penagini *et al.*, 1986), capsules (Khan *et al.*, 1981), or granola bars (McIvor *et al.*, 1986). The use of modified guar gum formulation which remained fluid before ingestion, but developed its viscosity on contact with gastric acid has also been reported by Simons *et al.* (1982). This formulation proved to be more palatable than the unmodified version. The mode of administration of guar gum does not appear to influence its effectiveness greatly. On an equal weight basis, guar gum hydrated in milk, soup or fruit juice and guar gum incorporated into crisp bread were equally effective at reducing cholesterol in hyperlipidaemic subjects. Semi-hydrated guar gum given in the form of bread was not so effective, but this may have been related to its lower palatability and the small size of the subject group used.

The relationship between the amount of guar gum consumed and its effect on blood lipids has not been studied. In one study, 36 g guar gum powder/d induced a mean fall of 16 per cent in the plasma cholesterol level of the group (Jenkins *et al.*, 1975), whereas in the later study a daily dose of 9 g guar gum in capsule form induced a meal fall of 10 per cent (Khan *et al.*, 1981). These results suggest that there is diminished benefit to be obtained by increasing the consumption guar gum above a certain dose. An optimum dose of guar gum has not yet been proposed. However, doses of guar gum in excess of 15 g/d are required in order to achieve a significant long-term effect. This value was suggested in an attempt to explain the conflicting results obtained by various groups for the long-term effectiveness of guar gum as a treatment for hypercholesterolaemia. Use of 15 g guar gum/d observed an attenuation of its effect after 12 weeks compared with that seen at 6 weeks. However, other groups using slightly larger doses have claimed that the effect is sustainable for several months, even up to 1 year.

The hypocholesterolaemic effect of guar gum is evident within 2 weeks of daily consumption (Jenkins *et al.*, 1975; Khan *et al.*, 1981; Penagini *et al.*, 1986). After this there may be further small decrements for another 2 weeks, but then the effect seems to stabilize. This is the case for both hypercholesterolaemic and normolipidaemic subjects. Unlike whole pulses, guar gum appears to reduce the cholesterol levels of both groups to similar extents when expressed on a mg/l basis. In the studies reviewed, the mean reduction in plasma cholesterol experienced by the subjects was approximately 300 mg/l (range 230-460 mg/l), regardless of the starting lipid level of the group or the protocol followed. Thus, when expressed as a percentage of the starting lipid level, normolipidaemic subjects experienced greater reductions than hypercholesterolaemic subjects. This was not the case for locust-bean gum, which affected the plasma lipid levels of familial hypercholesterolaemic subjects to a greater extent than those of normals.

As in the case of whole pulses, considerable disparity was observed in individual responses to guar gum which may be attributed to differences in lipid metabolism between subjects (Turner *et al.*, 1990).

In studies where lipoprotein fractions have been measured, the reduction in plasma cholesterol seen as a result of guar gum administration is almost always due to a reduction in LDL-cholesterol. No significant changes in HDL- or VLDL-cholesterol have been reported. Locust-bean gum reduced HDL-cholesterol significantly, but as in the case of whole pulses, the HDL: LDL ratio was maintained unchanged. Triacylglycerol levels have also remained unchanged by treatment with these viscous gums, only being reduced in one study (Gatti *et al.*, 1984).

A study reported the results of a metabolic study using ^{125}I-labelled LDL to investigate the cholesterol-lowering effect of guar gum (Turner *et al.*, 1990). Patients with primary hypercholesterolaemia received 30 g guar gum/d for 6 weeks, after which their LDL and IDL levels were reduced by 11.5 and 10.7 per cent, respectively, due to a 39 per cent increase in the fractional catabolism of apolipoprotein B. There was also a slight increase in the production rate of apo B. These changes are similar to those seen with the bile acid-binding resin cholestyramine, and the authors suggest that guar gum may act in a similar way. By reducing the reabsorption of bile acids in the small intestine such resins stimulate a compensatory synthesis of hepatic LDL receptors in order that the liver can assimilate sufficient cholesterol for the production of new bile acids.

The idea that guar gum binds steroids in the small intestine of man appears to rely heavily on extrapolation from studies of pectin, which, although similar in some ways to guar gum, is a chemically distinct polymer. Some evidence has been provided that both substances can enhance faecal steroid excretion quite considerably, but there have been few other studies on this phenomenon in humans (Kingman, 1991).

Soybean Polysaccharides

Unlike guar gum, soybean polysaccharide concentrates have not been shown to reduce the cholesterol levels of normolipidaemic subjects, and may even raise them (Schweizer *et al.*, 1983; Tsai *et al.*, 1983). Nevertheless, some forms may be of benefit in the management of hyperlipidaemia. Concentrated cell-wall material from soybean cotyledons (25 g/d) given to mildly hyperlipidaemic subjects caused a 5-11 per cent decrease in total cholesterol compared with a starch placebo. When given at the same level to primary hyperlipidaemic subjects as an adjunct to a standard lipid-lowering diet, this material reduced the mean total cholesterol by an additional 130 mg/l over that seen with the standard diet alone (Lo *et al.*, 1986). In both cases LDL-cholesterol levels were reduced in proportion to the reduction in total cholesterol. Triacylglycerol levels were unaffected. In contrast, by using a slightly different soybean-polysaccharide concentrate, significant reductions were observed in serum and VLDL-triglycerides and VLDL-cholesterol in the absence of any effect on LDL- or HDL-cholesterol levels, when this preparation was fed to hyperlipidaemic subjects at a level of 11.4 or 15 g/d (Sasaki *et al.*, 1985). The reasons for the discrepancies between the two studies are not known.

Steroid excretion in relation to soybean polysaccharide consumption has been studied, but only in experiments where plasma lipids have been unaffected. No change in faecal steroid excretion was seen resulting from their dietary supplementation which, nevertheless, increased faecal wet weight. Twenty one per cent increase was observed in the excretion of bile acids by a group of normal subjects consuming a never-dried soybean pulp for 3 weeks (Schweizer *et al.*, 1983). Faecal wet weight was also increased. However, there was no effect on total, LDL- or HDL-cholesterol levels. It seems that the effects of soybean polysaccharides on plasma lipids in humans are inconsistent, and that the inconsistencies may depend on the chemical and physical characteristics of the particular concentrate used.

Studies using Soybean-Protein Preparations

Epidemiological studies have suggested that the incidence of coronary heart disease is correlated positively with consumption of animal protein and negatively with that of vegetable protein. Consequently the effects of animal and plant proteins on lipid metabolism have been studied widely. The ready availability and versatility of soybean protein had made this the obvious choice in clinical studies, for which it has been used almost exclusively as the archetypal plant protein. When considering the outcome of such studies it is important to recognize that soybean protein is available in various forms of different composition. In particular, the protein content of soybean protein preparations ranges from as little as 400 g/kg to as much as 920 g/kg.

Many investigators have used soybean protein isolates which are produced by isoelectric precipitation. These are the purest products, comprising at least 900 g protein/kg, the remainder being mainly ash. Others have used soybean protein concentrates, containing approximately 700 g protein/kg, which are produced from defatted soybean flakes by removing much of the sugar content. Both isolates and concentrates may be texturized to imitate meat, but such analogues should be distinguished from 'textured soybean-protein' which is made directly from the defatted flake and contains only 400-600 g protein/kg. Some investigators have chosen to use textured products containing a large proportion of non-protein constituents, mainly carbohydrate in origin, as their source of plant protein in clinical studies. Indeed, such products have been used to have great effect in the management of hypercholesterolaemia. However, because many soybean-protein preparations are so impure it has been difficult for researchers to identify the contribution of soybean protein *per se* to cholesterol reduction in humans (Kingman, 1991).

It has been shown unequivocally that proteins of differing origin can have marked effects on cholesterolaemia in laboratory animals, notably rabbits (Lovati *et al.*, 1990). However, considerable differences have been exposed in the responses of rabbits and humans to identical diets, so that extrapolation from such studies is of little value. Following a critical review of early human experiments in this area, it was concluded that very little change in plasma cholesterol occurred as a direct result of substituting vegetable proteins (mainly soybean) for animal proteins in human diets (Sacks *et al.*, 1983). Indeed several closely controlled studies have shown that low-lipid diets containing casein or meat as their principal protein source can be just as effective at reducing cholesterol levels as those containing soybean protein.

Attempting to resolve the question of whether plant and animal proteins affect cholesterol metabolism differently in humans, volunteers were fed for 1 month on liquid-formula diets containing either soybean protein isolate or casein (Grundy and

Abrams, 1983). It was shown that these two proteins did not differ in their effect on plasma cholesterol in normolipidaemic people when the diet was low in cholesterol. However, this is not altogether surprising. Studies in normolipidaemic subjects have generally demonstrated little, if any, change in plasma total or LDL-cholesterol in response to soybean-protein preparations of all types. Studies showing major reductions in human plasma cholesterol attributable to soybean-protein diet have, almost exclusively, involved hyperlipidaemic subjects. In fact the initial lipid level of the subject and the amount of dietary cholesterol consumed appear to be major determinants of the efficacy of a soybean-protein diet with regard to plasma cholesterol reduction (Kingman, 1991). The effects of soybean-protein and casein-based liquid-formula diets on the cholesterol levels of primary hypercholesterolaemic subjects have not yet been studied; however, normocholesterolaemic subjects receiving a dietary cholesterol supplement of 500 mg/d have been shown to respond differently to the two proteins. In contrast to the previous observations with low-cholesterol diets, it was found that when the diet was cholesterol-rich, the LDL-cholesterol level of subjects consuming soybean protein was 16 per cent lower than that of subjects consuming casein (Kingman, 1991).

In studies using solid foods, soybean-protein isolates have only been shown to be hypocholesterolaemic in cases of moderate to severe hyperlipidaemia. A 13 per cent reduction in plasma cholesterol of subjects with a mean starting level of 3210 mg/l, after 7 weeks on a soybean-protein diet has been reported by Wolfe *et al*. (1981). Similarly, a diet containing a soybean-protein isolate reduced the cholesterol concentrations of primary hyperlipidaemics with moderate hypercholesterolaemia to a small but significant extent, whereas it did not affect plasma lipids in normolipidaemic subjects (Goldberg *et al.*, 1982). Mildly hyperlipidaemic subjects were not responsive to soybean-protein isolate in another study (Shorey *et al.*, 1981).

Impure soybean-protein preparations have been reported to be more effective than soybean-protein isolates at reducing cholesterol. Two products in particular, Temptein (Miles Laboratories, Elkhart, Ind, USA) and Cholsoy (Gipharmex, Milan, Italy) containing 600 and 520 g protein/kg respectively, have repeatedly been shown to reduce cholesterol in hyperlipidaemic subjects, both in controlled and uncontrolled situation (Verrillo *et al.*, 1985; Lovati *et al.*, 1987). Subjects consuming these products have experienced reductions in total cholesterol of up to 35 per cent over several months. The effectiveness of these impure soybean preparations in comparison with purified protein isolates suggests that the protein element is not the only, or even perhaps the principal, determinant of the cholesterol-reducing effect attributed to soybean-protein preparations. Cholsoy contains approximately 300 g carbohydrates/kg of which (g/kg) 40 is raffinose, 50 stachyose and 160 NSP, (Verrillo *et al.*, 1985) all of which could conceivably influence cholesterol metabolism.

Not surprisingly, the effects of soybean-protein preparations on the metabolism of lipoprotein fractions are very similar to those of whole pulses. Reductions in total cholesterol are largely due to reductions in LDL-cholesterol, and there is a concomitant decrease in the amount of circulating apoprotein B (Goldberg *et al.*, 1982). The reduction in LDL seen in response to soybean-protein isolate was specifically in the LDL_2 subfraction (Meinertz *et al.*, 1989).

Most investigators have reported no change in the concentration of VLDL in the plasma, although isolated studies have identified small changes in the composition or turnover of this fraction when subjects are consuming a soybean-protein preparation. In the liquid-formula-diet, soybean-protein led to reductions in VLDL-cholesterol and triacylglycerols in comparison with casein, but only in subjects with initial hypertriglyceridaemia (Grundy and Abrams, 1983). Conversely, a significant increase in the concentration of VLDL-cholesterol was observed in five hyperlipidaemic subjects consuming a textured soybean-protein diet, in the absence of any effect on triacylglycerols (Wolfe and Giovannetti, 1985). In a study using dishes prepared from whole soybeans, increase was noted in both the synthesis and the fractional catabolism of VLDL, but these caused no overall change in plasma concentrations of total, LDL- or VLDL-cholesterol (Huff *et al.*, 1984).

HDL-cholesterol is generally unaffected by a soybean-protein diet. Increased HDL-cholesterol has only been reported in two studies, both of which have been in normolipidaemic subjects receiving a cholesterol-rich diet (van Raaij *et al.*, 1981; Meinertz *et al.*, 1989). The increase, specifically identified in the HDL_2 subfraction, was not associated with a reduction in triacylglycerols. Indeed, reductions in triacylglycerols attributable to a soybean-protein diet appear to be independent of changes in cholesterol level, and are confined to those subjects with initial hypertriglyceridaemia (Verrillo *et al.*, 1985).

Despite the abundance of research into the effects of soybean-protein preparations on cholesterol metabolism, their effect on the excretion of steroids in the faeces has received little attention. In two of the three studies that have included this aspect, the diet used did not result in a reduction in plasma total, LDL- or VLDL-cholesterol. Thus, it is not surprising that no change in the output of steroid molecules was observed. In the third study, reductions were reported in total cholesterol of 10-28 per cent in six of seven type II hyperlipidaemic subjects receiving a diet containing Temptein for 3 weeks. In this case, there was no change in the excretion of either neutral or acidic steroids in the faeces. As a result, it was suggested that the non-digestible (*i.e.* carbohydrate) fraction of Temptein was probably not involved in the hypocholesterolaemic effect (Kingman, 1991).

Possible Mechanisms for the Hypocholesterolaemic Effect of Legumes

Clinical investigations into the cholesterol-lowering effect of legumes have usually been approached from a therapeutic, rather than a mechanistic angle. Thus, human studies have sought and found answers to such questions as 'How much?' 'How long?' and 'Who will benefit?', but not to questions such as 'How?', and 'Why?' The answers to these latter questions have been sought rather through animal experimentation. Many individual components of legume seeds, once isolated and fed to experimental animals, have been shown to reduce cholesterol levels in the plasma. These components have been reported to be protein, lipid, NSP, plant sterols, saponins, and isoflavones. Animal experiments suggest that the effect of legume seeds on lipid metabolism represents the sum of a number of different events acting in concert to reduce plasma cholesterol. It is likely that this is also the case in humans.

However, the results of animal experiments are not always applicable to the human situation, and it is probably true to say that the mechanisms involved in the hypocholesterolaemic effect of legumes in humans are still not known for sure.

Effects of Lipoprotein Metabolism

The principal change that occurs in response to a diet rich in legumes or their derivatives is that of reduced LDL in the absence of any change in plasma VLDL. Specific LDL reduction may be the result of one of two metabolic changes, *i.e.* (a) increased LDL-receptor activity or (b) reduced synthesis of LDL, either of which may be secondary to events occurring in the gut lumen.

Increased LDL-Receptor Activity

LDL receptors are synthesized in response to a need for cholesterol, and are down-regulated by a sufficiency, either supplied from the circulation or available from *de novo* synthesis. An increase in LDL-receptor activity, therefore, indicates that the tissues require cholesterol, and this may be because they are unable to synthesize adequate cholesterol for their needs, or because they have been depleted; for example, if they have been required to convert cholesterol into other steroid molecules for export.

The most popular hypothesis to explain the cholesterol-reducing effect of legumes, and indeed many other foods containing NSP, is that of steroid binding. According to this hypothesis several components of the legume seed, notably NSP and saponins, bind biliary steroids in the small intestine and inhibit their reabsorption during the enterohepatic cycle. New bile acids are thus required and these are synthesized from cholesterol. In this manner, cells are depleted of their cholesterol and synthesize LDL-receptors in order to obtain more. The net result is an increase in LDL-receptor activity. Recent evidence suggests that this mechanism, which is responsible for the effects of steroid-binding resins like cholestyramine, may also be responsible for the cholesterol-reducing effect of guar gum. It is conceivable that whole pulses and other legume polysaccharides with sufficient affinity for bile acids could influence lipid metabolism in a similar way. However, at present there is not enough evidence from human studies of lipid turnover or steroid excretion to conclude that this is so.

In a study, steroid-binding hypothesis was dismissed as an explanation for the hypocholesterolaemic effect of navy beans (*Phaseolus vulgaris*) followed by the bean diet resulted in a 30 per cent decrease in their subjects' output of acidic faecal steroids. It was proposed instead that the soluble NSP present in the beans was fermented in the colon producing short-chain fatty acids, notably propionic acid. These molecules are absorbed and taken into the liver where they have an inhibitory effect on the enzyme HMG-CoA reductase, thus reducing *de novo* cholesterol synthesis. According to reports of the effects of proprietary HMG-CoA reductase inhibitors, reducing cholesterol synthesis results in a compensatory increase in LDL-receptor activity and, hence, a reduction in plasma cholesterol (Ma *et al.*, 1986).

There is strong evidence in rats to suggest that propionic acid can inhibit cholesterol synthesis (Chen *et al.*, 1984). It has also been shown that dietary propionate reduces total plasma cholesterol in pigs, although in this case the reduction has been associated with reduced HDL-cholesterol as well as LDL-cholesterol (Thacker *et al.*, 1981). The outstanding question is whether or not the NSP present in legumes is fermented to propionate by human gut flora in sufficient quantity to affect plasma cholesterol level. It has been demonstrated that the molar ratios of acetic, propionic and butyric acids produced by cultures of human faecal bacteria are dependent on the substrate used. For example, the main end-product of pectin fermentation is acetate, whereas starch is fermented more readily to butyrate. Using porcine faecal flora, it has been shown that both raffinose and pea fibre are relatively good substrates for the production of propionate. This lends weight to the idea that the end-products of the fermentation of legume carbohydrates may influence lipid metabolism *in vivo*. If this were the case, species-specific differences in effectiveness could be due to the differing compositions of their oligo- and polysaccharide components. So far the individual carbohydrate fractions of legumes have received little attention in human experimental work.

There is recent evidence to suggest that soybean protein preparations can also increase LDL-cholesterol activity in hyperlipidaemic subjects, possibly by inhibiting the down-regulation of LDL receptors (Lovati *et al.*, 1987). This hypothesis is supported by the consistent observation that soybean-protein preparations are only effective in situations where plasma cholesterol levels are already raised, *i.e.* where there is already some down-regulation of LDL receptors. At present the specific amino acid or peptide components responsible for the effect have not been identified.

Reduced Synthesis of LDL

The turnover of LDL in response to a diet rich in pulses has not yet been studied in man. However, in pigs, it has been reported that legumes were influencing the synthesis, rather than the clearance of LDL from the plasma. Under normal circumstances all LDL is derived from VLDL via IDL. However, not all VLDL particles become LDL particles. Large VLDL particles tend to become VLDL remnants, whereas small VLDL is metabolized to IDL, which has the potential to become LDL. Thus, any manipulation that alters the size of VLDL particles on secretion could also influence the number of circulating LDL particles without affecting the absolute amount of VLDL in the plasma.

A low-fat diet has been reported to reduce the proportion of VLDL converted to LDL without affecting the turnover of VLDL itself and, thus, resulted in a lower plasma cholesterol level. In contrast, a diet rich in polyunsaturated fatty acids was found to reduce synthesis of both VLDL and LDL. The former observation suggests that a diet high in fat will favour the production of small (*i.e.* LDL-forming) VLDL, and it is interesting to note that legumes are particularly effective at reducing cholesterol levels when the background diet is high in fat (Mathur *et al.*, 1968). If there is a component in legumes that can alter the secretion of VLDL in favour of large particles, it has not yet been identified

Effects on Insulin Secretion

In addition to their effects on plasma lipids, diets rich in leguminous seeds are associated with improved control of carbohydrate metabolism, particularly in diabetes.

Following a meal containing legumes or certain legume derivatives, post-prandial glucose absorption and insulin secretion are reduced and delayed in comparison with other starchy foods. The attenuated glucose response to legumes may occur for several reasons. In the case of substances such as guar gum, the mixing of lumen fluid is inhibited by the presence of a viscous material (Black burn *et al.*, 1984), whereas for starchy legumes the phenomenon is probably related to the nature of the starch and its entrapment within thick cell walls. Reduced insulin secretion occurs as a natural consequence of the delayed glucose absorption. Insulin is known to stimulate the activity of HMG-CoA reductase and, hence, the *de novo* synthesis of cholesterol. Thus, reducing the absolute amount of insulin circulating in the plasma could potentially reduce cholesterol synthesis and plasma cholesterol. It has recently been shown that reductions in post-prandial plasma glucose and insulin, achieved simply by increasing the frequency of meals (nibbling rather than gorging) are associated with significant reductions in LDL-cholesterol and apolipoprotein B in human subjects (Jenkins *et al.*, 1989), but it is uncertain whether the magnitude of the reduction in plasma insulin as a consequence of legumes in the diet is sufficient to effect a change in plasma cholesterol. In diabetes, elevated plasma cholesterol is a common complication which is thought to be secondary to accumulation of triacylglycerol-rich lipoproteins due to impaired activity of lipoprotein lipase. A low-glycaemic-index diet was associated with significant reductions in plasma total and LDL-cholesterol and triacylglycerol levels in patients with hypertriglyceridaemic conditions, but not in those with normal triacylglycerol levels (Jenkins *et al.*, 1987). These results suggest that the effect of a low-glycaemic-index diet on cholesterol metabolism is indeed linked to its effect on carrying lipoproteins. However, legumes have also been shown to reduce plasma cholesterol independently of changes in triacylglycerols.

In relation to the influence of legume proteins on cholesterol metabolism, it has been suggested that glucagon secretion may be stimulated by arginine, an amino acid in which soybean protein is rich, and that this might be the means by which legume proteins affect plasma cholesterol. However, in testing this hypothesis, it was found that, although the peak glucagon secretion following arginine infusion was increased by soybean protein, it was increased even further by casein (Noseda *et al.*, 1982). Thus, there seems to be little basis for this particular hypothesis for the cholesterol-lowering property of soybean protein.

Overall, it can be suggested that legume seeds and certain legume derivatives, eaten frequently, are able to reduce the level of LDL-cholesterol in the plasma, particularly when this is abnormally high for genetic or dietary reasons. However, the mechanisms responsible for the effect are still not fully understood. Although the specific reduction of LDL-cholesterol is common to whole pulses, legume polysaccharides and soybean-protein preparations, it seems that the metabolic processes underlying this reduction may be different for all three products. The compositional complexity of legumes has been a major obstacle to researchers, making it difficult to control for all potentially active components in experimental diets, and to predict metabolic areas for specific consideration.

In studies using animal models, progress has been made by isolating potentially hypocholesterolaemic components and incorporating these into formula diets. This approach is impractical in humans because of such considerations as palatability and fundamental nature; for example, determination of the effects of leguminous diets on steroid balance, of which there is a dearth. If the metabolic sequelae of eating a leguminous diet can be determined, some indication of the component responsible for the effect might be obtained. Much more information about the specific effects of leguminous diets on sterol balance, lipoprotein kinetics and hormone secretion is required before the mechanism responsible for the hypocholesterolaemic effect of legumes and their derivatives can be elucidated.

Chapter 14
Diet, Fat and Cancer

Cancer is a term used for diseases in which abnormal cells divide without control and are able to invade other tissues. All cancers begin in cells, the body's basic unit of life. Our bodies are always making new cells: so we can grow, to replace worn-out cells, or to heal damaged cells after an injury. This process is controlled by certain genes. All cancers are caused by changes to these genes. Changes usually happen during our lifetime, although a small number of people inherit such a change from a parent.

How a Normal Cell Becomes Cancer

To understand cancer, it's helpful to know what happens when normal cells become cancer cells. Cells in different parts of the body may look and work differently but most reproduce themselves in the same way. Normal body cells grow and divide and know to stop growing. Cells are constantly becoming old and dying, and new cells are produced to replace them. Normally, cells divide in an orderly and controlled manner. Hence, normal cells grow and multiply in an orderly way. Over time, they also die. During the early years of a person's life, normal cells divide more quickly until the person becomes an adult. After that, cells in most parts of the body divide only to replace worn-out or dying cells and to repair injuries.

However, sometimes this orderly process of growth and division of a cell goes wrong. The genetic material (DNA) of a cell can become damaged or changed, producing mutations that affect normal cell growth and division. When this happens, cells do not die when they should and new cells form when the body does not need them. Cancer cells develop because of damage to DNA. This substance is in every cell and directs all of the cell's activities. Most of the time when DNA becomes damaged by things in the environment, like, chemicals, viruses, tobacco smoke or too much sunlight, wrong food habits, etc., either the cell dies or is able to repair the DNA. In cancer cells, the damaged DNA is not repaired. People can inherit damaged DNA, which accounts for inherited cancers. Hence, unlike the normal cells, cancer cells just continue to grow and divide out of control and don't die. The extra cells may form a mass of tissue called a tumor. Not all tumors are cancerous; tumors can be benign or malignant.

Benign tumors aren't cancerous. Benign tumors rarely are life threatening and do not spread to other parts of the body. They can often be removed, and, in most cases, they do not come back. Cells in benign tumors do not spread to other parts of the body.

Malignant tumors are cancerous. When it first develops, this malignant tumour is confined to its original site. If these cells are not treated they may spread into

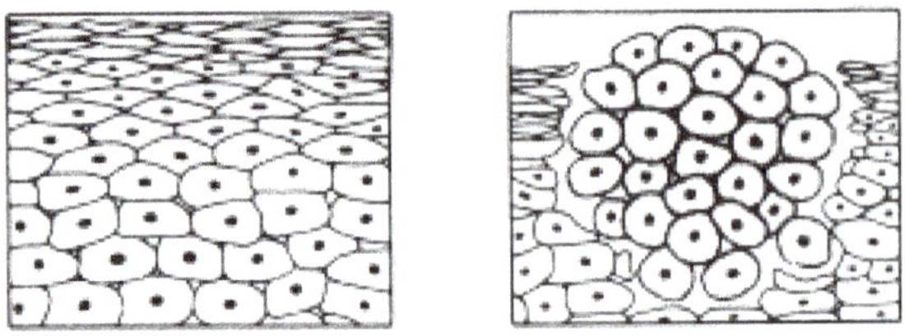

Normal cells   Cells forming a tumour

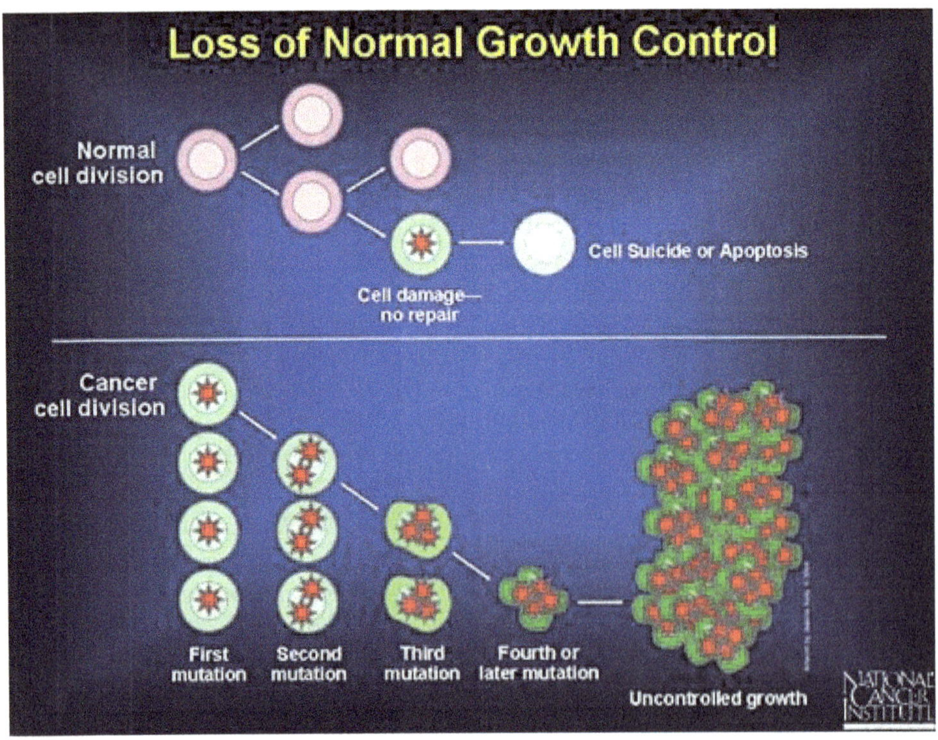

Source: Image from Understanding Cancer Series: Cancer

surrounding tissue and to other parts of the body. When these cells reach a new site they may continue to grow and form another tumour at that site. This is called a secondary cancer or metastasis. Cancer cells can spread to other parts of the body through the blood and lymph systems. Some cancers do not form tumors. For example, leukemia is a cancer of the bone marrow.

Types of Cancer

It is important to realize that cancer is not just one disease but many diseases. Cancer can begin almost anywhere in the body. There are more than 200 different types of cancer. Most cancers are named for the organ or type of cell in which they start–for example, cancer that begins in the colon is called colon cancer; cancer that begins in basal cells of the skin is called basal cell carcinoma. Sarcomas begin in the connective tissue, such as muscle, fat, cartilage, or bone.

Cancer types can be grouped into broader categories. The main categories of cancer include:

Carcinoma

A *carcinoma* is a cancer which is derived from the lining cells, or epithelium, of an organ. There are 4 major types of epithelium in the body (Glandular, squamous, transitional, and pseudostratified). Some types are only found in a few select organs such as the lung (pseudostratified) or urinary bladder (transitional). Carcinomas can arise from any of these epithelial types. For example, breast carcinoma is most commonly derived from the lining cells of the milk producing glands. A carcinoma with a glandular growth pattern is an *adenocarcinoma*. Common adenocarcinomas include prostate, colon, and breast. A carcinoma with a growth pattern resembling the squamous lining cells is termed a *squamous cell carcinoma*. Common squamous cell carcinomas are found in the esophagus and skin. However, any of these organs may have either type of carcinoma arising from it, although these latter diagnoses are exceedingly rare.

Sarcoma

A *sarcoma* is a cancer derived from the soft tissues of the body. Soft tissues include the fat, muscle, nerves, and connective tissue support. Although not usually soft, it also includes bone and cartilage.

Leukemia

Cancer that starts in blood forming tissue such as the bone marrow and causes large numbers of abnormal blood cells to be produced and enter the blood.

Lymphoma and Myeloma

Cancers that begin in the cells of the immune system.

Central Nervous System Cancers

Cancers that begin in the tissues of the brain and spinal cord.

Sometimes cancer will spread to the lymph nodes. A lymph node is a tiny, bean-shaped organ that filters the flow of lymph, the clear fluid that plays a role in the body's immune system. Lymph nodes are located in clusters in different parts of the body, such as the neck, groin area, and under the arms. Cells from malignant tumors can also break away and travel to other parts of the body, where they can continue to grow. This process is called metastasis. Metastatic cancer is named for the part of the body where it started. For example, if breast cancer spreads to the lungs, it is called metastatic breast cancer, not lung cancer.

What Causes Cancer?

There is no one single cause of any disease including cancer. One can only talk about cofactors, causative agents and life situations that like pieces of puzzle come together and promote disease of cancer. There are hundreds of cofactors and causative agents that each have casual relationship to poor immunity, poor health, accumulation of toxins inside body, poor thoughts and each one have been mistakenly called cause of cancer. Most important cofactors are lack of knowledge, poor thoughts, lack of consciousness, lifestyle, diet, exposure to toxins, life situations etc. We can recognize the largest pieces of this puzzle, while some smaller pieces, that all together may cover an area as big as that area covered by the large pieces of the cancer puzzle, often stay unrecognizable. Our body, mind and spirit are one with our environment. Anything that disturbs balance inside our body, mind, spirit, or our relationship with environment promotes cancer.

"Every interference or intervention which disturbs man's biological-dynamic balance, his place in the cosmic scheme of things, in the dipolar field current of Electro-magnetic powers which surrounds the world, and its creatures, and which govern the entire cosmos, every interference with these far reaching relationships, promotes the disease of cancer (Bugwig, J)." No two persons in the world have exactly the same set of cofactors, thoughts and life situations. Significantly different set of cofactors, thoughts and life situations can promote or cause the same kind of cancer in two different persons. Almost identical set of cofactors, thoughts and life situations can cause different kind of cancer in two different persons.

There are about 200 different types of cancer affecting all the different body tissues. What affects one body tissue may not affect another. For example, inhaling of tobacco smoke may cause lung cancer. Over exposure to skin to the sun can cause a melanoma. But the sun shall not cause lung cancer and smoking would not cause melanoma.

The causes of cancers are 'multifactorial'. In other words, there is no single cause for any one type of cancer. Some of the important causes of cancers are described as under:

Carcinogens

A 'carcinogen' is something that can help to cause cancer. Tobacco smoke is a powerful carcinogen. But it is not must that everyone who smokes shall get lung cancer.

Aging

Most types of cancer become more common as we get older. This is because the changes that cause a cell to become cancerous in the first place take a long time to develop. There have to be a number of changes to the genes within a cell before it turns into a cancer cell. The changes can happen by accident when the cell is dividing or they can happen because the cell has been damaged by carcinogens and the damage is then passed on to future 'daughter' cells when that cell divides. The longer we live, the more time there is for us to accumulate these genetic mistakes in our cells.

Aging is in good part due to the oxidants also produced as by-products of normal metabolism. These oxidants, such as superoxide and hydrogen peroxide, are the same mutagens produced by radiation, and cause damage to DNA, proteins, and lipids. The DNA in each cell of a normal rat receives on average about 100,000 oxidative lesions per day. DNA repair enzymes constantly, remove this damage, but they do not keep up: a young rat has about one million oxidative lesions in the DNA of each cell, which increases to about two million in an old rat. A human cell receives about ten times less damage than a rat cell, in agreement with the higher cancer rate and shorter lifespan of a rat (Ames, 1997). The degenerative diseases of aging such as cancer, cardiovascular disease, cataracts, and brain dysfunction, are increasingly found to have, in good part, an oxidative origin.

Genetic Makeup

There have to be a number of genetic mutations within a cell before it becomes cancerous. Sometimes one is born with one of these mutations already. This does not mean that he or she will get cancer. But with one mutation from the outset, it makes it more likely statistically that one will. It is called as 'genetic predisposition' of a person to cancer. The BRCA1 and BRCA2 breast cancer genes are examples of genetic predisposition. Women who carry one of these faulty genes have a higher chance of developing breast cancer than women who do not.

The Immune System

People having problems with their immune systems are more likely to get some forms of cancer. This group includes people who have had organ transplants and take drugs to suppress their immune systems to stop organ rejection; those who have AIDS; and those who are born with rare medical syndromes which affect their immunity.

Viruses

Viruses can help to cause some cancers. But this does not mean that these cancers can be caught like an infection. What happens is that the virus can cause genetic changes in cells that make them more likely to become cancerous. These cancers are linked with cervical cancer, the genital wart virus, HPV, primary liver cancer, Hepatitis B virus and Human T cell leukemia virus. Many people can be infected with a cancer-causing virus, and never get cancer. The virus only causes cancer in certain situations. Many women get a high risk HPV infection, but never develop cervical cancer.

Aluminum Salts

Aluminum salts used in antiperspirants have been linked to elevated risk of breast cancer. According to a study, aluminum may affect the breast cancer risk by interfering with estrogen functions.

Low Doses of Radiation:

Radiation such as x-ray is a risk factor for a variety of cancers. Experts representing their respective interests have been debating over the risk of exposure to low-dose radiation. A new study confirmed that even tiny amounts of radiation raise risk of solid cancers, a notion that has been rejected by the medical industry for decades.

Day to day environment: The following environmental factors may increase the chances of causing cancer:

- Tobacco smoke
- The sun: Sun exposure, which is a major source of vitamin D, reduces risk of advanced breast cancer among women with light skin pigmentation.
- Natural and manmade radiation
- Work place hazards
- *Asbestos*: Past occupational exposures might cause about 2 per cent of current human cancer, a major part being asbestos exposure in smokers, and industrial or synthetic chemical pollution.
- *Living in a city*: A new study suggests that women living in urban areas are more likely to have dense breasts than those who live in the suburbs, meaning that the city women may have a higher risk of breast cancer as previous studies showed that dense breasts are associated with higher risk of the disease.

Antibiotics

Use of antibiotic may increase risk of developing breast cancer in a dose-dependent manner, according to a study published in October, 2007 of Pharmacoepidemiology and Drug Safety. The study led by researchers from King Saud bin Abdulaziz University for Health Sciences in Riyadh, Saudi Arabia showed use of antibiotics increased risk of breast cancer by 50 to 79 per cent, depending upon the number of prescriptions an individual received during one to 15 years prior to the diagnosis of the disease. But this does not mean that antibiotics are definitely the cause for breast cancer. It is possible that those who use antibiotics often have a weak immune system that makes them more susceptible to cancer.

Obesity

Obesity causes a host of medical problems. That obesity increases risk of diabetes, hypertension and ischemic heart disease is well-known. But that obesity can also significantly increase cancer risk is even more chilling news; a 2008 meta-analysis of hundreds of cancer studies shows that 14 to 20 per cent of cancer deaths were related to obesity. Evidence is strongest for cancers of the endometrium, breast (post-menopause) and kidney. Obesity possibly also increases the risk of cancer of the colon.

The traditional image of a cancer patient is of a thin, wasted person; so one tends to rationalise that a jolly, plump person would never get cancer. But the truth is otherwise. Among men, those with a Body Mass Index five points above the normal run an increased colon cancer risk of over 55 per cent. Women with a similar increase in BMI have a more than 50 per cent increased risk of developing uterus or breast cancer. In both sexes, being overweight increases the risk of cancer of the oesophagus, kidney, gall bladder, colon and pancreas. Obese people may have increased risk of bowel cancer because they tend to have higher blood sugar levels. It also increases risk of various types of leukemia and lymphomas.

Researchers are not sure exactly why obesity increases risk of these cancers. Breast cancer is hormone linked. Its development is affected by amounts of the sex hormones oestrogen and testosterone. Fatty tissue produces an enzyme called 'aromatase'. Aromatase affects the balance between these hormones and this may explain why being obese affects the risk of breast cancer. Although obesity increases breast cancer risk in postmenopausal women, it lowers breast cancer risk if woman is premenopausal. But risk of breast cancer increases strongly with age, and being obese increases the risk of several cancers as well as other diseases.

Another factor that researchers at the National Cancer Institute, Bethesda, pointed out is that there seems to be a global immune impairment in the obese. Even vaccines do not work as well in them. An impaired immune system is fertile ground for carcinogenesis. In the case of food-pipe cancers, the link may be a little more straight-forward. The obese always have more acid refluxing back into the food-pipe from the stomach. This initially results in inflammation and heartburn; but later, the cells turn cancerous. The scientists don't have all the answers; but clearly being fat increases the cancer risk. So it is important to maintain a healthy body weight throughout life. A diet of vegetables, fruit juices, roughage and exercising–both part of any sensible weight management programme themselves have an anti-cancer effect; not to mention the salutary effects on the heart, blood pressure, glucose metabolism and so on.

Breastfeeding

Women who breastfeed their first baby can reduce their risk of breast cancer even if the first birth occurs later in life, according to a study presented at a news conference on April 16 at the 2007 Annual Meeting of the American Association for Cancer Research held in Los Angeles.

Diet

Cancer experts estimate that changes in the diet could prevent about one in three cancer deaths in the western world. In the western world, due to more consumption of many types of animal fats and less dietary intake of fresh fruit and vegetables, risk of cancer is increased. But how exactly one should alter the diets is not clear. Sometimes foods or food additives are blamed for directly causing cancer and described as 'carcinogenic'. This is often a distortion of the truth. Sometimes a food is found to contain a substance that can cause cancer but in such small amounts that we could never eat enough of it to do any harm. And some additives may actually protect us.

Moderate Exercise

Researchers found that regular moderate physical activity such as housework provides a better protection against breast cancer than more strenuous but less frequent sporting activity. Women with breast cancer can drastically increase their odds of survival if they do moderate physical exercise after diagnosis, which is equivalent to walking one more hour per week.

Diet, Cancer Risk and Research

Our diets are made up of hundreds of different types of foods, containing thousands of nutrients and chemicals. Some of these protect us against cancer, while others increase risk. We all eat different types of foods in different amounts, which confuse the picture even more. As well as that, there are more than 200 types of cancer. So trying to find out how diet affects cancer risk is extremely difficult.

There are many research studies going on at the moment across the world to try to answer more questions about diet and cancer. The ongoing International study in Europe, called EPIC which stands for European Prospective Investigation into Cancer and Nutrition, is being done on 500,000 people in 10 countries. Over many years, the researchers are recording these people's food intake, monitoring their health records and noting who gets cancer and who doesn't. Then they may be able to link certain factors in the diet with the risk of getting particular cancers. It is the largest study into diet and cancer ever conducted.

The results of EPIC could have huge implications for the prevention of cancer. To start with, the researchers are looking into common cancers such as breast, lung, bowel, prostate and stomach cancer. But the size of this study means that researchers will also be able to look into the possible role of diet in rarer cancers. The results of the study will have implications for cancer prevention everywhere. The results will be presented at international conferences and published in journals available to researchers and health officials throughout the world.

I. Foods and Nutrients that might be Protective

There has been a lot of interest in whether eating certain foods might reduce risk of certain types of cancer. Despite a great deal of research, the scientists haven't found any convincing links. There is some evidence that eating plenty of fruit and vegetables can protect against cancer. The evidence is strongest for cancers of the upper digestive system, such as the mouth, oesophagus and stomach.

Restricted Calories

Elaine Hsieh and colleagues at UC Berkeley published a study in the May, 2005 issue of the American Journal of Physiology-Endocrinology and Metabolism showing that a 30 percent reduction in calories would result in an 89 percent reduction in the proliferation of breast cells. Faster cell proliferation could make cells more prone to errors leading to cancer cells. Less calorie intake may reduce cancer risk.

High Dietary Fiber

Fruit and vegetables contain a wide variety of nutrients and are high in fibre. Scientists are working to find out about which of these nutrients protect against cancer. It is also well known that that bowel cancer is less common in people who eat lots of fibre. One EPIC study showed that people who ate the most fibre had 40 per cent lower risk of bowel cancer than those who ate the least.

Eating fiber-rich vegetables, fruit and whole grain foods may reduce risk of breast cancer in pre-menopausal women, but not in postmenopausal women, according to a UK study, which found that those who ate the highest amounts to total dietary fiber cut their risk of breast cancer by 50 percent.

High Glycemic Index Diet

According to study published by Stephanie and colleagues (April 20, 2005 issue of the International Journal of Cancer) showed that consumption of high glycemic index (GI) or high carbohydrate diets may increase the risk of breast cancer in postmenopausal women.

Vitamins and Dietary Antioxidants

It is argued that some of the vitamins such as vitamins C, E, A and carotenoids which are also good sources of dietary antioxidants play major role in protection against cancer. But the world's population is receiving inadequate amounts of them, at a great cost to health.

Men with low vitamin C intake have low vitamin C in their seminal fluid and much more oxidative damage to the DNA in their sperm. Male smokers are particularly at risk as they have depleted antioxidant pools as cigarette smoke is extremely high in oxidants. A smoker must eat two to three times as much vitamin C as a non-smoker to maintain an equal plasma level, yet smokers tend to eat worse diets than non-smokers. Indeed, male smokers have a considerably higher risk of having children with birth defects and childhood cancer.

A study led by researchers at Sookmyung Women's University in Seoul, Korea found some biological basis for the ascorbate induced apoptosis in human breast cancer cells. Ascorbate (vitamin C) has been shown to inhibit cell growth and induce cell deaths in a variety of cancer cells including human breast cancer cells, according to the background information provided by the researchers in their study report, which was published in the October 18, 2007 issue of Oncology Reports.

Pro-vitamin E, a precursor of vitamin E known as alpha-tocopheryl succinate may be used to effectively treat breast cancer with high levels of human epidermal growth factor receptor (HER2), an Australian study suggests.

The main source of dietary antioxidants and vitamins is fruits and vegetables. Humans should eat 5 portions of fruits and vegetables per day which most of us do not eat. Epidemiological studies show that the incidence of most types of cancer is double among people who eat few fruits and vegetables as compared to those who eat about five portions per day. A study by Dr. Rui-Hai Liu at Cornell and colleagues suggested eating apples may reduce the risk of breast cancer in humans. The study of rats showed that the number of tumors was reduced by up to 61 percent when rats were fed the amount of extract from six apples a day.

Vitamin D

Vitamin D has been linked to reduced risk for a variety of cancers including breast cancer. It's reported that using high doses of vitamin D can cut breast cancer risk by up to 70 percent. Women with advanced-stage breast cancer appear to have significantly lower levels of vitamin D, according to a study conducted by researchers at the Imperial College, London. However, researchers were not sure whether lower levels of vitamin D cause the cancer or vice versa.

Iron

High levels of free iron either released from iron reservoirs in the body or from dietary intake may increase risk of developing breast cancer, according to a review article published in the October 2007 issue of Cancer Causes Control. In the review of 83 research reports, Drs Geoffrey C. Kabat and Thomas E. Rohan from Albert Einstein College of Medicine proposed that iron overload and disruption of iron homeostasis resulting in an increase in free iron may increase the oxidative stress and cause damages that eventually lead to breast cancer.

Calcium

A new Australian animal model study showed that calcium deficiency due to low dietary intake or vitamin D deficiency increases the rate of calcium absorption back into the bone, promoting breast cancer tumor growth in bone.

Cabbage and Sauerkraut

Results from the U.S. component of the Polish Women's Health Study showed an association between cabbage and sauerkraut consumption, and a constituent called glucosinolate, and lower risk of breast cancer.

Soy and Broccoli

3, 3-Diindolylmethane and genistein found in broccoli and soy, respectively may help prevent the spreading of breast cancer and ovarian cancer, according to a study by researchers at the University of California, Los Angeles. Studies have linked eating such foods as broccoli and soy to reduced risk for some types of cancer, but it is not well understood how these foods could possibly provide such protection against cancer. Soy isoflavones may not raise markers for breast cancer in postmenopausal women and could protect them against the disease, suggests an animal study.

Grapefruit

Eating too much grapefruit too often may drastically increase the risk of breast cancer, according to a new epidemiologic study conducted by the University of Southern California and published in the British Journal of Cancer Advance online publication (July, 2007). Evidence revealed early through *in vitro* and *in vivo* studies suggests that grapefruit inhibits CYP3A4, which is involved in the metabolism of estrogen and increases plasma estrogen concentration, increasing risk of breast cancer.

Green tea and Mushroom

Use of green tea extract and a mushroom extract may suppress progression or invasiveness of metastatic breast cancer, according to a study published in the April 2007 issue of International Journal of Oncology suggests.

Whole Wheat

Baby girls born to mothers who eat lots of whole wheat during pregnancy may have a reduced risk of breast cancer, suggests a study published in the Nov 15, 2006 issue of International Journal of Cancer.

Turmeric

Curcumin in turmeric, a yellow spice widely used in Indian cuisine, has long been touted for its health benefits. A study recently found that turmeric may have the potential of stopping the spread of breast cancer.

Oleic Acid in Olive Oil

Women who used a Mediterranean diet full of olive oil have a lower risk of breast cancer, according to a study published in the Journal Annals of Oncology. Researchers attributed the lower risk to oleic acid, which was found to suppress the activities of a common cancer-causing oncogene called HER-2/neu. Oleic acid in olive oil protects against breast cancer.

Dietary and Adipose Fat

Due to high fat intake in the diet, more calories are deposited in the form of fat in the adipose tissues of our body. Adipose fat increases breast cancer risk and boosts breast cancer growth. Reducing dietary fat intake may cut the risk of a breast cancer recurrence in women who have been treated for early-stage breast cancer, according to a trial published in the Journal of the National Cancer Institute.

Fish Oil

Omega-3 fatty acids in fish oil have been associated with a reduced risk of breast cancer. Dietary intake of omega 3 fatty acids such as docosahexaenoic acid (DHA) and eicosapentaenoic acid (EPA) may curb the growth of breast cancer cells.

II. Foods and Nutrients that might Increase Risk

It is also possible that other foods and nutrients might increase risk. Again it has proved difficult to show any firm links, apart from alcohol. The strongest evidence we have is probably for high intakes of red or processed meat increasing risk.

Alcohol

It is known now that alcohol can increase the risk of a number of cancers. It increases risk of mouth cancer, throat cancer, cancer of the food pipe (esophagus), liver cancer, breast cancer and bowel cancer according to a review of 156 previous studies. The review (Alcohol ups cancer risk) was published in the Journal of Thrombosis and Haemostasis.

Western Diet

Meat and sweets are two treats for the westerners. Researchers found those who were in the quartile with the highest intake of meat and sweets were 30 percent more likely to have breast cancer than those who were in the quartile with the lowest intake of meat and sweets, according to a study published in the July 16 2007 issue of Cancer Epidemiology, Biomarkers and Prevention.

Red and Processed Meat

Eating red meat may be associated with higher risk for hormone receptor-positive breast cancers in premenopausal women. Bowel and stomach cancer are more common in people who eat lots of red and processed meat. Red meat includes all fresh, minced and frozen beef, pork, lamb or veal. Processed meats have been preserved in some way other than freezing and include bacon, ham, salami, sausages, spam, corned beef, black pudding and tinned meat.

The way of cooking meat may also increase cancer risk. There are chemicals made when red and processed meats are cooked at high temperatures, such as on a barbeque. These chemicals can damage the body cells, making them more likely to become cancerous.

Barbecued Meat

A study published in the May, 2007 issue of Epidemiology suggests that eating grilled, barbecued and smoked meat for a long period may raise the likelihood of developing breast cancer in postmenopausal women.

Dairy Products

There are other aspects of diet where the evidence is much less clear. Some studies have shown that dairy products reduce bowel cancer risk. Other research shows that dairy products might increase the risk of prostate cancer. It is too early to be sure. There doesn't seem to be any reason to cut down on dairy foods, but it is probably best to choose lower fat dairy products.

Food Additives

There are many different substances added to commercially prepared foods. But these are not all bad. Some additives stop food from going off and so can help to keep us healthy. A good example of this is a toxin called aflatoxin that comes from a mould. It grows on stored food in hot and humid countries, especially on peanuts. This is known to help cause liver cancer so anything that stops the mould from getting into the nuts is helping to prevent cancer.

Most additives are not thought to affect cancer risk. Colours, flavours and sweeteners are constantly investigated by researchers and if any are thought to be a real risk, they may be withdrawn. Sometimes there is a scare about a particular additive. Some years ago saccharin was claimed to be a carcinogen. Researchers had found that when it was fed to rats in huge quantities, the rates of cancer in the rats increased. We are very unlikely to eat so much saccharin and so it is unlikely to cause cancer in people, but far fewer foods contain it now than did a few years ago.

Other additives can be a cancer risk. Pickled foods may increase risk of cancer of the stomach and esophagus, particularly if they are very salty. This may explain why there are such high rates of stomach and esophageal cancer in Japan, where salty, pickled foods are popular.

Contaminants

This means chemicals in foods or drinks that are not meant to be there. They could form as a by-product of the manufacturing process, for example. Nitrosamines are chemicals found in cured meats (bacon and ham, for example) and in very small amounts in beer. Nitrosamines have been shown to be carcinogenic so the amount in such foods should be cut as much as possible. In brewing, one cause of nitrosamines is a reaction between pollution in the atmosphere and the malted barley that is one of the main ingredients of the beer. The brewing industry has tried to cut the levels of nitrosamines in beer as much as possible. Levels are now much lower than they used to be, but it hasn't been possible to get rid of them completely.

Smoking and barbecueing foods so that they are slightly burnt on the outside causes chemicals called polycyclic aromatic hydrocarbons to form. These chemicals are known to help cause cancer. So in barbecueing or cooking over a high heat could increase the cancer risk of meat and fish. But few research studies have shown this.

Frying and baking meat at high temperatures can create chemicals called heterocyclic amines. These may increase risk of cancer of the bowel and esophagus, but this isn't certain. Acrylamide, another chemical that may cause cancer, has been found in foods such as crisps and chips. This is formed during thermal processing in starchy foods. But there isn't proof yet that these chemicals cause cancer in humans and so there are no grounds for telling people to change cooking or eating habits because of these chemicals. But according to a US study published in a recent issue of the International Journal of Cancer, it has been reported that young children who eat French fries frequently may be more likely to develop breast cancer in their later life.

A new study led by Henrik Frandsen, a senior scientist at the Technical University of Denmark and the Danish Cancer Society and colleagues showed that high dietary intake of acrylamide may increase the risk of breast cancer.

Animal cancer tests, which are done at the maximum tolerated dose (MTD), are being misinterpreted to mean that low doses of the chemicals tested and found positive are thereby relevant to human cancer. Animal cancer tests are mainly done on synthetic chemicals and industrial pollutants, yet half of all natural chemicals that have been tested at the MTD are rodent carcinogens.

It is argued that the explanation for the high frequency of positive results in animal cancer tests is that high dose animal cancer tests are mainly measuring increases in cell division due to cell killing and compensatory cell division; this is a high dose effect that does not occur at low doses.

In any case 99.9 per cent or more of the chemicals we eat are natural. For example, 99.99 per cent of the pesticides we eat are natural chemicals that are present in plants to ward off insects and other predators. More than half of those natural pesticides tested in high dose animal tests are rodent carcinogens. There are about 10,000 or so different natural pesticides in our diet, and they are usually present at enormously higher levels than synthetic pesticides.

Cooking food also generates thousands of chemicals. There are over 1000 chemicals reported in a cup of coffee. Only 26 have been tested in animal cancer tests and more than half are rodent carcinogens; there are still a thousand chemicals left to test. The amount of potentially carcinogenic pesticide residues consumed in a year is less than the amount known of rodent carcinogens in a cup of coffee.

The reason we can eat the tremendous variety of natural chemical rodent carcinogens in our food is that animals are extremely well defended against all chemicals by many general defense systems. These enzymes, *e.g.*, DNA repair and glutathione transferases which defend against reactive compounds such as mutagens are all inducible; more of them are made when they are in use. They are equally effective against natural and synthetic reactive chemicals. Thus, animals are extremely well defended against low doses of chemicals. One does not expect, nor does one find, a general difference between synthetic and natural chemicals in their carcinogenicity, and though less well studied, the same would be expected for mutagenicity, teratogenicity, and acute toxicity.

The effort to eliminate synthetic pesticides because of unsubstantiated fears about residues in food will make fruits and vegetables more expensive, decrease consumption, and thus increase cancer rates. The levels of synthetic pesticide residues are trivial in comparison to natural chemicals, and thus, their potential for cancer causation is extremely low.

Cleaning Chemical

A study carried out on mice as reported in the Journal of Applied Toxicology observed that a chemical called 4-nonylphenol, present in cleaning materials, textiles, plastics, paper and clothing causes breast cancer in mice.

Hormones

In a monograph, an International Agency for Research on Cancer concluded that estrogen-progestogen hormone replacement therapy (HRT), used by millions of women around the world, causes breast and endometrial cancers.

Two factors are critical in the formation of mutations: lesions in DNA, formed when DNA is damaged, and cell division, which converts DNA lesions to mutations. Agents increasing either lesions or cell division increase mutations and as a consequence increase cancer incidence. Hormones stimulating cell division increase cancer incidence *e.g.*, levels of estrogen in breast cancer and testosterone in prostate cancer; hormones may be a risk factor in about 20 per cent of human cancer.

Dietary Fat and Cancer

For over two decades, oncologists have had a hunch that fat spells disaster but they had no real evidence. But in 2008, an article in the Lancet analysed over 2, 50,000 cancer patients across 200 studies. Without any shred of doubt, obesity was nailed as a culprit aiding and abetting cancer; and the figures are significant- an increased cancer-risk of 34 to 59 percent in the obese.

What exactly is the link between fat and cancer? There are no simple answers; but fatty deposits are a big source of hormones like oestrogen. Excess oestrogen can result in endometrial and breast cancer. Fat cells also result in high insulin-like growth factors. These have a role in cell multiplication; some of these chemicals unleash out-of-control cell multiplication and result in cancer. Fat cells produce chemicals that cause inflammation; and an out-of-control inflammatory response may turn into a cancerous response. Basically, the key cause seems to be cell growth and cell multiplication getting "out of control". Fatty tissue seems to produce chemicals that can affect the delicate balance of the immune system whose role it is to control cell multiplication, cell differentiation and cell death (Seshader, 2008).

Though death spells the 'end' for the body; for the body's own survival, cells have to die after their normal cell life-span and allow young new cells to replace them. Cells continuing beyond their "expiry date" and then going on to multiply could result in cancer. Chemicals produced by fat cells seem to aid the pro-cancer activities of such 'geriatric' cells.

Total Fat Intake and Cancer

In most parts of the developing world, fat intake on a population basis varies between less than 15 to 25-30 per cent total energy. Consumption of total fat, saturated fat and cholesterol tends to vary as a function of the amount and type of foods of animal origin consumed. In the developed world and in urban areas of the developing world, fat intake, on a population basis, varies from 30 per cent to over 40 per cent total energy, and much fat comes from foods of animal origin containing substantial amounts of saturated fat. The relationship between the risk of cancer and fat intake is often adjusted for total energy intake, so that fat is assessed not absolutely but as a proportion of total dietary energy (Willett *et al.*, 1997).

Fat has been studied extensively in the context of those cancers that are more common in the developed world, including those associated with obesity. The National Academy of Sciences report, Diet, Nutrition and Health (NAS, 1982), concluded that, of all the dietary components it reviewed, the epidemiological evidence from correlation and some care-control studies, supported by experimental evidence, was the strongest and most suggestive for a casual relationship between dietary fat and cancer, particularly cancers of the breast and colon.

The panel has reached the following conclusions:

- ☆ There is a consistent pattern, suggesting that diets high in total fat possibly increase the risk of lung, colorectal, breast and prostate cancers.

Evidence	*Decreases Risk*	*No Relationship*	*Increases Risk*
Convincing			
Probable		Cholesterol Breast	
Possible		Monounsaturated fat: Polyunsaturated/ vegetable fat: Breast	Total fat: Lung Colon, rectum[a] Breast[a] ProstateSaturated/animal fat: LongColon, rectum Breast Endometrium Prostate Cholesterol: Lung Pancreas
Insufficient			Total fat: Ovary Endometrium Bladder Saturated/animal fat: Ovary Cholesterol: Endometrium

a: Risk of these cancers is convincingly (endometrium), probably (post-menopausal breast) or possibly (colon) increased by high body mass, risk of which is increased by diets high in fat

- ✰ Diets high in animal fat and/or saturated fat possibly increase the risk of lung, colorectal, breast, endometrial and prostate cancers.
- ✰ Diets high in cholesterol possibly increase the risk of lung and pancreatic cancers.

Diet, Nutrition, and the Prevention of Chronic Diseases (WHO, 1990) also concluded that diets containing large amounts of total fat were associated with an increased risk of cancers of the colon, prostate and breast, in order of the strength of evidence, and that obesity was associated with endometrial cancer.

The epidemiological evidence linking the fat content of diets with obesity has been reviewed by lissner and Heitmann (1995). Cross-cultural correlation studies show associations between the fat content of diets and the body mass index (BMI) of populations: in general, the higher the proportion of fat in the diet, the greater the incidence of obesity and vice versa (Keys, 1970). Fat is the most energy-dense constituent of diet and it is generally accepted that diets high in fat increase the risk of obesity and therefore of obesity-related diseases, including cardiovascular disease and adult-onset diabetes (Royal College of Physicians, 1983; NAS, 1989; WHO, 1990; Department of Health, 1994). It is therefore, reasonable to conclude that high-fat diets increase the risk of obesity-related cancers.

Diets high in fat increase the risk of obesity; therefore, high-fat diets are an indirect risk factor for cancers, the risk of which is increased by obesity. As already noted, the evidence that obesity increases the risk of endometrial cancer is convincing, and obesity probably also increases the risk of postmenopausal breast and renal cancers. Obesity possibly also increases the risk of cancer of the colon.

In most parts of the developing world, most fat consumed is of plant origin, and fat intake on a population basis varies between less than 15 to 25-30 per cent total energy. Consumption of total fat, saturated fat and cholesterol tends to vary as a function of the amount and type of foods of animal origin consumed. In the developed world and in urban areas of the developing world, fat intake, on a population basis, varies from 30 per cent to over 40 per cent total energy, and much fat comes from foods of animal origin containing substantial amounts of saturated fat.

Diets high in fat increase the risk of obesity; therefore, high-fat diets are an indirect risk factor for cancers, the risk of which is increased by obesity. As already noted, the evidence that obesity increases the risk of endometrial cancer is convincing, and obesity probably also increases the risk of postmenopausal breast and renal cancers.

Saturated Fat and Cancer

Up to the 19th century, fat was relatively expensive and butter was a luxury. The poor lived mainly on potatoes and bread, which were cheap, supplemented whenever possible with whatever source of protein and fat they could afford. Not surprisingly, mortality was high amongst the poorer classes. To fill the gap in the market, cheap substitutes for butter began to be produced in the last quarter of the Victorian era. Made from cheaper fats and coloured yellow to mimic the look, if not the taste of butter, they were called margarine. And this started, quite slowly at first, a radical change in the types of fat we had.

Originally margarines were made of beef suet, milk and water. Later the recipes changed to include lard, whale oil and the oils of olive, coconut, ground nut and cottonseed. By the middle of the 20th century an emulsion of soya bean and water was substituted for the milk and margarines could be made entirely of inexpensive oils from vegetable sources. In all these forms, margarine was the poor relation to butter. Now a days, the polyunsaturated fats used to make margarine are generally obtained from vegetable sources: sunflower seed, cottonseed, and soybean. As such they might be thought of as natural foods. Usually, however, they are pressed on the public in the form of highly processed margarines, spreads and oils and, as such, they are anything but natural.

In the 1920s a new disease had suddenly 'taken off' all over the industrialized world. By the 1940s it had become a leading cause of premature death and nobody knew why. In 1950, an American scientists hypothesized that cholesterol might be to blame. The idea that saturated fat causes cancer began to form in the 1950s, when another American Ancel Keys stated that saturated fat raised cholesterol levels and caused heart disease. In 1953, Ancel Keys, compared levels of this disease in seven countries with the amounts of fat in those countries. To reduce the risk of a heart attack, Ancel Keys recommended cutting down on the vegetable oils and margarines. However, it was discovered that vegetable oils, which are composed largely of unsaturated fats and oils, tended to lower blood cholesterol levels, while saturated fats tended to raise them. And by that time, it had been decided, largely by majority vote, that raised cholesterol increased the risk of a heart attack. And so was born the 'Diet-Heart' hypothesis, for the new disease was coronary heart disease. In the article on causes of coronary heart disease, this idea is badly mistaken. However, many scientists embraced this idea and, by the 1970s, saturated fat acquired a strong reputation as the "bad fat" – even though it is medically known that saturated fat is necessary for many body functions.

In 1977, the US Senate Select Committee on Nutrition and Human Needs, chaired by Senator George McGovern, released its Dietary Goals for the United States (**The McGovern Committee report).** The Dietary Goals stated categorically that "the overconsumption of fat, generally, and saturated fat in particular. have been related to six of the ten leading causes of death." in the United States.

The McGovern Committee report claimed that a high fat diet caused cancer. The report said saturated fat and cancer particularly breast cancer and colon cancer were closely linked. It urged for Americans to substitute polyunsaturates for saturated fat from animal sources, use margarine and corn oil instead of butter, lard and tallow. The rest of the world followed America's example.

With the advent of the 'Prudent Diet' in the USA in 1982, and COMA's introduction of 'healthy eating' in Britain two years later, the fats in our diet changed even more dramatically: we were told to avoid animal fats such as butter and lard, which have a larger proportion of saturated fats, in favour of largely polyunsaturated vegetable margarines and cooking oils. Now margarines could be priced to rival butter. Recently, margarines have been developed specifically to lower cholesterol levels, and prices have risen again. Benecol, made from tree bark is considerably more expensive than butter.

In 1989, the petroleum-based solvent, benzene, that is known to cause cancer, was found in Perrier mineral water at a mean concentration of fourteen parts per billion. This was enough to cause Perrier to be removed from supermarket shelves. The first process in the manufacture of margarine is the extraction of the oils from the seeds, and this is usually done using similar petroleum-based solvents. Although these are then boiled off, this stage of the process still leaves about ten parts per million of the solvents in the product. That is 700 times as much as fourteen parts per billion.

The oils then go through more than ten other processes: degumming, bleaching, hydrogenation, neutralization, fractionation, deodorisation, emulsification, interesterification,. that include heat treatment at 140-160C with a solution of caustic soda; the use of nickel, a metal that is known to cause cancer, as a catalyst, with up to fifty parts per million of the nickel left in the product; the addition of antioxidants such as butylated hydroxyanisol (E320). These antioxidants are again usually petroleum based and are widely believed to cause cancer.

The hydrogenation process, that solidifies the oils so that they are spreadable, produces *trans* fatty acids that rarely occur in nature. The heat treatment alone is enough to render these margarines nutritionally inadequate. When the massive chemical treatment and unnatural fats are added, the end product can hardly be called either natural or healthy.

Review of Researches Done on Relationship between Intake of Saturated Fat and Cancer

Saturated fat and cancer are widely believed to be closely linked. Many doctors, nutritionists and health authorities believe that a high intake of saturated fat increases the risks of cancer just as they believe that saturated fat increases the risks of heart disease.

Epidemiological evidence on saturated/animal fat and cancers at these various sites comes from: for lung cancer, two cohort, four case-control and an ecological study; for breast cancer, nine cohort, seventeen case-control and two ecological studies; for ovarian cancer, three case-control and an ecological study; for endometrial cancer, from four case-control studies; for prostate cancer, from six cohort studies, seven case-control studies and three ecological studies. The balance of evidence from case-control and cohort studies suggests that diets high in saturated fat and/or animal fat possibly increase the risk of these cancers, with the exception of ovary, for which the evidence is suggestive, but currently insufficient. Five cohort and 14 case-control studies have examined saturated fat intake and the risk of gallbladder cancer. 11 of 19 studies found evidence of increased risk with higher intakes; 6 showed no association, and the one other study reported a decrease in risk. Diets high in saturated/animal fat possibly increase the risk of colorectal cancer.

As closer examination of the disease patterns tells us, however, that there is no positive relationship between saturated fat and cancer.

Until early last century, people ate large amounts of saturated fat and used it as their main form of cooking oil, pork lard in China, butter in Europe, ghee in India, coconut oil in the tropics etc. Yet cancer was rare. The rate of cancer began to rise sharply only in recent decades when the consumption of saturated fat actually fell. Thus, we need to seriously re-consider the idea that saturated fat and cancer are closely related.

Among the scientists who testified before the McGovern Committee was Dr Fred Kummerow of the University of Illinois. He disagreed with the view that there were links between saturated fat and heart disease, as well as links between saturated fat and cancer.

Dr. Fred Kummerow pointed out that the real harm was caused by trans fat in products like margarine. He also warned against soft drinks, which contained large amounts of sugar. And, Dr. Fred Kummerow pleaded for a return to traditional foods rich in saturated fats. However, the testimony of Dr. Fred Kummerow was buried in the voluminous McGovern Committee report. His views and the scientific evidence he presented were largely ignored.

At the time the McGovern Committee released its Dietary Goals for the United States, Ms. Mary Enig was a graduate student at the University of Maryland. She was familiar with the research of Dr. Fred Kummerow, noted that the McGovern Committee report claiming a strong link between saturated fat and cancer contradicted many real life situations:

- ☆ In America, the consumption of saturated fat had been declining steadily since the turn of the century, yet the cancer rate was rising sharply.
- ☆ Greece had the same level of dietary fat intake as Israel, but only one-fourth the breast cancer rate.
- ☆ Spain had a slightly higher dietary fat intake than France or Italy, but only one-third the mortality rate from breast cancer.
- ☆ Puerto Rico, with a high animal fat intake, had a very low rate of breast and colon cancer.

- ☆ The Netherlands and Finland both have the same level of animal fat intake *i.e.* about 100 g per person per day. But the Netherlands has twice the rate of both breast and colon cancer. The difference was that people in the Netherlands consumed 53 grams of vegetable fat per person compared to 13 g in Finland. This seemed to suggest that there is a stronger link between vegetable oil, or polyunsaturated fat and cancer, than between saturated fat and cancer.
- ☆ A study in Cali, Columbia found a fourfold excess risk for colon cancer in the higher economic classes, which used less animal fat than the lower economic classes.
- ☆ A study on Seventh-Day Adventist physicians, who avoid meat found they had a significantly higher rate of colon cancer than non-Seventh Day Adventist physicians.

Ms Mary Enig analyzed the US Department of Agriculture data that the McGovern Committee had used and she reached an opposite conclusion:

- ☆ **There is a a strong positive correlation between total fat / vegetable fat and cancer.**
- ☆ **There is a strong negative correlation or no correlation between animal fat or saturated fat and cancer deaths.**

In other words, Ms Mary Enig found that the use of vegetable oils seemed to predispose to cancer while animal fats seemed to protect against cancer.

More recent research by Prof Walter Willett at the Harvard School of Public Health provides further evidence that there is no real connection between a high fat diet and cancer. Nor is there any link between saturated fat and cancer. Walter Willett's research at Harvard includes the Nurses Study II, which monitors the long-term health condition of nearly 116,000 women, and the Health Professionals Study, which monitors the long-term health condition of 52,000 men.

These studies reveal that the type fat has a far greater effect on cancer risks than the amount of fat. In other words, quality matters more than quantity. The website of the Harvard University School of Public Health reports:

Fat and Breast Cancer

Initially, international comparisons showed higher breast cancer rates in countries with higher per capita fat intake. But as more detailed studies were performed over the next couple of decades, the apparent link between total fat intake and breast cancer has faded.

Fat and colon cancer: As with breast cancer, international comparisons initially suggested an association between total dietary fat intake and colon cancer risk. But later studies contradicted these earlier findings and revealed instead an association that was weak at best.

However, Harvard researchers found that although fat and saturated fat intake did not seem to increase colon cancer risk, high consumption of red meat appears to increase colon cancer risks.

Fat and Prostate Cancer

Here, the evidence is contradictory. There is some evidence that diets high in animal fat and saturated fat increase prostate cancer risk. However, some studies have also shown no association, while others have implicated unsaturated fats.

Fat and other Cancers

In the Nurses' Health Study, Harvard researchers found that a high intake of trans fats increased the risk for non-Hodgkin's lymphoma and that a high saturated fat intake increased the risk for endometrial cancer.

Although the Harvard website did not specially mention a lack of correlation between saturated fat and cancer, its findings can be taken to include saturated fat as part of overall fat intake.

One of the problems with earlier scientific studies on saturated fat and cancer is that the researchers often do not take into account trans fats. Even Walter Willett and his team of Harvard researchers failed to make this distinction until the 1990s. Once they took trans fats into account, they discovered that trans fats are often the real culprits in causing heart disease, cancer, diabetes, obesity and other modern, degenerative diseases.

Before the 1990s, Epidemiologist Walter Willett at Harvard University found, like most other researchers, that saturated fat "caused" heart disease and cancer. But in the early 1990s, his researchers contacted Ms Mary Enig for data on trans fats. Working with the refined data, Walter Willett confirmed, in the Nurses Health Study II, that nurses with higher rates of cancer were those who consumed more margarine and vegetable shortenings, not those who ate butter, eggs, cheese and meat. In other words, he no longer found any link between saturated fat and cancer, but he now found a strong link between trans fats and cancer. This correlation between trans fat and cancer was never published, but was reported at the Baltimore Data Bank Conference in 1992. Unfortunately, even many present day research studies continue not to make any distinction between saturated fat and trans fat. And so we continue to get reports every now and then about links between saturated fat and cancer, heart disease and various other diseases. As more researchers work with better and more accurate data, a clearer picture will emerge showing that, just as there was no link between saturated fat and cancer a hundred years ago, there is no link today. The problem is not saturated fat which even protects against cancer in certain cases. In fact, even trans fats that occur naturally in the milk and meat of cows and other grass-fed animals are known to protect against cancer. The real problem is with artificial trans fats, and other types of artificial foods.

Trans Fat and Cancer

Trans fats are created when manufacturers add hydrogen to vegetable oil. Manufacturers hydrogenate liquid oils to make them semi-solid. In the process, some hydrogens in the fats get rearranged. Scientists refer to fats with the ordinary arrangement as "cis." The new ones are called "trans". Margarine and vegetable shortening may also be made with partially hydrogenated oil. Trans fats are food additives in the sense that they're mainly added to the food supply by manufacturing processes, although small amounts of trans fats are present naturally in animal fat (Nutrition Action Health letter, March, 1988 by Elaine Blume). Much of the anxiety over trans fats stems from their reputation as "unnatural." Yet ruminants, such as cows and sheep, hydrogenate oils in one of their several stomachs. So although most of the trans fat people consume today is man-made, about 5 to 20 percent comes from beef, lamb, and dairy products.

These "partially hydrogenated oils" are used most often for deep frying food, and in baked goods. Trans fats are the "hydrogenated" and "partially hydrogenated" fat ingredients in cake mixes, store baked cookies, pie crusts and donuts, in chewy candies, French fries, fried chicken and in supermarket peanut butter. Hydrogenation increases shelf life and saves big bucks by making it possible to store fats longer at room temperature. And it gives cakes, cookies and pie crusts a fake buttery texture and moist "mouth feel," which consumers like.

Most scientists now agree that eating trans fats can be very harmful to health. These fats have been found to lower people's HDL (good) cholesterol and raise LDL (bad) cholesterol. According to Brian Olshansky, a cardiologist and University of Iowa Health Care professor of internal medicine 'Trans fatty acids may help preserve food so that it tastes good, but our body can't break them down and use them correctly. Normal fats are very supple and pliable, but the trans fatty acid is a stiff fat that can build up in the body and create havoc.'

Trans fats are harmful in tiny quantities. Trans fats can clog linings of blood vessels and surfaces in the brain. Trans fatty acids are linked to obesity, heart disease, diabetes, high cholesterol and even to sudden cardiac death.

Despite the rumors, there is little good evidence that trans fats cause any more harm than other fats. Though new questions can always be raised, some of the standard accusations can be laid to rest. Does Trans Equla Trouble? In the Goldbecks' Guide to Good Food, Nikki and David Goldbeck stated that trans fats "are suspected of interfering with fat metabolism, disrupting normal heart functions, enhancing fatty deposits in the arteries, inhibiting the production and utilization of substances in the body which influence the immune system, and reducing the body's ability to rid itself of carcinogens, drugs, and other toxins." Other authors have raised similar concerns.

Although some human studies suggest that trans fats do raise blood cholesterol, most of these had serious flaws. Several, for example, used an unusual fat with two trans groups. This fat is not present to a significant extent in commercial margarines or oils.

Only a few studies were well designed, and these showed that hydrogenated (trans-containing) and non-hydrogenated fats produced similar cholesterol levels. However, even in the weaker studies, trans fats did not raise cholesterol as much as saturated fats. "In general," said Fred Mattson, a noted researcher at the University of

California in San Diego, "studies showed trans fats to have the same effect on human blood lipid levels as cis fats."

Abour cancer worries, iIn (1978), Mary Enig and others at the University of Maryland examined the rise in vegetable fat intake since 1910. This rise, they asserted, was linked to an increase in the number of people who developed or died of cancer, especially breast and colon cancer, during that period. The trans fats in vegetable fats, suggested the scientists, could best account for the "significant positive correlation" with cancer rates.

At most, associations of this type can only provide clues about the cause of a disease. In no way do they prove cause and effect. But this particular analysis had serious flaws. For example, experts pointed out that most cancer rates, including deaths from colon cancer, had remained essentially stable during much of the period in question. What's more, the authors failed to consider other changes in America's eating habits over more than half a century. Commenting on the paper, John C. Bailar III, editor-in-chief of the Journal of the National Cancer Institute, concluded, "Evidence for a [cancer-causing] role of the trans fatty acid component is no better and no worse than for countless other dietary components."

In most animal studies, trans fats don't increase the incidence of tumors. But non-hydrogenated corn, safflower, and sunflower oils, which contain high levels of polyunsaturated fats, are relatively strong tumor promoters, at least in animals. Unfortunately, few people are familiar with these studies. Instead, many have heard of the cancer "correlation," but not of its flaws. So the rumor that trans fats cause cancer persists. Animal studies showed that trans fats, like other fats, may become incorporated into the membranes that surround all cells in the body. Some fear that the incorporated trans fats might alter the normal passage of substances into and out of cells, perhaps permitting carcinogens to enter cells with greater ease.

Olshansky has recommended his patients not to eat products with trans fatty acids and to keep away from processed foods and fast foods until they improve. Go for what's fresh instead, he said, citing a study published in the *Journal of the American Medical Association* that showed eating fresh food can lower blood cholesterol as much as taking a statin medication.

The American Heart Association recommends getting less than 1 per cent of the daily calories from trans fats. Product labels are now required to list the amount of trans fat in a serving. But many fried foods and baked goods that are laden with trans fats are served in restaurants, and they don't come with nutrition labels. To avoid trans fats, it's best to limit the overall daily fat intake. Usually, when the total amount of fat consumed is more, the amount of trans fat is increased as well. If total fat intake is reduced from 13 per cent to less than 10 per cent of the daily calories, probably the amount of trans fat intake shall also not exceed.

Is Any Trans Fatty Acid *good*?

Some scientists and health advocates say that some naturally occurring trans fats, found in the meat and especially the milk of ruminant animals and in some plant oils are actually healthy. In grass-eating animals, these trans fats are formed as a normal part of the digestive processes by bio-hydrogenation of dietary fatty acids by microbial enzymes in the rumen (Strax, 2006, *University of Iowa Health Center; Mark Moyad; PUBMED).*

According to Olshansky, one good trans fat is CLA (conjugated linoleic acid). Conjugated linoleic acid (CLA) differs from the normal form of linoleic acid only in the position of two of the bonds that join its atoms. Conjugated linoleic acid has one other difference from the usual form – it is not found in vegetables but in the fat of ruminant animals. The best sources are dairy products and the fat on red meat, principally beef (Lin *et al.*, 1998). But this small difference has been shown to give it powerful anti-cancer properties. Scientists have reported that even at concentrations of less than one percent, CLA in the diet is protective against several cancers including breast cancer, colorectal cancer and malignant melanoma.

CLA actually improves the immune system and reduces the risk of cancer. Most of the reported evidence for anti-cancer benefits of CLA is about colon cancer. Recent research puts the brakes on enthusiasm. A team of researchers in Aberdeen, writing in 2004, said: "Recent reports, albeit in the minority, that CLAs, particularly the trans-10, cis-12 isomer, can elicit pro-carcinogenic effects in animal models of colon and prostate cancer and can increase prostaglandin production in cells. warrant further investigation and critical evaluation in relation to the many published anti-cancer and anti-prostaglandin effects of CLAs."

Studies on Relationship between Polyunsaturated Fat and Cancer

The total amount of fats in our diet today, according to the MAFF National Food Survey, is almost the same as it was at the beginning of this century. What has changed, to some extent, is the types of fats eaten. At the turn of the century we ate mainly animal fats that were largely saturated and monounsaturated. Now we are tending to eat more polyunsaturated fats, it's what we are advised to do. The vegetable oils and the solid margarines made from them came on the market in large amounts after 1930 as the new and huge oil seed industry was being established. These new fats such as sunflower seed oil and the margarines made from them sold for about half the price of the animal fats, butter and lard and they quickly replaced butter and lard in the diet in the Western World. Then in 1955 the medical establishment come out saying that these new vegetable fats were good and and the saturated animal fats, butter and lard were bad. What with the low cost of these new vegetable fats and with the medical establishment telling us that they were the good fats, butter and lard were greatly reduced in the diet in favor of the new polyunsaturated vegetable fats,

In 1991, two studies, from USA (Carroll, 1991) and Canada, (France and Brown, 1991) found that linoleic acid, the major polyunsaturated fatty acid found in vegetable oils, increased the risk of breast tumours. This, it seems, was responsible for the rise in the cancers noted in previous studies. Experiments with a variety of fats showed that saturated fats did not cause tumours but, when small amounts of polyunsaturated vegetable oil or linoleic acid itself was added, this greatly increased the promotion of breast cancer.

Body cell walls are made of cholesterol, protein and fats. The graph below demonstrates that the human body's fat make-up is largely of saturated and monounsaturated fatty acids. We contain very little polyunsaturated fat. Cell walls have to allow the various nutrients that body cells need from the blood, but stop harmful pathogens. They must be stable. An intake of large quantities of polyunsaturated fatty acids changes the constituency of cholesterol and body fat. Cell walls become softer and more unstable.

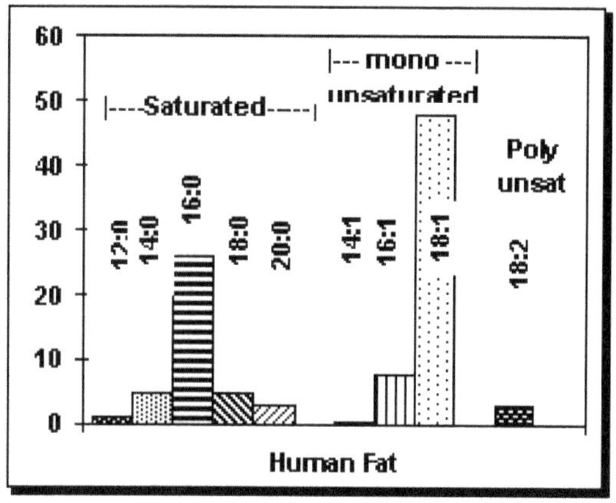

Polyunsaturated Fats Suppress the Immune System

Polyunsaturated fats (PUFs) are greatly immunosuppressive, and anything that suppresses the immune system is likely to cause cancer. The first person to suggest that polyunsaturated fats cause cancer was Dr R A Newsholme of Oxford University, England (Newsholme, 1977). What Newsholme wrote was that when our bodies get sufficient nutrition, our diet includes immunosuppressive PUFs which make us prone to infection by bacteria and viruses. When we are starved, however, our body stores of PUFs are depleted. This allows our bodies' immune systems to recover which, in turn, allows us to fight existing infection and prevent other infections. He was making the point that the immunosuppressive effects of PUFs in sunflower seeds are useful in treating autoimmune diseases such as multiple sclerosis, (Miller *et al.*, 1973) and that the same fatty acids could be used to suppress the immune system to prevent rejection of kidney transplants.

It was during the early days of kidney transplantation that doctors first encountered the problem of tissue rejection as their patients' bodies destroyed the alien transplanted kidneys. If transplantation were to be a success, they had to find a way to suppress the immune system. Newsholme had said that there was no better way to immunosuppress a renal patient than with sunflower seed oil. So kidney transplant doctors fed their patients linoleic acid (Uldall *et al.*, 1974) which is the major polyunsaturated fatty acid in vegetable oils. But the transplant doctors were then astonished to see how quickly their patients developed cancers; some cancers were up to twenty times as frequent as was expected.

This was in line with heart trials using diets that were high in PUFAs which reported an excess of cancer deaths from as early as 1971(Pearce and Dayton, 1971). By the early 1980s, we were being exhorted by doctors and nutritionists to eat more PUFAs because they were 'good for us' despite the fact that *Oncology Times* carried a paper in January 1980 from the University of California at Davis that mice fed PUFAs were more prone to develop melanoma. In May 1980, the same publication carried a similar report from Oregon State University which said that PUFAs fed to cancer-prone mice increased the numbers of cancers formed.

In 1989 there was a report of a ten-year trial at a Veterans' Administration Hospital in Los Angeles. In this trial half the patients were fed a diet which had double the amount of PUFAs as compared to saturated fats. In half of the patients on the high PUFA diet there was a fifteen percent increase in cancer deaths compared to the saturated fat group. The authors of the report said that the PUFAs had been the cause of the increase in cancer deaths. The *British Medical Journal* carried an editorial in its 6 October 1973 issue which asked if PUFAs were carcinogenic. It came to the conclusion that they were.

Wayne Martin likes to tell a story which suggests just how cancer-causing are PUFAs. In 1930 in the USA, eighty percent of men smoked cigarettes and the tar content of cigarettes was much higher than it is today. The death rate at that time from lung cancer was very low. In 1955 doctors decided that PUFAs were good in terms of heart disease protection. After this lung cancer deaths increased so dramatically. By 1980 although the number of American men who smoked had dropped to only thirty percent, three times as much PUFA was being eaten and there were sixty times as many lung cancer deaths (Nauts, 1984).

In 1990, Martin called Newsholme's Oxford University office but by then Newsholme had retired. Martin spoke to his successor to find that they were still treating autoimmune diseases with PUFAs. By then they were using fish oil. The doctor said the reason for the fish oil was that the degree of immunosuppression increased with the degree of unsaturation and fish oil was much more unsaturated than sunflower oil. Martin asked the doctor why they were not talking about PUFAs causing cancer. The doctor replied that if he did that he would be run out of Oxford.

Carcinogens, background radiation, ultraviolet radiation from the sun, particles in the air we breathe and the food we eat continually attack us all. Normally, the immune system deals with any small focus of cancer cells so formed and that is the end of it. But linoleic acid suppresses the immune system. With a high intake of margarine, therefore, a tumour may grow too rapidly for the weakened immune system to cope thus increasing our risk of a cancer.

Reviews Regarding Causation of Cancer by Polyunsaturated Fats

Since 1974, the increase of polyunsaturated fats has been blamed for the alarming increase in malignant melanoma (skin cancer) in Australia (Mackie, 1974). Are Australians going out in the sun any more now than they were fifty years ago? They are certainly eating more polyunsaturated oils: in Australia in 1995, people used to remove the cream from milk and replaced it with vegetable oil. Victims of the disease have been found to have polyunsaturated oils in their skin cells. Polyunsaturated oils are oxidised readily by ultra-violet radiation from the sun and form harmful 'free radicals'. These are known to damage the cell's DNA and this can lead to the deregulation we call cancer. Saturated fats are stable. They do not oxidise and form free radicals.

Malignant melanoma is also said to be increasing in this country. Does the sun cause this? In Britain the number of sufferers is so small as to be relatively insignificant. Even so, it is not likely that the sun is to be blamed since all the significant increase is in the over-seventy-five-year-olds. People in this age group tend to get very little sun. That the sun is not to blame is confirmed by other findings:

- ☆ Melanoma occurs ten times as often in Orkney and Shetland than it does on Mediterranean islands.
- ☆ It also occurs more frequently in areas that are *not* exposed to the sun.
- ☆ In Scotland, for example, there are five times as many melanomas on the feet as on the hands; and in Japan, forty per cent of pedal melanomas are on the soles of the feet (Karnauchow, 1995).

Many laboratories have shown that diets high in polyunsaturated fatty acids promote tumours. Cancer promotion is not the same as cancer causing. The subject is complex; suffice to say here that promoters are substances that help to speed up reproduction of existing cancer cells.

It has been known since the early 1970s that it is linoleic acid that is the major culprit. As Professor Raymond Kearney of Sydney University put it in 1987: 'Many laboratories have shown that a greater proportion of polyunsaturated fats are superior to diets rich in saturated fats in promoting the yield of experimental mammary tumours. In such studies, omega-6 linoleic acid appeared to be the crucial fatty acid.' and 'Vegetable oils (*e.g.* Corn oil and sunflower oil) which are rich in linoleic acid are potent promoters of tumour growth' (Kearney, 1987).

A study of 61,471 women aged forty to seventy-six, conducted in Sweden, looked into the relation of different fats and breast cancer. The results were published in January 1998. This study found an inverse association with monounsaturated fat and a positive association with polyunsaturated fat. In other words, monounsaturated fats protected against breast cancer and polyunsaturated fats increased the risk. Saturated fats were neutral (Wolk *et al.*, 1998). *Flora* margarine, the brand leader, is thirty-nine percent linoleic acid; *Vitalite* and other 'own brand' polyunsaturated margarines are similar. Of cooking oils, sunflower oil is fifty percent and safflower oil seventy-two percent linoleic acid. Butter, on the other hand, has only a mere two percent and lard is just nine percent linoleic acid. Linoleic acid is one of the essential fatty acids. We must eat some to live, but we do not need much. The amount in animal fats is quite sufficient.

Because of the heart disease risk from trans-fats in margarines, in 1994 the manufacturers of *Flora* changed its formula to cut out the trans fats and other manufacturers have since followed. But that still leaves the linoleic acid. There are a number of problems with the fats present in the standard diet. First of all, the balance between inflammation-producing omega-6 fats and inflammation-suppressing essential omega-3 fats has tilted drastically toward the former. Secondly, unnatural trans-fats are widely used in deep-frying and in the manufacture of commercial baked goods such as crackers. Avoid polyunsaturated food oils with high omega-6 content, such as corn, safflower, sunflower or soybean oil. These oils promote tumor growth in animal tests. This may be because of their high content of omega-6 fatty acids, which cause the body to product prostaglandins which stimulate tumor growth. Also, polyunsaturated fat is prone to oxidation, which generates free radicals. Polyunsaturated fats are so immunosuppressive that one researcher has even used them as immunosuppressive therapy to stop rejection of organ transplants. Saturated fats were not found to have this effect. This is the last thing any cancer patient needs! One should avoid corn, safflower, soy and sunflower oils. One should also avoid all synthetic trans fats in any quantity. These are toxic, altered fats made by processing polyunsaturated oil with hydrogen, changing the chemical structure and creating substances with chemical bonds in positions not found in nature. They cannot be processed properly by the human body, and they incorporate into cell membranes causing changes in cell function. Trans fats are a major cause of heart disease and place a further burden on the already weakened body of a cancer patient.

A recent study found an increased risk of prostate cancer linked to trans-fat consumption. In 2000, researchers in Toronto and Vancouver, Canada, reported the results of a study of 263 men with prostate cancer. After adjustment for clinical stage, tumor grade, and other factors, prostate cancer patients who ate the most monounsaturated fat (found in olive and canola oils) survived longest. Their risk of dying was 70 percent lower, compared to subjects with the lowest intake of monounsaturates. The study also found a slightly higher risk associated with saturated fat intake and animal fat, although this was not large enough to be clinically significant.

Use monounsaturated oils such as extra-virgin olive oil or canola oil in salads or as dressing for vegetables, and natural saturated oils such as butter and unrefined coconut oils for cooking. Frying damages oils and is not recommended for cancer patients. Fish oil supplements, which contain essential omega-3 fats, are highly recommended at the dose of one gram EPA/DHA per day. Eat fatty fish such as sardines or mackerel at least twice a week for a natural source of omega-3 fat. Flaxseed oil can be metabolized by the body into omega 3 fatty acid, but this metabolic process works poorly in many people, so is not recommended as a first choice.

In this study, conclusions drawn by the researchers were:

Saturated fats and animal fats are usually blamed for all manner of diseases in Western society. But look at the facts:

- ✰ In the 19th-century, when animal fats were all that was available, cancers were rare (as was heart disease).
- ✰ Polyunsaturated fats and oils are used to suppress the immune system, such immunosuppression is known to cause cancers to start and promote cancer.
- ✰ In this last century there has been a change in favour of polyunsaturated fats and oils – and cancer rates have soared.

Unfortunately, as polyunsaturated fatty acids are also essential to the body; we must have some. So a proper balance must be struck. Whether the dramatic increase in the numbers of cancers in the last century was as a result of a similarly dramatic rise in our intake of polyunsaturated vegetable oils is not known – but the evidence strongly favours such a conclusion.

Under the circumstances, it seems prudent to get what linoleic acid we need from animal sources. Or to restrict polyunsaturated oil consumption so that linoleic acid is no more than three percent of the total fat intake.

Monounsaturated Fat

There is a small amount of evidence to suggest that monounsaturated fat, as such, might influence cancer risk. Overall, evidence regarding intake of monounsaturated fat and the risk of breast cancer is mixed: a pooled analysis of cohort studies showed no relationship, but a combined analysis of case-control studies showed increased risk. Ecological studies suggest no relationship. Diets high in monounsaturated fat possibly have no relationship with the risk of breast cancer.

Cholesterol and Cancer

Seven prospective and seven case-control studies have been fairly consistent in reporting no material relationship between cholesterol intake and the risk of breast cancer. Diets high in cholesterol possibly have no relationship with breast cancer.

The evidence regarding dietary cholesterol and lung cancer is somewhat mixed. One of four cohort studies and three of five case-control studies showed increases in risk with higher intakes. The evidence is supported by ecological and experimental data.Evidence from four out of seven case-control studies reported an increased risk of pancreatic cancer with higher intakes of cholesterol; the remaining studies were null. Three case-control studies each reported increased risk of endometrical cancer with increased intake of cholesterol.

Omega-3 Fatty Acids

Speaking on the "Dietary fats and cancer", Dr. B.R. Lokesh of Central Food Technological Reseacrh Institute (CFTRI), Mysore, stated that there are 3 million cancer patients at any given time in India and at least one million new cases are added annually, while 2.5–3 lakh people die annually due to cancer. Dr. Lokesh mentioned altered membrane fluidity, modulation of hormone levels, intracellular communication and subversion of immune system could be the possible mechanisms through which fats promote carcinogenes. He presented data on consumption of n-3 oils and their modulatory effects on prostaglandin (PG) levels, especially PGE2 (prostaglanolin G2). He reported that presence of n-3 rich oils in cell culture medium makes the cells sensitive to chemotherapeutic agent like adriamycin. He observed that n-6 fatty acids promote cancer, while n-3 fatty acids have inhibitory effect.

He concluded that saturated fat and n-6 PUFA promote cancer cell growth. It acts through immunosuppressive pathway and production of PGs of 2 series. Oils with neutraceuticals (tocotrienols) may be helpful in view of their inhibitory effect, n-3 PUFA should be included in diet. He ended the talk by posing a question–what should be an ideal level of n-3 level in Indian diet to combat cancer?

Chapter 15

Fat Substitutes

Despite fat's bad reputation, it is a very important nutrient. Fat is a difficult substance to replace because it has many important functions. A major nutrient, it is important for proper growth and development and maintenance of good health. Fats carry the fat-soluble vitamins A, D, E, and K and aid their absorption in the intestine. They are the only source of the essential fatty acids linoleic and linolenic acids. They are an important source of Kcal for many adults and for infants and toddlers, who have the highest energy needs per kg of body weight of any age group. Fat provides 9 Kcal per g, compared with 4 Kcal per g from protein and carbohydrates.

As a food ingredient, fat is important in food preparation and consumption because it gives taste, consistency, stability, and palatability to foods and helps us feel full so we stop eating. Fat absorbs the essence of spices and flavors and allows people to experience their full aroma. In other words, fat is one of the main reasons people enjoy food. But there are limits on the amount we should eat because of fats' link to heart disease, cancer and overweight.

Saturated fat and cholesterol are the substances in fat that contribute to the formation of plaque, which clogs arteries, leading to heart disease. Hence, now a days, the health conscious people look for low-calorie, low-fat, and diet foods and beverages. In a survey, it was found that 72 percent of respondents who said they look for "light" foods said they are most attracted to food products claiming to be "reduced in fat." Therefore, manufacturers are also responding by adding more and more reduced-fat foods to their product lines.

No doubt consumers are concerned about nutrition, and they want to moderate the fat in their diet but there are challenges to overcome. Nutrition, price, convenience, and product safety are important, but taste is the key driver behind food selection for most people. And many consumers still think that less fat means less taste. Fat substitutes were developed to help meet consumers' expectations about taste while providing fewer Kcal from fat.

Since the late 1980s, fat-free and reduced-fat foods have become widely available. While not all new products survive the competitive marketplace, thousands of new reduced-fat and fat-free products have been introduced each year since 1990. In part, these new reduced-fat food products are not only the result of consumer demand but they are also a response to public health concerns and initiatives.

What are Fat Substitutes and how they are Used?

Fat substitutes are ingredients that mimic one or more of the roles of fat in a food. Substitutes, or fat replacers, provide the sensory and functional qualities normally provided by fat. For example, fat provides moistness in baked goods, texture in ice cream, and crispiness in potato chips. Because fat has so many diverse functions in foods, it is virtually impossible to replace it with a single compound or process. The ingredients used in place of fat depend on how a food product will be eaten or prepared. For instance, not all fat-substitute ingredients are stable when heated, so the type of fat substitute used in a fat-free salad dressing may not work well in a muffin mix.

Fat substitutes have been developed to decrease the quantity of fat in foods and help people lower their fat intake. Some fat replacers are used as "fat substitutes" or "fat analogs" and replace fat in a food. Others are used as "fat mimetic" to partially replace fat and impart the sensory qualities of fat (taste and feel in the mouth). Some evidence suggests that people who include fat-modified products in their diet may have a reduced fat and calorie intake and improved nutrient profile compared with people who don't use any fat-modified products.

Classification of Fat Substitutes/Replacers

Fat substitutes can be categorized on the basis of nutrient sources, functional properties, and use in food. Many fat substitutes are simply old ingredients used in new ways. For example, the Food and Drug Administration (FDA) approved polydextrose for use as a moisture-binding agent in the early 1980s, but more recently it has been used as a fat substitute. Carrageenan has been used since the early 1960s as an emulsifier, stabilizer, and thickener, but is now commonly used to replace fat in foods, as is guar gum, which has been used as a thickener for nearly a hundred years.

Some fat substitutes are newer to the food supply, though they are made from familiar ingredients. For example, microparticulated protein is made from milk, egg, or whey protein. Other fat substitutes are new ingredients made from combinations of basic molecules.

They are classified into three categories based on their nutrient source:

1. Carbohydrate-based fat substitutes use plant polysaccharides in place of fat.
2. Proteins and microparticulated proteins are used as fat replacers.
3. Fat-based fat replacers act as "barriers" to block fat absorption.

Table 15.1: Common Fat Substitutes

Carbohydrate-based	*Protein-based*	*Fat-based*
Cellulose	Microparticulated protein	Caprenin
Dextrins	Modified whey protein concentrate	Salatrim
Fiber		Emulsifiers (mono- and diglycerides)
Gums		Sucrose polyester (Olestra)
Inulin		
Maltodextrins		
Oatrim		
Polydextrose		
Polyols		
Starch/modified food starch		
Z-Trim		

Carbohydrate Based Fat Substitutes

Carbohydrate-based fat substitutes are the most common. They are very versatile and found in many types of food products. Most carbohydrate-based fat substitutes are GRAS substances as affirmed by FDA. Although their original intent was to perform certain technical functions in food that would improve overall quality, some carbohydrate-based fat replacers are now used specifically to reduce a food's calorie content. They provide from zero to 4 Kcal per g. When used to replace fat, they may significantly lower the calorie content of a food. They are used in a variety of foods, including dairy-type products, sauces, frozen desserts, salad dressings, processed meats, baked goods, spreads, chewing gum, and sweets. Some of these ingredients are only partially digestible. However, when consumed at expected levels, most carbohydrate-based fat substitutes have no digestive effects. Guar gum is an example of a carbohydrate-based fat substitute. Some of the carbohydrate based fat substitutes include:

Gums

They are also called hydrophilic colloids or hydrocolloids. Examples include guar gum, gum arabic, locust bean gum, xanthan gum, carrageenan and pectin. Carrageenan, a seaweed derivative, was approved for use as an emulsifier, stabilizer and thickener in food in 1961. Its use as a fat replacer became popular in the early 1990s.

Gums are virtually non-caloric, provide thickening, sometimes gelling effect and can promote creamy texture. They are used in reduced-calorie, fat-free salad dressings and to reduce fat content in other formulated foods, including desserts and processed meats.

Cellulose

Avicel, for example, is a cellulose gel introduced in the mid-1960s as a food stabilizer. It is a non-caloric purified form of cellulose ground to microparticles which, when dispersed, form a network of particles with mouth feel and flow properties similar to fat. Cellulose can replace some or all of the fat in dairy-type products, sauces, frozen desserts and salad dressings.

Maltodextrins

This four kilocalorie per g gel or powder is derived from carbohydrate sources such as corn, potato, wheat and tapioca. It is used as fat replacer, texture modifier or bulking agent. Its applications include baked goods, dairy products, salad dressings, spreads, sauces, frostings, fillings, processed meat, frozen desserts, extruded products and beverages.

Polydextrose

It is a reduced calorie (1 Kcal/g) fat replacer and bulking agent. It is a water soluble polymer of dextrose containing minor amounts of sorbitol and citric acid. It is approved for use in a variety of products including baked goods, chewing gums, confections, salad dressings, frozen dairy desserts, gelatins and puddings. Litesse (polydextrose) came in the market in 1981 as a humectant, which helps retain moisture.

Dextrins

This four Kcal/g fat replacer can replace all or some of the fat in a variety of products. Food sources for dextrins include tapioca. Applications include salad dressings, puddings, spreads, dairy-type products and frozen desserts.

Fiber

Fiber can provide structural integrity, volume, moisture holding capacity, adhesiveness and shelf stability in reduced-fat products. Applications include baked goods, meats, spreads and extruded products.

Nu-Trim is a beta-glucan rich fat replacer made from oat and barley using an extraction process that removes coarse fiber components. The resulting product can be used in foods and beverages such as baked goods, milk, cheese and ice cream, yielding products that are both reduced fat and high in beta-glucan.

Oatrim is a water-soluble form of enzyme treated oat flour containing beta-glucan soluble fiber and used as a fat replacer, bodying and texturizing ingredient. It provides reduced Kcal (1-4 Kcal/g) and is used in baked goods, fillings and frostings, frozen desserts, dairy beverages, cheese, salad dressings, processed meats and confections.

Inulin

This reduced-calorie (1-1.2 Kcal/g) fat and sugar replacer, fiber and bulking agent is extracted from chicory root. It is used in yogurt, cheese, frozen desserts, baked goods, icings, fillings, whipped cream, dairy products, fiber supplements and processed meats.

Protein-Based Fat Substitutes

Protein-based fat substitutes came along in the early 1990s. These and fat-based replacers were designed specifically to replace fat in foods. Protein-based fat substitutes are not as numerous as carbohydrate-based ingredients, but they have many applications and can be used in many products, including cheese, yogurt, sour cream, ice cream, mayonnaise, and salad dressing. Protein-based fat substitutes cannot be used for deep-frying.

Whey protein concentrate is a protein-based fat substitute. One form, Microparticulated Protein Product (MPP), such as Simplesse and Trailblazer, is made from whey protein or milk and egg protein. Simplesse is made from egg white and milk protein blended and heated in a process called microparticulation, in which the protein is shaped into microscopic round particles that roll easily over one another. The aim of the process is to create the feel of a creamy liquid with the texture of fat.

These fat replacers provide 1 to 4 Kcal per g, depending on their water content, and are approved for use in frozen dessert-type foods. FDA has agreed that whey-based MPP conforms to FDA's definition of whey protein concentrate, such as the fat replacer Dairy-Lo, a GRAS substance. Therefore, whey-based MPP can be used in other foods, including reduced-fat versions of butter, sour cream, cheese, yogurt, salad dressing, margarine, mayonnaise, baked goods, coffee creamer, soups, and sauces. Another type of protein-based fat replacers, called protein blends, combine animal or vegetable protein, gums, food starch, and water. They are made with FDA-approved ingredients and are used in frozen desserts and baked goods.

Fat-Based Fat Substitutes

The last category of fat substitutes includes those that are fat-based. Because they are made from fat, they often come closest to providing fat's taste and cooking properties. Olestra is an example of a fat-based fat replacer. FDA approved Olestra (brand name Olean), made by Procter and Gamble Co. of Cincinnati, in January 1996, for use in preparing potato chips, crackers, tortilla chips, and other savory snacks. It is a fat-based fat substitute made from sucrose (table sugar) and fatty acids from vegetable oils. Olestra has properties similar to those of naturally occurring fat, but it provides zero Kcal and no fat. That's because Olestra is indigestible. It passes through the digestive tract but is not absorbed into the body. This is due to its unique configuration: a center unit of sucrose (sugar) with six, seven or eight fatty acids attached. It has the potential to inhibit absorption of some fat-soluble nutrients in the digestive tract, and, to offset any possible effects, products made with Olestra have appropriate amounts of vitamins A, D, E, and K added. Olestra's configuration also makes it possible for the substance to be exposed to high temperatures, such as frying-a quality most other fat replacers lack.

As promising as Olestra sounds, it does have some drawbacks. Studies show that it may cause intestinal cramps and loose stools in some individuals. Also, according to clinical tests, Olestra reduces the absorption of fat-soluble nutrients, such as vitamins A, D, E, and K and carotenoids, from foods eaten at the same time as Olestra-containing products. Tests by Procter and Gamble show that no reduction in absorption of fat-soluble vitamins will occur when proper levels of vitamins are added for compensation to Olestra-containing foods.

To address these concerns, FDA approved Olestra on conditions that vitamins A, D, E, and K be added to Olestra-containing foods and that Procter and Gamble continue studies on consumption and long-term effects of Olestra. To provide consumers with information about Olestra's possible effects, FDA also required that the following interim labeling statement appear on products made with Olestra: "This product contains Olestra. Olestra may cause abdominal cramping and loose stools. Olestra inhibits the absorption of some vitamins and other nutrients. Vitamins A, D, E and K have been added." As limited studies have been conducted in children, teens and elderly on the effect of Olestra, it is not recommended for consumption by these populations until more comprehensive researches have been performed.

Other Replacers

Some other fat-based replacers are being considered or developed such as Salatrim (which stands for short and long-chain acid triglyceride molecules) is the generic name for a family of reduced-calorie fats that are only partially absorbed in the body. Salatrim provides 5 Kcal per g. A petition seeking FDA's affirmation that Salatrim is GRAS, was filed in June 1994. An example of its use is in Hershey Co.'s reduced-fat baking chips, semi-sweet chocolate flavor. Caprenin, another Procter and Gamble product, is a 5-calorie-per-g fat substitute for cocoa butter in candy bars. A petition seeking FDA's affirmation that Caprenin is GRAS was filed in 1991.

Emulsifiers are fat-based substances that are used with water to replace all or part of the shortening content in cake mixes, cookies, icings, and vegetable dairy products. They give the same Kcal as fat but less is used, resulting in fat and calorie reductions. Other fat replacers are being developed, according to the Calorie Control Council and other organizations. They include DDM (dialkyl dihexadecylmalonate), a fat-based substance that is not absorbed into the body and can be used in frying and baking. Frito-Lay Inc. has been studying this fat substitute since 1986, although it has not yet petitioned FDA for approval.

Also on the horizon is a fat substitute made by combining starches or gums with small amounts of oil. Opta Food Ingredients Inc. received an exclusive license from the U.S. Department of Agriculture for the process, called Fantesk. This fat replacer would give foods the taste and texture of regular fat but provide less than 0.5 g of fat per serving.

In some cases, the FDA has approved fat-reduction ingredients as food additives. To be approved, food additives are tested extensively to assess their safety and level of use among different population groups. Examples of fat substitutes approved as food additives include carrageenan, Olestra, and polydextrose.

In other instances, fat-reduction ingredients are "generally recognized as safe" (GRAS). GRAS ingredients are made from common food components and are considered by experts to be safe. Examples of GRAS fat substitutes include guar gum and maltodextrin.

Can Fat Substitutes Help to Reduce Dietary Fat?

In theory, the perfect fat replacer is one that contributes everything fat does in a food but without the Kcal, saturated fat, and cholesterol. The question remains: Can fat-reduced products actually reduce people's overall calorie intake and have a significant impact on their total fat intake?

Now a days, food manufacturers are making it easier for fat-conscious consumers to have their cake and eat it, too and their cheeses, chips, chocolate, cookies, ice cream, salad dressings, and various other foods that are now available in lower fat versions. These products can help adult consumers reduce their fat intakes to recommended levels while allowing them to enjoy foods traditionally high in fat. A diet high in fat can contribute to heart disease and some forms of cancer and, because fats are calorie-dense, to excessive body weight.

Several studies have shown that using reduced-fat versions of food products can significantly reduce the amount of fat that people eat. For some people, eating less fat may lead to eating fewer Kcal and, eventually, to weight loss.

A common misconception about reduced-fat foods is that they also are low in Kcal. For many products, however, this is not the case. Most reduced-fat foods have had other ingredients added to replace the texture or flavor provided by fat, so that while the Kcal may be slightly lower in a fat-reduced product, the difference between it and a full-fat product may not be significant. With fat-modified products, as with all foods, portion size and Kcal still count.

Fat-modified foods can fit into a healthy eating plan. According to the American Dietetic Association, they offer a safe, feasible, and effective means to maintain the palatability of diets that are controlled in fat or Kcal. But they are only one of the many tools that can be used to achieve nutrition goals. Foods with fat substitutes should be consumed as part of an overall healthful eating plan.

Research Studies on Fat Substitutes

i) Reducing Dietary Fat

Can these fat replacers help consumers make positive dietary changes? Can they help those who are overweight lose weight? A possible concern about fat replacers is: Can foods claiming to be reduced in fat inadvertently influence people to eat more? It may be too early to say, and studies to date give varying answers.

Individuals with a higher education level and a perception of a strong relationship between diet and disease reported higher rates of Olestra use. Overweight and obese individuals were more likely to be Olestra users than were normal-weight individuals, but having diabetes was negatively associated with Olestra use. In a double-blind, placebo-controlled, within-subject crossover study, 20 to 35 g of Olestra was covertly substituted for conventional fat, and subjects had ad libitum access to additional fat, which allowed the investigators to determine if the replacement of conventional fat with a substitute would reduce fat and energy intake (Hill *et al.*, 1998). During the 2 weeks of Olestra feeding, subjects consumed 8 per cent less total energy and had an 11 per cent lower intake of fat than during the 2-week conventional fat feeding period. The total deficit achieved with the substitution was only 2616 kcal over the 14-day study period (Hill *et al.*, 1998).

In a study of lean non-dieting men, one group ate breakfasts of conventional fat foods, while the other ate Olestra-containing foods. Those who ate the Olestra-containing foods made up their usual daily calorie intake by eating more carbohydrate-containing foods. The study, sponsored partly by Procter and Gamble and published in a 1992 issue of the American Journal of Clinical Nutrition (Volume 56), suggested that a diet of reduced-fat foods can help reduce fat intake without affecting total Kcal.

In a single-meal feeding study, substituting Olestra for regular fat reduced intake by 450 kcal, but neither the participants' subjective ratings of post meal hunger nor the amount of food consumed during the subsequent meal changed (Lawton *et al.*, 1998). One-year follow-up data from the Olestra Post-Marketing Surveillance Study indicate that individuals in the highest consumption category (≥2 g/d) did not significantly reduce total energy intake, although they reduced the percentage of Kcal from fat by 2.7 per cent and that from saturated fatty acids by 1.1 per cent. Analysis of the dietary intake data indicated that higher intake of Olestra-containing products was associated with higher intake of vegetables, fiber, protein, and sodium (Patterson *et al.*, 2000).

Fat intake also was decreased in a study of 96 men and women "habitual snackers." One group was fed potato chips prepared with Olestra, while the rest ate potato chips prepared with conventional frying oil. The group fed Olestra chips ate on average 29 g less fat and 270 fewer Kcal a day than those fed regular chips–even though those who knew they were eating fat-free chips ate 10 g of chips more than those who ate regular chips. This study, done at Pennsylvania State University, also was partly sponsored by Procter and Gamble.

In other study conducted at Pennsylvania State University, women were fed the same yogurt labeled either "high-fat" or "low-fat." The group fed the low-fat-labeled version ate more in a lunch that followed the yogurt than the group eating the high-fat-labeled yogurt. As a result, the group eating what they thought was low-fat yogurt took in more Kcal than the other group. "It appeared that these women regarded the low-fat label as a license to overeat," wrote Debra Miller, a doctoral student in biobehavioral health and nutrition at Pennsylvania State, in an article she wrote for Weight Control Digest.

Still, reduced fat foods appear to be an important part of a fat-reduction diet, according to a study involving the Women's Health Trial. The study, designed to determine the role of low-fat diets in the prevention of breast cancer, found that eating "specially manufactured" low-fat foods was one of the most easily adopted dietary practices for those who received prior dietary instruction. Avoiding meats and giving up fats as flavorings (for example, eating bread without butter or margarine) were among the most difficult practices to adopt.

In using reduced-fat foods, the American Dietetic Association cautions consumers to realize that fat-free doesn't mean calorie-free. The Kcal lost in removing regular fat from a food can be regained through sugars added for palatability, as well as fat replacers, many of which provide Kcal too. Consumers should refer to the Nutrition

Facts panel on the food label to compare Kcal and other nutrition information between fat-reduced and regular-fat foods.

Many nutrition experts agree that, used properly, fat replacers can play an important role in improving diets. But, as with any diet or food, they emphasize variety and moderation to ensure a healthy intake.

ii) Potential Effects on Health and Nutritional Status

The potential physiological effects of fat substitutes on health and nutrient status vary. Some research suggests that individuals who consume a diet that is reduced in fat and calories and includes use of fat-modified products have a better overall nutrient profile than do individuals who do not use any fat-modified products.

Health- and weight-conscious consumers are expected to welcome fat-free products that taste like the real thing. In fact, a recent survey by the Calorie Control Council of USA, An Association of Low-Calorie and Diet Food Manufacturers, found that 57 percent of adult Americans believe there is a need for fat substitutes.

According to the 1988 Surgeon General's Report on Nutrition and Health, high intake of fat is associated with increased risk for obesity, some types of cancer (breast, colon, prostate, rectum, ovaries, and endometrium), and possibly gallbladder disease. Studies also show strong evidence of a relationship between high saturated fat intake and a high blood cholesterol level, which is a risk factor for coronary heart disease. The report also states that because obesity is a risk factor for several chronic diseases, it is important to maintain a desirable weight. Obesity increases the risk of high blood pressure and, consequently, stroke. It also increases blood cholesterol and may, by itself, be a risk factor for coronary heart disease.

It remains to be seen, however, whether consumers will, indeed, become healthier by using products with fat substitutes. According to the June 15, 1990, issue of The Medical Letter, a professional publication on drugs and therapeutics, no clinical studies have shown that use of either Simplesse or Trailblazer leads to weight reduction or decreases blood lipid (fat) concentrations.

Data from the CSFII from 1989 to 1991 and 1994 to 1995 indicate that adults who used fat-reduction strategies had lower intake of total fat, saturated fat, cholesterol, and energy and were more likely to meet the dietary guidelines than those who did not use fat-reduction strategies (Kennedy *et al.*, 1999; Peterson *et al.*, 1999; Lichtenstein *et al.*, 1998). The micronutrient intake of persons who used several strategies to reduce fat intake was comparable to that of individuals who used only full-fat products (Peterson *et al.*, 1999).

Data from the children participating in the CSFII suggest that the use of fat-modified products could help children reach dietary recommendations, but concomitant reductions in total energy and vitamin E intake may occur (Peterson *et al.*, 1997). However, these data were obtained from dietary intake data and were collected before Olestra became available in 1998.

Short-term data suggest that use of fat substitutes has few adverse or positive effects (Sigman-Grant, 1997; Patterson *et al.*, 2000). Longer-term studies will determine the potential impact of fat substitutes on preventing or treating obesity. Factors that affect energy balance specifically, *i.e.* portion control and physical activity, are likely to have a greater impact on weight than does use of fat-modified products. Thus, substitution of low-fat for full-fat products may not be effective in lowering body weight if other strategies for weight control are not implemented.

Some nutritionists are concerned that people who eat products made with fat substitutes will feel freer to eat more of other high-fat foods, rationalizing that they are "saving" on those made with substitutes. Another possibility experts anticipate is that people will eat more fat-free double-dip ice cream cones, leaving less room for the more nutritious foods they need.

A more basic, as yet unanswered, question is whether non-fat foods will satisfy as well as the traditional foods they replace and, therefore, whether they will really help people reduce fat consumption.

Lisa Lefferts, staff scientist with the Washington-based consumer advocacy group Center for Science in the Public Interest, points to the experience with sugar substitutes: "We're eating four times the amount of sugar substitutes as we were in 1975, but sugar consumption has gone up as well, so clearly sugar substitutes are not substituting for sugar." Lefferts says that the effect of fat substitutes on the diet is unclear. "Fat substitutes such as Simplesse are a step in the right direction," she says, "but we would encourage that their use be monitored in order to assess their true impact."

FDA, too, has questions about the impact of fat substitutes in the food supply. "There are two categories of fat substitutes to consider," says Walter Glinsmann, M.D., associate director for clinical nutrition. "Products like Simplesse are processed from substances already in the diet, and they are digested and used by the body in the same way as the original substances. Others, like Olestra, are new, undigestible molecules never before in the food supply."

The possible health effects of consuming large amounts of a novel substance must be carefully researched and reviewed before such a product can be marketed. When fat intake is about 30 to 40 percent of the daily caloric intake and that half of that fat is derived from foods in which the fat can be replaced with a substitute, one should take a hard look at the potential health effects.

Some of the questions to be considered are:

- ☆ If the materials are absorbed in the body even in very small amounts, are they toxic?
- ☆ If they are not absorbed, how do they affect gastrointestinal functions? For example, could they interfere with the absorption of nutrients or drugs?
- ☆ Are the substitutes suitable for general use or only for sub-populations of the general public?

Literature reviews indicate that few if any health issues have been raised about adverse impact of the carbohydrate-based or protein-based fat substitutes, which seem to have little or no effect on digestion, absorption, or metabolism of other nutrients.

Fat-based substitutes derived from modifying length or number of fatty acids also seems to have no effect. These substitutes include caprenin and salatrim, as well as mono- and di-glycerides.

Within the fat-based group, the safety research has focused primarily on Olestra, which may affect nutritional status by its effects on absorption of fat-soluble nutrients. In the gastrointestinal tract, fat-soluble nutrients can partially partition into Olestra and be excreted. Factors that affect the level of partitioning include:

(*a*) Degree of fat solubility (the more fat soluble nutrient, the more it will be partitioned into Olestra),

(*b*) Relative amount of Olestra to nutrient (partitioning increases as the amount of Olestra per measure of nutrient increases), and

(*c*) Timing of Olestra and nutrient consumption (partitioning can occur when Olestra and the fat-soluble nutrients are in the gut at the same time).

The manufacturer had compiled partitioning coefficients for fat-soluble nutrients in 382 foods. The affected nutrients included phytosterol and carotenoids, with reduced absorption rates of <10 per cent and 6 per cent to 10 per cent, respectively (Cooper *et al.*, 1997). Little is known about potential interactions with pharmacological agents and ingredients in food products that can affect fat-soluble nutrient motility and absorption rates in the gastrointestinal tract.

In an 8-week, randomized, controlled parallel study, Olestra reduced serum concentrations of carotenoids, α-tocopherol, 25-hydroxy-ergocalciferol, and phylloquines in a dose-response manner. However, Olestra did not affect other nutrients, lipids, or prothrombin time or concentration (Schlagheck *et al.*, 1997; Patterson *et al.*, 2000). Specified amounts of fat-soluble vitamins A, D, E, and K must be added by the manufacturer to offset the effects of Olestra.

The results of several studies indicate that Olestra intake affects the composition of the stool and its softness (McRorie *et al.*, 2000; Balasekaran *et al.*, 2000; Jandacek *et al.*, 1999; Freston *et al.*, 1997). Intake of Olestra did not increase objective measures of diarrhea (stool output of >250 g/d, liquid or water stool, or >3 bowel movements per day) (McRorie *et al.*, 2000). However, consumption of 40 g of Olestra in ≈5 oz of chips (15 chips are ≈1 oz) can increase fecal fat excretion and result in a misdiagnosis of malabsorption (Balasekaran *et al.*, 2000). Consumption of Olestra does not seem to exacerbate quiescent inflammatory bowel disease (Zorich *et al.*, 1997). Continued monitoring of consumption patterns and health biomarkers is needed to determine the longer-term effects of Olestra.

Fat Labeling

Products labeled fat free and low fat must contain <0.5 and ≤3 g of fat per serving, respectively. Reduced or less fat may be used on the labels of products that contain 25 per cent less fat than regular (full-fat) products. The fat labeling claims do not provide any indication of the caloric content of the food item. However, products containing one third fewer Kcal or one half the fat of the reference food may be labeled as light. If

≥50 per cent of Kcal in a food are derived from fat, the fat content of the reduced-fat version must be reduced by 50 per cent. The terms calorie free and low calorie only can be used on products with <5 and ≤40 Kcal per serving, respectively, and reduced or fewer Kcal only can be used on products that have ≤25 per cent of the Kcal in the regular product.

Table 15.2: Synthetic Fat Substitutes and their Regulatory Status

Fat substitute	*Chemical composition*	*FDA approval*	*Potential application*
Polydextrose texturiser	Modified glucose polymer	GRAS	Bulking agent, humectants,
Caprenin	Structured medium chain triacylglycerol	GRAS	Cocoa butter equivalent
Salatrim, Benefat	Two medium-chain fatty acids and one long chain fatty acid in a triacylglycerol	GRAS	Cocoa butter equivalent
Olestra, Oleaan	Sucrose fatty acid polyester	Approved Jan. 1996, July 2004	Savoury snacks, pre-packaged ready-to-eat popcorn
Sucorse fatty acid esters		Approved	Emulsifier
Sorbestrin	Cyclic sorbitol fatty acid polyesters	No approval	Frying or baking oil, salad dressings
Polyglycerol	Polyglycerol fatty acid esters	No approval	Shortenings, margarines, confectionaries
Retrofat	Trialknoxytricarballylate	No approval	Shortenings, mayonnaise
Trialkoxy citrate	Ester bonds reversed from triacylglycerol	No approval	Similar to corn oil
Trialkoxy glycerol ethers	Dialkyl glycerol ethers, glycerolmonoester diethers	No approval	Vegetable oils
Dialkyl dihexa-decylmalonate	Fatty alcohol dicaroxylic acid esters of malonic acid and alkylmalonic acid	No approval	Mayonnaise, margarine, salad dressing
Polysiloxane, phe-nylmethyl polysil-oxane and phenyl-dimethypolysiloxane	Organic derivatives of silica	No approval	Functionality similar to soybean oil
Esterified propoxy-lated glycerol	Polyetherpolyol fatty acids	No approval	Vegetable oil
Jojoba oil	Linear esters of C20:1 and C22:1	Toxic?	Edible oils
Membrane lipids	Extracts of Halobacterium halobium	Expensive?	Fat-like material

From Swanson (2006) GRAS= Generally Recognized as Safe notice

Source: Ann. Nutr. Metab. 2009; 55: 273-300.

Safety Regulation of Fat Substitutes

Table 15.2 depicts the synthetic fat substitutes and their regulatory status till date. Although fat substitutes in the market are considered safe by the U.S. Food and Drug Administration (FDA), their long-term benefits and safety are not known. The cumulative impact of using multiple fat substitutes as they increase in the marketplace is unknown. Still, within the context of a healthy dietary pattern, fat substitutes, when used judiciously, may provide some flexibility in dietary planning, although additional research is needed to fully determine the longer-term health effects.

Under FDA regulations, fat replacers usually fall into one of two categories: food additives or "generally recognized as safe" (GRAS) substances. Each has its own set of regulatory requirements. Food additives must be evaluated for safety and approved by FDA before they can be marketed. They include substances with no proven track record of safety; scientists just don't know that much about their use in food.

Manufacturers of food additives must test their products, submit the results to FDA for review, and await agency approval before using them in food. GRAS substances, on the other hand, do not have to undergo rigorous testing before they are used in foods because they are generally recognized as safe by knowledgeable scientists, usually because of the substances' long history of safe use in foods. Many GRAS substances are similar to substances already in food. Examples of GRAS substances used as fat replacers are cellulose gel, dextrins, guar gum, and gum arabic.

Chapter 16

Recommended Fatty Acid Ratios in Dietary Fats for Good Health

Nutrition is the relationship of foods to the health of the human body. The foods we consume should provide our bodies with the nutrients necessary for good health. The basic premise of any good diet is variety, balance and moderation in what we eat, on a regular basis. Good nutrition from eating a healthy diet is the foundation of any wellness programme. The Goal is to eat the right ratios of the macronutrients *i.e.* carbohydrates, proteins and fats at a total caloric rate that will either maintain the present body weight, or achieve the ideal body weight over a reasonably long period of time.

Poor nutrition is the result of consuming too little, too much, or the wrong kinds of food, on a regular basis. Food science, a root cause of poor nutrition, transforms natural whole foods into garbage that fills the belly while developing excessive human appetites for fat, sugar, and salt. Avoiding poor nutrition simply means refusing to eat junk and fat rich foods. Therefore, the question arises is 'what are the right ratios of the macronutrients *i.e.* carbohydrates, proteins and fats?' In the ideal diet, carbohydrates, proteins and fats should provide 55, 15 and 30 percent of the calories in the daily diet (Table 16.1). In this chapter, our main emphasis shall be on ideal amount of fat and type of fat to be taken in the daily diet.

Fat, a naturally occurring substance in food, plays an important role in nutrition. It is one of three main macronutrient groups that supply calories in food. Fat includes what we commonly call "oils" and "fats". Dietary oils (fats) are essential for the body. They are an excellent source of energy and almost all foods contain fat in

Table 16.1: Dietary Patterns of the Natural Health Perspective Daily Diet.

	Defect	*Ranges of Diet*					
		Min	*TypicalDiet*	*Ideal Diet*	*Modified Diet*	*Max*	*Excess*
Carbs		41%	50%	55%	45%	55%	67%
Protein		10%	16%	15%	20%	15%	
Fat		25%	34%	30%	35%	35%	39%
Total	n/a	n/a	100%	100%	100%	n/a	n/a
UFA		16%	n/a	n/a	n/a	23%	
SFA		7%	16%	7%	7%	11%	
MUFA	12% 8		11%	18%	21%	22%	
PUFA		3%	7%	5%	7%	7% 2,5	11%
Fat Total	n/a	n/a	34%	30%	35%	n/a	n/a

The ratio of protein, carbohydrate, and the types of fat in what we eat is the key to optimal health.

Defect–Consumption at a level so low that the result clearly is Negative.

Excess–Consumption at a level so high that the result clearly is Negative.

Min–Consumption at a low level where few if any Negatives have generally been reported.

Max–Consumption at a high level where few if any Negatives have generally been reported.

Carbs–Carbohydrates.

Protein–Reports, such as in Journal of Nutrition 2000; 130: 2889-2896, of "oxidative stress" in "adequate / low protein" diets are due mostly to clearly excessively high levels of carbohydrates and excessively low fat levels. Up the FAT to a recommended 30 per cent low fat diet and most "oxidative stress" will disappear with an "adequate protein" diet. Excessive protein in the diet results in excess "Protein Oxidation."

The Typical Diet that is consumed widely today or the average American diet.

The Ideal Diet is for, so called, NORMAL individuals who weigh 200 pounds or less and who are SATURATED FAT sensitive individuals. These individuals are susceptible to the adverse effects of Saturated Fat on their blood cholesterol levels. The majority of the population is SATURATED FAT sensitive.

The Modified Diet is for, so called, SUGAR sensitive individuals. These individuals generally weigh more than 200 pounds. They are more susceptible to the adverse effects of dietary sugars than the population of normal body weight is.

Persons with known coronary-artery disease, high triglycerides blood levels, diabetics, extremely obese individuals, and those with Syndrome-X are likely to be sensitive to sugars in the diet.

Everybody responds to sugar in their diet. Sugar Sensitive individuals exhibit an extreme response to all forms of Sugars. This extreme response is generally considered an ABNORMALITY.

SFA = Saturated Fat

MUFA = Monounsaturated Fat

PUFA = Polyunsaturated Fat

UFA = Unsaturated Fat (*i.e.*, total Monounsaturated and Polyunsaturated Fat)
Most of this table is NOT supposed to add up to 100 per cent. This table quantifies the acceptable High and Low ranges of the specific parts of a diet that characterizes the Natural Health Perspective diet.

varying amounts. Certain fatty acids are even vital for good health. They promote absorption of fat soluble vitamins, facilitate the production of hormones, support vital organs and protect us from cold. Apart from making the food more tasty and palatable, fat acts as an excellent heat transfer media in cooking, frying and baking applications.

Unfortunately we are drowned in heavy consumption of saturated fats which has been linked to heart disease. Moderation should be the key and the choice should be with the lowest levels of saturated fats. Lin Yutang, a Chinese writer has very rightly quoted 'Our lives are not in the lap of the gods, but in lap of our cooks'. How well one cooks is not just a matter of taste but health as well.

Ever wondered how restaurants make their food taste so good. The secret lies behind the use of butter, oil, animal fat, salt and sweeteners. Butter is the, simplest, easiest and quickest way to make things taste rich and wonderful. Ever paused to ponder over love affair with fried foods? The key is oil, lots of oil. We Indians are used to using too much of oil. Many recent studies have linked the consumption of saturated fat with an increased risk of heart attack. The best option is to explore ways to cook without oil, like healthy sauté, steaming, broil etc. If we find it hard to forego oil, then be prepared to cut this down drastically and finally be wise in the selection, usage and storage of oils. Today food companies have come a long way in their ability to improve the properties of vegetable oils at the manufacturing level. There are refined and conditioned oils in the marketplace, including oils from plant hybrids that are high in certain types of fat such as MUFA, which are less susceptible to damage from heating. To know the right proportion of various types of fats in the diets, it is important to first know the various types of fatty acids present in various types of fat and oils. Such brief information is given as under:

Composition of Fat

Fats and oils are made up of basic units called fatty acids. Each type of fat or oil is a mixture of different fatty acids.

Saturated Fatty Acids (SFA)

They are found mainly in animal sources such as meat and poultry, dairy fat, vegetable oils like Coconut oil, Palm kernel oil and Palm oil. Saturated fats are usually solid at room temperature. Oils rich in SFA are known as saturated oils.

Monounsaturated Fatty Acids (MUFA)

These are found mainly in vegetable oils such as Canola, Olive, Mustard and Groundnut oils. They are liquid at room temperature. Oils rich in MUFA are known as Mono unsaturated oils. The American Heart Association (AHA) suggests that MUFA rich diet reduces risk of heart diseases. High MUFA diet lowers total and LDL Cholesterol without affecting the HDL Cholesterol level and also lowers triglycerides.

Polyunsaturated Fatty Acids (PUFA)

These are found mainly in vegetable oils such as Safflower, Sunflower, Corn, Soya and Cottonseed oils. Polyunsaturated fats are also the main fats found in seafood.

They are liquid at room temperature. Specific polyunsaturated fatty acids, such as linoleic acid (omega-6) and alpha-linolenic (omega-3) acid, are called essential fatty acids. These are not synthesized in our body but are vital as they are necessary for cell structure and making hormones. Essential fatty acids hence are obtained from foods we consume. Oils rich in PUFA are known as polyunsaturated oils.

Ideal Balance among Various Fatty Acids

It is well known that dietary saturated fatty acids (SFA) increase the risk for CHD while monounsaturated fatty acids (MUFA) and polyunsaturated fatty acids (PUFA) decrease the risk for CHD via the modification of fasting lipids. Since all dietary sources of fat are composed of a combination of SFA, MUFA nad PUFA, it is best to characterize dietary fats as ratio of SFA: MUFA: PUFA. In fact, the SFA: MUFA: PUFA ratio in any given region or population is relatively homogeneous due to common food sources, food accessibility, food preparation and processing, dietary culture and tradition. For example, dietary fatty acid compositions (SFA: MUFA: PUFA) obtained directly or derived from existing national/regional reports are: 1:1.7:0.4 in Greece, 1:1.0:0.5 in USA, and 1:1.5:1 in the mainland of China. The research done at Sun Yat-sen University showed that the composition was 1:1.7:1.2 among type 2 diabetic patients in Guangzhou, a city in Southern China (Sun Yat-sen University, ClinicalTrials.gov Identifier, 2007). Various research workers and Heart associations have recommended different proportions of SFA, MUFA and PUFA which are discussed as under:

I. Studies done by Hayes and his Co-workers

Within the concept of a 'balance' among classes of SFA, MUFA and PUFA is the issue of which specific SFA or PUFA are best. According to Hayes (2002), the ideal ratio of SFA: MUFA: PUFA should be 1:1.5:1.

i) Saturated and Trans Fatty Acids

Many studies have suggested that saturated fatty acids raise total cholesterol (TC), low density lipoprotein (LDL) and high density lipoprotein (HDL), and that PUFA lower them. But certain SFA (as consumed in our daily diet) are better than others in terms of their impact on the LDL/HDL ratio. Fats rich in 12:0 + 14:0 (*e.g.*, milk fat, coconut oil and palm kernel oil) raise LDL the most. Stearic acid (18:0) is not very prevalent in saturated fats, but it is neutral in its effect on blood cholesterol when consumed in natural fats. The most common SFA is palmitic acid (16:0), so-named because it represents the major SFA in palm oil. The 16:0 SFA is present to some degree in essentially all fats and is by far the most prevalent SFA in our diet. Considering the influence on the lipoprotein profile, 16:0 is intermediate, that is, it can be neutral when placed on a triglyceride molecule with MUFA, PUFA or 18:0, or cholesterol-raising when attached along with 12:0 + 14:0. In high amounts, 16:0 can even raise TC and LDL when substituted for 18:0, MUFA or PUFA in people who already have elevated TC or who eat large amounts of cholesterol. Accordingly, the general advice has been to remove as much SFA from the diet as possible. But this is not practical because the manufacture of many food products requires SFA (or some facsimile thereof, such as trans fatty acids (TFA), and extreme removal of dietary SFA is not prudent because their deletion from the diet surprisingly exerts an adverse effect on the LDL/HDL ratio. Even the 'less than 7 per cent of calories' now proposed by NCEP and American Heart Association can prove deleterious if total fat is allowed to drift toward 40 per cent en. So what should be the approach to saturated fat, and what is the best dietary combination of SFA? In recent years one mistaken answer has been to utilize synthetic SFA manufactured by 'hardening' vegetable oils through hydrogenation. This process makes a stiff, plastic fat that is rich in so-called trans fatty acid (TFA). But it turns out that certain of these TFA can be worse than any of the individual natural SFA because they not only raise LDL but also lower HDL, leading to an unfortunate and exaggerated increase in the LDL/HDL ratio (unfortunate in terms of cardiovascular risk). Trans fatty acids also increase a highly atherogenic lipoprotein in the LDL fraction called lipoprotein (a).

An alternative to this predicament is to provide a reasonable level of SFA in our diet by careful selection of naturally available SFA. According to Hayes (2002), the research with monkeys and humans indicates that the guidelines are best tempered by the original AHA Step I diet (30 per cent en from dietary fat and 1:1:1 for SFA: MUFA: PUFA) and that the best SFA are 16:0 and 18:0 from natural fats. This conclusion is derived from carefully analyzing all aspects of the NCEP/AHA recommendations coupled with analysis of the available lipoprotein data in relevant studies involving the controlled intake of dietary fat in humans and experimental animals.

ii) Balance among Polyunsaturated Fatty Acids

In selecting PUFA, the issue of whether to include linoleic acid (18:2 n-6), linolenic acid (18:3 n-3) or longer n-3 fatty acids like eicosapentanenoic acid and docosapentaenoic acid must be considered. Both n-6 and n-3 families are essential fatty acids and both are important to health, especially cardiovascular health. The linoleic acid level has the greatest impact on regulating the LDL/HDL ratio, whereas linolenic acid and its longer derivatives have a major influence over the clotting mechanism, as well as stabilizing the heart against abnormal beating (arrhythmia) that can lead to sudden death. Diets enriched in 18:3 n-3 or 22:6 n-3 have been shown to exert a significant anti-CHD effect in humans, both in clinical and epidemiological studies. The best dietary fat would contain an ideal balance (7:1) of n-6 linoleic to n-3 linolenic acids. This balance is not available in partially hydrogenated margarines, in which most of the n-3 linolenic acid has been destroyed by processing, and is also unlike most vegetable oils that contain only a small amount of this important fatty acid.

iii) Dietary Cholesterol

Dietary cholesterol is very important in this scenario, as evidenced by the NCEP/AHA dietary recommendations to reduce the daily intake to below 300 or 200 mg depending on individual risk. In fact, dietary cholesterol increases the body's sensitivity to SFA, so that maximizing its removal can substantially reduce much of the negative influence of SFA on the lipoprotein profile. PUFA, on the other hand, are the major fatty acids able to actually offset the negative impact of dietary cholesterol because linoleic acid (18:2 n-6) enhances the removal of plasma LDL, the main lipoprotein that is increased by dietary cholesterol (Hayes, 2002).

iv) Monounsaturated Fatty Acids

From the results of most of the research studies, MUFA have been found to be essentially neutral in terms of their lipoprotein profile, and therefore, are perhaps the best source of fatty acids to use as 'filler' in the dietary fat load. This is true to some extent, but the critical issue remains as to how much SFA and PUFA should be consumed to achieve the best LDL/HDL ratio. A high MUFA intake at the expense of PUFA and SFA did not counter the presence of dietary cholesterol very well and led to an increased LDL/HDL ratio relative to a balanced SFA: MUFA: PUFA ratio that allowed for a higher PUFA intake in cynomolgus monkeys when Hayes (2002) compared olive oil and various oil blends. Thus, fat blends incorporate a better fatty acid balance than olive oil alone.

v) Lipoprotein Profile

How the individual (normocholesterolaemic vs hypercholesterolaemic) fits into this story is an important consideration. Obviously, more research is needed, but it appears that the fundamental response to the AHA balanced fatty acid diet is similar in both types of individuals. That is, a 1:1.5:1 balance in SFA: MUFA: PUFA appears to be important to both groups for generating the ideal LDL/HDL ratio. In absolute terms, the response by the hypercholesterolaemic individual is more dramatic, but the person with a normal cholesterol value responds in the same manner, just not to the same degree (Hayes, 2002).

II. Brandeis–PORIM Patent

The novel finding from Nutritional Research at Brandeis University and Palm Oil Research Institute of Malaysia is that the 1:1:1 balance in SFA: MUFA: PUFA recommended over the years by the AHA actually induces the best lipoprotein profile in animals and humans. This seems to be true for all levels of fat intake normally consumed in Western diets (20–40 per cent of total calories). Significant deviation from 1:1.5:1, such as too low SFA or too high MUFA or PUFA, induces a less desirable lipoprotein profile, even if the total plasma cholesterol is lower. The tested fat blends of Hayes (2002) were specifically designed to adhere to this 1:1.5:1 balance while removing all TFA. Several human studies and epidemiological reports indicate that trans fats are 'equal to or worse than' the SFA they were designed to replace. In fact, some of the deleterious effects attributed to SFA over the years were very probably the result of substitution by TFA. Future research will undoubtedly examine this possibility. The following published reports serve to substantiate the above points.

Both SFA and PUFA are required for the Optimal LDL/ HDL Ratio

The first report tested the hypothesis that providing either too few SFA or PUFA in the diet could be detrimental to the HDL or LDL level, respectively (Sundram *et al.*, 1995). Three fats were fed in the whole-food diets of 23 young men with normal cholesterol values, providing two-thirds of the daily fat load from supplemented dietary oils (31 per cent fat energy). The dietary fat was initially balanced as in the AHA Step I with a 10:13:8 ratio of SFA: MUFA: PUFA in the final diet, followed by a high-MUFA low-SFA (6:17:8) or high-SFA, low-PUFA (13:14:4) diet. The first represented a blend of soybean oil, palm oil and canola oil whereas the other two fats were supplied as canola oil or palm olein. All three fats produced about the same normal TC value, but the AHA blend produced the highest HDL and lowest LDL, so that the LDL/HDL ratio was significantly enhanced by the AHA balanced blend of SFA: MUFA: PUFA. Therefore, neither too low SFA nor too low PUFA is adequate, and MUFA are no substitute for either. Rather, one needs a balance of PUFA (to lower LDL) and SFA (to raise HDL) for the best TC and LDL/HDL profile, at least when following an AHA Step I diet at 30 per cent en fat. The 8:12:8 balance for SFA: MUFA: PUFA inherent in the current NCEP and AHA guidelines for 30 per cent en from fat appears to be the best advice for the average individual (Hayes, 2002).

High PUFA or High SFA cause Lipoprotein Imbalance

The second study (Lottenberg *et al.*, 1996) reports data that closely resemble that of Sundram *et al.* (1995). The run-in diet, which was 'AHA Step I' generated the best LDL/HDL ratio because the HDL level was significantly higher than with the other two diets. The other diets were either much more saturated (palm oil) or much more polyunsaturated (sunflower and olive oils) than the AHA recommended balance of 1:1.3:1. Because the subjects were hypercholesterolaemic, the SAT diet raised LDL significantly, unlike in the report of Sundram *et al.* (1995) where subjects were normolipaemic. This rendered the LDL/HDL ratio for the SAT diet much worse. But the polyunsaturated fat (PUFA) diet contained too much 18:2 and not enough SFA. Although it lowered LDL to a level equal to that found with the AHA Step I balanced fatty acid profile of the run-in diet, it also lowered HDL. The latter result was very similar to the Schaefer data where too much PUFA also seriously depressed HDL (Schaefer *et al.*, 1981). On the other hand, the SAT diet provided too much 16:0, which raises LDL in hypercholesterolaemic individuals. Therefore, the AHA Step I diet at 30 per cent en fat and 1:1.3:1 generates the highest HDL and best LDL/HDL ratio, even in hypercholesterolaemic subjects.

PUFA Intake is Critical for the Best LDL/HDL Ratio

Another study (Jones *et al.*, 1987) addressed two questions: (i) whether a low fat diet (20 per cent fat energy) would improve relatively normal TC values in 31 adult women; and (ii) whether it matters much if dietary fatty acids are balanced between SFA: MUFA: PUFA in either a high-fat (40 per cent en) or a low fat (20 per cent en) situation (*i.e.*, considerably above or below the AHA Step I diet objective of 30 per cent fat energy, but with or without the 8:12:8 balance in SFA: MUFA: PUFA that the AHA endorses). Several results were apparent. The dietary polyunsaturated to saturated fatty acid ratio (P/S) was 0.3 in group I (n = 15) and 1.0 in group II (n = 16). Fatty acid balance had little effect on LDL or HDL at 40 per cent en, primarily because the basal (group I) intake of PUFA (6 per cent en) was close to the amount of 18:2 required for normal lipoprotein metabolism under the circumstances. But the suggested AHA balance (P/S 1.0) did tend to improve the LDL/HDL ratio slightly at this high-fat intake. However, when consuming the low-fat diet, the balance in fatty acids was exceedingly important because a 1:1:1 ratio prevented the substantial decline in HDL seen with group I, where the typical American fat imbalance (P/S 0.3) resulted in higher LDL and lower HDL. This undesirable impact on LDL and HDL in group I occurred primarily because the absolute intake of PUFA (3 per cent en) was too low for adequate lipoprotein metabolism when total fat supplied only 20 per cent en. The LDL/HDL ratio was much improved by feeding the 1:1:1 fatty acid balance at the low-fat intake (group II) because the 6 per cent en from PUFA was now adequate in absolute terms (*i.e.*, grams 18:2/day). Therefore, with dietary fat somewhere between 40 per cent en and 20 per cent en, the proper balance in fatty acid intake becomes exceedingly important for generating the optimal LDL/HDL ratio, that is, the lowest LDL and highest HDL values. As in the report of Sundram *et al.* (1995) it would appear that a controlled intake of 18:2 PUFA is required to allow for the greatest decline in LDL without also lowering HDL. The particular type of SFA fed in this study was not specified, although an amount of SFA equal to the PUFA resulted in a favourable LDL/HDL response.

Fatty Acid Balance can Selectively Lower LDL but not HDL

A report by Schwandt *et al.* (1982) addressed the issue of whether improving the fatty acid balance in the diet of 30 normolipaemic men fed a typical Western diet (fat = 37 per cent en) would enhance their lipoprotein profiles, even after 3 months of comparison feeding. The hypothesis was tested by switching from a P/S ratio of 0.3 to a ratio of 1.0 that is, adopting the AHA balance in SFA: MUFA: PUFA of 1:1:1, even if not including the reduced fat intake recommended by the AHA (30 per cent en). The average entry TC was upper-normal (200 mg/dL) and the level of PUFA intake (5.6 per cent en) is very typical of the USA today. Balancing the P/S to 1.0 by shifting 6 per cent en from SFA to PUFA caused a significant decline in TC and LDL without depressing HDL. This resulted in significant improvement in the LDL/HDL ratio. Thus, similar to a subsequent trial (Weisweiler,1985) balancing the dietary fatty acid intake over a significant period of time is important, even with a somewhat elevated level of dietary fat (37 per cent en) in normolipaemic subjects, if one wants to lower LDL-C without depressing HDL-C.

Fatty Acid Valance is more Critical than Amount of Fat

Research conducted by Weisweiler *et al.* (1985) evaluated the importance of dietary fatty acid balance on the lipoprotein profile of 22 nuns (22–55 years, mostly postmenopausal) who had mildly elevated TC (224 mg/dL) at entry (Weisweiler,1985). They were fed three dietary fats for 6 weeks each: first, a high level, saturated fat (42 per cent en, P/S = 0.16); second, that same level of fat with a balanced fatty acid profile (P/S, 1.0), which was accomplished by decreasing SFA (exact profile not provided) and increasing PUFA. The third fat was close to AHA Step I (32 per cent en with a 1:1:1 balanced fatty acid profile) similar to the SFA: MUFA: PUFA balance in the second fat rotation. The results suggest that if one begins with a very unfavourable P/S ratio (0.16 because PUFA was too low) in a high-fat diet (42 per cent en), balancing the P/S ratio according to AHA guidelines improves the TC and LDL/ HDL ratio. The new balance between SFA and PUFA decreased LDL and increased HDL. However, dropping the fat intake to 32 per cent en with the AHA balance in place did not improve TC or the LDL/HDL ratio further. Therefore, in the 30–40 per cent en range, a balance (adequate PUFA, adequate SFA) seems more critical than total fat. The particular type of SFA was not detailed in this report. Other studies have found that decreasing 12:0 + 14:0 is more important than decreasing 16:0 + 18:0 if the best LDL/HDL ratio is to be achieved at a lower SFA intake (Hayes, 2002). Thus, the approximately equal balance of SFA: MUFA: PUFA (1:1.3:1) as recommended by NCEP and AHA is a very important basic consideration at any fat intake for maintaining the best LDL/HDL ratio.

Too High PUFA or Too Low Fat Depresses both LDL and HDL

Schaefer *et al.* (1981) have demonstrated what happens to LDL and HDL in normolipaemic (n = 11) and hyperlipaemic (n = 19) subjects fed a very saturated, high-fat diet (P/S 0.2, 40 per cent en) or a very polyunsaturated, high-fat diet (P/S 2.0, 40 per cent en). Subjects were compared to an almost fat-free saturated fat diet (P/S 0.2, 3 per cent en). The questions addressed were: (i) does the response to fat by normocholesterolaemic subjects differ from hypercholesterolaemic subjects? and (ii) does the lipoprotein profile benefit more from a high-PUFA approach to diet modification, or is it better to drastically reduce the fat intake with a high-carbohydrate diet without concern for the fatty acid balance?

The results showed that a high PUFA diet (P/S 2.0) decreased both LDL and HDL in all subjects. Removing essentially all the fat decreased both LDL and HDL still further. The LDL/HDL ratio did not improve with either tactic or the general response was similar for both groups of subjects (*i.e.*, normolipaemics and hyperlipaemics).

Therefore, although a very high-PUFA diet will decrease TC and LDL-C in both normolipaemic and hyperlipaemic subjects, the decline in HDL-C is also substantial. The LDL/ HDL ratio does not improve. As shown by Weisweiler *et al.* (1985) if one wishes to maintain HDL and lower LDL to improve the LDL/HDL ratio, a balance between SFA and PUFA is important. The same decrease in LDL-C obtained with very high PUFA can be achieved if the SFA: MUFA: PUFA ratio is balanced, but this balanced approach does not depress HDL.

Fatty Acid Balance is Especially Critical in Low-Fat Diets

The objective of a study by Nelson *et al.* (1995) was to determine whether the lipoprotein profile would be altered by decreasing fat intake from a high level (39 per cent en) to a low level (22 per cent en) if the P/S ratio was held constant and balanced at about 1.0.(Nelson, 1995). Most studies show that switching to a high carbohydrate, low-fat diet lowers TC, including both LDL and HDL. Nine normolipaemic men were evaluated in a metabolic ward, but the SFA: MUFA: PUFA ratios were not totally equal between the diets and were either 1.2:1.5:1.0 (high-fat) or 1.0:1.4:1.0 (low-fat), providing P/S ratios of 0.8 and 1.0, respectively.

The results revealed that the TC, LDL-C, and HDL-C were not significantly affected by the low-fat, high-carbohydrate diet, although they tended to be slightly lower than the high fat period. Therefore, a high-carbohydrate, low-fat diet does not necessarily mean that HDL will decline, provided that the balance between SFA and PUFA is maintained. However, the tendency toward slightly lower HDL at 22 per cent en suggests that the 30 per cent en AHA Step I level might better sustain HDL1 or that the MUFA intake was allowed to drift up too far relative to SFA and PUFA during the low fat intake. The LDL/HDL ratio might have been improved at low fat (and even at high fat) if the overall balance between SFA: MUFA: PUFA fatty acids had been maintained closer to 1:1:1 for both diets. The dietary P/S ratio is therefore important at any fat intake, but is an especially important determinant of the lipoprotein response at low fat intake (<20–25 per cent en) because it dictates the absolute availability of 18:2. At low fat intakes, a low P/S ratio (<0.5) greatly limits the 18:2 needed to meet metabolic requirements for normal lipoprotein metabolism, especially for lowering the LDL but also for raising HDL. In fact, a SFA: MUFA: PUFA ratio of 1:1.3:1 appears to be superior in such cases.

HDL can Increase when Total Fat Intake Decreases

It is generally agreed that replacing fat with carbohydrate is associated with a decline in TC, but unfortunately HDL-C also tends to decrease. One of the first studies to show that this does not necessarily occur if fatty acids are balanced was a subgroup from the Oslo study (Hjermann *et al.*, 1979). The original study revealed that reducing total fat, especially SAT and monounsaturated fat, and dietary cholesterol intakes to about 30 per cent en and <300 mg/day, respectively, greatly reduced TC and LDL-C without decreasing HDL-C in 18 000 men. To examine this more closely, 23 diet responders from the original cohort were compared with 23 controls who continued to eat the high-fat baseline diet. Both groups had identically elevated initial blood lipid values. The test group was instructed as to how dietary fat should be lowered from 44 per cent en to about 30 per cent en by focusing on removal of SAT. In the process, a good balance of SFA: MUFA: PUFA was achieved, decreasing from an imbalanced 18:19:7 to 8:12:8. The data demonstrate sharp declines in TC, LDL-C and triglycerides (200 vs 129 mg/dL) with an equally sharp increase in HDL-C (from 42 to 50 mg/dL). Thus, removing SFA and MUFA from a high-fat diet decreased LDL-C sharply, but also increased HDL-C when the P/S ratio was rebalanced to 1.0 and the total balance in SFA: MUFA: PUFA approximated 1:1.3:1.

A High-Mono Diet is not as Favourable as a Low-Mono Diet

The original AHA recommendation called for an even balance between SFA: MUFA: PUFA at 30 per cent en from fat. Recently, AHA has recommended a 50 per cent increase in MUFA at the expense of SFA and PUFA. However, a human study on eight normolipaemic men demonstrated the potential downside of exaggerating the MUFA: PUFA ratio too much (Chang and Huang, 1990). The men were fed either 0.5 or 3.0 MUFA: PUFA ratios in two diets in which the P/S ratio was constant at 1.0. The high-MUFA diet produced a TC that was identical to the Low-MUFA diet, but LDL-C was elevated ($P < 0.05$) when intake of SFA and PUFA got too low. HDL was also lower, so that the LDL/HDL ratio was significantly higher. In addition, the high-MUFA diet induced a 20 per cent rise in triglycerides. Thus, the high-MUFA diet was inferior to the low- MUFA intake, indicating that a proper balance in SFA: MUFA: PUFA is important for generating the best LDL/HDL ratio. Whereas keeping the P/S ratio at around 1.0 may be the most critical relationship, it would appear that MUFA should not exceed 1.5 times the relative abundance of PUFA and SFA.

A High-Mono Diet is Inferior to a Balanced SFA : MUFA : PUFA Ratio

The objective of a study in cynomolgus monkeys was to explore the relative importance of the SFA: MUFA: PUFA balance in regulating TC and the LDL/HDL ratio when consuming 30 per cent en and less than 300 mg/day cholesterol (equivalent to human AHA Step I diets) (Hayes and Pronczuk, unpubl. data, 1999). Similar to the human results just cited (Chang and Huang, 1990) and compared to an American fat blend derived from butter and canola oil, an unfavourable imbalance developed in the LDL/ HDL ratio when dietary SFA and PUFA were about equal but too low relative to MUFA. Specifically, AHA Step 1 diets (diets 1X and 1H), with P/S ratios close to 1.0, represented blends of four and three oils, respectively. The third test diet was olive oil alone with a fairly favourable P/S ratio of 0.75. The TC response and the LDL/HDL ratio were much improved when the relative intakes of SFA: MUFA: PUFA were fully balanced by either of the Step 1 diets, that is, the specific oil blend did not make a difference. Therefore, while the dietary P/S ratio is a rough indicator of how a fat will affect the plasma LDL/HDL ratio, it would appear that an approximate balance of SFA: MUFA: PUFA is also critical, at least at a 30 per cent en fat intake.

Progressive Removal of SFA Lowers both LDL-C and HDL-C

This study examined the effect of a two-step selective removal of SFA (4.5 per cent en each step) from a diet initially containing 34 per cent en as fat, while keeping MUFA and PUFA constant (Mustad *et al.*, 1997). Even though the P/S ratio increased to 1.0 in the process, MUFA intake was twice that of the other two fatty acid classes when the low-fat diet (providing 25 per cent en as fat) was achieved. LDL-C was decreased to the extent of 12 per cent when 9 per cent en as SFA was decreased, but at the same time, HDL-C was also depressed proportionally. Therefore, this study concluded that indiscriminate removal of SFAs (individual SFA not identified) and their replacement by MUFA lowers total cholesterol without improving the LDL-C/ HDL-C ratio, at least when the MUFA intake substantially exceeds that of SFA or PUFA.

SFA are Best Represented by 16 : 0 and 18 : 0 Fatty Acids

When reducing dietary SFA, does it matter which SFA are removed? The study conducted by Pronczuk (1999) had revealed that removal of fats containing 12:0 + 14:0 (leaving 16:0 + 18:0-rich fats) leads to a greater reduction in TC and LDL-C and results in an improved LDL/HDL ratio. This is because 12:0 + 14:0-rich fats tend to increase LDL. Thus, when balancing the SFA: MUFA: PUFA ratio in a fat blend, it is preferable to utilise a 16:0 + 18:0-rich fat as the SFA source rather than one rich in 12:0 + 14:0, in terms of generating the best LDL/ HDL ratio (Hayes, 2002).

Thus, dietary fat composition does, indeed, have a major impact on the plasma lipid profile. However, beyond the typical call for a better balance between SFA and PUFA, it is apparent that MUFA figures in the final outcome if one attempts to induce the best plasma LDL/HDL profile in humans. According to Hayes (2002), between dietary fat intakes of 20–40 per cent en, the ideal balance would seem to approximate 1:1.3:1 for SFA: MUFA: PUFA.

III. Recommendation by WHO/ other Heart Associations

As per recommended dietary guidelines of WHO/ Japanese Heart Association/ American Heart Association the ideal ratio of SFA: MUFA: PUFA should be 1:1.5:1.

The World Health Organization (WHO) recommends polyunsaturated fatty acid (PUFA)/saturated fatty acids (SFA) ratio of 0.8 to 1.0 and linoleic acid (Omega6) alpha linolenic acid (Omega3) ratio of 5-10 in the diet. Earlier, the American Heart Association used to recommend use of oils having an equal proportion of saturated, monounsaturated and polyunsaturated fats in the past. The most recent recommendations according to the National Research Council, Washington DC are 10 per cent saturates, 12 to 13 per cent for monounsaturates, not more than 7 to 8 per cent for polyunsaturates. Japan's Ministry of Health and Welfare suggests fatty acid ratio of saturated/monounsaturated/ polyunsaturated as 1:1.5:1 and a 4:1 ratio of omega 6 to omega 3 fatty acids.

The WHO Diet Model

In western populations during the 1970s and 1980s, the consumption of dietary fats has been reported in the high range of 36-43 per cent kcal (Rizek *et al.*, 1983; James, 1988). WHO dietary guidelines for CHD prevention (WHO, 1986; WHO, 1990), contained somewhat similar dietary messages as the AHA prudent diet with respect to total fat, SEA and cholesterol intakes, although the 1:1:1 ratio of the three major families of fatty acids implied in the AHA prudent diet nor any PUFA/SFA ratio was mentioned, in order to avoid any promotion of a progressive Increase in the consumption of PUFA in some populations. WHO has also indicated in its 1990 report that the 30 per cent kcal total fat should be regarded as an Interim goal for nations with high fat intakes, and that further benefits would be expected by reducing fat intake towards the lower limit of 15 per cent of total energy.

Thus, both WHO and AHA then recommended 30 per cent kcal total fat as a realistic dietary target, with an intermediate goal of 30-35 per cent kcal from fat, to address the health problems associated with high total fat intakes in these communities (AHA, 1988; James 1988, WHO, 1990; James and Ralph, 1992). In addition, WHO also recommended lower and upper limits for population average Intakes for several nutrients including total fat, SFA, PUFA and cholesterol etc (1990). Of interest, the initial 1986 WHO upper limit for dietary PUFA of 10 per cent kcal was reduced to 7 per cent kcal in 1990 following reports of adverse effects associated with high intakes of PUFA (Shepherd *et al.*, 1978).

In an October, 1993 Up-date of Fats and Oils in Human Nutrition by a WHO Expert Group in Rome, the above WHO diet model remained essentially unchanged. However, according to WHO (1993), there were two issues that warranted attention.

One was the statement that "In non-sedentary populations a range of fat intake from 15 to about 35 per cent of dietary energy is compatible with good health as long as the supply of essential fatty acids, fat soluble vitamins and other essential nutrients is adequate, and the saturated fatty acids provide less than 10 per cent of energy."

In 1993, however, a WHO Expert Committee advocated instead 35 per cent kcal total fat as the upper limit for "active individuals who were in energy balance" and

Chronology of FAO Expert Consultations on Fats and Oils

- ☆ The first expert consultation on Fats and Oils in Human Nutrition was held in 1977.
- ☆ A second expert consultation on the subject was held in 1993, with the subsequent report of the consultation being published in 1994.
- ☆ There have been many developments in the field in the intervening fourteen years, and the 1994 report and recommendations need to be critically reviewed and updated where necessary.
- ☆ The main purpose of the expert consultation will be to review the scientific data in order to update human nutrient intake values for fats and fatty acids, and to provide internationally valid recommendations.
- ☆ FAO and WHO held an expert consultation on fats and fatty acids in human nutrition in the last quarter of 2008. The specific objectives of the expert consultation were to:
- ☆ Review the scientific evidence to determine, based on a set of agreed-upon criteria, nutrient requirements for total fat and fatty acids for different life stages (infants, children, adolescents, adults, the elderly, pregnancy and lactation).
- ☆ Assess the risk to adequate growth, development and maintenance of health from insufficient intake of total fat and fatty acids.
- ☆ Assess the risks and health effects of excessive intakes of fat and fatty acids, in particular, total fat, saturated fatty acids and trans fatty acids.
- ☆ Assess the risks and benefits associated with particular aspects of dietary fat and provide recommendations based on a review of this body of scientific evidence.

whose intake of EFA and other nutrients was adequate, and the level of SFA did not exceed 10 per cent kcal. No mention was made of the ultimate goal of 20-30 per cent kcal dietary fat contained in the earlier WHO recommendations (WHO, 1986 and 1990). The previous minimum fat intake of 15 per cent kcal was retained but the general upper limit of 30 per cent kcal total fat was then recommended instead for "sedentary individuals". It appeared then that there was a discrepant shift towards higher upper limits for total fat intake advocated by the 1993 WHO Expert Committee. The introduction of upper limits for total fat according to two activity levels of individuals, although apparently technically sound, tended to complicate the recommendations.

The most recently convened expert meeting was the Joint FAO and WHO Expert Consultation on Fats and Fatty Acids in Human Nutrition, held in Geneva, Switzerland, from Nov. 10-14, 2008 and its recommendations are given as under:

Recommendations of FAO/WHO in 2008

An overview of recommendations given by the FAO/WHO Expert Consultation (2008) for fat and fatty acids has been given in Table 3 (Kornsteiner, E. M. 2009). The FAO/WHO Expert Consultation (2008) came to the following agreements:

- ☆ Individual SFA lauric (C12:0), myristic (C14:0), palmitic acid (C16:0), and stearic acid (C18:0) have different effects on plasma cholesterol levels. Lauric, myristic, and palmitic acids increase LDL-cholesterol levels compared with stearic acid.
- ☆ There is convincing evidence that substituting SFAs C12:0– C16:0 with PUFAs reduces LDL-cholesterol levels and the TC/ HDL-cholesterol ratio. This effect can also be observed, but to a lesser extent, by substituting these SFAs with MUFAs.
- ☆ There is convincing evidence that exchanging SFAs (C12:0– C16:0) with mainly refined carbohydrates reduces LDL and HDL cholesterol levels, but has no effect on the TC/HDL-cholesterol ratio.
- ☆ There is convincing evidence that substituting (C12:0-C16:0) with trans fatty acids decrease HDL-cholesterol levels and increases the TC/HDL-cholesterol ratio.
- ☆ Based on the results of epidemiological studies and trials on CHD (events and death) it was also agreed that:
- ☆ There is convincing evidence that substituting SFAs with PUFAs reduces the risk of CHD.
- ☆ There is probable evidence that substituting SFAs with mainly refined carbohydrates does not impair the risk of CHD, but may support the development of metabolic syndrome.
- ☆ There is insufficient evidence that substituting SFAs with mainly whole grain carbohydrates does not impair the risk of CHD.

A. FAO/WHO Recommendations for SFAs

- ☆ The intake of SFA should not exceed a MAL of 10 per cent E to keep cholesterol levels in a normal range and to reduce the risk of CHD.

B. Dietary Recommendations for MUFAs

The FAO/WHO Expert Consultation (2008) came to the following agreements:

- ☆ There is convincing evidence that substituting carbohydrates with MUFAs raises HDL-cholesterol levels.
- ☆ There is possible evidence that substituting carbohydrates with MUFAs improves insulin sensitivity.
- ☆ There is convincing evidence that substituting SFAs (C12:0-C16:0) with MUFAs lowers LDL-cholesterol levels and the TC/HDL-cholesterol ratio.

Table 16.2: Dietary Recommendations for Fat and Fatty Acid Intake.

Total fat, %E	AMDR	20–35	con[1]; pro[2]; ins[3]
	MAL	35	
	MIL	15	
SFAs, %E	MAL	10	con[4–7]; pro[8,9]; ins[10]
MUFAs, %E	AMDR	by difference[a,b]	con[4,11]; pos[12]
Total PUFAs, %E	AMDR (LA + ALA + EPA + DHA)	6–11	con[4,7]
	MAL11	pos[13]	
	MIL (to prevent deficiency)	3	con[14]; pos[15]
	MIL (to prevent chronic diseases)	6	
n–6 PUFAs, %E	AMDR (LA)	2.5–9	con[4,7]; pos[15]
Average LA requirement	2		
Individual LA level	2.5	con[14]; pos[15]	
n–3 PUFAs	AMDR (n–3c), per cent E	0.5–2	con[14]; pos[15]
	Minimum requirement (ALA), %E	0.5	
	AMDR (EPA + DHA), g/day	0.250–2[d]	
	MAL[e], g/day	3	con[16]; pro[17],[18]; pos[19]; ins[20]
TFAs, per cent E	UL (from ruminants and industrially produced sources)		

a Total fat [per cent E] – SFAs [per cent E] – PUFAs [per cent E] – TFAs [per cent E]; b can amount up to 15–20 per cent E; c ALA + n–3 long-chain PUFAs; d for secondary prevention; e including supplements.

ALA = -Linolenic acid; AMDR = acceptable macronutrient distribution range; con = convincing; DHA = docosahexaenoic acid; E = energy; EPA = eicosapentaenoic acid; ins = insufficient; LA = linoleic acid; MAL = maximum level; MIL = minimum level; MUFAs = monounsaturated fatty acids; PUFAs = polyunsatura- ted fatty acids; pos = possible; pro = probable; SFAs = saturated fatty acids; TFAs = trans fatty acids; UL = upper level.

1 con: Energy balance, dietary patterns, and optimal nutrient intakes are important for healthy body weight, apart from macro- nutrient distribution expressed in per cent E.

2 pro: No relation with coronary heart disease (CHD) events, fatal CHD.

3 ins: Association between total fat intake and body weight.

4 con: Substituting SFAs (C12:0–C16:0) with PUFAs and MUFAs reduces LDL-cholesterol levels and the TC/HDL cholesterol ratio.

5 con: Substituting SFAs (C12:0–C16:0) with mainly refined carbohydrates reduces LDL- and HDL-cholesterol levels, but has no effect on the TC/HDL-cholesterol ratio.

6 con: Substituting SFAs (C12:0–C16:0) with TFAs decreases HDL-cholesterol levels and increases the TC/HDL-cholesterol ratio.

7 con: f Risk of CHD events when PUFAs replace SFAs.

Contd...

Table 16.2–*Contd...*

8 pro: Increased SFA intake results in increased weight.

9 pro: Substituting SFAs with mainly refined carbohydrates does not impair the risk of CHD, but may support the development of metabolic syndrome.

1 con6,21, pro22

10 ins: Substituting SFAs with mainly whole grain carbohydrates does not impair the risk of CHD.

11 con: Substituting carbohydrates with MUFAs raises HDL-cholesterol levels.

12 pos: Substituting carbohydrates with MUFAs improves insulin sensitivity.

13 pos: d Lipid peroxidation with high consumption levels, especially when tocopherol intake is low.

14 con: Essential.

15 pos: Specific minimum required to prevent deficiency.

16 con: Strong inverse relationship is present between n–3

LCPUFAs or fish intake and risk of CHD.

17 pro: Fish intake probably decreases colorectal cancer risk.

18 pro: n–3 LCPUFAs and fish oil have probable benefits for depression.

19 pos: n–3 LCPUFAs and fish oil have possible benefits for bi- polar disorder, cognitive decline, aggression, hostility, anti-social behavior and age-related maculopathy.

20 ins: n–3 LCPUFAs and fish oil have insufficient benefits for

Alzheimer's disease, schizophrenia, and Huntington's disease.

21 con: d Risk of CHD events.

22 pro: d Risk of fatal CHD and sudden cardiac death

C. FAO/WHO Dietary Recommendations for MUFAs

MUFA intake is calculated by: total fat intake (MIL 15 per cent E, MAL 35 per cent E) minus SFAs (MAL 10 per cent E) minus PUFAs (MIL 3 per cent E; MAL 11 per cent E) minus TFAs (UL 1 per cent E). For this reason, MUFA intake can show a wide range depending on the total fat intake and dietary fatty acid pattern.

D. Dietary Recommendations for PUFAs

The FAO/WHO Expert Consultation (2008) considered that there was convincing evidence showing that substituting SFAs with PUFAs reduces the risk of CHD.

Dietary Recommendations for n-6 and n-3Fatty Acids

FAO/WHO Dietary Recommendation for LA Intake

It is recognized that only new data on humans are available for the establishment of the LA requirement, which has the effect that most authorities do not set an average LA requirement. However, animal and human studies have demonstrated that the prevention of deficiency signs (*e.g.* in rats reduced growth, scaliness of skin, necrotic tail) occurs by an estimated daily requirement of 1-2 per cent LA of total energy. Therefore, an average LA requirement of 2 per cent E and an individual LA level of 2.5 per cent E are given. On the one hand, this requirement seems to be very low but on the other hand, the requirement of a young healthy adult is around 6.5 g LA/day [Deutsche Gesellschaft für Ernährung, 2000] corresponding to about 2 per cent E of LA which can be very close to the intake in a normal diet (6.8g/day French women) (Burdge and Calder, 2005). Under the condition that the maximum intake levels of PUFAs (MAL 11 per cent E) and n-3 fatty acids (MAL 2 per cent E) are taken into consideration, the resulting acceptable range for n-6 fatty acids (LA) can range between 2.5 and 9 per cent E. The lower value corresponds to the prevention of deficiency symptoms, whereas the higher value can be part of a healthy heart diet by lowering LDL and TC levels, and therefore, the risk of CHD.

FAO/WHO Dietary Recommendations for AA Intake

AA is not essential for a healthy person, who gets enough LA (12.5 per cent E) from their normal diet.

FAO/WHO Dietary Recommendation for N-3 Fatty Acid Intake

It was estimated that 0.5-0.6 per cent E ALA per day prevents deficiency symptoms. The n-3 fatty acid intake can range between 0.5-0.6 per cent E. The minimum dietary requirement of ALA for adults to avoid deficiency symptoms is 0.5 per cent E, whereas the higher value 2 per cent E (ALA) plus n-3 LCPUFAs, EPA and DHA (AMDR 250-2000 mg) can be part of a healthy heart diet probably preventing CHD and possibly some cancers and degenerative diseases of ageing. The MAL for n-3 LCPUFA is by 3g/day, because high supplement intakes of n-3 LCPUFAs have been demonstrated to reduce cytokine production and increase lipid peroxidation. High supplement intakes of n-3 LCPUFAs (13g/day) have been demonstrated to reduce cytokine production (Meydani, 2000; Vedin *et al.*, 2008; Sanders, 2009), whereas the requirement for antioxidants is increased (Elmadfa and Scwalbe, 1989).

Dietary Recommendations for Trans Fatty Acids Intake

The Food and Drug Administration estimated the average adult's daily ruminant trans fatty acid intake in the USA, which is about 1.5g for men and 0.9 g for women. The average intake of both men and women is about 1.2 g, which correspond to 0.5 per cent E. If similar average intake values from industrially hydrogenated fat could be anticipated, then the trans fatty acid intake from all sources should be limited to 1 per cent E.

Food-Based Dietary Guidelines

Moderate dietary fat intake can increase the risk of heart diseases in a population with a low fat intake (20 per cent E) [Suh *et al.*, 2001]. Therefore, promoting an acceptable macronutrient range of dietary fat between 20 and 35 per cent E may not be advisable for all population groups and should be done with caution, especially when no signs of deficiency are obvious. Therefore, the minimum fat intake should be greater than 15 per cent E, while paying attention to an adequate intake of essential fatty acids. The absorption of fat-soluble vitamins can also be achieved with very low amounts of fat (*e.g.* 12 per cent E for carotenoids) [Ribaya-Mercado *et al.*, 2007]. The total fat intake can range between 20 and 35 per cent E with focus on the energy balance and diet quality. Higher fat intakes are associated with raised saturated fat, cholesterol, and total energy intake. The intake of SFA should be below 10 per cent E, whereas trans fatty acids should be 1 per cent E to balance cholesterol levels in a normal range [Department of Health and Human Services, 2005; Deutsche Ge- sellschaft für Ernährung, 2006].

Therefore, lean cuts of meat and poultry should be preferred in comparison to sausages rich in fat (*e.g.* salami), crumbed and fried fish, and meats. These animal products can provide significant amounts of SFA. They can be part of a balanced diet, but only in small amounts. The intake of lean meat and the removal of visible fat can help to limit total fat intake as well as SFA and cholesterol intake [National Health and Medical Research Council, 2003].

Conversely, fatty fishes, which are rich in the longer chain derivates of n–3 fatty acids, are recommended, especially for people who are at risk of CHD. Fish, but especially fatty fish like sardines, salmon, tuna, herring, and mackerel, are part of a healthy diet and are recommended in least 2 meals per week [National Health and Medical Research Council, 2003].

The majority of the fat should come from plant oils, which are excellent sources of PUFAs and MUFAs. Good sources of the essential n–6 PUFAs (LA) are vegetable oils, including soybean oil, corn oil, sesame oil, sunflower oil, groundnut oil, rice bran oil, cottonseed oil and safflower oil, whereas soybean oil, rapeseed oil, mustard oil, walnut oil, and flaxseed oil are rich in the n–3 PUFAs (ALA). n–3 LCPUFAs (EPA and DHA) are available from fish. Vegetable oils that are rich in MUFAs include canola, olive, sunflower (product of new breeding techniques or by blending PUFA-rich oils with MUFA-rich ones to end up with high oleic oil), and nuts oils [Kornsteiner *et al.*, 2006; Boskou and Elmadfa, 2009, in press; Farhoosh *et al.*, 2009].

IV. The AHA Prudent Diet'

In the early 1980s, the AHA recommended the prudent diet to lower plasma cholesterol levels in the general American population (Poleman and Peckenpaugh, 1991), with the following main dietary messages:

- reduce total fat to <30 per cent kcal
- reduce cholesterol intake to <300 mg per day
- limit SFA to <10 per cent kcal
- dietary fat composed of approximately equal parts of saturated, monounsaturated and polyunsaturated fat

It must be emphasized that these dietary recommendations were made for a general population that was consuming high amounts of total fat (average about 42 per cent kcal) and cholesterol (450 mg/head daily) (Gallo, 1983). The 30 per cent kcal cut-off selected was probably considered a realistic dietary goal for the general American population at the time.

The 1SFA: 1MUFA: 1PUFA ratio recommended by AHA appeared sound initially, since it suited the concept of a balance of dietary fatty acids and also fitted nicely with the upper limit of 30 per cent kcal for total fat, and a maximum of 10 per cent kcal for each of the SEA, MUFA and PUFA (Step I diet). Now the amount of total fat intake and proportions of various fatty acids have been revised and updated.

V. Recommendation of Therapeutic Lifestyle Changes (TLC) Diet by AHA

The American Heart Association (AHA) no longer uses the terms "Step I" and "Step II" in reference to heart -healthy diets. These terms, however, still appear in some older materials and journal articles. In June, 2006, AHA released new Dietary Recommendations. The Step I diet restricted total fat to no more than 30 percent of total calories, saturated fat to no more than 10 percent of total calories, and cholesterol to less than 300 mg/day. It was intended as the starting point for patients who had high cholesterol levels. The Step II diet goals were lower for saturated fat (less than 7 percent) and cholesterol (less than 200 mg/day). They were intended for people already at the Step I goals or for patients with a high-risk cholesterol level (240 mg/dL or higher) or who had had a heart attack.

TLC Diet and Fat Recommendations

The American Heart Association now endorses "Therapeutic Lifestyle Changes (TLC)" diet according to which the recommended intake of nutrients especially fat should be as given as reported in the Table 16.3.

TLC diet recommends the following amounts of MUFA, PUFA, SFA and total fat in the daily diet:

MUFA

The TLC diet recommends the substitution of MUFA fat for saturated fats at an intake level of up to 20 per cent of total energy intake because MUFA fats lower LDL cholesterol levels relative to saturated fats without decreasing HDL cholesterol or TG levels. It is recommended that plant oils and nuts be used because they are the best sources of MUFA fats.

PUFA Fats

PUFA fats, in particular linoleic acid, reduce LDL cholesterol levels when used instead of saturated fats. However, they can also bring about small reductions in HDL cholesterol when compared side by side with MUFA fats. The TLC Diet recommends liquid vegetable oils, semi liquid margarines, and other margarines low in trans fatty acids be used because they are the best sources of PUFA fats, intakes can range up to 10 per cent of total energy intake.

Total Fat

In view of the fact that only saturated fats and trans fatty acids increase LDL cholesterol levels, serum levels of LDL cholesterol are unrelated to total fat intake per se. For that reason, the ATP III suggests it is not crucial to limit total fat intake for the

Table 16.3: Recommended Nutrient Intake in TLC Diet

Nutrient	*Recommended Intake as Per cent of Total Calories*
Total Fat[1]	25-35 per cent
Saturated fat	Less than 7 per cent
Polyunsaturated fat	Up to 10 per cent
Monounsaturated fat	Up to 20 per cent
Carbohydrate[2]	50-60 per cent of total calories
Protein	Approx. 15 per cent
Cholesterol[3]	Less than 200mg/day
Total calories	Balance energy intake and expenditure to maintain desirable body weight and prevent weight gain

1. The 25–35 per cent fat recommendation allows for increased intake of unsaturated fat in place of carbohydrates in people with the metabolic syndrome or diabetes.
2. When saturated fats are replaced with carbohydrates, LDL cholesterol levels are reduced. On the other hand, very high intakes of CHOs (60 per cent total energy intake) are associated with a reduction in HDL cholesterol and an increase in serum TG. Increasing soluble fibre intake can sometime reduce these responses. On an average, increasing soluble fibre to 5-10g/day is accompanied by an approx. 5 per cent reduction in cholesterol.
3. Carbohydrate should come mainly from foods rich in complex carbohydrates. These include grains (especially whole grains), fruits and vegetables.
4. Options include adding 10–25 grams of viscous (soluble) fiber; 2 g/day of plant-derived sterols or stanols. Soy protein may be used as a replacement for some animal products.
5. Daily energy expenditure should include at least moderate physical activity (contributing about 200 Kcal a day).

The essential components of TLC diet are:

Component	*Recommendation*
LDL Raising nutrients	
Saturated fats*	Less than 7 per cent of total calories
Dietary Cholesterol	Less than 200mg/day
Therapeutic options for LDL-lowering	
Plant stanois/sterols	2g/day
Increased viscous (soluble) fibre	10-25g/day
Total calories(energy)	Adjust total calorie intake to maintain desirable body weight/prevent weight gain
Physical activity	Include enough moderate exercise to expand at least 200 kcal per day

* Trans fatty acids also raise LDL and should be kept at a low intake.

specific goal of reducing LDL cholesterol levels, provided saturated fats are decreased to goal levels.

People who have high cholesterol because they eat too many fatty foods may be able to lower their cholesterol 10 per cent to 20 per cent with diet changes alone, while others may only achieve a 5 per cent to 8 per cent reduction. Those who are most successful using diet changes to lower their cholesterol are those who lose excess weight. Diet changes are usually the first step in lowering cholesterol before medicines are added.

The Therapeutic Lifestyle Changes (TLC) diet is recommended by the National Cholesterol Education Programme of the U.S. National Institutes of Health. The diet's main focus is to reduce the amount of saturated fat we eat because it elevates the blood cholesterol. One can reduce the saturated fat in the diet by limiting the amount of meat and milk products. Choose low-fat products from those food groups instead. Replace most of the animal fat in the diet with unsaturated fat, especially monounsaturated oils, such as olive, canola, or peanut. Monounsaturated fat lowers LDL ("bad") cholesterol if it is substituted for saturated fat and keeps HDL ("good") cholesterol up.

Other Recommendations

The TLC diet also includes recommendations on soluble fiber and phytosterol, both of which are known to lower cholesterol levels. Soluble, or viscous, fiber includes oatmeal, psyllium, pectin, and bran. Phytosterols, also known for their ability to lower cholesterol. Current recommendations for soluble fiber consumption are 10 to 25 grams daily, whereas two grams a day of phytosterol intake is recommended. Additionally, the TLC diet recommends that salt intake be limited to 2400 milligrams a day.

The TLC diet might seem complicated because of the many guidelines given for each main nutrient. However, it basically encourages eating a heart-healthy, balanced diet and lowering cholesterol through decreased fat intake and increased consumption of fiber.

Chapter 17

Trends in Production and Consumption Patterns of Oilseeds, Oils and Fats: World Scenario

Vegetable oils, besides being a cooking and frying medium also serve as an important source of energy in the daily diet of both rural and urban inhabitants. These oils are obtained from crops commonly designated as oilseeds. Oilseed crops are grown primarily for the oil contained in the seeds. The oil content of oilseed crops ranges from about 20 per cent for soybeans to over 40 per cent for sunflowers and rapeseed (canola). The major world sources of edible seed oils are soybeans, sunflowers, rapeseed, cotton and peanuts. Seed oils from flax (linseed) and castor beans are used for industrial purposes.

The demand for vegetable oils has increased rapidly in the past decade, catapulted by a combination of factors, including: i) increasing demand sparked off by higher consumption for edible oils, particularly in emerging countries such China and India caused by, among other things, population growth, improving living standards and changing diets; ii) the development of the biofuels industry (and more specifically biodiesel) around the world, particularly in the EU, USA, Brazil, Argentina, China and India, iii) price increases which have been due to varying factors *e.g.*

increase in oil prices, low stock worldwide, droughts, and speculation, iv) changing weather patterns which can have major geographical impacts and can be, potentially, quite large.

There are two major markets for vegetable oils: i) food which represents over 80 per cent, and ii) industrial uses including biodiesel. The main driver for expansion is still the growing demand for edible oils for the food market, although an important part of this demand comes from the biodiesel sector.

Trends in Area, Production and Yield of Oilseeds

In recent decades, the oilcrops sector has been one of the most vibrant in world agriculture. Over the past 20 years the sector grew at 4.3 percent per annum compared with an average of 2.3 percent per annum for all agriculture. The major driving force has been the growth of food consumption in developing countries, mostly in the form of vegetable oil but also direct consumption of soybeans, groundnuts, etc., as well as in the form of derived products other than oil. Food demand in developing countries has accounted for around 40 percent of the increases in world output during the last two decades (with output measured in oil content equivalent). China, India and a few other countries represent the bulk of this increase. In addition, the strong growth in demand for protein products for animal feed has been a major supporting factor in the buoyancy of the oil crops sector.

The rapid growth of the oil crops sector illustrates the synergy of the two fastest rising components of food demand: demand for oils favouring all oil crops with the potential for rapid production expansion (*e.g.* oil-palm), and that for livestock products favouring oil crops with high protein oil meals for feed (*e.g.* soybeans). In addition, support policies of the European Union (EU) also helped shift world production of oilseeds in favour of rapeseed and sunowerseed.

Overall, four oil crops (oil-palm, soybeans, rapeseed and sunowerseed) now account for 75 percent of world production. For several countries, including some major producers, these fast expanding oil crops were once hardly cultivated at all, or only in insignicant amounts.

- ☆ 168 million tonnes of oilseeds and oil bearing crops were gathered in 2010.
- ☆ This volume represents a signicant increase compared to the level two decades ago.
- ☆ Soybeans, rapeseed and sunflower are the major oil crops in temperate zones, while palm oil fruit is the major oil bearing crop in the tropics, increasingly cultivated in Southeast Asia.

Looking at the previous years' major world oilseed production, it indicates that there is an, increasing trend in the area, production and yield of oilseed crops *viz.*, groundnut, soybean, rapeseed and mustard, sesame, sunflower, linseed, safflower and castor worldwide when comparing their figures of 1986 to 2005. During 2006, area in fact decreased slightly under oilseed crops, however there was a slight increase in production. While there has been significant growth between 2002-03 and 2004-05 from 330.26 million tonnes to 381.29 million tonnes, the next two years have not

Table 17.1: World Major Oilseeds Production (2002-2012)

Oilseeds	*2002-03*	*2003-04*	*2004-05*	*2005-06*	*2006-07*	*2007-08*	*2008-09*	*2009-10*	*2010-11 Estimated*	*2011-12 Forecast*	*Change 2011-12 Over 2010-11 (per cent)*
											(In Million Tonnes)
Soybean	197.03	186.77	215.95	218.04	226.78	220.0	211.8	259.7	265.3	240.0	-9.5
Rapeseed	32.91	39.43	46.14	48.55	46.78	48.6	58.4	61.4	60.9	60.6	-0.5
Groundnut	30.83	32.78	33.39	33.71	31.59	35.4	35.4	34.9	36.9	36.4	-1.6
Sunflower	23.93	26.76	25.30	29.77	30.54	29.1	34.2	32.8	33.2	38.0	14.5
Palm Kernel	7.76	8.43	9.51	9.98	10.85	11.2	11.6	11.7	12.6	13.0	3.8
Cottonseed	32.67	35.60	45.40	42.51	43.77	44.1	41.3	40.4	43.5	46.6	7.1
Copra	5.12	5.38	5.59	5.79	5.19	5.0	5.2	5.8	4.9	5.6	15.2
Total	330.26	335.16	381.29	388.33	395.50	393.4	397.9	446.3	457.3	440.2	-3.7

Source: USDA.

Note: The split years bring together northern hemisphere annual crops harvested in the latter part of the first year shown, with southern hemisphere annual crops harvested in the early part of the second year shown. For tree crops, which are produced throughout the year, calendar year production for the second year shown is used.

Oilseed Sector 2011-12

☆ Area under oilseed cultivation	26-27 Million hectares
☆ Average yield	1100 Kgs
☆ Output of 9 cultivated oilseeds	30.1 Million tonnes
☆ Output of Cottonseed and Copra	11.0 Million tonnes
Total 41.1 Million hectare	
☆ Production of vegetable oils	8.12 Million tonnes
☆ Demand of veg. oils (Edible)	16.7 Million tonnes
☆ Import of Veg.oil 2011-12 (Nov-Oct) (Edible)	9.4 Million tonnes

E)

☆ Per capita consumption (2011) 13.5 Kg

☆ Per capita consumption is rising by 3 to 4 per cent per annum.

seen such a growth. Soybean and cottonseed were major contributors to the growth between 2002-03 and 2004-05 while in 2011-12, the major contributors are soybean and rapeseed (Table 17.1, Figure 17.1). Country-wise area and production under major oilseeds in the world are given in Table 17. 2.

In recent years, oilseeds production has rapidly expanded under the yield growth and demand characteristics linked to the more income elastic-products (Figure 17.2). Production of the five major oilseeds crops rose from 159.4 million hectares (m ha) in 1996 to peak at 198.7 m ha in 2006 before declining to 192.8 m ha in 2007. According

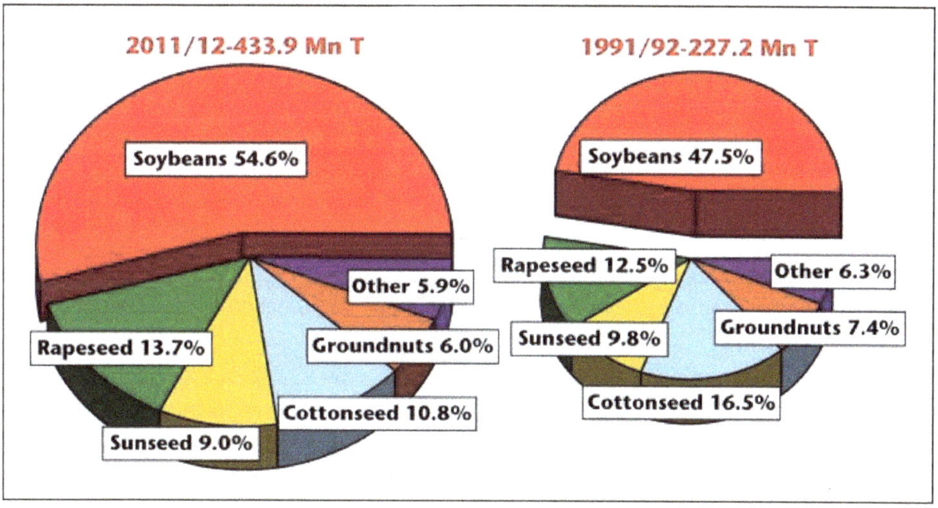

Figure 17.1: World Production (year 2011/12 vs 1991/92) of 10 Oilseeds (Soybeans, cotton seed, rapeseed, sunflower seed, groundnuts (shelled), sesame seed, palmkernels, copra, linseed and castor seed)

Table 17.2: World Major Oilseeds, Area, Yield and Production

Coountry	Area (Million Hectares)	Yield (MT/Hect)	Production (Million Tonnes)
United States	36.99	2.62	97.03
Brazil	22.17	2.63	58.33
Argentina	18.60	2.52	46.79
Paraguay	2.36	2.14	5.04
Bolivia	1.15	2.02	2.32
Uruguay	0.46	1.74	0.79
China	27.55	2.05	56.55
India	32.50	0.92	29.80
Pakistan	3.83	1.30	4.99
Russian Federation	6.92	1.18	8.15
Ukraine	4.90	1.32	6.45
Uzbekistan	1.42	1.69	2.40
Canada	6.60	1.93	12.75
France	2.02	2.76	5.59
Germany	1.46	3.67	5.37
United Kingdom	0.58	3.30	1.90
Czech Republic	0.35	2.81	0.99
Hungary	0.71	2.33	1.65
Poland	0.60	2.67	1.60
Italy	0.33	2.73	0.90
Australia	0.99	1.12	1.11
Turkey	1.25	1.73	2.17
Nigeria	2.04	1.04	2.11
South Africa	0.67	1.47	0.98
Indonesia	1.41	1.46	2.06
Romania	1.29	1.46	1.88
Others	19.55	1.01	19.78
Total World	198.69	1.91	379.46

Major Oilseeds: Soybean, Sunflower, Rapeseed, Cottonseed and Groundnut

to FAO, increase in oilseed production in 2007-08 was less than 2 per cent over the previous year. Production figures reached 395.2 million metric tons in 2009, with three major producers *i.e.* United States, Brazil and China which accounted for 64 per cent of this world production.

Global oilseed production remained virtually unchanged in 2010. Production increased in the United States, Canada, India, Ukraine, Indonesia, Brazil, Argentina,

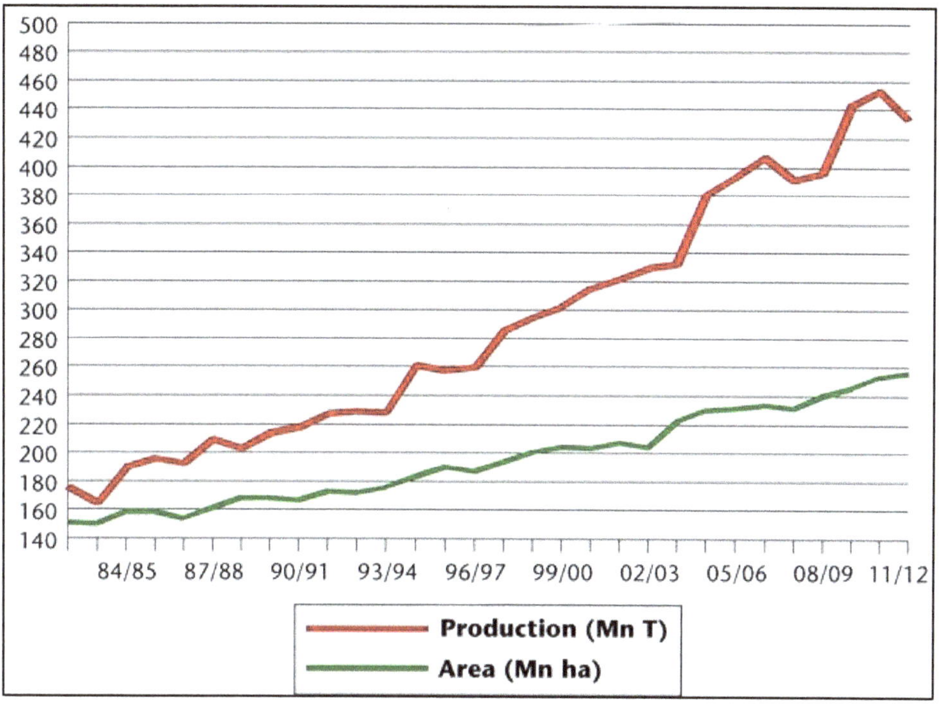

Figure 17.2: World Area and Production of the Major 10 Oilseeds (Soybeans, cotton seed, rapeseed, sunflower seed, groundnuts (shelled), sesame seed, palmkernels, copra, linseed and castor seed)

and Australia, and declined in the European Union, Pakistan, Russia, and China (Figure 17.3).

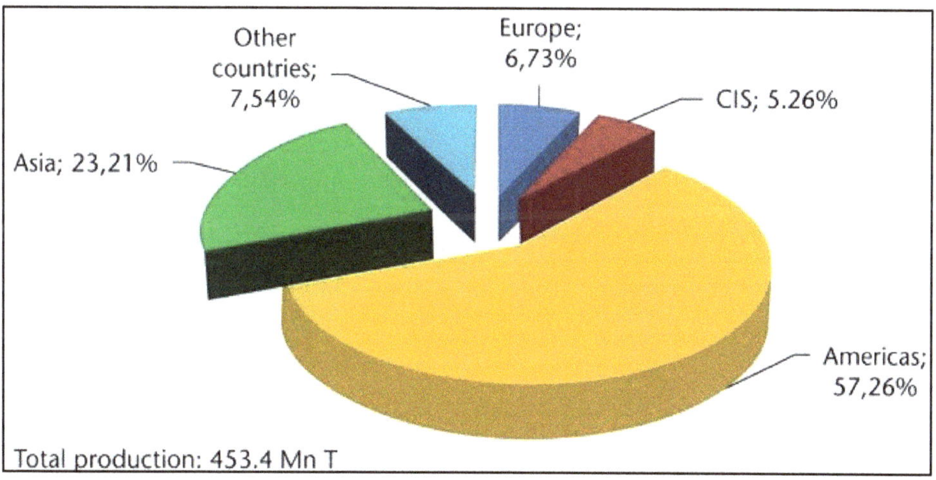

Figure 17. 3: World Production of Oilseeds by Main Regions (Year 2011)

Following last season's exceptional decline, world oil crop production is forecast to recover in 2012/13, possibly hitting a new record of 474 million tonnes. Unlike in the last season, when it fell by over 3 percent, global production is anticipated to rise by 5 percent in 2012/13, sustained by a strong recovery in global soybean output. By contrast, cotton, rape and sunowerseed, which yielded record harvests last season, are expected to experience a sizeable decrease.

In future, world oilseed's production is expected to expand by 23 per cent over the 2011-2020 period, marking a strong slowdown in growth relative to the past (Table 17.3). The anticipated production increase is based equally on higher plantings and yield improvements. The United States (USA) has long been the leader in oilseeds production. China, second before 2002, was replaced by Brazil in order of production, and is currently followed by Argentina, India, the EU-27 and Canada. The share held by Latin American and Eastern European producers is likely to increase at the expense of China and the US.

Annual yield improvement is expected to slow down, compared to the last decade, and the productivity gap between developing and developed countries will diminish only marginally. The growth in oilseed plantings is also projected to slow down markedly in both developed and developing countries due to high marginal costs of area expansion, environmental constraints and sustained profitability of competing crops. Two thirds of global area expansion should take place in the developing world; growth is expected to be concentrated in Brazil, India and China (Figure 17.4). Among developed countries, some further area expansion is expected in Canada, Australia and among Eastern European producers, whereas in the US and the EU plantings should grow marginally (OECD/FAO, 2011).

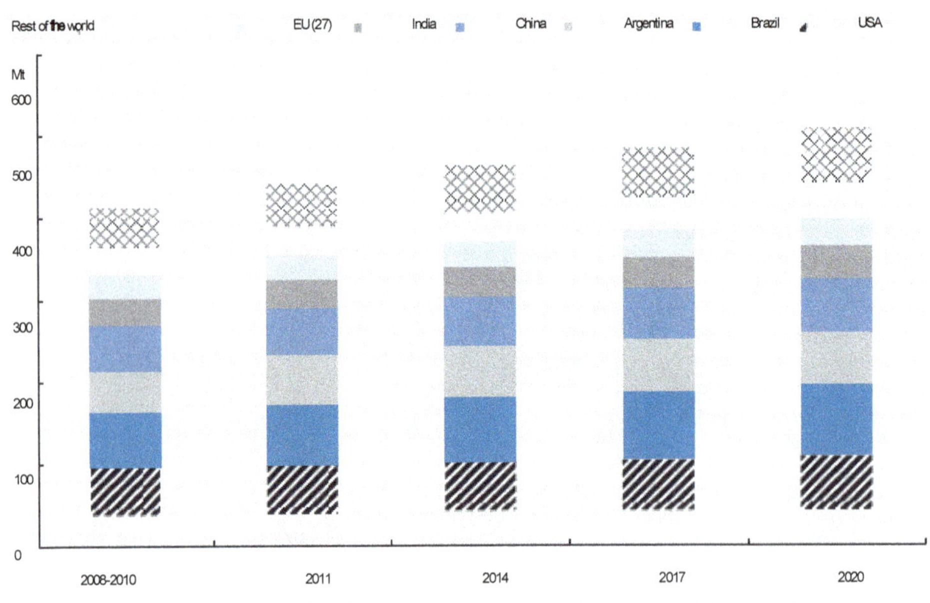

Figure 17.4: Oilseed Production to be Dominated by Few Market Players

Evolution of global oilseed production over the projection period

***Source:* OECD and FAO Secretariats.**

Table 17.3: World Oilseed Projections

		Avg 08/09-10/11est	11/12	12/13	13/14	14/15	15/16	16/17	17/18	18/19	19/20	20/21
OILSEED (crop year)[1]												
OECD[2]												
Production	mt	146.3	150.8	153.1	153.6	155.8	157.3	160.7	163.3	166.7	167.5	170.5
Consumption	mt	129.6	132.5	134.3	135.2	136.4	137.6	139.6	140.9	142.8	143.8	145.5
Crush	mt	115.2	118.3	120.1	120.7	121.8	122.9	124.9	126.1	128.0	129.0	130.6
Closing stocks	mt	15.4	15.6	15.1	15.1	15.6	15.5	15.3	15.4	15.5	15.5	15.6
Non-OECD												
Production	mt	267.4	290.3	295.8	301.6	307.2	312.2	316.7	321.2	326.2	331.2	336.6
Consumption	mt	281.2	302.6	309.5	314.3	320.3	326.2	332.4	337.9	344.2	349.3	355.7
Crush	mt	226.6	245.8	251.8	255.5	260.5	265.2	270.3	274.5	279.7	283.7	288.8
Closing stocks	mt	24.5	29.3	29.0	29.1	29.3	29.5	29.4	29.5	29.6	29.6	29.9
WORLD												
Production	mt	413.7	441.1	448.8	455.1	463.0	469.5	477.5	484.5	492.9	498.8	507.2
Area	mha	203.3	217.9	220.0	221.5	223.4	225.2	227.4	229.4	231.8	233.1	235.1
Yield	t/ha	1.9	2.0	2.0	2.1	2.1	2.1	2.1	2.1	2.1	2.1	2.2
Consumption	mt	410.8	435.0	443.9	449.5	456.7	463.8	472.1	478.8	487.0	493.2	501.2
Crush	mt	341.8	364.1	371.9	376.1	382.3	388.1	395.2	400.7	407.7	412.7	419.5
Other use	mt	18.2	18.1	18.1	18.5	18.5	18.7	18.7	18.9	19.0	19.0	19.1
Exports	mt	94.8	115.2	116.3	116.6	118.8	120.5	122.2	123.2	124.9	125.3	127.0
Closing stocks	mt	39.9	44.9	44.2	44.2	44.9	45.0	44.8	44.9	45.1	45.1	45.5
Price[3]	USD/t	445.8	455.4	455.2	460.8	462.7	468.0	474.5	475.8	473.6	483.3	477.9

Contd...

Table 17.3–*Contd...*

Avg 08/09-10/11est			*11/12*	*12/13*	*13/14*	*14/15*	*15/16*	*16/17*	*17/18*	*18/19*	*19/20*	*20/21*
VEGETABLE OILS (marketing year)												
OECD[2]												
Production	mt	31.1	32.2	32.8	32.9	33.3	33.7	34.3	34.7	35.3	35.7	36.3
Consumption	mt	44.0	45.7	47.3	48.2	49.1	50.0	50.7	51.6	52.4	53.3	53.9
Closing stocks	mt	3.2	2.9	2.8	2.8	2.8	2.8	2.9	2.9	2.9	2.9	2.8
Non-OECD												
Production	mt	106.6	114.0	117.5	120.5	123.7	126.9	130.2	133.4	136.7	139.9	143.2
Consumption	mt	95.7	103.7	105.8	108.0	110.8	113.6	116.5	119.3	122.3	125.1	128.2
Closing stocks	mt	11.3	11.1	11.4	11.6	11.6	11.6	11.8	11.9	12.2	12.3	12.6
WORLD												
Production	mt	137.7	146.3	150.2	153.4	157.0	160.6	164.5	168.1	172.0	175.5	179.5
Of which palm oil	mt	45.7	49.3	51.1	52.9	54.7	56.5	58.3	60.2	62.1	64.0	65.8
Consumption	mt	139.7	149.4	153.0	156.2	159.9	163.6	167.2	170.9	174.7	178.4	182.1
Food	mt	112.6	123.6	126.0	128.1	130.6	133.2	136.0	138.6	141.4	144.0	147.0
Biofuel	mt	18.4	18.8	19.8	20.7	21.8	22.7	23.4	24.4	25.2	26.2	26.8
Exports	mt	54.3	61.6	62.6	64.4	66.1	67.9	69.6	71.7	73.7	75.8	77.7
Closing stocks	mt	14.4	14.0	14.2	14.4	14.5	14.5	14.7	14.8	15.1	15.2	15.5
Price[5]	USD/t	921.6	1 022.9	1 026.7	1 026.7	1 036.8	1 049.4	1 063.0	1 066.8	1 082.9	1 081.0	1 086.5

1. Beginning crop marketing year
2. Excludes Iceland but includes EU6 members that are not members of the OECD (Bulgaria, Cyprus, Latvia, Lithuania, Malta and Romania).
3. Weighted average oilseed price, European port.
4. Weighted average price of oilseed oils and palm oil, European port.

Source: OECD/FAO Agricultural Outlook, 2011-2020 and FAO Secretariats.

Trends in Production of Oils and Fats

The major vegetable oils and fats produced for edible purpose and comparison in the trend of their production over the last 20 years has been presented in Figure 17.5. Vegetable oil production globally has increased continuously in the past decades. Total vegetable oil (coconut, cottonseed, olive, palm, palm kernel) production during 2006-07to 2009-10 in the world indicates a slight increasing trend (Table 17.4). The major contributors were Indonesia, Malaysia, China, USA and EU.

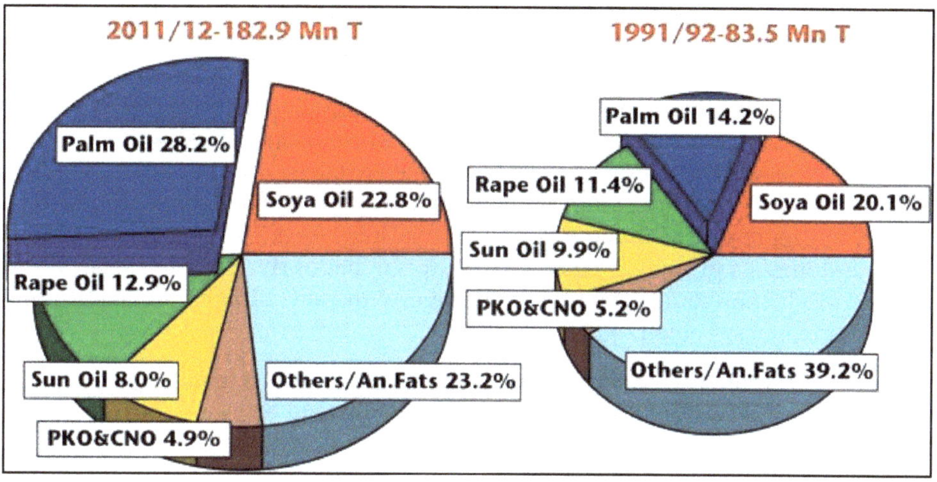

Figure 17.5: World Production (year 2011/12 *vs* 1991/92) of 17 Oils and Fats: Soya oil, palm oil, rapeseed oil, sunflower oil, cotton oil, groundnut oil, sesame oil, corn oil, olive oil, palmkernel oil, coconut oil, butter as fat, lard, fish oil, linseed oil, castor oil, tallow and grease

Table 17.4 Main vegetable and palm oils, average growth from 1987 to 2007

	Million tonnes/year	*per cent /year*
All vegetable oils	3.86	5.2
Palm oil	1.47	8.1
Soybean oil	1.22	5.7
Rapeseed oil	0.52	4.8
Sunflower oil	0.20	2.5
Palm kernel oil	0.17	7.6
Cottonseed oil	0.10	2.5
Olive oil	0.07	3.2
Peanut oil	0.08	2.1
Coconut oil	0.02	0.8

Source: www.fas.usda.gov/psdonline.

Table 17.4 shows the annual growth of world production of vegetable oils together with the percentage annual increase from 1987 through 2007. During 1975 – 2007, while production of sunflower oil and other lower share oils was fairly stable, rapeseed oil, soybean oil and especially palm oil production increased remarkably over the same period. As can be appreciated, palm tops the increase with over 8 per cent annually, followed by palm kernel with 7.6 per cent, and soybean oil with 5.7 per cent. It should be noticed that such increases date well back before the surge for biodiesel.

The 2012/13 crop forecasts translate into a 3 percent increase in global oils/fats production to 187 million tonnes, which compares with a stagnation last season and buoyant growth rates in preceding years. Oil extraction from annual oil crops is anticipated to grow by about 3 million tonnes. The increase reects a strong expansion in global soy oil production (5.4 million tonnes or 13 percent above 2011/12), whereas sunower, rapeseed and cottonseed oil are expected to fall short of last season's record. As to perennial oil crops, oil palm is anticipated to add 2.8 million tonnes to global oil production, representing an about average annual increase of 5 percent. As in previous years, Indonesia's growth is expected to outpace that of rivaling Malaysia. Global olive oil production could suffer a sharp decline, with total output estimated to fall by 0.7 million tonnes (Table 17.5).

Table 17.5: World Vegetable Oils Supply and Distribution (Commodity View) (million metric tonnes)

	2008/09	*2009/10*	*2010/11*	*2011/12*	*Feb 2012/13*	*Mar 2012/13*
Production						
Oil Coconut	3.54	3.63	3.83	3.56	3.52	3.52
Oil Cottonseed	4.75	4.6	4.97	5.27	5.23	5.28
Oil Olive	2.78	3.08	3.25	3.39	2.87	2.87
Oil Palm	44.02	45.87	47.92	50.7	53.33	53.83
Oil Palm Kernel	5.17	5.5	5.55	5.91	6.25	6.25
Oil Peanut	5.08	4.74	5.04	5.07	5.29	5.29
Oil Rapeseed	20.59	22.55	23.51	24.29	23.52	23.8
Oil Soybean	35.88	38.82	41.29	42.4	43.41	43.18
Oil Sunflowerseed	11.95	12.12	12.29	15.08	13.81	13.75
Total	133.76	140.9	147.64	155.67	157.23	157.76
Imports						
Oil Coconut	1.66	2.29	1.79	1.82	1.84	1.83
Oil Cottonseed	0.06	0.07	0.05	0.07	0.06	0.06
Oil Olive	0.55	0.52	0.55	0.62	0.64	0.64
Oil Palm	34.06	35.32	36.11	38.5	39.79	40.41
Oil Palm Kernel	2.35	2.4	2.43	2.54	2.71	2.66
Oil Peanut	0.14	0.19	0.2	0.16	0.17	0.17
Oil Rapeseed	2.43	2.91	3.31	3.99	3.51	3.52

Contd...

Table 17.5–*Contd...*

	2008/09	*2009/10*	*2010/11*	*2011/12*	*Feb 2012/13*	*Mar 2012/13*
Oil Soybean	9.07	8.62	9.24	8.17	8.79	8.57
Oil Sunflowerseed	4.06	3.73	3.65	5.58	5.46	5.56
Total	54.38	56.04	57.34	61.45	62.96	63.42
Exports						
Oil Coconut	1.48	2.17	1.71	1.85	1.77	1.77
Oil Cottonseed	0.16	0.11	0.15	0.19	0.12	0.17
Oil Olive	0.64	0.68	0.75	0.84	0.69	0.69
Oil Palm	34.93	35.75	37.05	39.1	40.79	41.2
Oil Palm Kernel	2.61	2.62	2.81	2.53	3.08	3.08
Oil Peanut	0.2	0.19	0.18	0.19	0.22	0.22
Oil Rapeseed	2.44	2.74	3.42	3.96	3.75	3.8
Oil Soybean	9.15	9.14	9.53	8.52	9.08	8.87
Oil Sunflowerseed	4.55	4.49	4.58	6.42	6.22	6.09
Total	56.15	57.89	60.17	63.6	65.72	65.89
Domestic Consumption						
Oil Coconut	3.35	3.96	3.81	3.7	3.68	3.67
Oil Cottonseed	4.74	4.6	4.77	5.15	5.25	5.26
Oil Olive	2.91	2.96	3.02	3.07	3.09	3.09
Oil Palm	42.71	44.79	46.77	49.06	51.79	52.38
Oil Palm Kernel	4.9	5.06	5.25	5.63	5.8	5.75
Oil Peanut	4.94	4.88	5.04	5.07	5.25	5.25
Oil Rapeseed	20.29	22.6	23.49	23.78	23.74	23.8
Oil Soybean	36.17	38.13	40.76	41.76	43.62	43.35
Oil Sunflowerseed	10.68	11.59	11.55	12.94	13.33	13.42
Total	130.69	138.57	144.46	150.16	155.54	155.95
Ending Stocks						
Oil Coconut	0.79	0.57	0.67	0.5	0.42	0.41
Oil Cottonseed	0.2	0.16	0.27	0.26	0.17	0.17
Oil Olive	0.64	0.6	0.63	0.73	0.46	0.46
Oil Palm	4.82	5.46	5.68	6.73	7.2	7.39
Oil Palm Kernel	0.67	0.9	0.82	1.11	1.19	1.18
Oil Peanut	0.25	0.1	0.12	0.09	0.08	0.08
Oil Rapeseed	1.14	1.25	1.16	1.71	1.3	1.43
Oil Soybean	3.09	3.27	3.52	3.81	3.32	3.34
Oil Sunflowerseed	1.72	1.49	1.29	2.59	2.28	2.39
Total	13.32	13.81	14.15	17.51	16.42	16.85

Source: OECD/FAO, 2012

Led by developing countries, global vegetable oil production is expected to increase by over 30 per cent by 2020. However, in terms of annual growth rate, production slows down compared to the last decade. In Malaysia and Indonesia, where land restrictions and environmental regulations should become more binding, combined palm oil output will, nonetheless, expand by almost 45 per cent, raising their share in global output to 36 per cent. Other major expected sources of vegetable oil production growth are China, Argentina, the EU and Brazil. Also noteworthy is the expansion projected for Canada, the Russian Federation and the Ukraine. Only modest growth is expected in the US and India (OECD/FAO, 2011).

For all fats and oils, world production will remain concentrated in a few countries. About 80 percent of world production is accounted for by 11 countries, of which 4 are developed and 7 are developing countries (Figure 17.6). This percentage is expected to increase further during the projection period.

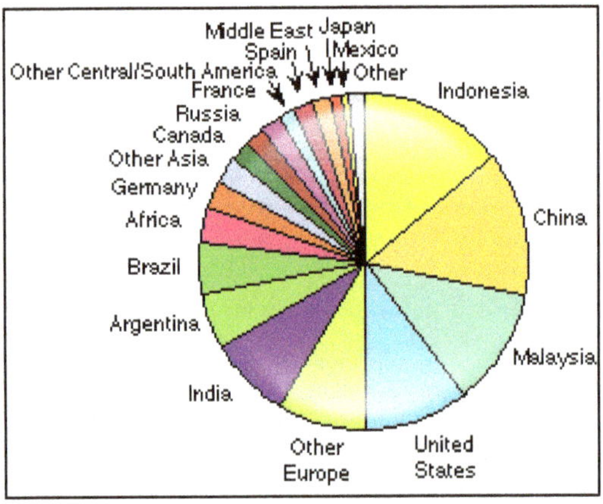

Figure 17.6: World Production of Fats and Oils (2011)

Global production of the major fats and oils is led by Asia. Indonesia is the world's largest producer, accounting for over 44 per cent of the world's palm oil production, the major type of vegetable oil produced. China produces a nearly equivalent volume of fats and oils, and is a larger producer of soybean and canola oils. Malaysia ranks third in world production because of its place as the second-largest world palm oil producer. India also produces large volumes of canola and butter. Overall, Asia accounts for over 50 per cent of world fats and oils production (Figure 17.6).

Trends in Consumption and Demand of Oils and Fats

Oilseeds consumption includes two parts: oilseed oils and oilseed meals. World supply of oil-bearing crops is used mainly for processing into oil, about 78.5 per cent ; for direct food, 10.5 per cent ; for seed, 2 per cent ; for feed, 5 per cent ; for industrial use almost 1 per cent and waste 2.9 per cent. The consumption of vegetable oils falls into two major applications: i) food industry, and ii) industrial uses, including biodiesel, which is a more recent trend.

The predominant use is for food with over 80 per cent of the market, with the industrial and biodiesel markets far behind. Thus, the rapid demand for vegetable oils has been sparked off by the food market rather than the industrial or biodiesel sectors, contrary to general belief. Although there is a growing role for industrial uses, the food industry is expected to be the dominant factor in the future for reasons already stated above.

As in previous years, consumption growth in developing countries is expected to be almost double that in developed country. Total consumption of fats and oils has increased from 79.31 million tons in 1996-97 to 157.47 million tons in 2011-12 (Figure 17.7). In 2008/09, developing Asia alone accounted for almost half of global oil/fat consumption, with utilization climbing to new records both in China and India, because of increasing population, rising incomes and a lower base level of consumption. The growth in these countries was projected to average 2.8 percent (compared to 1.8 percent in developed countries), and their share of the market was increased marginally from 60 percent to 62 percent by 2010. In per capita terms, growth is anticipated to be highest in transition countries, where the turnaround in income will encourage higher consumption. Among developed countries, significant consumption growth is only expected for the European Union. Disparity among countries in the consumption levels of oils and fats will remain, with developing countries consuming on an average per capita basis less than one-third of that of developed countries.

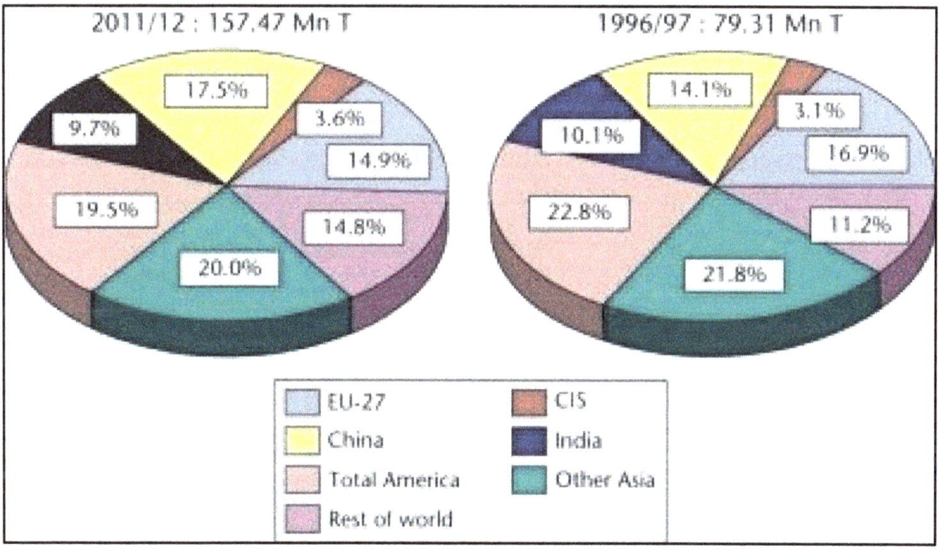

Figure 17.7: Consumption (Year 2011/12 *vs* 1996/97) of 13 Vegetable Oils by Major Countries (MnT)

Still developing countries are dominating the rise in vegetable oil consumption (Figure 17.7). World consumption is driven mainly by Asia, which accounts for 44 per cent of the world total (Figure 17.7). China and India together make up 32 per cent of the world total. China is the world's largest consumer of major oilseed oils, with its total oil consumption accounting for about 17.5 per cent of total world consumption in 2011-12. The following pie charts show world consumption of major fats and oils (Figure 17.8). Per capita consumption of fats and oils in 2011 in selected countries of the world has been depicted in Figure 17.9.

Comparison of Average Annual Growth Rates of Vegetable Oil Consumption

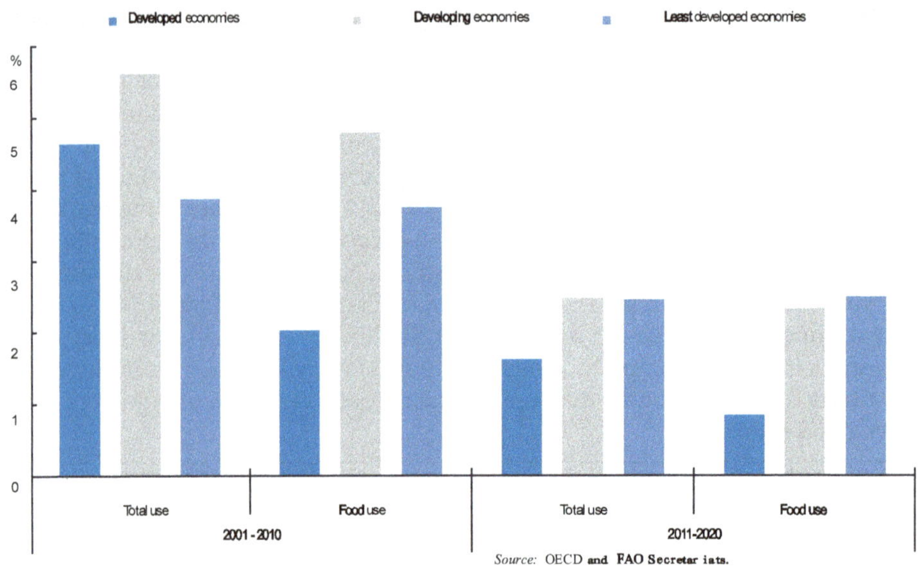

Figure 17.7: Developing Countries to Dominate the Rise in Vegetable Oil Consumption

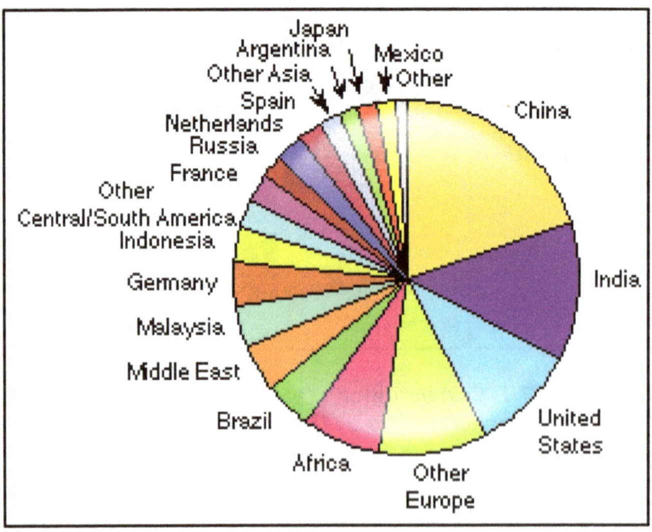

Figure 17.8: World Consumption of Fats and Oils-2011

In future, developing countries, in particular China and other Asian countries shall continue to dominate the rise in vegetable oil consumption (Figure 17.9). Oil consumption in some of the selected EU countries has been depicted in Figure 17.10. Biodiesel production is projected to contribute significantly to global consumption growth. While in China and India, growth occurs primarily in food use, in the EU and the US, the biodiesel industry is projected to represent a significant source of demand.

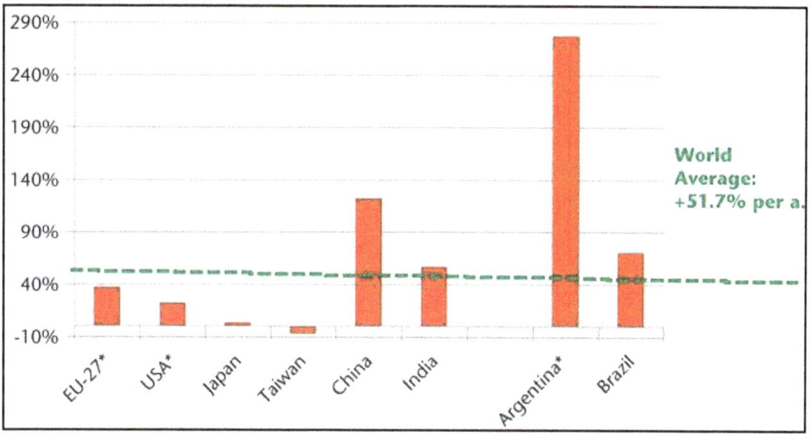

Figure 17.9: Per Capita Consumption in Year 2011 of 17 Fats and Oils of Selected Countries, Compared with World Average

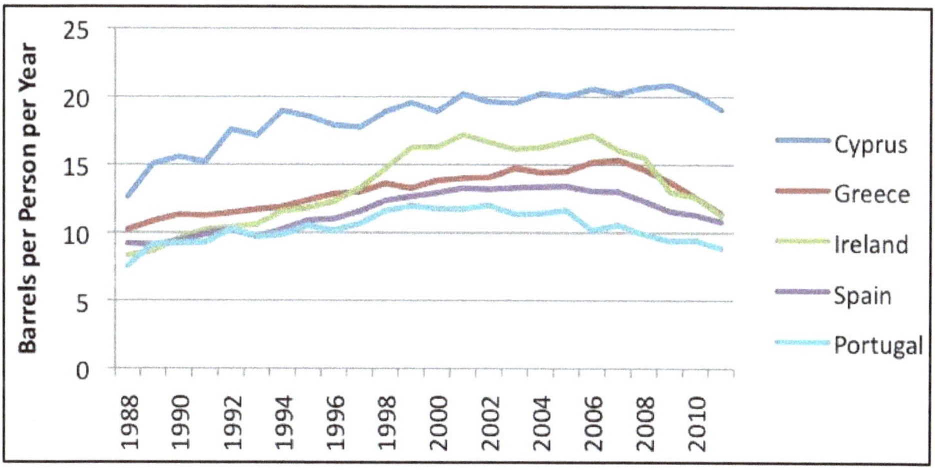

Figure 17.10: Per Capita Oil Consumption in EU Countries

In per capita terms, the discrepancy between edible oil intake in developed and developing countries is expected to narrow; however, looking at overall consumption (*i.e.* Food and non-food use), the lead developed countries have over developing ones should increase slightly (Figures 17.7, 17.11). Among least developed countries, positive income prospects should allow a reversal of the recent negative trend in per capita consumption. However, consumption levels are expected to take the full decade to return to levels recorded before the 2008-crisis (OECD/FAO, 2011).

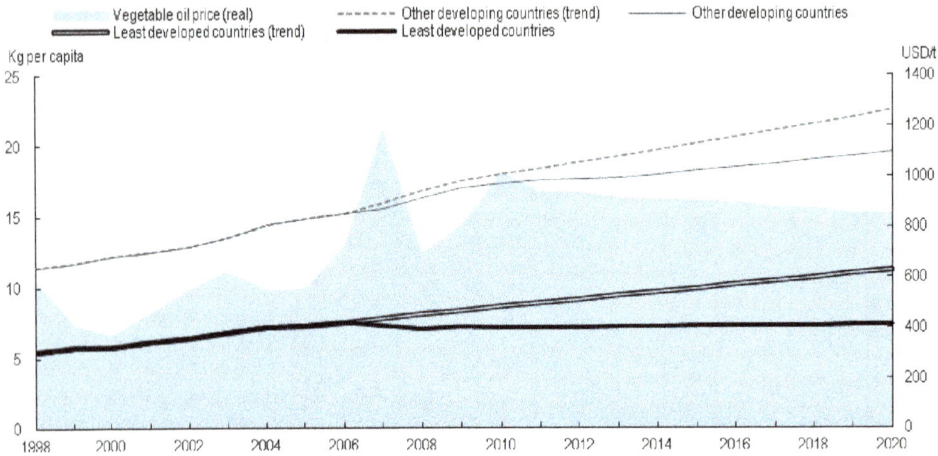

Figure 17.11: Per Capita Food Consumption and Real Price of Vegetable Oils

Overall, world fats and oils consumption is expected to grow at an average annual rate of 3.5–4 per cent, driven mainly by growth in Asia and steady increases in the United States and Europe. In Asia, China and India will continue to experience a growing population and economy, which will result in an increase in per capita demand for fats and oils. In the United States, Europe, and Central and South America, fats and oils demand for nonfood use, particularly biodiesel production is expected to continue to increase.

Types of Vegetable Oils in Demand for Consumption

Palm, soybean, canola and sunflower oil are the world's most widely used fats and oils, and together account for 72 per cent of total global consumption. Palm oil is the largest-volume oil used, surpassing soybean oil in the mid-2000s. In 1990, these four oils combined accounted for about 55 per cent of global fats and oils consumption, with soybean oil at 20 per cent of the world total, followed by palm oil with 14 per cent.

Palm oil is produced mainly by Indonesia and Malaysia. Demand for palm oil accounts for over 25 per cent of world demand for fats and oils, and is expected to grow at an average annual rate of more than 5 per cent. The main consumers include India, Indonesia and China, and the rest of Asia; Europe; and Africa. Chinese demand is mainly for soybean oil, followed by canola and palm oils. India is a major consumer of canola oil, as well as palm oil and butter. Both countries expect continued strong growth. Indonesia and Malaysia also contribute to overall consumption, especially in palm oil demand. Palm oil use has grown significantly as a result of its lower cost, edible properties, and supply availability.

Soybean oil is the dominant oil used in the United States, accounting for 45 per cent of total consumption. Biodiesel production will continue to drive U.S. growth.

Soybean oil accounts for over 63 per cent of total demand in Central and South America, and over 40 per cent of its use is for biodiesel production, especially in Argentina and Brazil. In Europe, soybean oil is used as a cooking oil but growth has been limited in food use and more recently by biodiesel production. Soybean oil use in Asia is also significant (about 20 per cent of the total) and strong growth of 4–5 per cent annually is expected. China is a large consumer.

Demand of Non-Food Uses of Vegetable Oil

Demand for non-food use (bio-fuel production) of vegetable oil should account for about 1/3 rd of global consumption growth. As a result, manufacturing plants have come up in significant numbers and from a production capacity of just about 6 million tonnes at the beginning of 2006, it is estimated to go upto over 20 million tonnes in future. Of course, use of vegetable oils for bio-fuels and the quantities will depend to a large extent on crude prices. But it is clear that large chunk of vegetable oils is being taken out of the global food use and this is going to have a profound impact on the vegetable oil availability and prices.

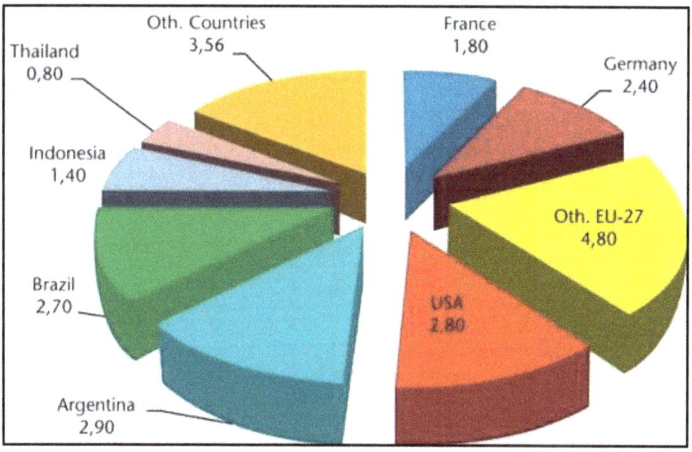

Figure 17.12: World Production of Biodiesel in Year 2012 (Forecast), in Mn T

Countries where the use of vegetable oils for biodiesel is estimated to grow further include Argentina, Brazil and the European Union (Figure 17.12). In the European Union, no less than 60 percent of overall rape oil utilization should be for biodiesel and also the importation of palm oils as fuel feedstock should continue. Also in Argentina and Brazil industrial demand for vegetable oils should rise further, thereby contributing to the fall in export availabilities. Europe uses large quantities of diesel and some countries, for instance Germany have even made blending of bio-diesel mandatory. Almost entire rapeseed crop in Europe is now going for making bio-diesel. In the US, while usage of bio-diesel is less than in Europe because they use more gasoline blended with ethanol, the use of soybean for bio-diesel is still increasing there too and the trend is catching up elsewhere also.

Usage of Oils/Fats for Biofuels in 2008/09

- ☆ USA - - 3.0 Mn T (vs. 2.4 Mn in 07/08)
- ☆ Brazil - - 1.4 Mn T (vs. 0.9)
- ☆ Argentina - - 1.0 Mn (vs. 0.5)

By 2020, biodiesel production accounts for 15 per cent of total consumption, compared to 10 per cent in 2008-10 base period. Higher mandatory use in developed countries but also rising biodiesel production in a number of developing countries drives this increase. In the EU, demand from the biodiesel industry is projected to nearly double by 2020. By 2020, vegetable oil use for biodiesel production is expected to account for more than half of the EUs total domestic consumption (Fig. 17.13). Although biodiesel driven demand is also projected to grow in the US and Canada, its role remains much smaller in those markets. As Argentina continues to develop its export-oriented biodiesel industry, by 2020 the latter should account for 72 per cent of domestic consumption supported by the system of differential export taxes in place (OECD/FAO, 2011). Overall demand for vegetable oil-based fuel should nonetheless continue to grow, driven by rising national blending requirements and continued support to producers.

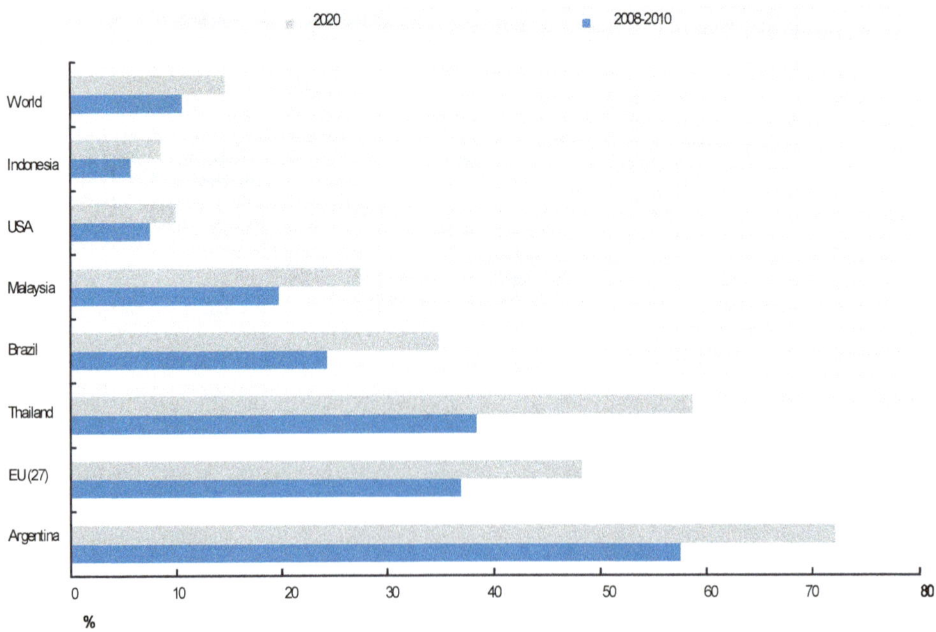

Figure 17.13: Biodiesel Production to Account for 16 per cent of Total Vegetable Oil Consumption

Share of vegetable oil consumption used for biodiesel production in selected countries

***Source:* OECD and FAO Secretariats.**

Trends in Trade of Oilseeds

With the increased production and consumption noted, oilseeds and oilseeds products have become one of the largest sectors in international trade (Figures 17.14 and 17.15). The amount of soybeans exported was the largest of the five major oilseed exports, increasing from 45.55 million tons in 1999 to 79.52 million tons in 2009. Exports of rapeseed, cottonseed, peanut and sunflower seed have been relatively stable between 1999 and 2008. The export of rapeseed was the second largest export in the world market, with lows of 4.11 million tons in 2002 and with the high export at 11.91 million tons in 2008.

The USA has been the premier exporter of oilseeds over the past several years, followed by Brazil, Canada and Argentina. Despite substantial production growth in the past 25 years and recent gains in export volume, the USA share of global exports has steadily decreased. The USA dominated world trade in unprocessed oilseeds in the mid to late 1970s, with a global market share of more than 70 per cent. Recently, however, it has fallen below 50 per cent (USDA, 2010). The main export markets for the USA are China, Mexico, Canada and Japan.

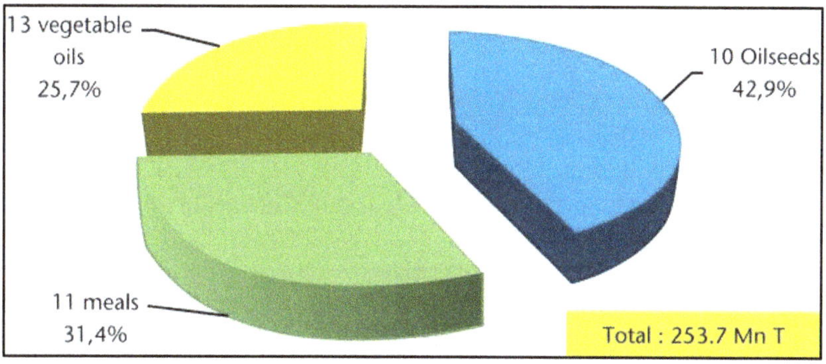

Figure 17.14: Share of Oilseeds and Products in Total World Exports in 2011 (in per cent). All non vegetable oils and meals are excluded.

***Source*: USDA (2012)**

In future, growth in world oilseeds trade is projected to slow down significantly. On the import side, developing countries will account for most of the slowdown. In particular China's imports should expand at a much slower pace than before. But the country will continue to dominate world trade, with purchases accounting for half of total global imports in 2020. Imported material continues to represent close to half of the oilseeds crushed in the country. In the EU, the volume of imports should remain more or less unchanged, as increased crushing demand is met by higher domestic production. All main oilseed exporters will experience poor export growth. In Argentina and Canada oilseed sales are expected to remain flat as crushing capacity and thus the exportation of higher-value oils and meals are expanded. Only some emerging exporters, notably Paraguay, the Ukraine, the Russian Federation and Uruguay should experience a significant expansion in seed exports.

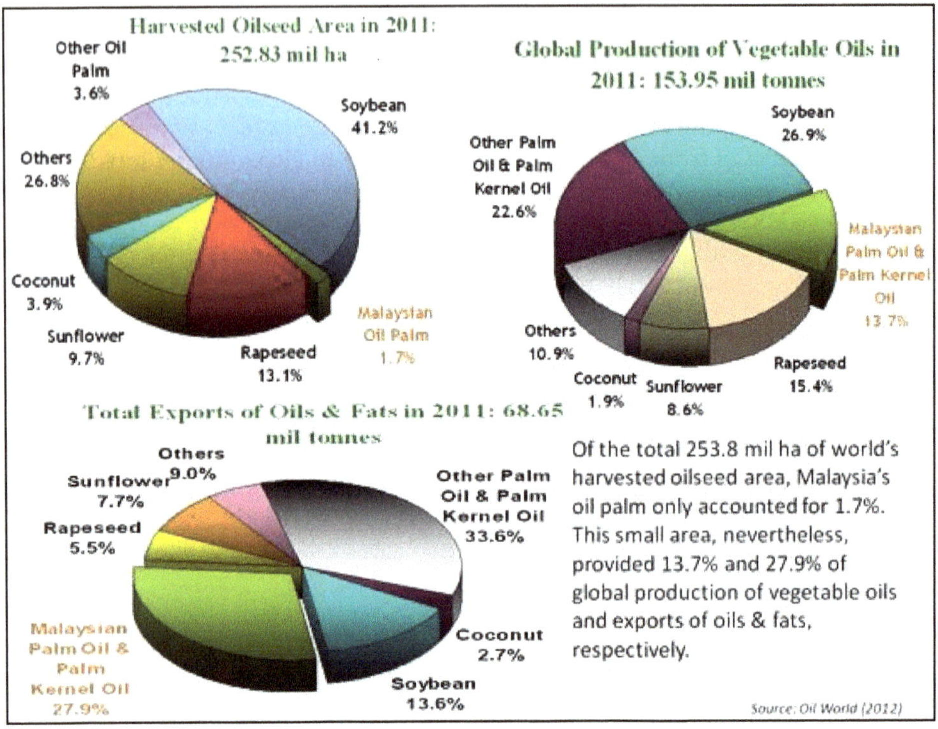

Figure 17.15: Trends in Trade of Oils and Fats in the World

Global export of oils and fats was projected to grow by about 15 million tonnes by 2010 compared to base period levels. With a highly concentrated profile of production by country, growth in production by a few countries was projected to represent the largest increase in exports, while increasing consumption of oils and fats by all countries implies an increasing diffusion of imports. In the base period, about 85 percent of exports were supplied by nine countries (four developed and five developing). This percentage was expected to grow during 2011-12, with an increasing share of Brazil and Argentina (soy oil), and Malaysia and Indonesia (palm oil).

The export share of the US fell from 18 percent to 12 percent by 2010. These data underscored an important aspect of oils and fats markets, namely that changes in trade were occurring mostly among the developing countries. Their export share may increase from 60 percent to 70 percent, and their import share from 61 percent to 65 percent. Western Europe and Africa are expected to increase their dependency on imported oils and fats.

World statistics regarding import, export and utilization of oils and fats during 2011-12 have been depicted in Table 17.6. Trade in oilseed products is expected to slow down markedly. Regarding vegetable oil exports, the combined share of Indonesia and Malaysia in total exports should climb to 68 per cent by 2020. Argentina is the third largest exporter with a world share of 9 per cent. About 65 per cent of the country's output is exported, in part due to the differential export tax system that favours sales of oilseed products. The US and Brazil, by contrast, are expected to remain the world's key suppliers of oilseeds. The Ukraine and the Russian Federation will continue to expand sales of both vegetable oils and oilseeds.

Developing countries in Asia led by India and China should account for almost 50 per cent of global vegetable oil imports in 2020. On average, in developing Asia, 45 per cent of consumption will come from imports (Figure 17.16). In India, where foreign purchases are estimated to expand nearly 50 per cent, the rate of import dependence rises to 62 per cent. China, in addition to covering a considerable part of its vegetable oil needs *via* the crushing of imported oilseeds, is set to expand edible oil imports by almost 35 per cent, which brings the share of imports in total consumption to 36 per cent.

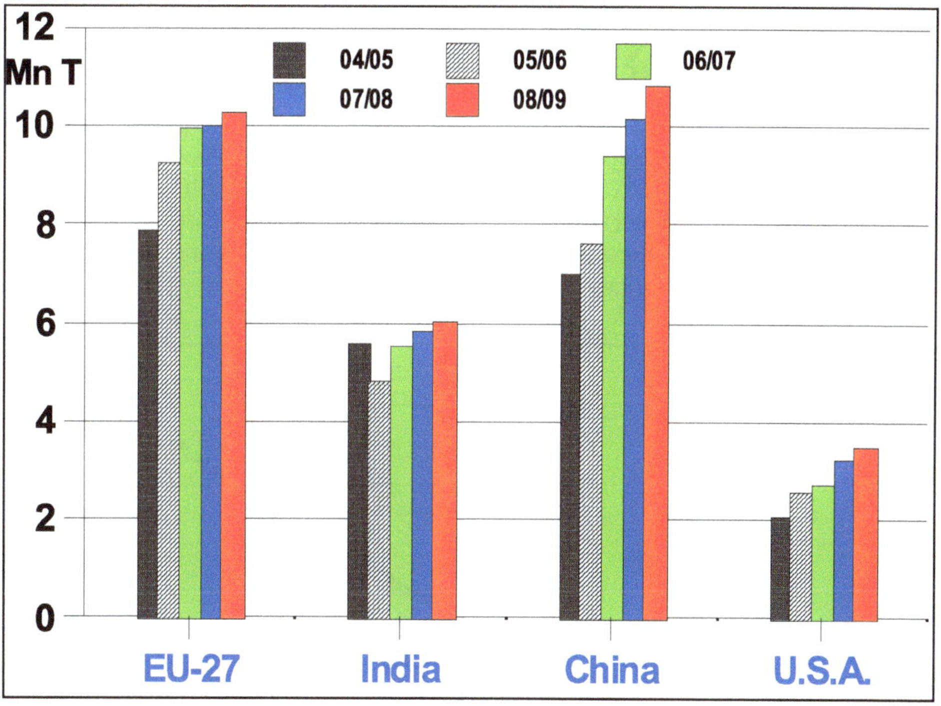

Figure 17.16: Imports of Key Countries

***Source*: Mielke, T. (Sept. 26, 2008 presentation on Global Impacts on India: Oilseeds and Products in Mumbai)**

In the EU, to meet both industrial and traditional vegetable oil demand, imports should rise by 42 per cent. This maintains the EU as the world's leading importer, which alone should account for almost 18 per cent of the market. The same holds for China, where, in addition to oils, oilseed imports (and subsequent crushing) will also be used to meet domestic consumption requirements.

Trend in Trade of Various Types of Oils and Fats

High prices of wheat, corn and beans have led to a titanic struggle for acres between cereals like wheat and rice, feed grains like corn and sorghum and oilseeds like soybeans, rapeseed and sunflower seed. Indeed, Palm oil is the only vegetable oil source which does not have to face this critical competition. The world will rely more and more on palm oil in the next years (Figures 17.17 and 17.18). Palm oil export boomed from 12 Mn T in 1997-98 to 35 Mn in 2008- 2009 (Figure 17.19). Palm oil share of world export was 55 per cent in 2008-2009 versus 39 per cent 10 years ago. There is an excess of world production of rapeseed and canola. Importer countries cannot absorb large export supplies. The exports of soybean oil, sunflower oil and rapeseed oil are no longer dynamic, due to higher demand in producing countries. Soya oil share is falling to 16 per cent, sunflower oil to 7.4 per cent and rapeseed oil to 4 per cent.

Price of Vegetable Oils

The 2008/09 season (October/September) started with low prices. After the extraordinary rise of 2007/08, by October 2008, the FAO price indices for oilseed, oils and meals had fallen back to the level recorded prior to the surge. The price decline was triggered by the prospect of improved crop output, combined with weak demand for oilseed products. In the case of oils/fats, the downturn in energy prices also contributed to the fall in prices.

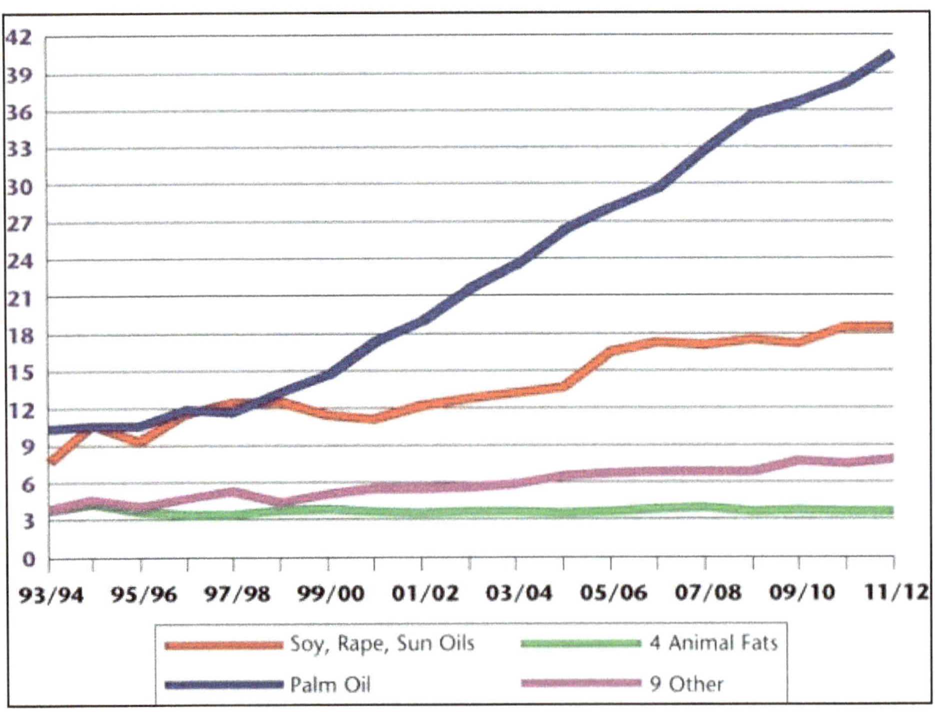

Figure 17.17: World Export of 17 Oils and Fats (in Mn T)

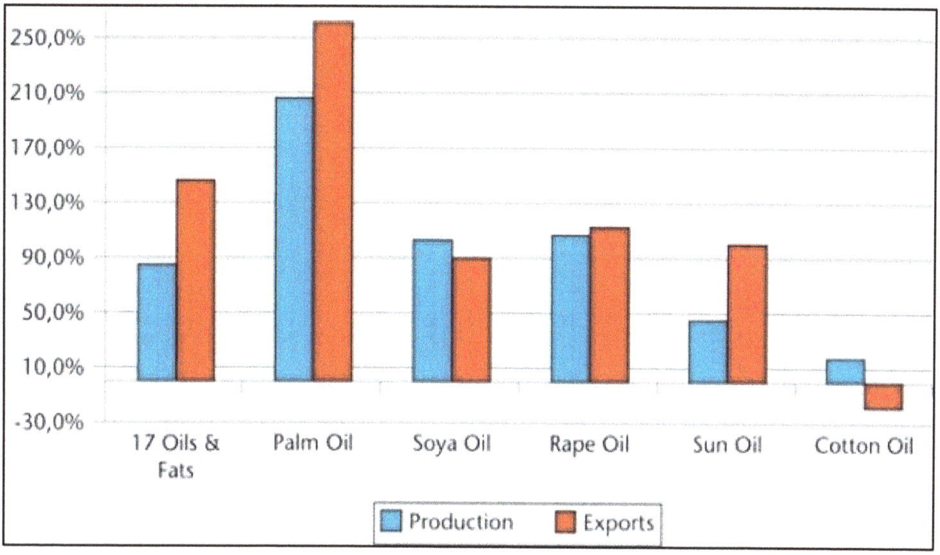

Figure 17.18: Growth of Production and Exports (2011 *vs* 1996) of 17 Oils and Fats and Selected Oils

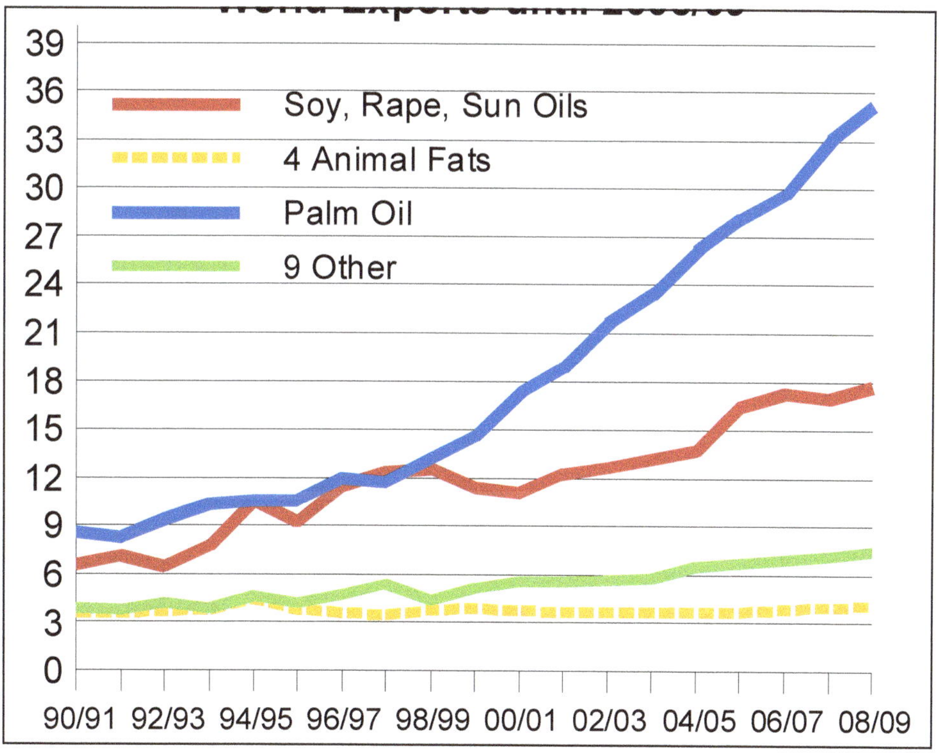

Figure 17.19: World Exports until 2008-09

***Source*: Mielke, T. (Sept. 26, 2008 presentation on Global Impacts on India: Oilseeds and Products in Mumbai)**

Table 17.6: Total Oils and Fats Statistics[1] (million tonnes)

	Imports			Exports			Utilization		
	07/08-09/10 Average Estim.	2010/11	2011/12 f'cast	07/08-09/10 Average Estim.	2010/11	2011/12 f'cast	07/08-09/10 Average Estim.	2010/11	2011/12 f'cast
ASIA	34.5	38.0	40.5	39.5	43.3	45.7	80.0	87.5	93.3
Bangladesh	1.2	1.4	1.4	–	–	–	1.5	1.6	1.7
China	10.6	10.6	11.4	0.5	0.5	0.5	30.1	33.3	35.7
of which Taiwan Prov.	0.4	0.4	0.4	–	–	–	0.8	0.9	0.9
India	8.0	8.7	9.5	0.5	0.5	0.5	17.3	18.6	19.7
Indonesia	0.1	0.1	0.1	17.9	19.9	21.0	5.7	6.9	7.9
Iran	1.2	1.6	1.3	0.2	0.3	0.1	1.6	1.8	1.8
Japan	1.1	1.2	1.2	–	–	–	3.1	3.1	3.1
Korea, Republic of	0.9	1.0	1.0	–	–	–	1.2	1.4	1.4
Malaysia	1.5	2.2	2.5	17.2	18.9	20.0	3.8	3.3	3.7
Pakistan	2.1	2.3	2.4	0.1	0.1	0.1	3.6	4.0	4.1
Philippines	0.5	0.6	0.7	1.1	1.0	1.1	1.0	1.2	1.1
Singapore	0.6	0.8	1.0	0.3	0.3	0.3	0.3	0.6	0.7
Turkey	1.2	1.3	1.5	0.3	0.4	0.5	2.3	2.3	2.6
AFRICA	7.5	8.2	8.4	1.2	1.3	1.4	13.1	14.2	14.5
Algeria	0.6	0.5	0.6	0.1	–	–	0.7	0.7	0.8
Egypt	1.6	1.6	1.9	0.1	–	0.1	2.0	2.1	2.2
Nigeria	0.8	1.1	1.1	0.1	0.1	0.1	2.5	2.8	2.9
South Africa	0.7	0.8	0.8	0.1	0.1	0.1	1.1	1.2	1.2
CENTRAL AMERICA	2.3	2.3	2.4	0.8	0.7	0.8	4.5	4.7	4.6
Mexico	1.2	1.2	1.3	0.2	0.1	0.1	2.9	3.0	3.0

Contd...

Table 17.6–*Contd...*

	Imports			*Exports*			*Utilization*		
	07/08-09/10 Average Estim.	*2010/11*	*2011/12 f'cast*	*07/08-09/10 Average Estim.*	*2010/11*	*2011/12 f'cast*	*07/08-09/10 Average Estim.*	*2010/11*	*2011/12 f'cast*
SOUTH AMERICA	2.3	2.6	2.7	9.7	9.1	8.8	12.0	14.5	15.7
Argentina	0.1	0.1	0.1	6.2	5.8	5.9	2.0	3.1	3.5
Brazil	0.4	0.5	0.6	2.1	1.9	1.5	6.4	7.4	7.9
NORTH AMERICA	4.0	4.5	4.8	6.1	7.0	6.5	17.2	18.4	19.0
Canada	0.5	0.5	0.6	2.3	3.2	3.2	0.9	1.0	1.1
United States of America	3.5	4.0	4.2	3.8	3.8	3.2	16.4	17.5	18.0
EUROPE	13.4	13.1	13.1	5.4	6.0	7.4	34.3	36.4	36.9
European Union	10.7	10.5	10.6	2.1	2.4	2.5	28.5	29.9	30.3
Russian Federation	1.2	1.2	1.1	0.8	0.5	1.4	3.6	4.0	4.1
Ukraine	0.5	0.4	0.4	2.2	2.8	3.1	0.9	1.0	1.0
OCEANIA	0.5	0.6	0.6	1.7	1.8	1.9	1.0	1.1	1.1
Australia	0.4	0.4	0.4	0.6	0.7	0.7	0.7	0.7	0.7
WORLD	64.5	69.1	72.4	64.5	69.2	72.5	162.2	176.7	185.3
Developing countries	44.4	48.6	51.6	51.7	54.9	57.2	104.5	115.6	123.0
Developed countries	20.1	20.5	20.9	12.8	14.3	15.2	57.7	61.1	62.3
LIFDCs	30.2	32.4	34.4	21.8	23.8	25.1	73.0	80.6	85.7
LDCs	4.3	5.0	5.0	0.4	0.5	0.5	7.3	7.9	8.0

1 Includes oils and fats of vegetable, marine and animal origin.

Source: OECD and FAO Secretariats.

Evolution of prices expressed in nominal terms (left) and in real terms (right)

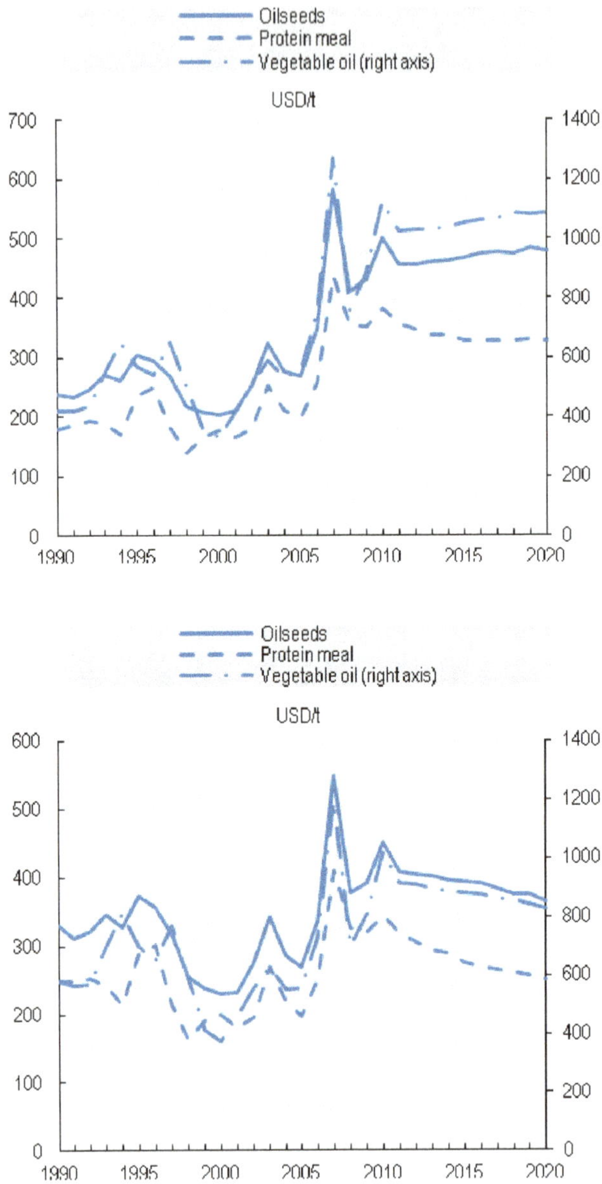

Figure 17.20: Oilseeds and Oilseed Products Prices to Remain above Historical Levels

***Note*: Oilseeds: Weighted average oilseed import price, Europe. Oilseed meal: Weighted average oilseed meal import Price, Europe. Vegetable oil: Weighted average export price of oilseed oils and palm oil, Europe.**

***Source*: OECD and FAO Secretariats.**

After a period of instability, in April 2009 prices in the oilseed complex started moving upward. Oil and fat prices took the lead, increasing as much as 14 percent over March 2009 (based on FAO's monthly price index). Meanwhile, the indices for oil meals and oilseeds grew by, respectively, 6 and 7 percent. In May, the upward trend in prices continued and all three indices rose well above the corresponding levels of 2007 (*i.e.* before the 2007/08 price rally started).

In future, world prices for oilseeds and oilseed products expressed in nominal terms are projected to remain well above levels recorded prior to the 2007-08 food crisis. After a short initial dip, oilseed and vegetable oil prices should rise in future (Figure 17.20).

Chapter 18

Trends in Production and Consumption of Oilseeds, Oils and Fats: Indian Scenario

Oilseed crops have been the backbone of agricultural economy of India from time immemorial. The Indian vegetable oil economy is the world's fourth largest after the US, China and Brazil, harvesting about 25 million tons of oilseeds against the world. Since 1995, Indian share in world production of oilseeds has been around 8-10 per cent. Oilseed crops form the second largest agricultural commodity after cereals occupying 14 per cent of the gross cropped area in our country (Hegde and Venkattakumar, 2007).

The diverse agro-ecological situations prevalent in the country favour cultivation of nine annual oilseed crops, which include seven edible oilseeds *viz,* groundnut, rapeseed-mustard, soybean, sunflower, safflower, sesame and niger and two non-edible oilseeds *viz,* castor and linseed. Oilseeds are being cultivated in all the agro-ecoregions of the country except island ecosystem.

Among the 20 different agro-ecoregions of the country, semiarid ecosystem is the most important one, covering more than 50 per cent of the oilseed area and 55 per cent of the total oilseeds production of the country. Central (Malva) highlands, Gujarat plains and Kathiawar peninsula are the most important ecosystems as far as area and production of oilseeds of the country are concerned. Central highland hot humid region, northern plains and central highlands including Aravallis hot semi-arid ecoregion follow this. Western plains, Kachchh and parts of Kathiawar peninsula, hot arid ecoregion and Deccan plateau, and hot semiarid ecoregions are also very important as far as the area under oilseeds is concerned.

Our country ranks first in area under groundnut, rapeseed-mustard, sesame, safflower and castor and also in production of sesame and castor. Oilseeds contribute 1.4 and 7 per cent to GDP and agricultural GDP, respectively. India has 15,000 oil mills, 711 solvent extraction units, and 264 vanaspati plants; and over 1,000 refineries employing more than one million people. It is estimated that 14 million farmers are involved in oilseed cultivation, while one million persons are involved in processing of oilseeds and oils.

Trends in Area, Production and Yield of Oilseeds

On the oilseed map of the world, India occupies a prominent position, both in regard to acreage and production. India is a leading producer of oilseeds and is estimated to account for around 6 per cent of the world's production of edible oils. India grows oilseeds on an area of over 26-27 million hectares (*kharif* and *rabi* combined), with productivity of around 1000 kg a hectare- half of the world average. The edible oil year is from November to October. About two-thirds of oilseeds are produced in the *kharif* season, with the major crops being soybean and groundnut. In the *rabi* season, mustard is the main crop. Though it has the largest cultivated area under oilseeds in the world, crop yields tantamount to only 50-60 per cent of the world's average.

Oilseed Sector 2011-12

☆ Area under oilseed cultivation	26-27 Million hectares
☆ Average yield	1100 Kgs
☆ Output of 9 cultivated oilseeds	30.1 Million tonnes
☆ Output of Cottonseed and Copra	11.0 Million tonnes
Total 41.1 Million hectare	
☆ Production of vegetable oils	8.12 Million tonnes
☆ Demand of veg. oils (Edible)	16.7 Million tonnes
☆ Import of Veg.oil 2011-12 (Nov-Oct) (Edible)	9.4 Million tonnes
E)	
☆ Per capita consumption (2011) 13.5 Kg	
☆ Per capita consumption is rising by 3 to 4 per cent per annum.	

In the early eighties, India imported 20-40 per cent of its edible oil requirements. Finding this to be a huge drain on its foreign exchange resources, the government launched the 'Oilseeds Technology Mission' (OTM) in 1986 to increase the production of oilseeds. Oilseeds production gained momentum with improving yields with the launching of the Technology Mission on Oilseeds by the Government in 1986. The Mission covered 183 districts in major oilseed growing states. Subsequently, in 1991 this scheme was extended to few more potential districts.

The primary sources of edible oil in India at that time were nine oilseed crops, of which groundnut, rapeseed-mustard and soybean accounted for the bulk. Technology inputs from the OTM were aimed at obtaining higher productivity from the land under these crops. The government also maintained a stable market and price environment through market interventions and by managing imports. This provided the necessary encouragement to farmers to increase acreage under oilseed crops. Since oilseed crops were mainly grown in rain-fed areas, the focus on oilseeds benefited rain fed area farmers who had been otherwise shut out from the gains of the earlier 'green revolution'. As a result, India recorded a spectacular increase both in area under oilseeds as well as output.

As a result, the dependence on import of edible oil was reduced to the extent of hardly 5 per cent in 1995-96 (Singh, 2007). During the OTM period, oilseed area increased by 50 per cent and yield by 80 per cent. It was a period of innovations, in bringing new area under oilseeds, application of technologies, input supplies, output pricing, development programmes, support policies etc (Mruthyunjaya, 2007). All the above mentioned measures taken together under OTM led to a rising edible oil output and most importantly, a remarkable stability in oilseeds and oil production. India even became a major exporter of oilseed meal and castor oil during this period.

In the initial years of OTM, The National Dairy Development Board (NDDB) established a large network of oilseed cooperatives with storage and processing capabilities. The procurement of oilseeds was also done with the initiative of NDDB, which provided better price support for oilseed growers. This kind of support provided by NDDB was crucial for the success of OTM till mid nineties (Hegde, 2007).

If we look at the trends in area, production and productivity of annual oilseeds during 1951-2010, it shows a compound annual growth rate of 1.57 per cent, 3.01 per cent and 1.42 per cent respectively. Nearly 41.9 per cent of the increased oilseed production was contributed by area expansion and 58.1 per cent by productivity improvement during the period 1985–86 and 2009–10 (Tables 18.1 and 18.2).

Oilseed Sector - Share of India

Vegetable oil sector turnover	US$ 23.0 bn. (Rs.125, 000Cr)
☆ Import and export from oilseed sector	US$ 12.0 bn. (Rs.65, 000 Cr)
2011-12	
☆ In world's oilseed production	8.0 per cent
☆ In world's oilmeal production	6.8 per cent
☆ In world's oilmeal export	6.5 per cent
☆ In world's production of veg. oils	5.2 per cent
☆ In world's vegetable oil import	13.6 per cent
☆ In world's edible oil consumption	10 2 per cent

Table 18.1: All India Area, Production and Yield of Nine Oilseeds

Year	Area (m. hect)	Production (m. tonne)	Yield (kg/hect)	Under Irrigation Per cent Coverage
1951-52	11.69	5.03	430	NA
1952-53	11.18	4.73	424	0.8
1953-54	10.99	5.37	488	1.0
1954-55	12.52	6.40	511	1.1
1955-56	12.09	5.73	474	2.4
1956-57	12.49	6.36	509	2.7
1557-58	12.66	6.35	502	3.5
1958-59	13.00	7.30	561	3.2
1959-60	13.95	6.56	470	3.1
1960-61	13.77	6.98	507	3.3
1961-62	14.77	7.28	493	3.6
1962-63	15.34	7.39	482	3.3
1963-64	14.82	7.13	481	3.7
1964-65	15.26	8.56	561	3.4
1965-66	15.25	6.40	419	3.7
1966-67	15.00	6.43	428	5.1
1967-68	15.67	8.30	530	5.0
1968-69	14.47	6.85	473	4.8
1969-70	14.81	7.73	522	6.1
1970-71	16.64	9.63	579	7.4
1971-72	17.27	9.08	526	7.7
1972-73	15.79	7.14	452	7.2
1973-74	16.90	9.39	555	8.8
1974-75	17.31	9.15	529	9.2
1975-76	16.92	10.61	627	7.9
1976-77	16.47	8.43	512	7.6
1977-78	17.17	9.66	563	10.4
1978-79	17.71	10.10	570	11.0
1979-80	16.94	8.74	516	12.6
1980-81	17.60	9.37	532	14.5
1981-82	18.91	12.08	639	15.4
1982-83	17.76	10.00	563	15.6
1983-84	18.69	12.69	679	17.0
1984-85	18.92	12.95	684	19.6
1985-86	19.02	10.83	570	17.3
1986-87	18.63	11.27	605	17.9

Contd...

Table 18.1–*Contd...*

Year	*Area (m. hect)*	*Production (m. tonne)*	*Yield (kg/hect)*	*Under Irrigation Per cent Coverage*
1987-88	20.13	12.65	629	20.6
1988-89	21.90	18.03	824	22.3
1989-90	22.80	16.92	742	22.1
1990-91	24.15	18.61	771	22.9
1991-92	25.89	18.60	719	25.5
1992-93	25.24	20.11	797	24.1
1993-94	26.90	21.50	799	22.8
1994-95	25.30	21.34	843	25.0
1995-96	25.96	22.11	851	26.0
1996-97	26.34	24.38	926	26.3
1997-98	26.12	21.32	816	24.3
1998-99	26.23	24.75	944	23.2
1999-2000	24.28	20.72	853	25.2
2000-01	22.77	18.44	810	23.0
2001-02	22.64	20.66	913	24.3
2002-03	21.49	14.84	691	22.7
2003-04	23.66	25.19	1064	24.5
2004-05	27.52	24.35	885	26.6
2005-06	27.86	27.98	1004	28.0.
2006-07	26.51	24.29	916	28.3.
2007-08	26.69	29.76	1115	27.1
2008-09	27.56	27.72	1006	27.1
2009-10	25.96	24.88	958	25.9
2010-11	27.22	32.48	1193	
2011-12*	26.44	30.01	1135	

* 4th Advance estimates

Note: Data for 1950-51 to 1969-70 relate to total of five major oilseeds *viz.* groundnut, castorseed, sesamum, rapeseed and mustard and linseed. After 1969-70 data also 'included soybean, sunflower, Nigerseed and saflower

Source: Directorate of Economics and Statistics, -Ministry of Agriculture, Govt. of India

The production of 9 oilseeds fell from 27.72 million tones in 2008-09 to 24.88 million tones in 2009-10, but rose to 30.25 million tones in 2010-11. In the case of soybean, the increase in output was sharp from 9.79 million tones in 2009-10 to 12.59 million tones in 2010-11 (Table 18.2).

The domestic achievements in oilseeds production are unparalled as there is six times increase in oilseeds production during the period 1950–2011, achieved under predominantly rainfed (72 per cent) agro-ecological conditions and it is even higher than the production increase in total food grains during this period (Hegde, 2012). Major gain in production came mostly from soybean, rapeseed–mustard, sunflower and castor (Table 18.3, Figures 18.1 and 18.2). There has also been large regional variation in area, production and productivity changes during the last two and a half decades. Only a few states like Haryana, Madhya Pradesh, Maharashtra, Rajasthan and West Bengal increased their oilseeds production both through area expansion and productivity improvement. State like Gujarat increased oilseeds production mainly through productivity improvement. In a state like Punjab, oilseeds production declined mainly in response to a sharp decline in area, whereas in state like Odisha both area and productivity declined sharply leading to large decline in oilseeds production.

Table 18.2: *Kharif* Oilseed Area during 2012-13 and 2011-12

Oilseeds	*2012-13 Area Lac Ha.*	*2011-12 Area Lac Ha.*	*+/- against 2011-12*
Groundnut	35.30	43.00	-7.70
Soybean	107.00	103.00	4.00
Sunflower	2.30	2.80	-0.50
Sesameseed	13.30	16.30	-3.00
Nigerseed	1.90	2.80	-0.90
TOTAL	159.80	167.90	-8.10

Table 18.3: Oilseeds Production (Million Tones)

Oilseed	*2008-09*	*2009-10*	*2010-11*
Groundnut	7.17	5.43	7.09
Castor seed	1.17	1.01	1.31
Sesame	0.64	0.59	0.78
Nigerseed	0.12	0.10	0.12
Rapeseed and mustard	7.20	6.61	7.42
Linseed	0.17	0.15	0.14
Safflower	0.19	0.18	0.15
Soybean	9.91	9.97	12.59
Sunflower	1.16	0.85	0.67
Total	27.72	24.88	30.25

Fourth advance estimates as on April, 2011 (oil year is from Nov.-Oct)

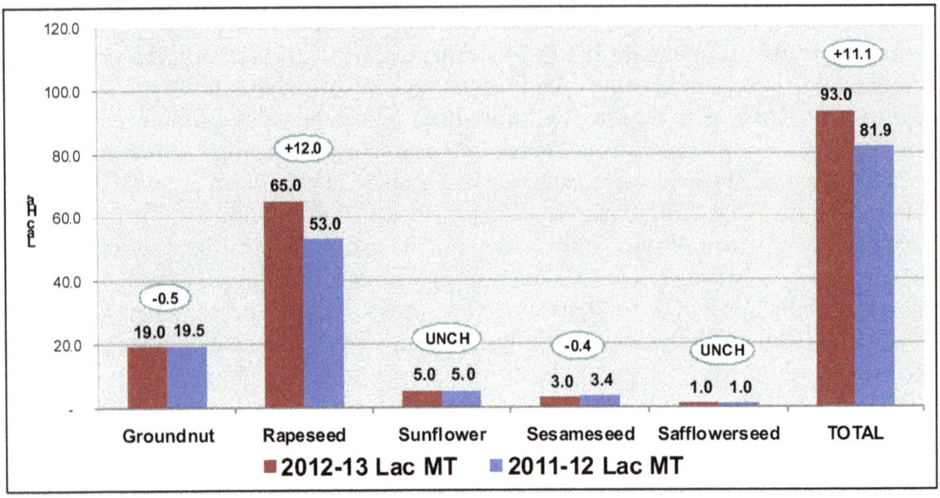

Figure 18.1: Estimate of *Rabi* Oilseed Crops during 2012-13 and Comparison with 2011-12.

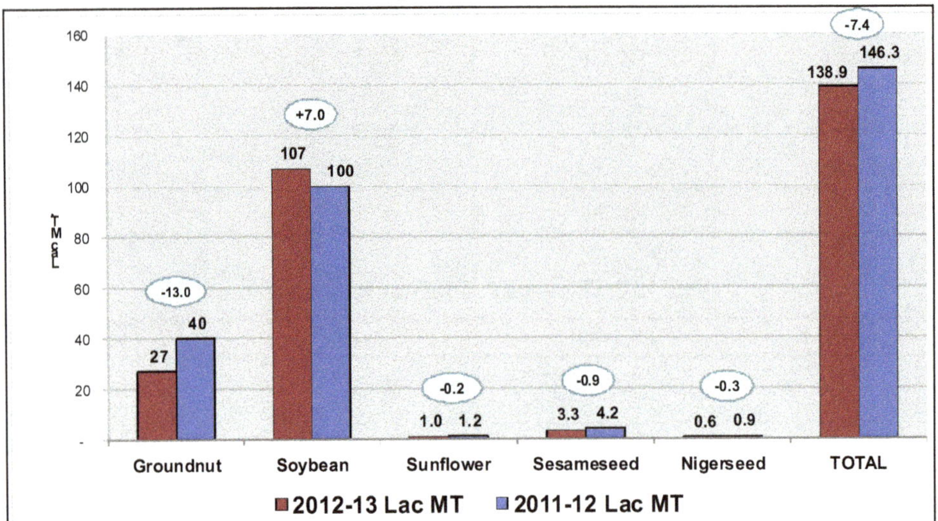

The *Kharif* Oilseeds crops may decreased by around 7.5 Lac MT during 2012-13 against 2011-12.

Soybean Crop may increases by 7.0 Lac T & GN Crop may decrease by 13 Lac T.

Figure 18.2: Estimate of *Kharif* Oilseed Crops during 2012-13 and Comparison with 2011-12.

Estimates and forecast for total oilseeds production during 2011-12 and 2012-13 are depicted in Table 18.4.

Table 18. 4: Estimates and Forecast for Total Oilseeds Production during 2010-11-2012-2013

Oilseeds ('000 metric tons)	*MY 2010/11*	*MY 2011/12*	*MY 2012/13*
	Revised	*Estimate*	*Forecast*
Beginning Stocks	3,425	1,740	1,302
Production	34,857	35,352	36,302
MY Imports	0	0	0
Total Supply	38,282	37,092	37,604
MY Exports	597	510	565
Crush	29,365	28,540	29,135
Food Use Dom. Cons.	1,710	1,760	1,910
Feed Waste Dom. Cons.	4,870	4,980	4,850
Total Dom. Cons.	35,945	35,280	35,895
Ending Stocks	1,740	1,302	1,144
Total Distribution	38,282	37,092	37,604

Source: Global Agricultural Information Network. USDA Agricultural Service.

Favourable weather and strong MY 2012/13 oilseed prices encouraged farmers to plant an additional 300,000 hectares, bringing the total oilseed area to 8.1 million hectares. Edible oil imports are expected to increase 11.3 percent to 10.1 million tons to meet rising demand for vegetable oils (USDA. Foreign Agricultural Service Gain Report, Feb., 2013).

The total area under oilseed cultivation in India is estimated to increase from 22 lakh hectare in 2001-02 to 30 lakh hectare in 2015-16, while average yield is likely to increase from 90 kg per ha to 100 kg per ha during the period. The total oilseed production is likely to increase to 50 lakh metric tons, according to the May 2012 report of the Asso-Com Grain Conference.

Area, Production and Yield Under Major Oilseed Crops

Mustard

Mustard seed is the second largest produced oilseed *i.e.* next to soybean in the world and. plays a significant role in total vegetable oil pool. It is the third leading source of edible oil after palm and soy oils. The global consumption of mustard seed has grown at 4.13 per cent CAGR in the past two decades and is currently 63.37 million tones (2011-12). China is the largest consumer, accounting for a 26 per cent share in global consumption, followed by Canada and India, with 11 per cent each. With respect to the consumption of mustard oil, Canada accounts for only 3 per cent share. However, 85 percent of the Canadian mustard oil production is exported globally, making it the world's largest exporter.

Mustard seed yields around 38 per cent oil, while the remaining 62 per cent is converted into cake, which is used as cattle feed. Being an important source of edible oil and protein meal, the world production of mustard seed has grown at a significant pace. The World production of rapeseed/mustard oilseed during 2012 was as under (Table 18.5):

Table 18.5: World Production of Rapeseed/Mustard Oilseed

Rank	*Country*	*Production (tones)*
1	Canada	186,400
2	Nepal	149,625
3	Ukraine	64,400
4	Myanmar	58,300
5	Russian Federation	36,410

Source: FAOSTAT Database 2012.

In India, mustard seed is the third largest produced oilseed after soy bean and groundnut. It is grown as a rabi crop, which is sowed during October-December and the harvesting begins from February onwards. The largest mustard seed producing states in India are Rajasthan (45 per cent), Haryana (13 per cent), Madhya Pradesh (13 per cent) and Uttar Pradesh (11 per cent). In Table 18.6, state-wise contribution and area covered for rapeseed and mustard have been depicted.

Table 18.6: State-Wise Contribution of Production and Area Covered (per cent) for Rapeseed and Mustard (2010-11)

State	*Area (Hectare)*	*Production (in tones)*	*Per cent Area Covered*	*Per cent of Production Contribution*
Andhra Pradesh	6922	16777	100	100
Assam	242815	142661	100	100
Chhattisgarh	48861	19974	100	100
Gujarat	222700	349200	100	100
HP	9363	4957	100	100
Maharashtra	7700	2860	100	100
Nagaland	22470	22490	100	100
Orissa	15925	3343	100	100
Punjab	29000	39000	100	100
Sikkim	5260	4164	100	100
UP	600714	714257	100	100

Source: Ministry of Agriculture, GOI.

Coming back to Indian scenario of mustard seed production in India, it is likely to increase acreage to 52.24 lakh ha against 50.68 lakh ha (Solvent Extractors Association of India) in future. Government estimates 81.93 lakh ton production of rape seed and mustard production for 2012 -13.

As per Annual Report of USDA (Feb., 2013), rapeseed-mustard planting increased 140,000 hectares to 6.7 million hectares. An increase in the Minimum Support Price (MSP) for rapeseed-mustard by Rs 500 to Rs 3,000 a quintal for the 2013-14 marketing season encouraged higher planting. Based on the initial crop assessment for marketing year (MY) 2012/13, rapeseed-mustard production is expected to reach 6.8 million tons, an increase of 600,000 tons from the previous year (Table 18.7, USDA Foreign Agricultural Service Gain Report, Feb., 2013)

Table 18.7: Production of Rapeseed during 2010-2013

Oilseed, Rapeseed India	*2010/2011*		*2011/2012*		*2012/2013*		
	Market Year Begin: Oct 2010		*Market Year Begin: Oct 2011*		*Market Year Begin: Oct 2012*		
	USDA Official	*New Post*	*USDA Official*	*New Post*	*USDA Official*	*New Post*	
Area Planted	7250	7250	6700	6600	7000	6730	(1000HA)
Area Harvested	7250	7250	6700	6600	7000	6730	(1000HA)
Beginning Stocks	1180	1620	729	1060	354	778	(1000MT)
Production	7100	7100	6500	6,700	6700	7,100	(1000MT)
MY Imports	0	12	0	20	0	20	(1000MT)
My Imp. from U.S.	0	0	0	0	0	0	(1000MT)
MY Imp. from EU	0	0	0	0	0	0	(1000MT)
Total Supply	8280	8732	7229	7280	7054	7598	(1000MT)
MY Exports	0	2	0	2	0	2	(1000MT)
MY Exp. to EU	0	0	0	0	0	0	(1000MT)
Crush	6800	6800	6100	5,600	6000	6000	(1000MT)
Food Use Dom. Cons.	540	610	560	630	580	660	(1000MT)
Feed Waste Dom. Cons.	211	260	215	270	220	270	(1000MT)
Total Dom. Cons.	7551	7670	6875	6500	6800	6930	(1000MT)
Ending Stocks	729	1060	354	778	254	666	(1000MT)
Total Distribution	8280	8732	7229	7280	7054	7598	(1000MT)
CY Imports	0	0	0	0	0	0	(1000MT)
CY Imp. from U.S.	0	0	0	0	0	0	(1000MT)
CY Exports	0	0	0	0	0	0	(1000MT)
CY Exp. to U.S.	0	0		0		0	(1000MT)
TS=TD		0		0		0	

Source: Annual Report. Feb., 2013. Gain Report. Global Agricultural Information Network. USDA Agricultural Service.

Table 18.8: Production of Rapeseed Oil during 2010-2013

Oilseed, Rapeseed India	2010/2011 Market Year Begin: Oct 2010		2011/2012 Market Year Begin: Oct 2011		2012/2013 Market Year Begin: May2012		
	USDA Official	New Post	USDA Official	New Post	USDA Official	New Post	
Crush	6,800	6,800	6,100	5,600	6,000	6,000	(1000MT)
Extr. Rate, 999.9999	0	0.3937	0	0.4107	0	0.41	(Per cent)
Beginning Stocks	0	0	260	237	233	185	(1000MT)
Production	2,575	2,677	2,310	2,300	2,270	2,460	(1000MT)
MY Imports	5	16	98	0	30	0	(1000MT)
MY Imp. from U.S.	0	0	0	0	0	0	(1000MT)
MY Imp. from EU	0	0	0	0	0	0	(1000MT)
Total Supply	2,580	2,693	2,668	2,537	2,533	2,645	(1000MT)
MY Exports	20	2	10	2	10	2	(1000MT)
MY Exp. to EU	0	0	0	0	0	0	(1000

Source: Annual Report. Feb., 2013. Gain Report. Global Agricultural Information Network. USDA Agricultural Service.

Groundnut

Groundnut (*Arachis hypogea* L.) is believed to be native to South America and the Caribbean. The plant was introduced by the Portuguese into Africa, from where it was introduced into North America. It came to India during the first half of the 16th century from one of the Pacific islands of China, where it was introduced earlier from either Central or South America.

Developing countries account for 96 per cent of the global groundnut area and 92 per cent of the global production. Asia accounts for 58 per cent of the global groundnut area and 67 per cent of the groundnut production with an annual growth rate of 1.28 per cent for area, 2 per cent for production and 0.71 per cent for productivity.

World peanut production totals approximately 35.7 million tons during 2011, with India being the world's second largest producer after China (Table 18.9). For India, Gujarat accounts to 36 per cent of total production of groundnut. Indonesia is the major importer of groundnut from India with a 41 per cent share of Indian exports.

Groundnut is the single largest source of edible oils in India and constitutes roughly about 50 per cent of the total oilseeds production. Groundnut cultivation has increased from 6.8 million hectare from 1980-81 to 8 million hectare in the recent year. Area under groundnut cultivation has been depicted in Figures 18.3 and 18.4. Groundnut is mainly grown in five states, Andhra Pradesh, Gujarat, Tamil-Nadu, Karnataka and Maharashtra and together they account for more than 90 percent of the crop's total area (Table 18.10). The states Andhra Pradesh and Gujarat, account for more than half of the cultivated area. Andhra Pradesh and Gujarat State share 28 and 24 percent of the total groundnut area, respectively, in the country. Tamil Nadu and Karnataka share about 15 per cent each of the total cultivated area. About 8 per cent of the total groundnut area in the country is in the State of Maharashtra. Among the major groundnut growing states, (Andhra Pradesh and Gujarat), there has been consistent increase in area under groundnut cultivation in Andhra Pradesh. However in both the adjoining States of Gujarat and Maharashtra, the area under groundnut has shown continuous decreasing trend (Figures 18.3 and 18.4).

Table 18.9: World Groundnut Production in 2010-11

Country	*Area (000ha)*	*Production (000 MT)*	*Yield (kg/ha)*
China	5125	13,448	2623
India	8000	7500	938
Indonesia	683	1377	2016
Myanmar	730	730	1270
Pakistan	100	106	1060
Thailand	132	132	1517
Vietnam	240	400	1665

Table 18.10: State-Wise Groundnut Production in 2011-12

States	*2011-12 ('000 tones)*	*2010-11 ('000 tones)*	*Per cent Change*
Gujarat	17.75	18.7	-5.08
AP	5.5	6	-8.33
Tamil Nadu	3.5	2	75 per cent
Maharashtra	1.8	2	-10 per cent
Madhya Pradesh	1.8	1.5	20 per cent
Punjab, Haryana and UP	0.8	0.8	-
Others	10.6	10	6 per cent
India (total, with shell)	41.75	41	1.83 per cent

* Estimated.

Table 18.11 depicts the trend in growth rate in production of groundnuts in India from 1973-2012. Production increased from 5 million tones in 1980- 91 to 8.06 million tones during the year 1994-95. From 1993-94 onwards the production of groundnut is fluctuating between 7 to 9 million tones indicating the fluidity of production trends in groundnuts. The growth rate in production of groundnut recorded remarkable decrease during the year 2011-12 (Figure 18.5).

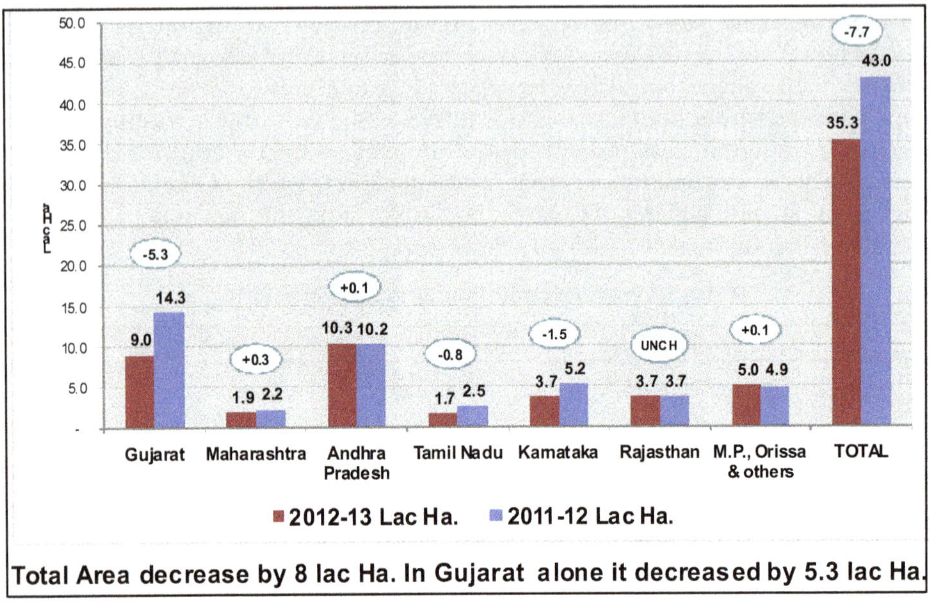

Figure 18.3: State-wise Groundnut Area

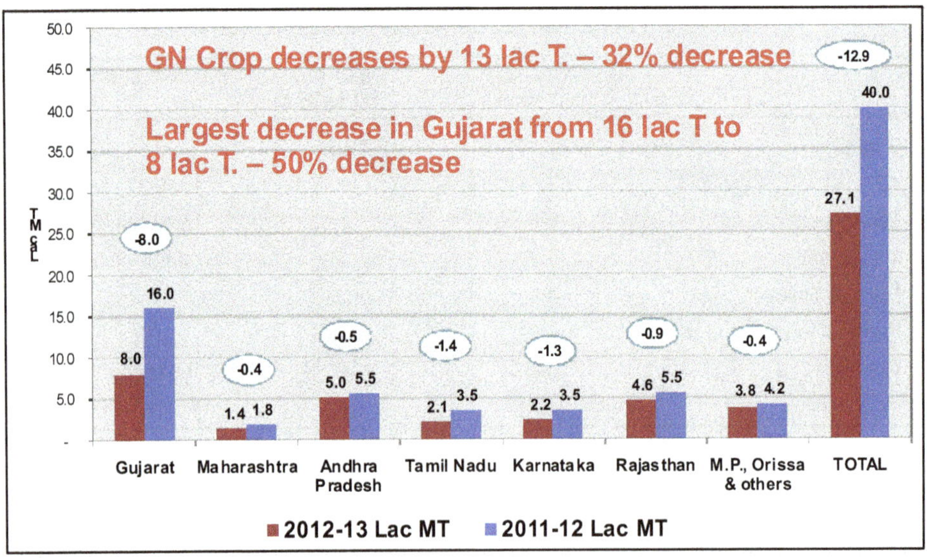

Figure 18.4: State-wise Groundnut Crop during 2012-13 and Comparison with 2011-12

The production of groundnut has been lowest during the recent years. This has been mainly due to the other oilseeds crops like soybean and sunflower gradually replaced this important oilseed crop. The production of groundnut has been declined mainly due to decrease in acreage under the crop.

Table 18.11: Trend in Growth Rate in Production of Groundnuts in India (1973-2012)

Market Year	*Production (1000 MT)*	*Growth Rate*
1972	1060	NA
1973	1242	17.17 per cent
1974	1310	5.48 per cent
1975	1491	13.82 per cent
1976	1319	-11.54 per cent
1977	1366	3.56 per cent
1978	1441	5.49 per cent
1979	1339	-7.08 per cent
1980	1177	-12.10 per cent
1981	1615	37.21 per cent
1982	1281	-20.68 per cent
1983	1608	25.53 per cent
1984	1520	-5.47 per cent
1985	1221	-19.67 per cent
1986	1360	11.38 per cent
1987	1363	0.22 per cent
1988	2080	52.60 per cent
1989	1882	-9.52 per cent
1990	1740	-7.55 per cent
1991	1655	-4.89 per cent
1992	2030	22.66 per cent
1993	1770	-12.81 per cent
1994	1910	7.91 per cent
1995	1700	-10.99 per cent
1996	2108	24.00 per cent
1997	1754	-16.79 per cent
1998	1675	-4.50 per cent
1999	1357	-18.99 per cent
2000	1420	4.64 per cent
2001	1901	33.87 per cent
2002	1360	-28.46 per cent
2003	1874	37.79 per cent
2004	1748	-6.72 per cent
2005	1557	-10.93 per cent
2006	1315	-15.54 per cent
2007	1675	27.38 per cent
2008	1545	-7.76 per cent
2009	1165	-24.60 per cent
2010	1300	11.59 per cent
2011	1165	-10.38 per cent
2012	1190	2.15 per cent

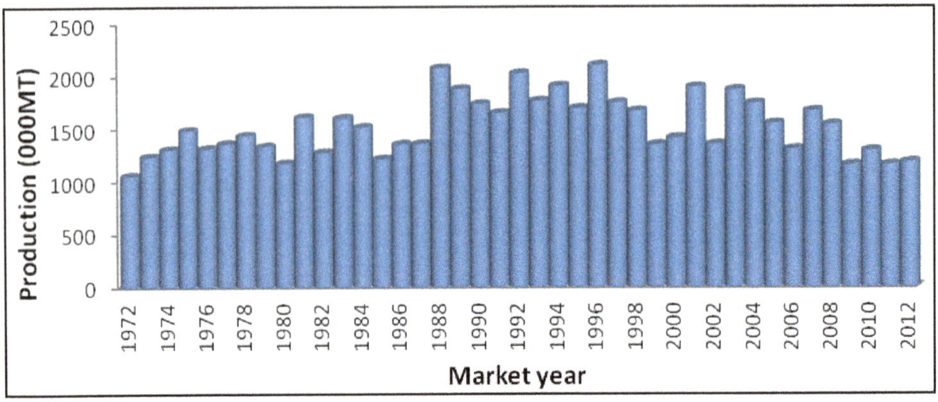

Figure 18.5: Trend in Growth Rate in Production of Groundnuts in India (1973-2012)
***Source*: USDA.**

The USDA forecasts India's 2012/13 peanut production at 4.95 million tones, down 0.85 million or 14.7 percent from last month and down 10 percent from last year. The area is forecast at 5.0 million hectares, down 0.6 million from last month or 11 percent, and down 0.3 million or 6 percent from last year. The yield is forecast at 0.99 tones per hectare, down 5 percent from last month and from last year. The dry soil moisture conditions coupled with hot temperatures in most peanut producing regions in Gujarat, Maharashtra and Madhya Pradesh are raising concerns about the 2012-13 area and yield prospects (Table 18.12, FAS/USDA, Feb. 2013).

According to Indian Oilseed and Produce Export Promotion Council (IOPEPC), India's ground nut production for 2012-13 is expected to be higher on the back of increased production in Gujarat at around 459,000 tons, pulling the price of the commodity in the domestic lower, This rise in production is higher by 56 per cent than last year's 294,000 tons. With the higher arrivals of ground nuts, prices have declined by Rs 60-70 per 20 kg to Rs 900-1050 per 20 kg. The higher arrivals and lower price is likely to relive the pressure over the mills as the most of the mills in the country were on the verge of closing down.

The current productivity of groundnut is more than a tonne per hectare. During the year 1993-94 it was only 934 kg per hectare. The productivity of groundnut in India is deplorable low mainly because of 80 percent of the crop is grown under rainfed conditions. Among different states producing groundnut, Tamil Nadu tops the list with 1500 kg/ha, which is half quintal more than the all India average (Kaushik, 1993). The decrease in productivity due to droughts and or insufficient monsoon rains during the pods formation *i.e.* September has also badly affected the production level of the crop during the period under study (Table 18.13). The other reasons for the fluctuations and variations in acreage and production of groundnut were price and non-price incentives announced by the Government from time to time for other competitive and short duration varieties of oilseeds crops such as soybean, sunflower and safflower crops. The future strategy for development of this crop should be centered on increasing productivity through introduction of short duration and

Table 18.12: Production of Peanut Oilseed

Oilseed, Peanut India	*2010/2011*		*2011/2012*		*2012/2013*		
	Market Year Begin: Oct 2010		*Market Year Begin: Oct 2011*		*Market Year Begin: Oct 2012*		
	USDA Official	*New Post*	*USDA Official*	*New Post*	*USDA Official*	*New Post*	
Area Planted	6,100	5,900	5,300	5,300	5,000	4900	(1000 HA)
Area Harvested	6,000	5,900	5,300	5,300	5,000	4900	(1000 HA)
Beginning Stocks	108	65	174	45	99	95	(1000 MT)
Production	5,850	5,500	5,500	5,500	5,000	4,650	(1000 MT)
MY Imports	0	0	0	0	0	0	(1000 MT)
My Imp. from U.S.	0	0	0	0	0	0	(1000 MT)
MY Imp. from EU	0	0	0	0	0	0	(1000 MT)
Total Supply	5,958	5,565	5,674	5,545	5,099	4,745	(1000 MT)
MY Exports	864	550	1,050	450	427	375	(1000 MT)
MY Exp. to EU	23	1	20	1	20	2	(1000 MT)
Crush	3,900	3,950	3,500	4,000	3,575	3,450	(1000 MT)
Food Use Dom. Cons.	620	600	625	580	615	450	(1000 MT)
Feed Waste Dom. Cons.	400	420	400	420	400	350	(1000 MT)
Total Dom. Cons.	4,920	4,970	4,525	5,000	4,590	4,250	(1000 MT)
Ending Stocks	174	45	99	95	82	120	(1000 MT)
Total Distribution	5,958	5,565	5,674	5,545	5,099	4,745	(1000 MT)
CY Imports	0		0	0	0	0	(1000 MT)
CY Imp. from U.S.	0		0	0	0	0	(1000 MT)
CY Exports	975	385	800	535	425	500	(1000 MT)
CY Exp. to U.S.	0	0	0	0	0	0	(1000 MT)
TS=TD		0		0		0	

Source: USDA Gain Report (Feb., 2013). Global Agricultural Information Network. USDA Agricultural Service.

drought resistant varieties through expansion of area under irrigation of provision of life saving irrigation during the dry spell of rainy season (Patil *et al.*, 2009).

The oil content of the seed varies from 44 to 50 per cent, depending on the varieties and agronomic conditions. Groundnut oil is edible and extensively used as a cooking medium, both as refined oil and vanaspati. According to USDA estimates, groundnut oil production is likely to be 1,173, 000 MT (Table 18.14).

In April, 2012, the price of ground nut oil in the domestic market rose to record heights of Rs 2100-2110 per tin though demand was lower due to lower availability of the commodity. The demand for the oil dipped due to higher prices. The consumers switched over to other oils like cotton seed oil, soy oil etc.

Table 18.13: Area, Production and Productivity Of Groundnut In Maharashtra State (1993-94 To 2006-07)

Sl.No.	Year	Areas in '00' ha.	Production '00' tones	Productivity Kg/ha.
1.	1993-94	5105	5123	1004
2.	1994-95	4740	4137	873
3.	1995-96	4229	4635	1096
4.	1996-97	4401	5578	1267
5.	1997-98	4167	4200	1008
6.	1998-99	4077	4746	1164
7.	1999-00	4065	3862	950
8.	2000-01	4037	3605	893
9.	2001-02	3725	3503	848
10.	2002-03	3509	3363	958
11.	2003-04	3241	3552	1096
12.	2004-05	3466	3588	1035
13.	2005-06	3367	2748	831
14.	2006-07	3416	2541	744

Source: 2009. B.N.Patil, Dr. S. R. Bhonde, D.N.Khandikar 2009. Trends in Area, Production and Productivity of Groundnut in Maharashtra. Financing agriculture. A National J. Agri and Rural Dev. (March-April issue 35-39).

Soybean

Soybean is the world's foremost provider of protein and oil. India is the fifth largest soybean producing country in the world after the US, Brazil, Argentina, and China (Table 18.15). India harvested about 9.8 million metric tones of soybean in 2011against the world annual production of 263.59 million metric tones (FAO, 2011). India is the third largest importer of soy oil in the world. India is one of the major exporters of soy meal to the Asian countries.

Soybean is the third largest oilseed crop in India next only to groundnut and rapeseed/mustard seed. It accounts for 25 per cent of the total oilseeds produced in the country in a year. It contributes about 13.3 lakh tones of oil (about 16 per cent) out of 82 lakh tones of vegetable oil currently produced in the country.

In India soybean is grown exclusively during the *kharif* (southwest monsoon season) under rain fed conditions. The ideal sowing window is early to mid-June and typically commences with the arrival of the monsoon. The harvesting of soybean in India commences around September and October. It is highly dependent on rain and a change in the rainfall pattern affects the production of soybean. The average size of soybean farm in our country is less than 2 hectares. The productivity is one third of the US or Brazilian farms. Indian soybean farmers are competing with the most efficient oil seed farmers in the world.

Table 18.14: Production of Peanut Oil

Oilseed, Peanut India	2010/2011 Market Year Begin: Oct 2010		2011/2012 Market Year Begin: Oct 2011		2012/2013 Market Year Begin: Oct 2012		
	USDA Official	New Post	USDA Official	New Post	USDA Official	New Post	
Crush	3,900	3,950	3,500	4,000	3,575	3,450	(1000 MT)
Extr. Rate, 999.9999	0.	0.3357	0.	0.3355	0.	0.34	(PERCENT)
Beginning Stocks	10	38	50	49	35	32	(1000 MT)
Production	1,300	1,326	1,165	1,342	1,190	1,173	(1000 MT)
MY Imports	0	0	0	0	0	0	(1000 MT)
MY Imp. from U.S.	0	0	0	0	0	0	(1000 MT)
MY Imp. from EU	0	0	0	0	0	0	(1000 MT)
Total Supply	1,310	1,364	1,215	1,391	1,225	1,205	(1000 MT)
MY Exports	4	4	20	2	0	10	(1000 MT)
MY Exp. to EU	0	0	0	0	0	0	(1000 MT)
Industrial Dom. Cons.	15	15	10	10	10	10	(1000 MT)
Food Use Dom.Cons.	1,241	1,296	1,150	1,347	1,200	1,050	(1000 MT)
Feed Waste Dom.Cons.	0	0	0	0	0	0	(1000 MT)
Total Dom. Cons.	1,256	1,311	1,160	1,357	1,210	1,060	(1000 MT)
Ending Stocks	50	49	35	32	15	135	(1000 MT)
Total Distribution	1,310	1,364	1,215	1,391	1,225	1,205	(1000 MT)
CY Imports	0	0	0	0	0	0	(1000 MT)
CY Imp. from U.S.	0	0	0	0	0	0	(1000 MT)
CY Exports	6	0	20	0	0	0	(1000 MT)
CY Exp. to U.S.	0	0	0	0	0	0	(1000 MT)
TS=TD		0		0		0	

Source: USDA Gain Report (Feb., 2013). Global Agricultural Information Network. USDA Agricultural Service.

Even though India's share in the world's total area under soybean is about one percent at present, development as well as the expansion of this crop in the country during the past years is rated as one of the striking occurrences in the agricultural development process. Soybean cultivation in India has steadily increased. It was a minor crop during the early 1970s but at present, it occupies third place in the oilseed production in India. Soybean experienced rapid development in terms of area and production expansion within a limited period. The area under soybean rapidly increased from 0.03 million ha in 1970 to 2.6 million ha in 1990 and to 5.7 million ha in 2000 (Directorate of Economics and Statistics, Government of India, 2012). Increased soybean production is mainly driven by increased area sown to the crop. Trends in growth rate of annual soybean production during 1970-2012 have been depicted in Table 18.15 and Figure 18.6. The progress in soybean production is most impressive, however, these growth figures belie the fact that the productivity continues to remain low and major steps are required to enhance production by increasing productivity rather than increasing area under the crop. The average soybean productivity for India has hovered around 1 t ha-1 during 1983–2000.

Table 18.15: India Soybean Oilseed Production by Year

Market Year	Production (1000 MT)	Growth Rate
1964	0	NA
1969	11	NA
1970	18	63.64 per cent
1971	20	11.11 per cent
1972	25	25.00 per cent
1973	30	20.00 per cent
1974	35	16.67 per cent
1975	70	100.00 per cent
1976	150	114.29 per cent
1977	180	20.00 per cent
1978	220	22.22 per cent
1979	350	59.09 per cent
1980	442	26.29 per cent
1981	467	5.66 per cent
1982	491	5.14 per cent
1983	614	25.05 per cent
1984	955	55.54 per cent
1985	1020	6.81 per cent
1986	891	-12.65 per cent
1987	898	0.79 per cent
1988	1547	72.27 per cent
1989	1806	16.74 per cent
1990	2602	44.08 per cent
1991	2492	-4.23 per cent
1992	3106	24.64 per cent
1993	4000	28.78 per cent
1994	3236	-19.10 per cent
1995	4476	38.32 per cent
1996	4100	-8.40 per cent
1997	5350	30.49 per cent

Contd...

Table 18.15–*Contd...*

Market Year	*Production (1000 MT)*	*Growth Rate*
1998	6000	12.15 per cent
1999	5200	-13.33 per cent
2000	5250	0.96 per cent
2001	5400	2.86 per cent
2002	4000	-25.93 per cent
2003	6800	70.00 per cent
2004	5850	-13.97 per cent
2005	7000	19.66 per cent
2006	7690	9.86 per cent
2007	9470	23.15 per cent
2008	9100	-3.91 per cent
2009	9700	6.59 per cent
2010	9800	1.03 per cent
2011	11000	12.24 per cent
2012	11500	4.55 per cent

In addition to the rapidity of this expansion, soybean development in India involves another facet: selectivity in its spread. The rise of M.P. as a soy state presents a concrete representation of this selective development, while Maharashtra presents another contrasting situation wherein a sudden boom was followed by an immediate extinction of the crop. Out of 814 thousand hectares under soybean in the country during 1983-84, about 616 thousand hectares were in the state of Madhya Pradesh in Central India. In fact, this state increased its area share from 24 percent in 1971-72 to

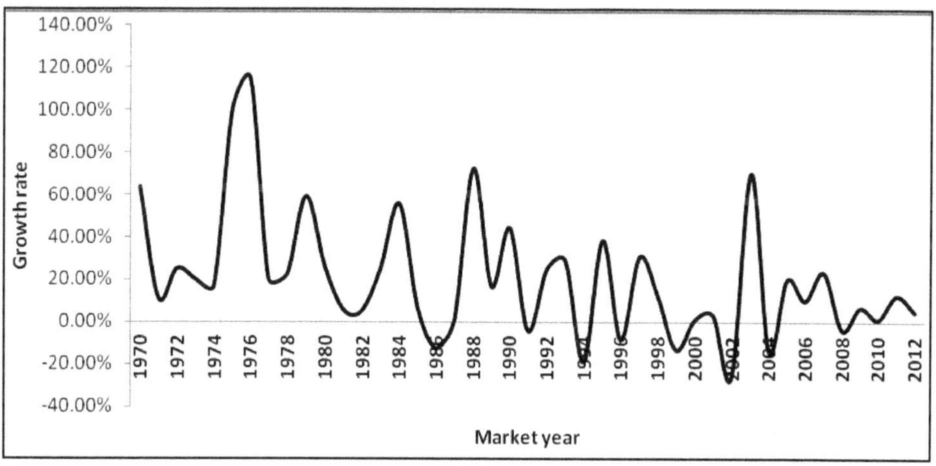

Figure 18.6: Annual Growth Rate of Soybean Oilseed Production (1970-2012) in India

***Source*: USDA**

about 77 per cent in 1983-84 of total area under soybean in the country. The concentrated selective developmental pattern of this crop is even more evident when we observe that 11 out of 45 districts in the state of Madhya Pradesh had an area share of 80 percent of the total soybean area of the state. The state of Madhya Pradesh experienced a 38-fold increase- in area and a similar increase in production during the period 1972–1983; Uttar Pradesh increased its area and production 10 and 8 times, respectively, while Maharashtra's soybean crop had become insignificant by 1983.

Madhya Pradesh is known as the soybean bowl of India, contributing 59 per cent of the country's soybean production, followed by Maharashtra with 29 per cent contribution and Rajasthan with a 6 per cent contribution (Figure 18.7). Andhra Pradesh, Karnataka, Chhattisgarh and other parts of India also produce the bean in small quantities. Rajasthan Government in its advance estimate had estimated the record area of soybean at 8.97 lakh hectares and production at 13.85 lakh tones in 2011-12. During the same period the area under soybean was 9.33 million hectares with a production of 10.5 million tones in India.

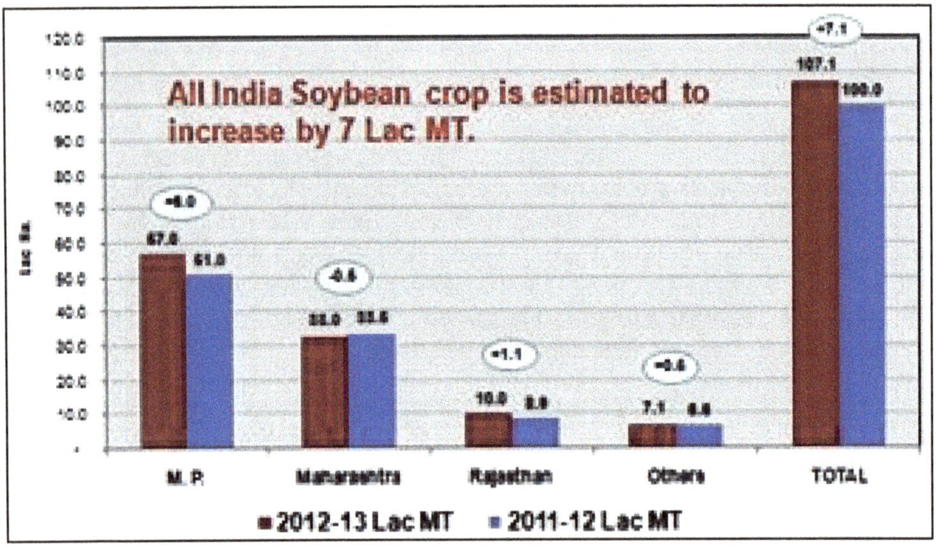

Figure 18.7: Estimates of State-wise Soybean Crop during 2012-13 and Comparison with 2011-12

Extensive Survey was undertaken by Soybean Processors Association of India (SOPA) along with other associate agencies in major districts of three Soybean Producing States of Madhya Pradesh, Maharashtra and Rajasthan as per the standard norms laid down by the Ministry of Agriculture, Government of India and its estimates for area, yield and production of soybean during 2011-12 were given (Table 18.16).

Despite increased acreage under soybean for 2012-13, the delay in monsoon rains across India has raised concern over the crop production (FAOSTAT, 2012). In India, both top two soybean producing states *i.e.* Madhya Pradesh and Maharashtra

Table 18.16: Area (Lakh Ha), Yield (kg/Ha) and Production (Lakh MT) of Soybean during 2011-12 in Various States of India

State	Kharif 2011			Kharif 2012		
	Area Sown	Yield	Production	Area Sown	Yield	Production
Madhya Pradesh	57.300	1076	61.666	58.128	1150	66.850
Maharashtra	30.613	1163	35.609	32.130	1243	39.950
Rajasthan	8.964	1393	12.489	9.870	1249	12.326
Andhra Pradesh	1.550	1050	1.628	1.950	1113	2.170
Karnataka	2.170	1070	2.322	2.000	1103	2.206
Chhattisgarh	1.500	1025	1.538	1.520	1155	1.756
Gujarat	-	-	-	0.830	1103	0.915
Rest of India	1.241	1010	1.253	0.520	1155	0.601
Total All India	103.338	1127	116.504	106.948	1185	126.775

Source: The Soybean Processors Association of India.

have so far received below average rains. India's soybean acreage is likely to rise by 7 per cent in 2012-13 (Tables 18.17 and 18.18). India is likely to produce 11.5 million metric tones against world production of 268 million metric tones in 2012-13. Globally, the availability of soybean is under concern over the bad weather condition especially in U.S, major exporter of the commodity (USDA, 2012).

Likewise soybeans, the rate of production of soy meal in India is on an increasing level with a production figure of 5 million tons. Soy oil is considered as one of the most important edible oil in the country. Indian production of soy oil is around 1 million tones annually and it accounts for about 18 per cent of total consumption of oils in the country. Trends in soyoil production and growth rate over the last about 45 years have been depicted in Figure 18.8.

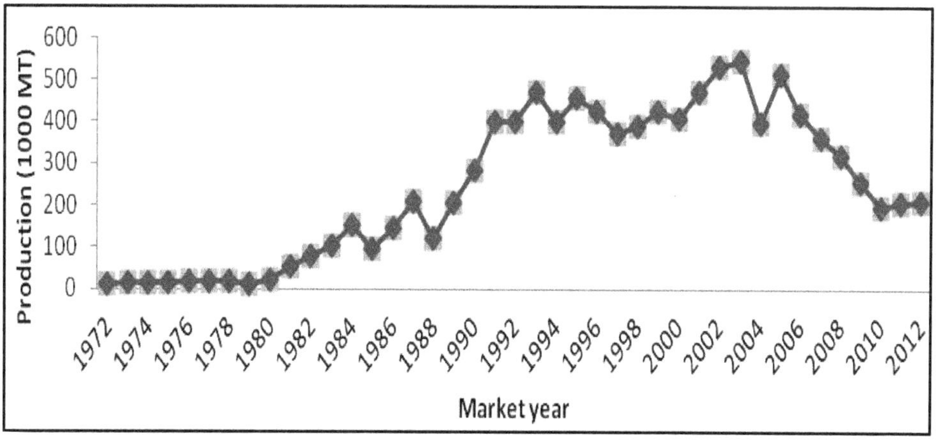

Figure 18.8: Trends in Production and Growth Rate of Soybean Oil in India (1972-2012)

***Source*: USDA**

Table 18.17: Soybean–Area, Yield and Production

Country/Region	*Area (Million hectares)*				*Yield (Metric tons per hectare)*				*Production (Million metric tons)*				*Change in Production*	
			2012/13 Proj.				*2012/13 Proj.*				*2012/13 Proj.*		*From last year*	
	2010/11	*Prel. 2011/12*	*Feb*	*Mar*	*2010/11*	*Prel. 2011/12*	*Feb*	*Mar*	*2010/11*	*Prel. 2011/12*	*Feb*	*Mar*	*MMT*	*Per cent*
World	103	102.9	108.9	108.75	2.56	2.32	2.47	2.46	263.59	238.73	269.5	268	29.27	12.26
United States	31	29.86	30.8	30.8	2.92	2.82	2.66	2.66	90.61	84.19	82.06	82.06	-2.14	-2.54
Brazil	24.2	25	27.5	27.5	3.11	2.66	3.04	3.04	75.3	66.5	83.5	83.5	17	25.56
Argentina	18.3	17.58	19.5	19.35	2.68	2.28	2.72	2.66	49	40.1	53	51.5	11.4	28.43
Paraguay	2.87	2.96	3.1	3.1	2.48	1.47	2.5	2.5	7.13	4.36	7.75	7.75	3.39	77.87
Bolivia	1.03	1.09	1.09	1.09	2.24	2.13	2.2	2.2	2.3	2.32	2.4	2.4	0.08	3.45
Uruguay	0.87	0.9	0.95	0.95	1.79	1.78	2	2	1.55	1.6	1.9	1.9	0.3	18.75
China	8.52	7.89	7.2	7.2	1.77	1.84	1.75	1.75	15.1	14.48	12.6	12.6	-1.88	-12.98
India	9.3	10.27	10.8	10.8	1.05	1.07	1.06	1.06	9.8	11	11.5	11.5	0.5	4.55

Source: FAOSTAT, 2012.

Table 18.18: Production of Soybean Oilseed

	2010/2011		2011/2012		2012/2013		
	Market Year Begin: Oct 2010		Market Year Begin: Oct 2011		Market Year Begin: Oct 2012		
	USDA Official	New Post	USDA Official	New Post	USDA Official	New Post	
Area Planted	9,300	9,300	10,300	10,270		10,600	(1000 HA)
Area Harvested	9,300	9,300	10,270	10,270		10,600	(1000 HA)
Beginning Stocks	1,695	1,695	600	630		460	(1000 MT)
Production	9,800	9,800	11,000	11,000		11,500	(1000 MT)
MY Imports	0	0	0	0		0	(1000 MT)
My Imp. from U.S.	0	0	0	0		0	(1000 MT)
My Imp. from EU	0	0	0	0		0	(1000 MT)
Total Supply	11,495	11,495	11,600	11,630		11,960	(1000 MT)
MY Exports	10	15	10	20		20	(1000 MT)
MY Exp. to EU	0	0	0	0		0	(1000 MT)
Crush	9,600	9,400	9,800	9,600		9,900	(1000 MT)
Food Use Dom. Cons.	480	500	500	550		600	(1000 MT)
Feed Waste Dom, Cons.	805	950	900	1,000		1,050	(1000 MT)
Total Dom. Cons.	10,885	10,850	11,200	11,150		11,550	(1000 MT)
Ending Stocks	600	630	390	460		390	(1000 MT)
Total Distribution	11,495	11,495	11,600	11,630		11,960	(1000 MT)
CY Imports	0	0	0	0		0	(1000 MT)
CY Imp. from U.S.	0	0	0	0		0	(1000 MT)
CY Exports	10	0	10	10		10	(1000 MT)
CY Exp. to U.S.	0	0	0	0			(1000 MT)
TS=TD		0		0		0	

Source: USDA Annual Report. Sept., 2012. Gain Report. Global Agricultural Information Network. USDA Agricultural Service.

Sunflower Seed

In India, sunflower as an oilseed crop was introduced in 1969 and is one of the fastest growing oilseed crops. Prior to which it was used mainly as an ornamental plant. Sunflower oil is popular as healthy cooking oil due to its health benefits while the meal is used in animal feed industry. Among sunflower products, meal is the most traded in world market.

The world sunflower seed production stood at 32.39 million tones from an area of 23.71 million hectares, accounting for 8.5 per cent of the total oilseeds production. The major uptrend in acreage and production started during 70s and 80s and the production outbreak started during the period when Russian federation and Ukraine added their acreages, with 14 per cent and 10 per cent along with Argentina adding another 17 per cent during 1992. Russia was the largest producer of sunflower occupying 18.9 percent of area with 13.3 percent of production in the world followed by Ukraine (13.9 per cent), India (8.7 per cent) Argentina (7.6 per cent), China (4.9 per cent), Romania (4.2 per cent), and France (2.6 per cent) during 2009-10. India produced 670, 000 MT of sunflower oilseed in 2012 and is expected to produce 700,000 MT in 2012-13 (Table 18.19).

Table 18.19: Production of Sunflower Oilseed

Oilseed, Sunflowerseed India	*2010/2011*		*2011/2012*		*2012/2013*		
	Market Year Begin: Oct 2010		*Market Year Begin: May 2011*		*Market Year Begin: May 2012*		
	USDA Official	*New Post*	*USDA Official*	*New Post*	*USDA Official*	*New Post*	
Area Planted	760	860	750	745	760	800	(1000HA)
Area Harvested	760	760	735	735	760	800	(1000HA)
Beginning Stocks	0	0	0	0	0	0	(1000MT)
Production	655	655	620	620	630	700	(1000MT)
MY Imports	0	0	0	0	0	0	(1000MT)
MY Imp. from U.S.	0	0	0	0	0	0	(1000MT)
MY Imp. from EU	0	0	0	0	0	0	(1000MT)
Total Supply	655	655	620	620	630	700	(1000MT)
MY Exports	6	0	5	0	4	0	(1000MT)
MY Exp. to EU	0	0	0	0	0	0	(1000MT)
Crush	550	590	580	530	590	600	(1000 MT)
Food Use Dom. Cons.	0	0	0	0	0	0	(1000MT)
Feed Waste Dom. Cons.	99	65	35	90	36	100	(1000MT)
Total Dom. Cons.	649	655	615	620	626	700	(1000MT)
Ending Stocks	0	0	0	0	0	0	(1000MT)
Total Distribution	655	655	620	620	630	700	(1000MT)
CY Imports	0	0	0	0	0	0	(1000MT)
CY Imp. from U.S.	0	0	0	0	0	0	(1000MT)
CY Exports	6	0	5	0	4	0	(1000MT)

Source: Annual Report. Feb. 2013. Gain Report. Global Agricultural Information Network. USDA Agricultural Service.

If we look at the trend in annual growth rate over the last few years (Figure 18.9), it shows a declining trend; area under sunflower cultivation and sunflower oilseed production has declined in India.

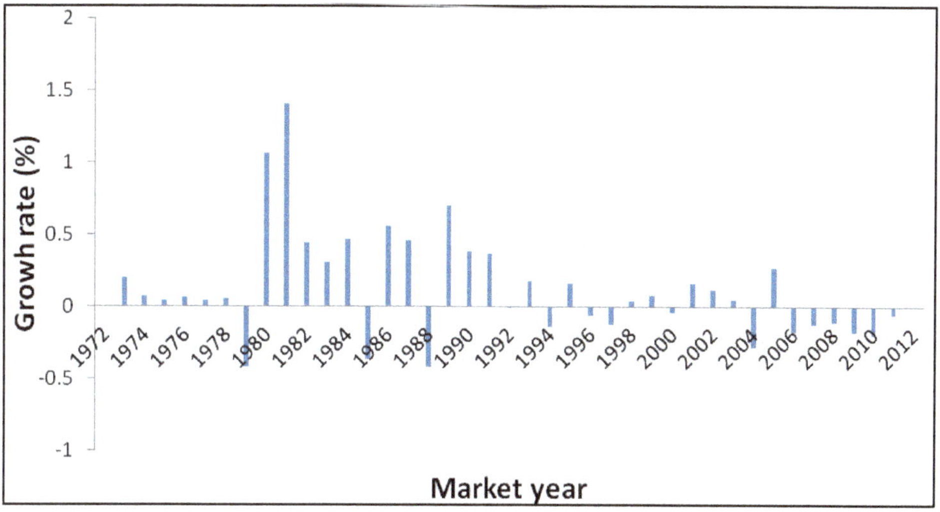

Figure 18.9: Annual Growth Rate of Sunflower Oilseed Production in India

***Source*: USDA**

Six states with Karnataka in the lead are the major producers of sunflower in the country. Karnataka with a production of 3.04 lakh tones from an area of 7.94 lakh hectares followed by Andhra Pradesh, Maharashtra, Bihar, Orissa and Tamil Nadu are major sunflower producing states of India (Figure 18.10). Sunflower production follows a systemic weather risk as about 80 per cent of the area is under rain-fed production. In terms of productivity, Bihar leads with 1402 kg/ha followed by Tamil Nadu with 1328.7 kg, although both the states have less than 25000 hectares under

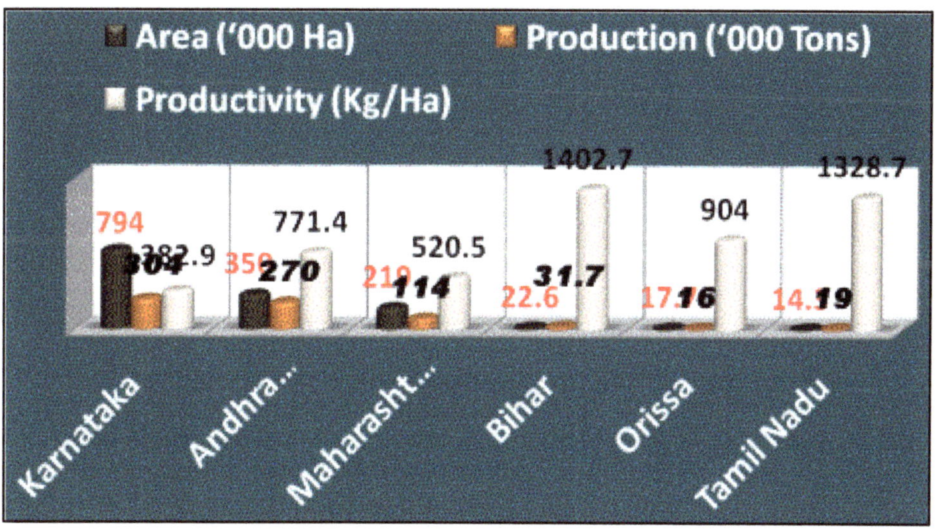

Figure 18.10: Area, Production and Productivity of Sunflower in Major Producing States

***Source*: FAOSTAT, 2009-10**

the crop which is mostly irrigated. The average productivity at all India level was 900 kg/ha depending on the climatic conditions and irrigation, which are critical factors for high yields.

Table 18.20: Commodity, Oil, Sunflowerseed, PSD

Oil, Sunflower Seed India	*2010/2011*		*2011/2012*		*2012/2013*		
	Market Year Begin: Oct 2010		*Market Year Begin: May 2011*		*Market Year Begin: May 2012*		
	USDA Official	*New Post*	*USDA Official*	*New Post*	*USDA Official*	*New Post*	
Crush	550	590	580	530	590	600	(1000 MT)
Extr. Rate, 999.9999	0.	0.3593	0.	0.3623	0.	0.3617	(PERCENT)
Beginning Stocks	121	143	100	231	137	437	(1000 MT)
Production	195	212	205	192	209	217	(1000 MT)
MY Imports	776	776	1,114	1,114	1,200	1,100	(1000 MT)
MY Imp. from U.S.	0	0	0	0	0	0	(1000 MT)
MY Imp. from EU	0	0	0	0	0	0	(1000 MT)
Total Supply	1,092	1,131	1,419	1,537	1,546	1,754	(1000 MT)
MY Exports	1	0	2	0	2	0	(1000 MT)
MY Exp. to EU	0	0	0	0	0	0	(1000 MT)
Industrial Dom. Cons.	0	0	0	0	0	0	(1000 MT)
Food Use Dom.Cons.	991	900	1,280	1,100	1,430	1,300	(1000 MT)
Feed Waste Dom. Cons.	0	0	0	0	0	0	(1000 MT)
Total Dom. Cons.	991	900	1,280	1,100	1,430	1,300	(1000 MT)
Ending Stocks	100	231	137	437	114	454	(1000 MT)
Total Distribution	1,092	1,131	1,419	1,537	1,546	1,754	(1000 MT)
CY Imports	871	660	1,125	871	1,200	750	(1000 MT)
CY Imp. from U.S.	0	0	0	0	0	0	(1000 MT)
CY Exports	0	0	0	0	0	0	(1000 MT)
CY Exp. to U.S.	0	0	0	0	0	0	(1000 MT)
TS=TD		0		0		0	

There is a considerable shift in acreage and production of sunflower in these six states of India. In 2000-01, Karnataka, Maharashtra and Andhra Pradesh were leading with 45 per cent, 31 per cent and 18 per cent, respectively covering almost 94 per cent of total acreage of sunflower in India which then found shifted to Karnataka accounting for 54 per cent in 2009-10 from the previous level of 45 per cent share (2000-01) followed by Andhra Pradesh with 24 per cent. Maharashtra reported substantial reduction in sunflower area between 2001 and 2009 registering 31 per cent and 15 per cent of sunflower area respectively. Country as whole has registered negative growth in sunflower area (Figure 18.9).

Prior to 1969, sunflower was grown as an ornamental plant and afterwards, it is being used as edible oil. Till now, maximum sunflower oil production was in 2003 (546,000 MT) and afterwards, there is a declining trend; it was only 209,000 MT in 2012 (Figure 18.11). In 2012-13, it is expected to be 217,000 MT (Table 18.20).

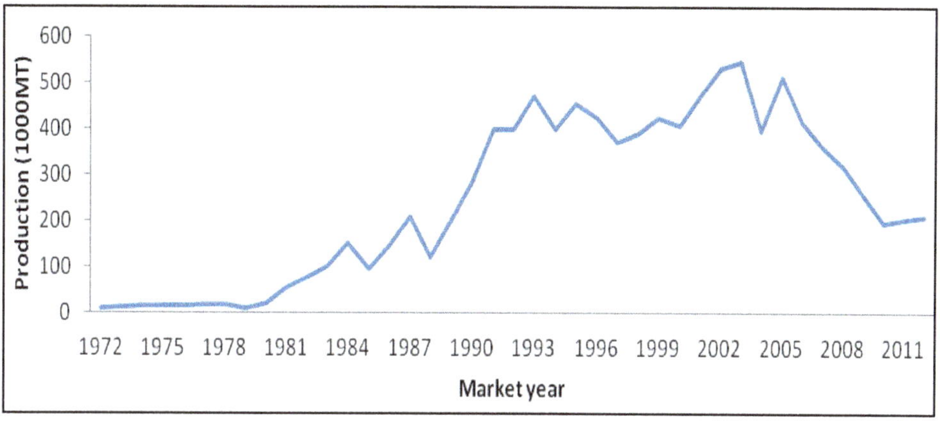

Figure 18.11: Sunflower Oil Production in India

***Source*: USDA**

Copra Oilseed

The coconut palm is one of the most useful plants in the world. It is grown in more than 80 countries of the world. In area under cultivation, India is ranked third; Indonesia is first with an overall of 385 million hectare. Sri Lanka is ranked second in international output with 7,223 nuts per hectare. India contributes about 15.46 per cent in area and 21 per cent in terms of production of coconut in the world. India has bagged second position in coconut production, while first position in productivity in 2012. As per the Asian and Pacific Coconut Community (APCC), India manufactures 15,730 million nuts annually, which is next to Indonesia with 16,498 million. India is the largest domestic consumer with 1,494.4 million nuts annually. Indonesia stands second at 996.5 million. India consumes 95 per cent of its net output and Indonesia consumes 60 per cent. Malaysia is the largest importer of coconut and coconut-based products since it imports 1,400 million nuts.

The major coconut growing states in India are Kerala, Tamilnadu, Karnataka, A.P., West Bengal, Maharashtra, Orissa, Assam, Goa, Daman and Diu, Lakshwadeep, Gujarat. Kerala tops in production accounting 39 per cent of total production in the country. Giving focus on productivity, Tamil Nadu comes in 1st position (14495 nuts/ha), West Bengal in 2nd position (14307 nuts/ha) and A.P. in 3rd position (12629 nuts/ha). Kerala being a major coconut producing state, its productivity is not so high (6951 nuts/ha).

Total production of coconut in India has been in a rising trend during the past decade (Table 18.21 and Figure 18.12). It has risen from levels of 5500 million nuts in the 1980s to 12500 million nuts in the 1990s. On all India basis, in 2008-09, total production and productivity rose to 15729.75 million nuts and 8303 nuts/ha, respectively. Higher productivity in Tamil Nadu was the main reason for this escalation in production.

Table 18.21: India Copra Oilseed Production (1990-2012)

Market Year	*Production (1000 MT)*	*Growth Rate*
1990	400	14.29 per cent
1991	450	12.50 per cent
1992	490	8.89 per cent
1993	550	12.24 per cent
1994	600	9.09 per cent
1995	610	1.67 per cent
1996	735	20.49 per cent
1997	718	-2.31 per cent
1998	710	-1.11 per cent
1999	720	1.41 per cent
2000	725	0.69 per cent
2001	700	-3.45 per cent
2002	725	3.57 per cent
2003	735	1.38 per cent
2004	750	2.04 per cent
2005	750	0.00 per cent
2006	620	-17.33 per cent
2007	700	12.90 per cent
2008	736	5.14 per cent
2009	736	0.00 per cent
2010	736	0.00 per cent
2011	736	0.00 per cent
2012	736	0.00 per cent

During 2012-13, copra production is estimated at 730, 000 MT with equivalent coconut oil production at 382, 000 MT (Tables 18.23 and 18.24). Maximum coconut oil production was in 2004-05 (462,000 MT). After that it started declining to 447,000 MT which remained at this level from 2008-2012 (Figs. 18.13 and 18.14).

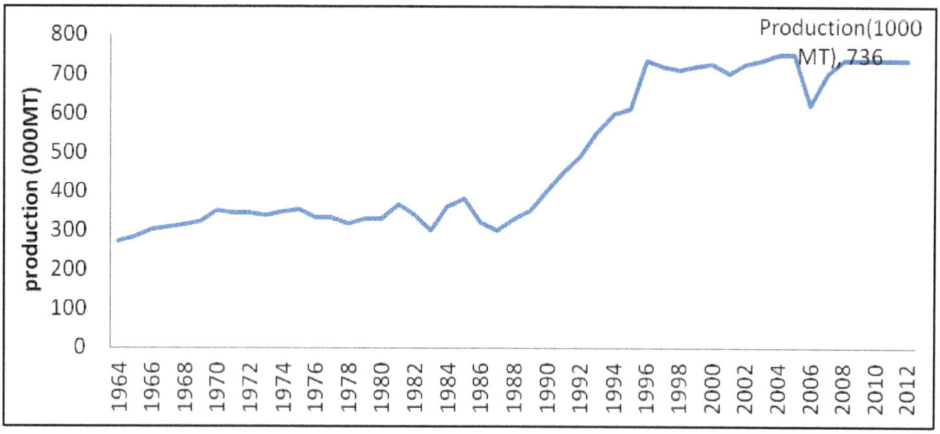

Figure 18.12: Trend in Copra Oilseed Production in India

***Source*: USDA**

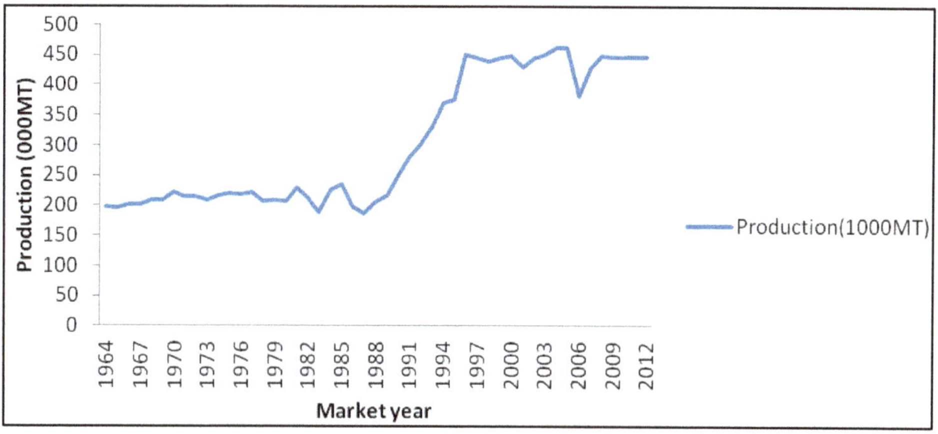

Figure 18.13: Coconut Oil Production in India

***Source*: USDA**

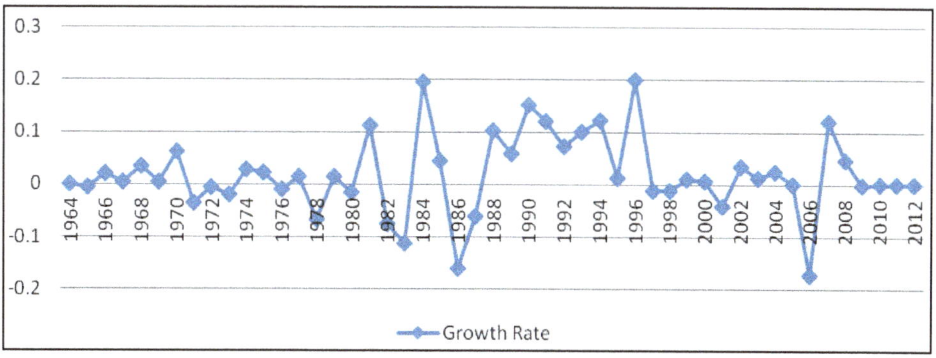

Figure 18.14: Annual Growth Rate in Coconut Oil Production in India

***Source*: USDA**

Table 18. 23 Production of Copra Oilseed

Oil, Copra India	*2010/2011*		*2011/2012*		*2012/2013*		
	Market Year Begin: Oct 2010		*Market Year Begin: May 2011*		*Market Year Begin: May 2012*		
	USDA Official	*New Post*	*USDA Official*	*New Post*	*USDA Official*	*New Post*	
Area Planted	0	0	0	0		0	(1000 HA)
Area Harvested	0	0	0	0		0	(1000 HA)
Beginning Stocks	0	0	0	0		0	(1000 MT)
Production	736	615	736	630		640	(1000 MT)
MY Imports	0	0	0	0		0	(1000 MT)
MY Imp. from U.S.	0	0	0	0		0	(1000 MT)
MY Imp. from EU	0	0	0	0		0	(1000 MT)
Total Supply	736	615	736	630		640	(1000 MT)
MY Exports	18	20	18	20		25	(1000 MT)
MY Exp. to EU	0	0	0	0		0	(1000 MT)
Crush	718	595	718	610		615	(1000 MT)
Food Use Dom. Cons.	0	0	0	0		0	(1000 MT)
Feed Waste Dom. Cons.	0	0		0		0	(1000 MT)
Total Dom. Cons.	718	595	718	610		615	(1000 MT)
Ending Stocks	0	0	0	0		0	(1000 MT)
Total Distribution	736	615	736	630		640	(1000 MT)
CY Imports	0	0	0	0		0	(1000 MT)
CY Imp. from U.S.	0	0	0	0		0	(1000 MT)
CY Exports	18	18	17	0		20	(1000 MT)
CY Exp. to U.S.	0	0	0	0		0	(1000 MT)
TS=TD		0		0		0	(1000 MT)

Source: USDA Annual Report. Sept, 2012. Gain Report. Global Agricultural Information Network. USDA Agricultural Service.

Major Constrains in Domestic Production of Oilseeds

- ☆ Low Productivity
- ☆ Small farm sizes
- ☆ Lack of varietal replacement
- ☆ Shifting of acreage from Oilseed to other crops
- ☆ Losses due to pests and diseases

Table 18.24: Production of Coconut Oil

Oil, Coconut India	2010/2011		2011/2012		2012/2013		
	Market Year Begin: Oct 2010		Market Year Begin: Oct 2011		Market Year Begin: Oct 2012		
	USDA Official	New Post	USDA Official	New Post	USDA Official	New Post	
Crush	718	595	718	610		615	(1000 MT)
Extr. Rate, 999.9999	1	0.6202	1	0.6213		0.6211	(PERCENT)
Beginning Stocks	2	22	1	19		18	(1000 MT)
Production	447	369	447	379		382	(1000 MT)
MY Imports	5	3	5	5		10	(1000 MT)
MY Imp. from U.S.	0	0	0	0		0	(1000 MT)
MY Imp. from EU	0	0	0	0		0	(1000 MT)
Total Supply	454	394	453	403		410	(1000 MT)
MY Exports	5	0	5	0		0	(1000 MT)
MY Exp. to EU	0	0	0	0		0	(1000 MT)
Industrial Dom. Cons.	225	175	225	180		190	(1000 MT)
Food Use Dom.Cons.	223	200	222	205		205	(1000 MT)
Feed Waste Dom. Cons.	0	0	0	0		0	(1000 MT)
Total Dom. Cons.	448	375	447	385		395	(1000 MT)
Ending Stocks	1	19	1	18		15	(1000 MT)
Total Distribution	454	394	453	403		410	(1000 MT)
CY Imports	5	3	5	10		10	(1000 MT)
CY Imp. from U.S.	0	0	0	0		0	(1000 MT)
CY Exports	5	0	0	0		0	(1000 MT)
CY Exp. to U.S.	0	0	0	0		0	(1000 MT)
TS=TD		0		0		0	

Source: USDA Annual Report. Sept, 2012. Gain Report. Global Agricultural Information Network. USDA Agricultural Service.

Trends in Production, Consumption and Demand of Fats and Oils

India is world's third largest edible oil economy, after China and US. The production of edible oils in India is dependent on the production and availability of oilseeds. While oilseeds production increased from 10.83 million tones (MT) in 1985-86 to 24.75 MT in 1998-99, yield per hectare increased from 570 kg to 944 kg during 1999 to 2003, oilseed output stagnated and also declined. As oilseeds are mostly sown in the non-irrigated regions of the country (*viz.*, Rajasthan, Gujarat, Maharashtra and Madhya Pradesh), its production suffers from high dependence on the monsoon.

Between 1986-87 and 2003-04, output of edible oils went up by 123 per cent, with an increase in yield per acre of 77.2 per cent and an increase in acreage by 25.8 per cent. Although there has been resurgence in oilseeds production in recent years, acreage under oilseeds has continued to remain below the all-time high of 26.34 million hectares achieved in 1996-97. The coincidence of decreasing acreage under oilseeds with increasing customs duty on crude palm oil, the main edible oil imported by the country, from 16.5 per cent in December 1999 to 80 per cent in 2005 clearly indicates the critical role that factors other than customs duty play in determining edible oils output in the country.

In 2011-12, total world production of oils and fat was 182.90 million tones out of which 51.49 million tones was contributed by palm oil while in India, the production was 8.12 million tones and the three major contributing oils were those extracted from rapeseed, soybean and cottonseed (Table 18.25).

Table 18.25: World and India Production of Oils and Fats (2011-12) (Quantity in Million Tones)

Oils and Fats	*World*	*India*
Palm oil	51.49	0.07
Soya oil	41.72	1.61
Rapeseed oil	23.64	1.92
Sunflower oil	14.63	0.22
Cottonseed oil	5.13	1.17
Groundnut oil	4.03	0.46
Other fats and oils	42.26	2.67
Total	182.90	8.12

Table 18.26: India's Oilseeds and Vegetable Oil Production (Quantity in Million Tones)

Year Nov.-Oct	*Oilseeds Production*	*Availability of Vegetable Oils*		
		Edible	*Non-edible*	*Total*
2011-12	30.01 (E)	7.34	0.78	8.12
2010-11	31.10	7.92	0.60	8.52
2009-10	24.88	7.26	0.51	7.77
2008-09	27.72	7.71	0.50	8.21
2007-08	29.76	7.75	0.49	8.24
2006-07	24.29	7.33	0.43	7.76
2005-06	27.98	7.56	0.47	8.03
2004-05	24.35	7.16	0.43	7.59
2003-04	25.18	7.21	0.38	7.59
2002-03	14.84	4.84	0.28	5.12
2001-02	20.66	6.37	0.35	6.72

In 2011-12, total 8.12 million tones vegetable oil was available out of which 7.34 MT was for edible purpose (Table 18.26). Vegetable oil production was only 5.12 MT in 2002-03 which rose to maximum *i.e.* 8.52 MT in 2010-11.

Table 18.27: Total Oils PSD

	MY 2010/11	*MY 2011/12*	*My 2012/13*
OILS ('000 metric tons)	*Revised*	*Estimate*	*Forecast*
Crush	29,365	28,540	29,135
Beginning Stocks	1,579	1,551	1,682
Production	7,443	7,123	7,345
MY Imports	8,281	9,555	9,710
Total Supply	17,303	18,229	18,737
MY Exports	7	5	22
Industrial Dom. Cons	530	580	625
Food Use Dom. Cons.	15,215	15,962	16,520
Feed Waste Dom. Cons.	0	0	0
Total Dom. Cons.	15,745	16,542	17,145
Ending Stocks	1,551	1,682	1,570
Total Distribution	17,303	18,229	18,737

Source: USDA Annual Report. Sept, 2012. Gain Report. Global Agricultural Information Network. USDA Agricultural Service.

Table 18. 28: Estimate of Availability of Domestic Edible Oils during 2012-13 and Comparison with 2011-12

Estimate of availability of domestic edible oils during 2012-13 and comparison with 2011-12

	Oils	*2012-13*	*2011-12*	*+/-*
		Lac MT.	*Lac MT.*	*against 2011-12*
1.	Groundnut	1.80	3.90	-2.10
2.	Soybean	17.10	16.50	0.60
3.	Rapeseed	21.10	17.30	3.80
4.	Others(Sun,Sesame, Safflower)	3.60	3.70	-0.10
5.	Cottonseed#	10.50	11.90	-1.40
6.	Secondary Sources.(Rice Bran, SE Oils,Copra and Misc. Oils)	14.30	13.40	0.90
	Total	68.40	66.70	1.70

Total edible oil production in 2012/13 is likely to be 7.3 million tones, 3 percent above the previous year (Table 18.27). Most of the increase is likely to be in rapeseed-mustard oil. Edible oil production for the marketing year 2011-12 was estimated at 7.1 million tones, which includes 2.3 million tons of rapeseed oil, 1.7 million tons of soybean oil, 1.3 million tons of peanut oil, and 1.2 million tons of cottonseed oil, and 600,000 tons of coconut, palm and sunflower oils (Table 18.28). Other minor edible oils such as rice bran oil, sesame seed oil, safflower oil and niger seed oil were not included (USDA, 2012).

According to the estimates by the Directorate of Vanaspati, Vegetable Oil and Fats (DVVF), in 2003-04, the net availability of edible oils from domestic production of 80.3 lakh tones of oils (edible and non-edible) from both primary and secondary sources was 71.4 lakh tones. In 2003-04, the balance of 9.2 lakh tones was used for export and industrial use. Export of oils was only about 3 lakh tones, including nearly one-lakh tones of groundnut oil. With production of 19.2 lakh tones, groundnut oil was the leading oil produced in the country followed by rapeseed/mustard oil and soybean oil which account for about 42 per cent of total production. Although domestic oilseeds production in 2004-05 was estimated to be marginally lower than that in 2003-04 (251.86 MT), net domestic availability of edible oils in 2004-05 (72.47 lakh tones) was expected to be of the same order as in the previous year (71.40 lakh tones). Net availability of edible oils increased from 73.30 lakh tones in 2006-07 to 77.5 lakh tones due to increased oilseed production during 2007-08 and 79.20 lakh tones in 2010–11 (Figure 18.15).

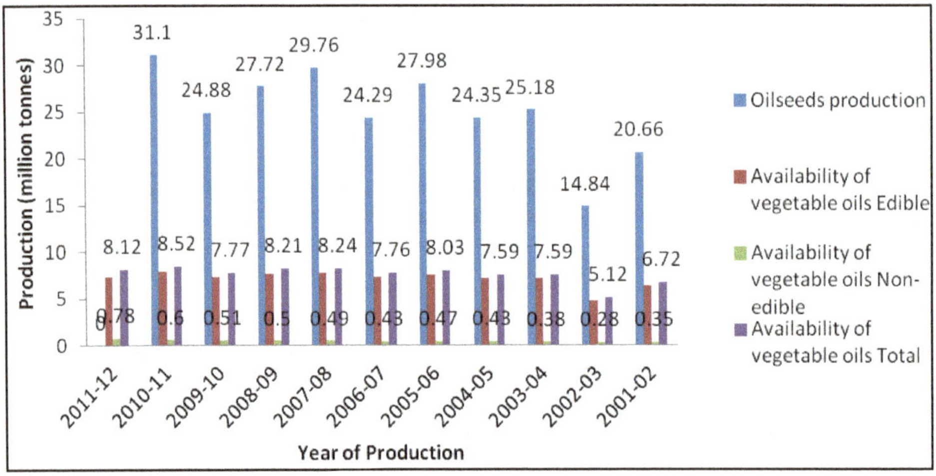

Figure 18.15: Indian Oilseeds and Vegetable Oil Production (Quantity in million tones)

***Source*: USDA**

In 2010-11, net availability of edible oils from all domestic sources was 97.82 lakh tons which decreased to 90.21 lakh tons in 2011-12. Availability of edible oils from domestic and import sources increased from 118.99 lakh tons in 2004-05 to 189.64 lakh tons in 2011-12 (Table 18.29).

Table 18.29: India's Oilseeds and Vegetable Oil Production (Quantity In In Lakh Tons)

Oil Year (Nov.–Oct.)	*Oilseeds Production* (In lakh Tons)*	*Net Availability of Edible Oils from all Domestic Sources (In lakh Tons)*	*Availability of Edible Oils (from domestic and import sources)** (In lakh Tons)*
2004-2005	243.54	72.47	118.99
2005-2006	279.79	83.16	124.07
2006-2007	242.89	73.70	119.75
2007-2008	297.55	86.54	140.88
2008-09	277.19	84.56	159.54
2009-10	248.83	79.46	154.10
2010-11	324.79	97.82	170.24
2011-12***	300.12	90.21	189.64
2012-13****	187.83 (kharif season)	-	-

Source: *: Ministry of Agriculture.

**: Directorate of Vanaspati, Vegetable Oils and Fats.

***: Based on 4th Advance Estimate (dated 16.07.2012) declared by Ministry of Agriculture.

****: Based on 1st Advance Estimate (dated 24.09.2012) declared by Ministry of Agriculture.

India's population is currently estimated at 1.15 billion and it is growing at the rate of 1.8 per cent per annum. India consumed around 14 million tonne of vegetable oil vis-à-vis China's consumption of 65.2 million tones per annum in 2011 (Figure 18.16). The country's consumption places India behind only China and the European Union in total edible oil consumption. With its large population and continued strong economic growth, India is likely to register strong gains in total and per-capita edible oil consumption in the future. India's per capita consumption of edible oil has increased from around 3 kg/yr in 1950 to 14.1 kg/annum in the 2011-12 but however,

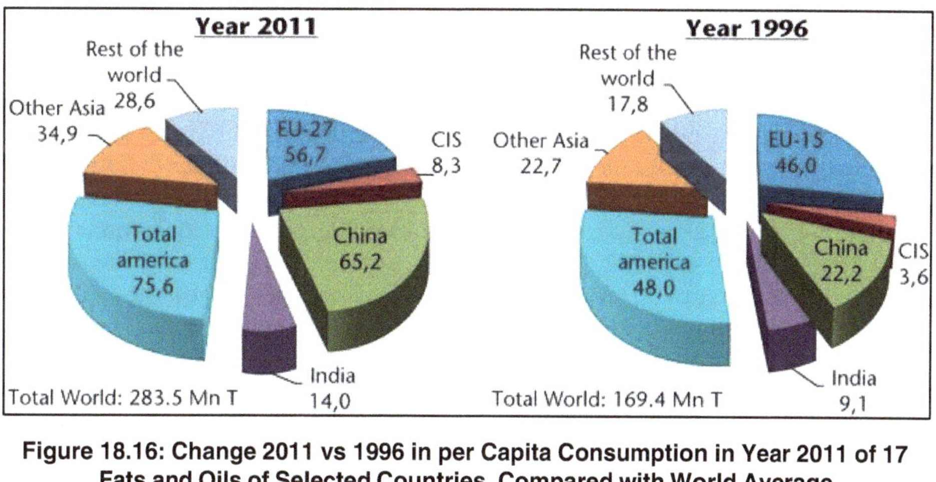

Figure 18.16: Change 2011 vs 1996 in per Capita Consumption in Year 2011 of 17 Fats and Oils of Selected Countries, Compared with World Average

this remains below the estimated world average of 21.6 kg and also when compared to the recommended level of 16 kg per person per annum.

Growing population, rising income levels and improved supply conditions will likely increase edible oil consumption in 2012/13 to 17.1 million tons, up 693,000 tons over the previous year (Figure 18.17, USDA, 2012). The surge in edible oil consumption was due to increased purchasing power of the middle class, which happened mainly due to the removal of import duty. India has been the biggest driver of consumption growth in this year. After the removal of import duty, we can state that the Indian vegetable oil market integrated with the world market.

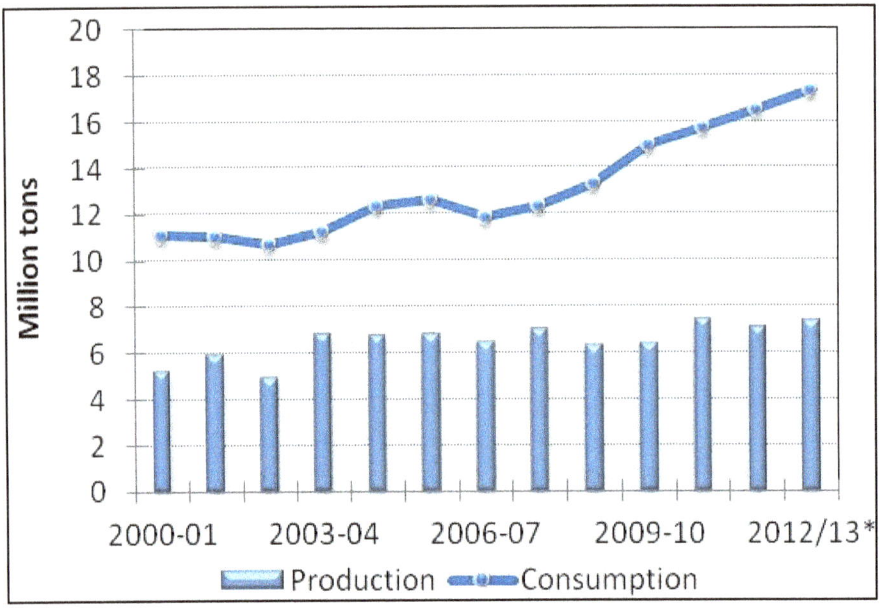

Figure 18.17: Growth and Consumption against Production of 17 Oils and Fats Over 2000-01 to 2012-13

***Source*: USDA Annual Report. Sept, 2012. Gain Report. Global Agricultural Information Network. USDA Agricultural Service.**

Table 18.30 depicts the consumption of various oils in our country. Palm oil and soy oil account for 46 per cent and 16.2 per cent of India's total edible oil consumption, respectively. Palm oil will continue to be the largest consumed edible oil. Considering its versatility in blending with other edible oils, relatively lower prices and increased usage across the vanaspati (partially hydrogenated vegetable oil) confectionary and margarine industries, the 2012/13 food use consumption is expected to increase to 7.4 million tons. After palm oil, soy, rapeseed and peanut oils are the largest edible oil segments in the Indian market, estimated at 2.8, 2.4 and 1.5 million tons respectively.

Demand of Edible Oils and Fats

As in past years, global demand for oils/fats, both for food and non-food purposes, is anticipated to expand significantly. During the coming years, world consumption

Table 18.30: Consumption of Various Oils in India (2011-12)

Oils	Domestic	Import	Total	Per cent
Palm oil	0.07	7.50	7.57	46
Soybean oil	1.65	1.01	2.66	16.2
Rapeseed oil	1.74	0.09	1.83	11.1
Sunflower oil	0.22	1.08	1.30	7.9
Cottonseed oil	1.19	-	1.19	7.2
Rice bran oil	0.85		0.85	5.2
Groundnut oil	0.39	-	0.39	2.4
Other	0.65	-	0.65	4.0
Total	6.75	9.67	16.42	100

Source: Solvent Extractors Association of India.

ESTIMATE OF CONSUMPTION FOR 2012-13 AND COMPARISON WITH 2011-12

	2012-13	2011-12
Population (Million)	1,256	1,244
Per Capita Consumption (Kg.)	13.60	13.20
Consumption Growth – Per Capita	3.10%	3.25%
Total Edible Oils Required Lac MT	171.00	164.20

Consumption growth during 2010-11 & 2009-10 was 4.70% & 4.00% respectively, but due to higher prices consumption growth has decreased to 3.25% in 2011-12 and estimate for 2012-13 is moderate growth of 3.10%.

is expected to increase by almost 6 million tones or 4 percent. An increasingly important demand factor is the fast growing use of oils/fats as fuels and as feedstock for biodiesel production.

Like at the global level, vegetable oils consumption is both income and price elastic in India too. Increase in per capita income pushes the demand for oil significantly. A similar effect is exercised by the price factor as well. In contrast to the pre-WTO period, the real price of vegetable oils had sharply declined in the subsequent period which enabled consumers to access larger quantities that were made possible through liberal imports. If per capita consumption of vegetable oils had stagnated at the level of 1991 or gone down, as had been the case with food grains, during the last two decades, then India would have faced no deficit in vegetable oils. This would imply no need for imports. However, as per capita consumption of edible oils has risen significantly, total demand in the country has risen at a very high rate and has created a big gap between domestic production and consumption, filled by liberal imports. The per capita oil consumption has surpassed the forecasts made earlier and may continue to increase at a blistering pace in the years to come, if the present conditions of vegetable oil price decline and income increase continue.

According to the National Council for Applied Economic Research (NCAER), the edible oil demand of our country is expected to go up to 20.16 kg/annum in the next 7 years, given 6 per cent rise in the per capita income and the edible oil demand between 22.8 (low estimate scenario) and 29.4 million tones (high estimate scenario). Keeping in view the growth in population and consumption estimates of demand of edible oils has been projected in Table 18.31. However, the recent demand projections made by Rabo bank for DAC, indicated that the edible oil demand may raise up to 14.8, 18.3 and 21.8 million tones by 2010, 2015 and 2020, respectively. This means, the present level of oilseed production of the country needs to be increased by three times to meet out the projected demand for edible oil.

Table 18. 31: Population and Consumption of Edible Oils

Year	*Population @1.8 per cent Growth*	*Consumption @4 per cent Growth*		*Consumption @5 per cent Growth*		*Consumption @6 per cent Growth*	
	(in Billion)	*Per Capita kgs*	*Million tones*	*Per Capita kgs*	*Million tones*	*Per Capita kgs*	*Million tones*
2009	1.19	12.37	14.75	12.73	15.18	13.1	15.61
2010	1.21	12.87	15.61	13.37	16.22	13.89	16.85
2011	1.24	13.38	16.53	14.04	17.34	14.72	18.18
2012	1.26	13.92	17.5	14.74	18.53	15.6	19.62
2013	1.28	14.48	18.53	15.48	19.81	16.54	21.17

Source: Solvent Extractors Association of India.

According to Hegde (2012), India needs to produce 17.84 MT of vegetable oils to meet the nutritional fat needs of projected population of 1685 million by 2050. This can be easily achieved from various sources like annual oil-seeds and also from supplementary sources of oil like rice bran, cottonseed, coconut, oil palm, corn, etc.

Supplementary Sources of Vegetable Oils

Contributing more than 25 per cent of the total vegetable oil consumption in the country, the minor and TBOs have considerable oil potential which needs to be fully tapped. Oil is obtained from rice bran, cotton seed, corn, coconut and oil palm, apart from seeds of underutilized plants like *Jatropha*, *tumba*, rubber seed, mango kernel, *neem*, *karanj*, *mahua*, *kusum*, *sal*, *simarouba*, *jojoba*, *cheura*, wild apricot, tung, etc. The current level of vegetable oils production from all these sources (2.767 Mt) could be further stepped up, given their tremendous potential (> 4.4 Mt; Table 18.32).

Table 18.32: Projected Production of Supplementary Sources of Vegetable Oils

Source	*Projected Production 2050 (lakh tones)*
Rice bran oil	22.44
Cotton seed oil	35.44
Coconut	10.00
Oil palm	32.00
TBOs	5.00*
Corn oil	3.00
Tobacco seed oil	0.02
Total	107.90
* Excluding TBOs	102.90

Processing of Oilseeds to Edible Oils

Edible oil processing consists of three operations:

1. Crushing and expelling (separating oil from the solids),
2. Solvent extraction (to chemically remove residual oil from the oilcake solids), and
3. Oil refining, if any.

In many countries, these three separate processing operations are conducted by one vertically integrated plant. In India, however, only a small share of oilseed production undergoes solvent extraction and oil refining. Instead, India's oilseeds processing sector is made up of the three groups viz *Ghanis*, solvent extractors and oil refiners engaged separately.

The village *Ghani* is a simple and straightforward oilseed crushing contraption. Solvent extraction consists of chemically extracting residual oil from oilcakes. While solvent-extracted oil has to be refined before consumption, even other oils can be refined for removing colour, odour and taste.

Indian processing industry suffers from several maladies like outdated technology, lower rates of utilization of installed capacity, low oil recoveries and high unit costs. The technical inefficiencies in oilseed production, on an average have been found to be 1/4 to 1/3 and even higher at the farm level/ processing unit level along with allocative and scale inefficiencies. The combined technical inefficiencies in the oilseeds sector (production and processing) have been found to be 1/2 to 1/3. If prevented/ minimized, the oilseed production of the country could be double than the existing (Mruthyunjaya, 2007). Under utilization of resources reflects a poor-resource base of the farmers and have implications for optimum utilization of inputs and production of outputs, both on farm and in processing unit to reduce allocative and scale inefficiencies.

Reservation of oilseeds output for small scale processing is depriving the farmers and consumers of the benefits of lower costs of modern processing technology, while putting up the costs for consumers. The fragmentation, low technical efficiency and excess capacity of India's oilseed processing industry are largely the result of regulatory and trade policies followed by the government (Hegde, 2007).

The cost of vegetable oil processing in India is very high as compared to the countries like China and USA mainly due to smaller capacities, low technical efficiency and low capacity utilization. The overall capacity utilization of both seed crushing as well as solvent extraction remains low due to large oilseed processing capacity installed. Additional inefficiency arises from non-integration of solvent extraction units with expeller units; as a result, significant amounts of expeller cake are not solvent extracted resulting in considerable losses of oil and meal products.

Vertical integration of expelling and solvent extraction alone can increase the oil recovery by more than a million tones worth about Rs.2500 crores annually (Prasad, 2007). Inspite of this, there is a lot of scope for the Indian vegetable oil industry for employing efficient technologies for oilseeds and oil processing to reduce the oil loss during the extraction and refining.

Oilseeds processing should be open for modern and efficient processors, just like paddy and wheat processing. Large-scale processing operations, typically 1200 tones a day should be promoted. The reservation of oilseed crushing and processing for small-scale industry should be removed (Shenoi, 2007).

The state governments' policy of offering incentives to new units exempting from sale tax renders old units and competing units in other states unviable and poor capacity utilization adds to the cost of processing, which needs to be set right through appropriate policy changes. This warrants immediate dereservation of the processing sector that can help in increasing the processing efficiency. Linkage mechanism can reduce the role of intermediaries in the oilseed sector thus, resulting in higher income to producers, lower cost of processing at the processors' level and finally cheap oil to the consumer. It will be a win-win situation to all the stakeholders.

There is a lot of scope for the industry to exploit the by-products obtained during vegetable oil processing for value addition. The by-products of vegetable oil processing like gums, soap-stock, spent bleaching earth, crude wax, deodorizer distillate are rich sources of various value added products like lecithin, glycolipids, oryzanol, fatty acids and their esters, tocopherols, tocotrienols, sterols, waxes, long chain fatty acids and fatty alcohols, squalene, steryl esters etc. Indian vegetable oil seed industry is now exploring the possibilities of value addition to these by-products and enhancing the returns from the by-products will be the real challenge for the oil industry.

There are uncommon opportunities to add value to different oilseeds and oils, which must be fully exploited, which will eventually enhance the competitiveness and sustainability of these crops (Hegde, 2007). Full value addition to castor oil before exports alone can fetch additional earning of Rs.20, 000 crores from the present level of Rs. 1000 to 1200 crores annually.

Status of Vegetable Oil Industry

Status of the vegetable oil industry as on April 2013 has been presented in the following Table 18.33.

Table 18.33: Status of the Vegetable Oil Industry (As on April, 2013)

Type of Vegetable Oil Industry	*No. of Units*	*Annual Capacity (Lakh MT)*	*Average Capacity Utilisation*
Oilseed Crushing Units	1,50,000 (Approx)	425 (In terms of Seeds)	10-30 per cent
Solvent Extraction Units	795	419 (In terms of Oil-bearing Material)	34 per cent
Refineries attached with Vanaspati Units	127	51 (in terms of oil)	45 per cent
Refineries attached with Solvent Units	226	37 (in terms of oil)	29 per cent
Independent Refineries	590	35 (in terms of oil)	36 per cent
Total Refineries	943	123 (in terms of oil)	37 per cent
Vanaspati Units	268	58 (in terms of Vanaspati, Bakery Shortening and Margarine)	19 per cent

Source: Directorate of Vanaspati, Vegetable Oils and Fats, Ministry of Food and Public Distribution.

Oilseeds crushing units include crushing units in the small-scale sector as also in the organised sector. The capacity utilisation generally ranges from an average of 10 per cent for the *ghanis* (small scale sector) to around 30 per cent in case of the expellers in the organized sector.

Indian rapeseed/mustard is reasonably import competitive at the farm/*mandi* level. But owing to the reservation of mustard oilseed processing (expeller) units in the micro and small-scale sectors, the average size of processing units for mustard oil has remained small besides having outdated technology. This makes the costs of processing high and mustard oil less import competitive (and many a times even protected). Therefore, de-reservation of the mustard/rapeseed expeller units (and also for groundnut processing units) from the small scale sector, along with emphasis on technology up gradation and modernization of the edible oil processing units to ensure their enhanced efficiency and capacity utilization leading to reduction in real costs of processing have been recommended.

Domestic Price of Oilseeds and Edible Oils

Oilseeds and edible oils prices had increased by about 43 per cent and 32 per cent respectively, between 1995-96 and 2004-05. These increases had been somewhat lower than the general price increase of about 53 per cent during the same reference period. The increase in the prices of oilseeds had been higher than that in edible oils partly as a result of deliberate policy of giving higher support prices to oilseeds to encourage diversification away from cereals such as rice and wheat.

Within oilseeds and edible oils, the price trends have displayed considerable divergences. For example, within oilseeds, the highest price increases of over 138 per cent took place in copra (coconut) followed by soybean and sunflower, while the lowest increase of 30 per cent was in rapeseed and mustard. The increases in edible oils prices have also shown considerable divergence, but, in general, the increase in oilseeds prices have been higher than the increase in edible oil prices in all cases, except in the case of rapeseed and mustard (Report of the Committee on Rationalisation of Customs and Excise Duties on Edible Oils and Oilseeds by Lahiri, A.K. 2006).

According to Dorab Mistry, Director of Godrej International, 2006 was a very successful year for the oils and fats industry. Production of oilseeds expanded and yet prices of vegetable oil rose by almost a third. Agriculture has for a long time suffered from low prices which led to low morale and mass migration from the countryside to the cities.

The wholesale prices of key edible oils like mustard, groundnut, soybean, sunflower and palmolein have risen sharply in the last few years due to rising domestic demand and inadequate oilseed production. The biggest rise in domestic wholesale price was seen in groundnut oil, where the price has increased by more than 60 per cent since 2008. According to the Food Ministry data, the wholesale prices of mustard oil, soybean oil and RBD palmolein had risen 24 per cent, 18 per cent and 19 per cent, respectively. Prices of edible oils rose sharply in 2008, and then declined in the subsequent year 2009.

Since 2010, the price of all major edible oils has risen by more than 25 per cent, attributed mainly to a rise in global crude price and a sharp increase in domestic demand (Table 18.34). Global prices of major edible oils such as crude palm oil, soybean oil, sunflower oil and RB palmolein have increased by 63 per cent, 59 per cent, 49 per cent and 48 per cent, respectively.

On the production front, the country is far from achieving self-sufficiency because of rising demand.

Table 18.34: Wholesale Price Trend of Edible Oil since 2008 in India

WHOLESALE PRICE TREND OF EDIBLE OIL SINCE 2008

Type of oil	2008	2009	2010	2011	2012 (Jan-Mar)
Mustard	Rs 6172	Rs 4984	Rs 5141	Rs 6390	Rs 7687
Groundnut	Rs 6752	Rs 6058	Rs 7515	Rs 8693	Rs 10,834
Soyabean	Rs 5746	Rs 4526	Rs 4697	Rs 6253	Rs 6825
Sunflower	Rs 6329	Rs 4249	Rs 5009	Rs 6498	Rs 6342
RBD Palmolein	Rs 4882	Rs 3752	Rs 4397	Rs 5645	Rs 5840

Rs /per quintal, year (Jan - Dec)

OILSEEDS PRODUCTION TREND

2008	2009-10	2010-11	2011-12
27.71 million tonne	24.88 mt	32.47 mt	30.06 mt

Source: Food ministry, agriculture ministry

Growing domestic consumption and larger crush of oilseeds in 2012/13 is expected to keep stocks relatively tight compared to current marketing year. Procurement of oilseeds by government agencies such as the National Agricultural Cooperative Marketing Federation of India (NAFED) is likely to be low as open market prices of major oilseeds in 2011/12 were higher than the government's minimum support price (Table18.35). Even privately held stocks are likely to remain low (USDA, 2012). While it is the job of commodity analysts and experts to forecast what the prices are likely to be, one can safely expect that owing to lower domestic crop and high international prices of vegetable oils, prices in India will remain firm.

Table 18. 35: Open Market Prices vis-a-vis Minimum Support Price

Commodity	*Minimum Support Price (Rs/100 kg)*			** Market Price*
	2011-12	*2010-11*	*2009-10*	
Soybean	1,650 (Black) 1,690 (Yellow)	1,400 (Black) 1,440 (Yellow)	1,350 (Black) 1,390 (Yellow)	2,100-2,800
Rapeseed/mustard	2,500	1,850	1,830	2,750-3,300
Peanut (in shell)	2,700	2,300	2,100	3,150-5,500
Sunflower seed	2,800	2,350	2,215	2,900-3,000

* Market prices during major centres 2011/12.

Source: Directorate of Agricultural Marketing, GOI.

There has been a conscious attempt in recent years to improve price parity of oilseeds (and also of pulses) through increase of Minimum Support Price (MSP) to encourage cultivation of these crops. However, despite such increase, there is still a substantial difference between the productivity per hectare at the current MSP between oilseeds/pulses on the one hand and wheat/rice on the other. At current MSP, per hectare productivity of wheat and rice is almost two to three times the productivity of oilseeds. Given the high differential between the per hectare productivity of oilseeds on the one hand and that of wheat/rice on the other, price mechanism as the only means of encouraging production of pulses and oilseeds is fraught with severe limitations. Increase in the MSP of oilseeds leads to corresponding increase in the market price of such products, which not only harms the interests of the consumers but also squeezes the margins of edible oils manufacturers. Substantial increase in MSP of oilseeds runs the risk of resulting in increased import of comparatively cheaper oilseeds/edible oils from abroad, and putting tremendous pressure on the Government procurement mechanism with subsidy implication. What is needed is a concerted attempt to increase the productivity of such crops (Report of the Committee on Rationalisation of Customs and Excise Duties on Edible Oils and Oilseeds by Lahiri, A.K. 2006).

Import of Vegetable Oils

Background

After the OTM programme had been in operation for several years, it resulted in near self-sufficiency in edible oil during 1994-95 in India. However, it was not palatable to the economic pundits as well as so-called 'market forces'. There were critics of this programme, notable among them being the World Bank. In a 1991 paper the bank argued that the government programme was economically costly, inefficient and unsustainable as production increases had been obtained in an environment where imports were controlled and domestic prices ruled higher than international prices. Its logic was that oilseed production in India did not have a 'comparative advantage'

- hence it was better off importing oil and spending its resources in other areas rather than on edible oilseed technology.

The World Bank in its 1997 report titled 'The Indian oilseed complex: Capturing market opportunities' considered the OTM programme to be a 'conditional success' and agreed that the technology inputs provided in a protected oilseeds market had indeed resulted in increasing the productivity and improving the cost competitiveness of Indian oilseeds as well as stabilized the production; however it still believed that the government's policy had left consumers in India bearing the cost, in terms of higher domestic prices of edible oil than international prices.

Ignoring the ground realities, and blindly following the World Bank's flawed prescription (under pressure, since India was restructuring its economy in accordance with the Structural Adjustment Programme), the country began the process of phased liberalization of edible oil imports from 1994-95 onwards. This was at a time when edible oil-exporting countries like Malaysia, Indonesia and Brazil were preparing to flood the Indian market with palm and soy oil. Two years later, the negative consequences of liberalizing the edible oil policy became clearly visible. With the country's edible oil import bill soaring to nearly US$ 1 billion during 1996-97, it was the Ministry of Agriculture that finally pressed the panic button.

Edible Oil Imports to Bridge Demand-Supply Gap

All is not well with India's edible oil economy. The country needs about 16.7 million tones of edible oils for its domestic consumption. The per capita availability of oils and fats (13.5Kg in 2011-12) is below the recommended level of 16 kg. Domestic vegetable oil production is about 8.12 million tones, which is not sufficient to meet domestic requirement. The demand for edible oils in India has been increasing at a fast rate. Despite efforts to raise edible oilseed production in the country, the growth in production could not keep pace with the growth in domestic demand. Thus, India meets the demand deficit through imports. India is the second largest consumer and importer of edible oil after China. India meets 60 per cent of its edible oil requirements through imports. Its annual consumption of 17-18 million tones relies extensively on imports.

With the domestic edible oil consumption growing at a healthy pace of 5.5-6 per cent per annum and the domestic oil production remaining stagnant, India's dependence on oil import is increasing steadily. Import of vegetable oils increased from 5.59 million tones in 2006-07 to 9.24 million tones in 2009-10 (Table 18.36). India imported 8.66 million tones of vegetable oils in 2008-09 and 2010-11, spending more than Rs 250,000 million. In 2011-12 oil year (Nov.-Oct.), it had imported 10.19 million tones of vegetable oil (Table 18.37). Palm oil constituted around 74.5 per cent of the total imports, with soy oil's share at 12 per cent. Other oils imported include sunflower seed oil and canola.

'The import of vegetable oils during 2012-13 is likely to increase by about 5-7 lakh tones and estimated in the range of 10.7 million tones to 10.9 million tones', Mumbai based SEA said in a statement. In 2012–13 also, the share of palm is expected to be a robust 80 per cent because of the large price disparity between the soybean oil and palm oil in the international market.

Table 18.36: Import of Vegetable Oils (Edible, Vanaspati and Non-Edible) (Quantity in Million Tones)

Vegetable Oils	*2010-11*	*2009-10*	*2008-09*	*2007-08*	*2006-07*
Edible oils	8.37	8.82	8.18	5.61	4.71
Vanaspati	-	-	0.02	0.05	0.25
Non-edible	0.29	0.42	0.46	0.65	0.63
Total	8.66	9.24	8.66	6.31	5.59

Import of vegetable oils is rising from year to year to bridge the demand and supply gap.

Table 18.37: Month-Wise Import of Vegetable Oil (Edible and Non-Edible) (Qty in MT) In 2010-11 and 2011-2012

Import of Vegetable Oil (Edible & Non-edible)						(Qty in MT)
Nov.'11 To Sept.'12	**2011-12**			**2010-11**		
Month	**Edible**	**Non-edible**	**Total**	**Edible**	**Non-edible**	**Total**
Nov.'11	827,684	27,679	855,363	652,262	16,655	668917
Dec.'11	654,714	15,198	669,912	730,194	22,494	752688
Jan.'12	647,693	12,286	659,979	691,780	29,417	721197
Nov-Jan (Q.1)	**2,130,091**	**55,163**	**2,185,254**	**2,074,236**	**68,566**	**2142802**
Feb.'12	873,313	3,356	876,669	538,172	11,709	549,881
Mar.'12	702,335	25,371	727,706	412,088	23,647	435,735
Apr.'12	897,404	27,930	925,334	458,119	17,004	475,123
Feb-Apr (Q.2)	**2,473,052**	**56,657**	**2,529,709**	**1,408,379**	**52,360**	**1,460,739**
May.'12	883,410	13,511	896,921	635,937	28,196	664,133
June.'12	769,885	13,430	783,315	828,959	33,591	862,550
July.'12	848,229	22,099	870,328	881,762	31,417	913,179
May-July (Q.3)	**2,501,524**	**49,040**	**2,550,564**	**2,346,658**	**93,204**	**2,439,862**
Aug.'12	882,269	14,749	897,018	785,518	31,922	817,440
Sept.'12	976,417	17,495	993,912	878,869	33,472	912,341
Total (Nov'11-Sept'12)	**8,963,353**	**193,104**	**9,156,457**	**7,493,660**	**279,524**	**7,773,184**

India's import of vegetable oils during February 2013 has been reported at 969,175 tons compared to 876,669 tons in February 2012, up by 10.55 per cent. According to one estimate, India may require 11 million tones in 2015 (Table 18.38). According to Jain (2009), the current sorry state of affairs is partially a result of our policies. If the current stagnation in production continues, we will be importing over 11 million tones by the year 2015 which would be 53 per cent share of the domestic demand. This, by no means, is a reassuring thought for a country the size of India because it compromises our food security.

Import of Major Vegetable Oils

India imports nearly 55 per cent of its annual vegetable oil requirement of 15.7 million tones from Argentina, Indonesia and Malaysia. India continues to import edible oils such as soybean oil, palm oil, sunflower oil and coconut oil (Figures 18.18 and Table 18.39).

Table 18.38: Edible Oil Demand and Import Projections

Parameter	*2010*	*2015*
Population (In Billion)	1.21	1.33
Total Demand of Edible Oils (million tones)	15.6	20.8
Domestic Supply of Edible Oils (million tones)	7.9	10.0
Import of Edible Oils (million tones)	8.0	11.0
Imports as Share of Demand	51 per cent	53 per cent

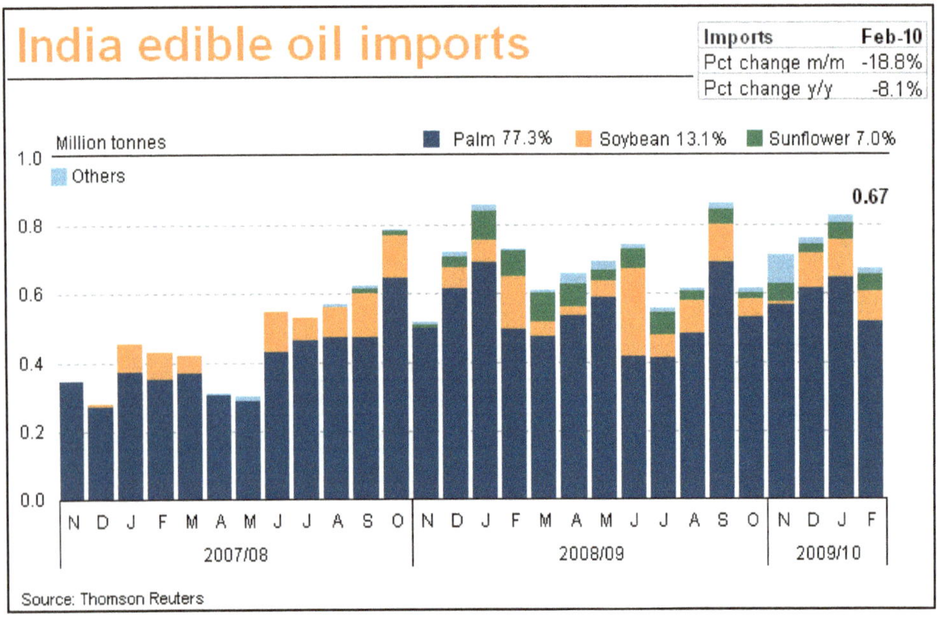

Figure 18.18: Import of Edible Oils in India

Palm Oil

Palm oil constitutes 80 per cent of all vegetable oil imports (Table 18.40). Purchases were a record 10.2 million tons in 2011-2012, according to the the Solvent Extractors' Association of India. During Nov.'12 to Feb.'13, palm oil import increased to 3,103,835 tons compared to 2,470,692 tons during the same period of last year. The country buys palm from Indonesia and Malaysia.

Soy Oil

India imports soybean oil from Brazil and Argentina. Soya imports were less than 100, 000 tones until 1997-1998. With the liberalization of imports and a sharp decline in the international prices of soybean oil, imports of soybean oil started rising rapidly. During the period from 2001 to 2005, India imported on average more than

Table 18.39: Import of Various Types of Vegetable Oils (Edible and Non-Edible) During Nov. and Dec. 2012

Edible Oils	*Nov.'12*	*Dec.'12*	*Nov.–Dec.'12*	*Nov.–Dec.'11*	*Per cent Change*
RBD Palmolein	76,519	137,475	**213,994**	217,091	
Crude Palm Oil	534,556	628,618	**1,163,174**	1,047,982	
Sunflower Oil	47,500	69,000	**116,500**	172,633	
Soybean Oil	14,160	21,960	**36,120**	15,387	
Rape Oil (Canola)	—	1,943	**1,943**	—	
Crude Palm Ker.Oil	3,499	16,998	**20,497**	27,805	
Coconut Oil	—	—	—	1,000	
Crude Olein	—	—	—	500	
Sub-Total	**676,234**	**875,994**	**1,552,228**	1,482,398	**(+) 4.71 per cent**
Non-edible					
P.K.F.A.D.	—	1,099	**1,099**	1,199	
P.F.A.D.	4,999	3,999	**8,998**	12,000	
C.P.K.O.	8,908	20,000	**28,908**	11,139	
C.P.S.	—	—	—	2,499	
RBD Palm Sterin	10,230	—	**10,230**	—	
Others	—	—	—	16,040	
Sub-Total	**24,137**	**25,098**	**49,235**	42,877	**(+) 14.82 per cent**
Grand Total	**700,371**	**901,092**	**1,601,463**	1,525,275	**(+) 5.00 per cent**

Source: The Solvent Extractors Association of India Letter dated 14.1.13 (PR038/2012-13).

one million tones of soybean oil annually. Maximum enhancement in annual growth rate in import of soy oil by India took place in 1997 (381.6 per cent) followed by 1998 (252.9 per cent), 1991 (225.0 per cent) and 2004 (123.6 per cent). In 2010, annual growth rate of soy oil import declined (-40.8 per cent) but again it increased in 2011 (1174, 000 tones; 24.2 per cent) and 2012 (1180, 000 tones; 0.51 per cent) (Figure 18.19).

Table 18.40 Import of Palm Oil by India (Quantity In '000 Tones)

Countries	*Jan./Dec. 2011*	*Jan/Dec. 2010*	*Jan/Dec. 2009*
Indonesia	5010	5435	5255
Malaysia	1677	1189	1541
Singapore	–	2	2
Thailand	49	21	28
Others	–	1	1
Total	6744	6648	6827

Source: Oil World.

Table 18.41 Import of Soybean Oil by India (Quantity In '000 Tones)

Countries	*Jan./Dec. 2011*	*Jan/Dec. 2010*	*Jan/Dec. 2009*
USA	–	161	146
Argentina	746	1284	693
Brazil	144	78	202
Paraguay	36	45	65
Thailand	8	–	–
Others	6.8	–	1
Total	941	1568	1107

Source: Oil World

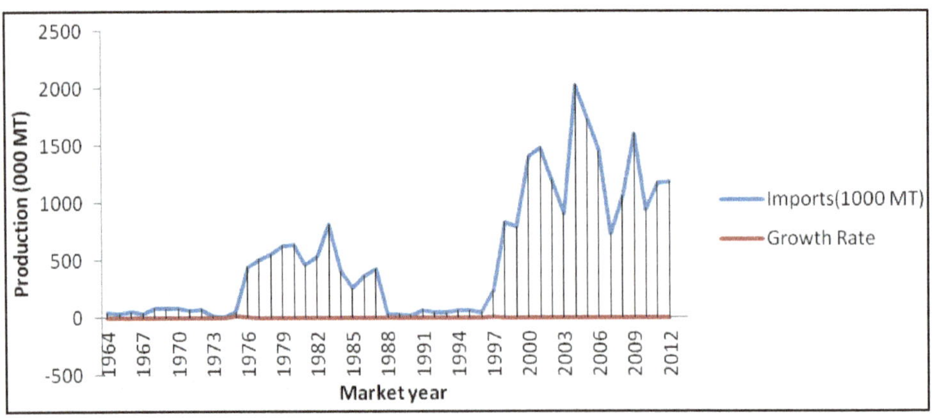

Figure 18.19: Indian Soy Oil Import and Annual Growth Rate from 1964-2012

***Source*: USDA**

Sunflower Oil

An important trend of recent years has been the increasing Indian imports of sunflower oil (Figure 18.20). If during the 2008/09 season its share in India's import of vegetable oils was 7 per cent, at the end of season 2011/12 it already was 11 per cent. During November 2011 to September 2012, the import of sunflower oil is reported at 1,049,181 tonnes compared to 739,173 tonnes during the same period of last year. The overall import of vegetable oils during November 2011 to September 2012 is reported at 9,156,457 tonnes compared to 7,773,184 tonnes, showing a growth of 17.80 per cent, noted SEA in its report (Business Standard, April 16, 2013). The sharp growth in imports of sunflower oil is attributed to attractive prices compared to soybean oil. Because of more import of sunflower seed oil, share of soybean oil in the Indian imports slightly decreased, and according to the results of the season 2011/12 for the first time there was less soybean oil purchased than sunflower oil (Table 18.42).

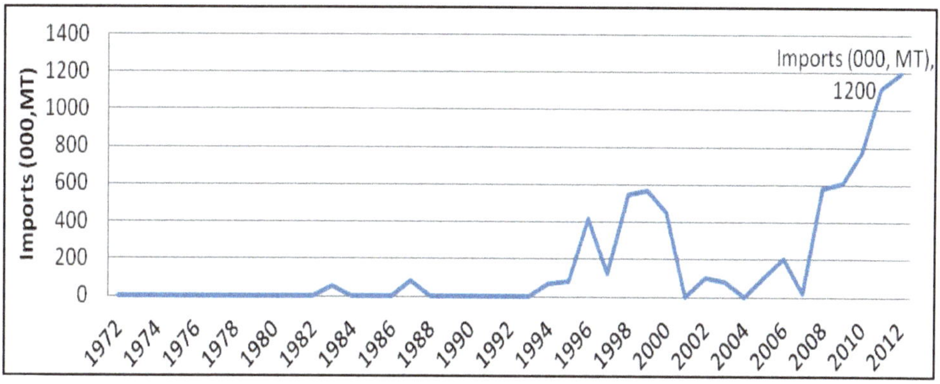

Figure 18.20: Sunflower Seed Oil Imports from 1972-2012

***Source*: USDA**

Table 18.42: Import of Sunflower Oil by India (Quantity in '000 Tones)

Countries	*Jan./Dec. 2011*	*Jan/Dec. 2010*	*Jan/Dec. 2009*
Russia	10	26	56
Ukraine	817	588	503
USA	-	11	-
Argentina	43	37	83
Others	1	1	1
Total	871	663	643

Source: Oil World.

Ukraine provides 100 per cent of the import of sunflower oil to India. According to UkrAgroConsult, Ukraine's share in sunflower oil shipments to India for the period of November 2011-October 2012 was 100 per cent against 96 per cent in 2010/11 (Figure 18. 21).

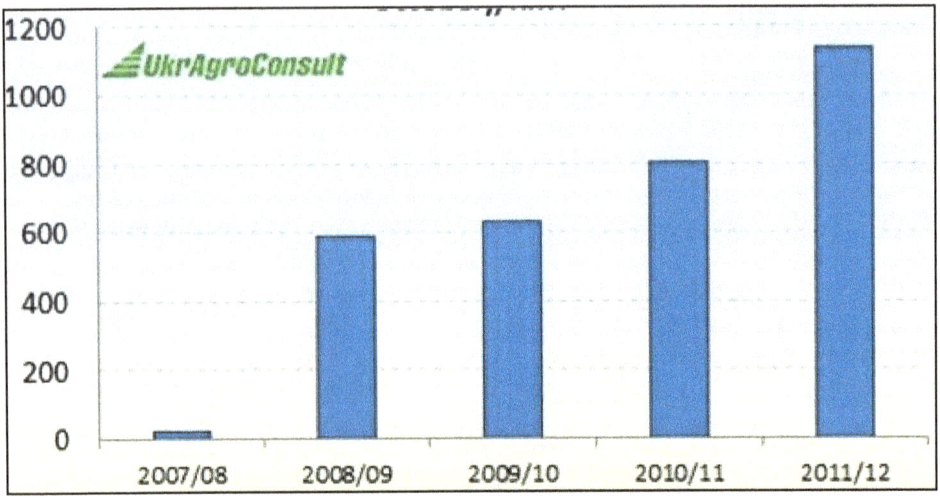

Figure 18.21: Import of Sunflower Oil to India
***Source*: UkAgroConsult (Nov. 12, 2012)**

Form of Vegetable Oils Imported

Edible oil imports, except that of palm and soybean oil, have been mostly in crude form. During 1996-2000, when import duties for crude and refined palm oils were uniform, the import of refined oils accounted for the larger chunk of palm imports. However, with fixation of differential import duties for crude and refined palm during the 2000s, crude palm import started to dominate the palm import basket (Figure 18.22). The share of crude oil in total oil import declined from a peak of over 97 per cent in 2001-02 to 81 per cent in 2003-04, when the duty differential between crude and refined palm oil was reduced to 5 per cent from April 2003. With the increase in the duty differential to 10 per cent from July 2004, there was an improvement in the share of crude oil to over 88 per cent in 2004-05.

Import Policies and their Implications

In 1994 the government, in a major policy shift, placed certain edible oil imports under the Open General License which meant that imports could be made freely after paying duty. This was probably in anticipation of the commitments that India had made in GATT (the pre-cursor to the World Trade Organization) relating to trade in agricultural commodities. Imports started increasing to satisfy some of the demand that could not be met earlier. Free imports (since 1994) have further lowered the entry barrier to the industry as crude or refined oil can be imported, packed and distributed doing away with the need of having manufacturing facility in the domestic market.

The World Trade Organization came into being in 1995 and adopted the agreements that had been reached by GATT members in the Uruguay Round. This included an agreement on agriculture that required reducing barriers to agricultural imports in the decade 1995-2004. As part of its obligations under WTO, the government removed quantitative restrictions on edible oil imports and replaced them with import

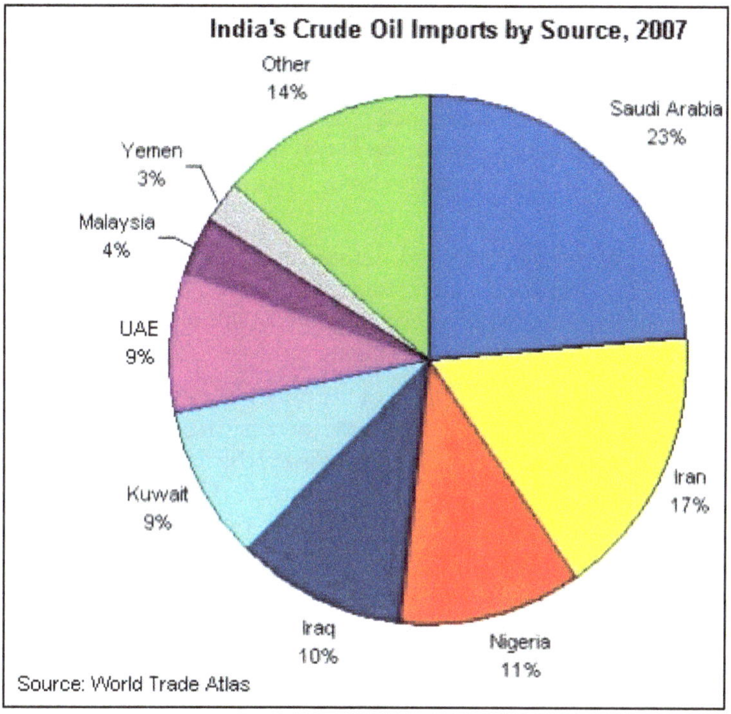

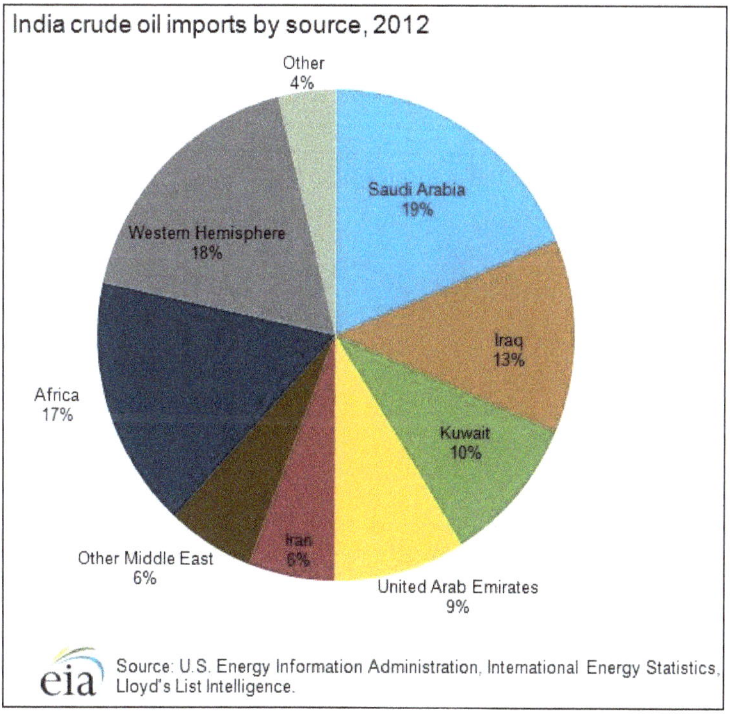

Figure 18.22: India's Oil Imports by Source, 2007and 2012

duties. In succeeding years, even the import duties were lowered rapidly, from 65 per cent in 1994 to 20 per cent in 1996 and 15 per cent in 1998. It must be pointed out that the duties applied by the government in this period were much lower than the upper bounds (300 per cent on crude and refined palm oil and RBD palmolein, for example) allowed by the WTO regime. The government was not disallowed from levying higher import duties; indeed it was only exercising its policy option by choosing lower import duties.

This lowering of duties combined with a sharp fall in international edible oil prices in 1999 led to a flood of cheap oil being imported into the country, initially in far greater quantity than the requirement. By 1998-99, imports reached the level of 4.3 million tones, a ten-fold increase in four years.

One argument advanced in support of the policy of free imports was the benefit that consumers got through low prices and the increase in per-capita consumption of edible oils as a result of the lower prices. However, the flood of cheap imported oil had a disastrous effect on India's edible oil farmers. Oilseed prices crashed and remained depressed for the next 3 years. In 1999, newspapers reported massive distress sales of oilseeds by farmers at prices much below the Minimum Support Price, with the government refraining from market intervention operations.

Not getting a remunerative price, farmers responded in the only way they could by reducing the acreage under oilseeds. Domestic edible oil production from primary oilseeds fell sharply in the period 1996-97 to 2002-03. The edible oil industry in India had come around a full circle from 1994; imports of edible oil were now firmly established and India had become the world's largest importer of edible oil.

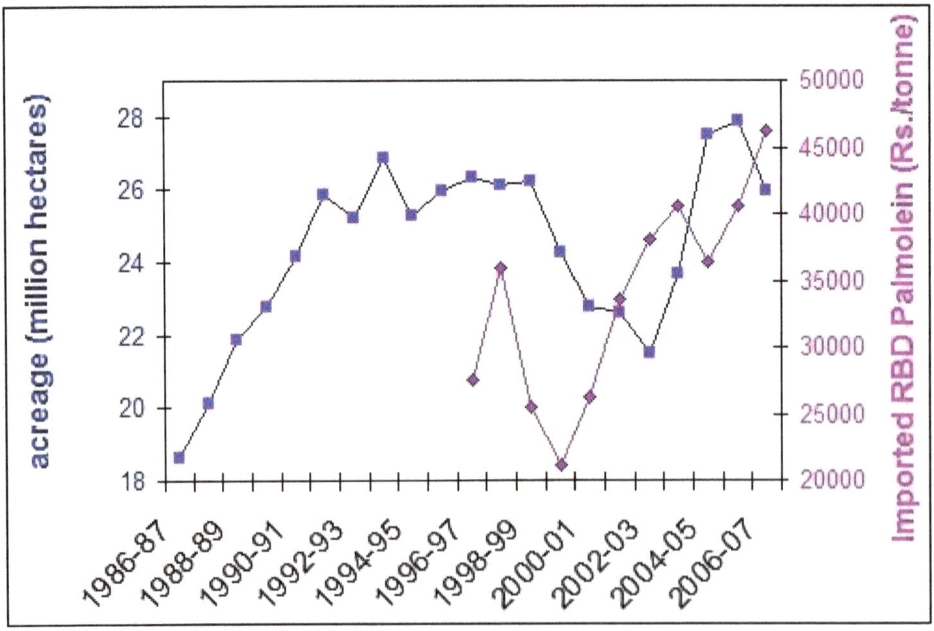

Figure 18.23: Oilseed Acreage and Price of Imported Oil

The above graph shows how the acreage under oilseeds is sensitive to the price of imported oil. As cheap imports rose, farmers planted less in India (Figure 18.23).

The edible oil policy of the post-WTO period introduced a large element of instability into domestic production by completely exposing it to international price fluctuations. After seeing a continuous increase in acreage up from 18 million hectares in 1986 to 27 million hectares in 1994, the area under oilseeds production has remained around 26-27 million hectares, falling at times of depressed international prices. Productivity of land under oilseeds has also remained stagnant at levels of a decade ago. The OTM became dormant, never recovering from the body blow it suffered from the post-WTO policy regime.

In the wake of the recent fall in international prices of edible oils, the government has re-imposed a 20 percent import duty on crude soybean oil with effect from November 18, 2008, while keeping the duty on refined oil unchanged at 7.5 per cent. Due to inflation concerns, the Centre had, on March 31, 2008, abolished import duties on crude edible oil and significantly reduced custom duties on refined edible oils at 7.5 per cent. The vegetable oil reference price has not been revised since December 2006.

With the recent fall in global prices of edible oils and the lower pace of off take from State Government/Union Territories, the Centre has deferred its plan to import edible oil for the Public Distribution System (PDS). On July 17, 2008, the GOI had formally launched the subsidized program of distribution of edible oils to the below-poverty-line population through the PDS. The program was intended to distribute one million tons of imported edible oils in MY 2008/09 through state governments involving a subsidy of Rs 15 billion ($312 million). Under the program, state trading enterprises (STE) such as PEC, MMTC, STC, and NAFED had imported around 350,000 tons of edible oils of which 240,000 tons had landed in the country and about 143,000 tons had been handed over to various State/Union Territories for distribution to ration card holders, to date.

Some Problems Related to Edible Oil Industry

1. An important economic decision in imports relates to the issue of whether to import oilseeds, or crude edible oil, or refined edible oils. Apart from differential import duties on oilseeds, crude oil and refined oil, other factors with a bearing on the decision include phytosanitary restrictions, differential freight cost because of varying volumes per unit of oil extracted, and storage quality of the product.
2. High imports of refined oil cause hardship to crushing mills. They are already suffering from lower crop output and lower availability of seeds. With rise in the volume of imported oil, refineries will also have less to refine. Local importers of edible oil make handsome gains by blending 'olein'–a cheaper alternative with almost all edible oils. This is illegal. Yet, 80 per cent (equivalent to the oil consumed in loose forms) of the edible oil sold contains 30 per cent olein, which is the liquid fraction of palm fruit and can be a severe health risk. It may even cause cardiovascular disease.

Only 20 per cent of an estimated 13.5 million tones of total consumption has been kept away from this evil. Low prices of these oils (around 15 per cent less than branded edible oil) attract consumers, particularly in rural areas.

3. Lack of assured market for oilseeds and timely and assured supply of quality seeds and raw material for processing have been found as important factors contributing to the poor performance of the oilseed industry. The standards set by the oil import countries after liberalization were very high, at times giving impression that they were used as trade barriers. But all said and done, exporting countries especially the developing and under developed countries were caught in the web of stringent quality parameters. Against such a background, it has become not an easy task for India to maintain its participation in oilseeds international trade. It is apparent that quite a good deal of domestic exercise has to be resorted to by India in the matter of quality upgradation. India needs to attain global competitiveness, that is to say ability to produce globally acceptable quality and at globally comparable cost (Subramanian, 2007).

FEW OBSERVATIONS

1. **Indian Oilseeds Yield/Ha. are very low in comparison with the World Average for the Oilseeds Crops grown in India. For GN it is 66%, for Soya 42%, for Rapeseed 45%, for Sunflower 55% and Sesameseed 88% of world average.**
2. **Edible Oilseeds area for said five Oilseeds increased from 205 Lac Ha in 2001-02 to 248 Lac Ha in 2011-12 i.e. on an average only 1.9% increase per year.**
3. **Domestic production of said Oilseeds increased from 190 Lac MT in 2001-02 to 228 Lac MT in 2011-12 i.e. average increase per year 1.8% only. That means productivity is stagnant.**
4. **Edible Oil Consumption increased from 101 Lac MT in 2001-02 to 164 Lac MT in 2011-12 i.e. average 5.6% increase per year.**
5. **Per capita consumption increased from 9.4 kg in 2001-02 to 13.2 kg in 2011-12.**
6. **Import of Edible Oils increased from 44 Lac MT in 2001-02 to 98 Lac MT in 2011-12 and import dependence increased from 44% to 60% during the same period.**

The Future Shock of Bio-Diesel on Edible Oil Industry

In recent years, the international edible oil markets have come around full circle from the price lows of the year 2000. Indian farmers have not added acreage under oilseeds from the mid nineties because of the unstable market environment and withdrawal of government support. This has led to a large gap in supply and demand that cannot be bridged quickly. India is in deep trouble now, being dependent on imports for 40 per cent of its requirements at a time of sky-rocketing prices. Wholesale prices (of imported RBD Palmolein) have been increasing for the last three years. The government is importing inflation and there is very little it can do in the short run besides reducing duties to zero per cent (it has already done this). The policy that reportedly favoured Indian consumers at the cost of farmers has come back to bite the consumers with a vengeance. But what does the future hold? Will market forces result in increasing edible oil production and hence bring down prices? Here, the situation appears extremely complex.

The demand for vegetable oil is becoming linked to the price of petroleum and to the geopolitical complexities of the crude petroleum market. The US and European countries are de-risking themselves from high dependence on imported crude petroleum by increasing the use of bio-diesel (made from vegetable oils) as fuel. Governments have started setting targets for petroleum companies for mandatory blending of bio-diesel with petro-diesel and these targets will be increased over time. Bio-diesel adoption and use will also be determined by government subsidies.

The demand and supply equation, and hence the price of edible oils will therefore be subject to the vagaries of government policy of the major petroleum importers, primarily the US and Europe, the international price of crude oil, as well as the requirements of the large edible oil importers like China and India.

In this 'mixed' economy of fuels and food, there is an urgent need for the government to formulate and implement a policy that will cater to the long term interests of Indian farmers as well as edible oil consumers. Indeed, now that 'agriculture' is being defined in the context of fuel as well, there may be some maneuvering room for India in the trade arena as well. If energy security needs provide justification for the US and Europe to take steps to limit their dependence on imports of crude petroleum oil, can India be faulted if, in the interests of its food security, it takes steps to limit its dependence on imports of edible oil, an essential food item in this country? (Kannan, Aug. 10, 2008).

Future Policy

Favourable policy framework for the oilseed sector is the basic pre-requisite for oilseed production. The policy must aim at increasing the efficiency and competitiveness of oilseed sector, which alone can lead to sustainable development in the market economy. In order to improve the trade competitiveness of oilseeds, India needs to pay attention for improving efficiency in cost of production, marketing and transport and processing of oilseeds. India needs to promote aggressively the export of niche oilseeds like castor oil, sesame seeds, groundnut and other oilseeds with specific attributes of consumer interest (Chand, 2007).

According to Hegde (2007), there is a need to adopt multi-pronged approach to meet out the challenges posed by the increasing demand for edible oil in the country. That approach will be increasing the oilseed production of the country through possible area expansion, improvement of the productivity of oilseed crops, increasing the global competitiveness of the oilseeds and oils through value addition, improving the processing efficiency of oilseeds and oils, solving the problems that pose in front of domestic marketing of oils, exploiting the supplementary sources of oils to the potential extent and liberalization of trade in the country's oilseeds economy.

The Government should encourage the industry to involve itself in the task of increasing oilseed productivity. Industry bodies can play in major role in this. The industry is all for taking a pro-active approach for increasing oilseed production and it is willing to invest into Oilseeds Extension Programme to provide to the farmers the necessary agri inputs to achieve higher productivity level. However, this needs to be encouraged by way of giving weighted Income Tax deduction of 200 per cent to companies undertaking Oilseeds Extension Programme. The private involvement in Oilseed Extension Programme will supplement Government's efforts and will go a long way in increasing oilseeds production and productivity in the country.

There has been a remarkable surge in the consumers' preferences for quality of oil world over (Singh, 2007). In recent years, the edible oil industry has taken initiatives to increase oilseed production. The state of Punjab has started contract farming on 1000 acres. The Solvent Extractors Association of Punjab is now in the process of finalizing a project with Punjab Agro-Industries Corporation under which sunflower, mustard, castor and others would be produced through contract farming (Mruthyunjaya, 2007). The initiatives taken by oil industry associations like Soybean Processors Association of India (SOPA) and The Central Organization for Oil Industry and Trade (COOIT) in laying out platforms wherein, the fruitful interaction between researchers, technocrats, industry representatives and consumers can take place are encouraging.

The Government may take a serious and immediate look at use of bio-technology for increasing oilseed productivity. Possibility of increasing the percentage of oil content can also be looked at, with the use of bio-technology.

Mr. Davish Jain President the Central Organisation for Oil industry & trade at the 30th All India Seminar on Rabi Oilseeds and Oils at New Delhi on 22nd March, 2009 said that currently time-bound plan of action is being prepared for the next five years, for submission to the Ministry of Agriculture, which aims at increasing average productivity of oilseeds from the current 1 tonne per hectare to at least 1.3 tones per hectare. The task of challenging but not unachievable as has been demonstrated by the scientists themselves, who have achieved yields higher by at least 50 per cent of current levels by using improved technology. The Government has recognized the urgent need to increase production and is willing to provide all help. The maiden efforts of working directly with the farmers and acting as an interface between them and the scientists and other stake holders, through COOIT's participation in FLD programme for rapeseed/mustard last year have brought in excellent results.

Both the government and industry should focus on increasing the productivity of oilseeds to overcome the over dependency on imported oils by maintaining the price of vegetable oil through the appropriate duty structure, which would translate into remunerative price for oilseeds to the farmers; paying more attention to improve the productivity rather oilseed area; paying attention to develop value-added products from the oilseeds; larger allocation of funds for raising the farm productivity through development and multiplication of high yielding varieties and weighted income tax deduction for oilseeds extension programmes to the private sector as granted to research organizations for research activity (Mehta, 2007). The country must aim to increase oilseed productivity to at least 1.5 t/ha by 2015 through a combination of multipronged strategies and policy support.

Steeply rising imports of edible oils (Rs 46,242 crores in 2011-12), need an urgent and bold policy decision. Developing oil palm on a million hectares that is identified as suitable for its cultivation is the main answer to bridging the gap between demand and supply of edible oils. The Commission has already submitted a separate report on that in January 2012, wherein it is analyzed and recommended that investing Rs 10,080 crores over the next six years can save the government an import bill of more than Rs 600,000 crores over the next 27 years. In view of this, the allocation of Rs 100 crores for current year for developing oil palm is woefully low looking at the need and savings it can yield. The Commission therefore recommends that at least Rs 2000 crores per year be allocated to develop oil palm in the country, and it should be taken up on a high priority, as it will benefit large numbers of farmers and consumers alike, and also save on the import bill.

The government should maintain a customs duty structure for edible oils to ensure a remunerative price to the farmers for their produce. This is very important because in a globalised economy, the oil prices are not in our control, they depend on demand-supply situation. The only mechanism to keep prices at a level for farmers to grow oilseeds is a proper duty regime.

The Central Organisation for Oil Industry and Trade (COOIT), the apex organisation of oilseed and edible oil industry, and trade, has demanded an immediate levy of import duty on crude edible oil. The move is required to restrict imports and protect Indian farmers. Both the manufacturers and solvent extractors have also been asking the government to immediately levy customs duties to protect domestic farmers. The centre, in March 2008, had removed import duty on crude edible oils from 40 to 50 per cent, while it announced a 7.5 per cent levy on all imported refined oils including expensive olive oil. The government should see that speculative imports do not prove to be a disincentive for farmers to pursue the goal of raising productivity to at least 1300 kg a hectare within five years. It should also think of creating an oilseeds development fund.

Strategies to Meet India's Oil and Fat Nutrition By 2050

To meet the challenges of oilseeds production in the post-WTO regime, there is need to adopt a multipronged strategy which involves enhancing oilseeds production through area expansion and productivity improvement through better adoption of improved technology, value addition to oilseeds and oils to increase their competitiveness, higher recovery of oils through efficient processing of oilseeds and oils, overcoming the constraints of domestic marketing of oilseeds and their products, and finally liberalizing trade in India's oilseeds economy.

If the country has to turn near self-reliant in the vegetable oils sector in the coming years, a comprehensive policy framework for the entire sector taking into consideration various demands and interests of all the stakeholders (consumers, industries, farmers and traders) with diverse interests is a pre-requisite. The policy must stimulate balanced growth of the vegetable oil sector which can be sustained over a long run and some of the major elements of such a policy frame work are as given under:

- ☆ All traditional oilseeds are reserved for the small-scale sector with an inefficient processing setup, losing more than one million tones of oil. There is a need to decontrol all these oilseeds to enhance efficiency of processing. India has large processing industry with low capacity utilization leading to high processing cost. Opening up all oilseeds to modern processing will lead to efficient processing, benefiting both producers and consumers.
- ☆ Although the government has been regularly announcing the minimum support price for oilseeds, effective market intervention by the National Agricultural Cooperative Marketing Federation (NAFED) to give price support was not forthcoming in most of the years and in several regions leading to distress sales and consequent low realization from oilseeds by the farmers and diversion of limited farm resources to more remunerative crops.
- ☆ India's liberalized import policy on vegetable oils is adversely affecting the domestic farmers, although consumers are benefited by cheaper availability of vegetable oils. Care has to be taken not to let low international prices affect the domestic market. Political and international pressures on the government to follow import friendly policy must be resisted.
- ☆ The oilseeds policy framework has to promote the goals of techno-economic efficiency and social equity through a creative combination of policies, which puts a premium on science and technology. Public policy should support greater involvement of the private sec-tor in providing inputs and services to the farmer, processor and trader. The tariff policy should strike an appropriate balance between the promotion of domes-tic production and of export, while safeguarding the interests of consumers through reasonable imports.

Chapter 19

Oil that Matters I

India accounts for 10 per cent of the world's edible oil consumption. Mentioning about the major oilseeds, groundnut, soy bean, and rape/mustard seeds account for 80 per cent of the total oilseeds grown in India. According to the United States Department of Agriculture (USDA), India was likely to produce about 7.4 million tonnes of vegetable oils in 2008-09 as against the requirement of 13 million tonnes, sufficient to meet only 46 per cent of the country's demand. The country will have to import the deficit vegetable oils to meet the domestic requirement (USDA, 2009). At present, India imports over 50 percent of its vegetable oil requirements.

Besides, vegetable oil seeds, livestock and fish are other important sources of oils and fats in Indian cooking. Since several studies in literature have directly implicated the amount and type of fat intake to specific diseases such as cardiovascular disease, cancer, high blood pressure and obesity, so one has to be very particular as to quantity as well as quality of fat in the diet to maintain good health. The quantity and quality of fats determine the intakes of various fatty acids in the total diet. Several studies have indicated that the hypocholesterolemic action of a dietary fat depends on the fatty acid composition and also to some extent on the micronutrients like tocopherols and tocotrienols present in them.

According to the American Heart Association, the optimum intake of fat for an adult is 25-35 per cent of its total caloric intake. Therefore, for an adult man consuming 2000 calories, the upper limit of total fat (visible and non-visible) is 78g per day. Apart from visible fat some amount of fat is present in food items like cereals, pulses, milk, eggs, meat etc. as invisible fat. From the data-base generated on fatty acid composition in Indian foods and National Nutrition Monitoring Bureau diet surveys, the daily invisible fat intake is estimated to be 15gm in rural poor and 25g in the urban middle and high-income groups. Thus, the daily requirement of visible fat intake works out to be somewhere between 20 to 50 g depending upon physical activity and physiological status.

In India, visible fat is taken from the animal fat and vegetable oils. These fat sources contain saturated, monounsaturated and polyunsaturated fatty acids. Hydrogenated fats contain trans fats too which are not healthy. Choice of healthy cooking oil is a controversial subject. Before selecting the right kind of fat source, it would be appropriate to discuss the various types of fats and oils available in the market which are generally used in the Indian meals. These are as under:

A. Animal Fat

Animal fats have been eaten by humans, and our ancestors, since the dawn of time. So our bodies have had plenty of time to get used to them. They are a highly efficient way of taking in dietary energy, and provided that their energy is burnt off through exercise and maintaining body temperature, they cause few problems.

Also, contrary to popular mythology, animal fats are not all saturated. Lard, for example, is composed of roughly equal amounts of mono-unsaturated and saturated fatty acids, and is very low in myristic acid, the main saturated fatty acid associated with cardiovascular disease. The more liquid poultry fats have even less saturated fat.

The harder animal fats such as beef fat and venison fat have a high proportion of longer chain saturates such as stearic acid, which is cholesterol neutral, and only traces of myristic acid. As for palmitic acid, a saturated fat which raises cholesterol is found in all animal fats. Our body readily converts surplus carbohydrate in our diets into palmitic acid for energy storage. Cutting our dietary intake of palmitic acid will, therefore, do little to lower levels of palmitic acid in our bodies so long as we eat a carbohydrate-rich diet.

Animal fats also contain cholesterol which is infamous as a cause of heart disease. However, dietary cholesterol only correlates weakly with blood serum cholesterol which in turn does not directly relate to cholesterol in tissues, or cholesterol laid down in a plaque on the inner surface of arteries which is what is really dangerous to health. The creation of arterial cholesterol plaque is also stimulated by oxidisation, often caused by free radicals and saturated fats provide some protection against free radicals.

Natural animal fats also contain other factors beneficial to health, such as tocopherols, natural anti-oxidants better known as Vitamin E, as well as other fat-soluble vitamins and mineral nutrients.

Recent scientific studies indicate that it is often carbohydrate, and especially refined carbohydrate, which should be removed from the diets, rather than fat generally and saturated fat in particular. For most of us (barring vegetarians) animal fats are a considerably superior alternative to hydrogenated vegetable fats. Another advantage of animal fats is that they tend to be chemically stable (unlike the polyunsaturated vegetable oils). They can therefore be used for frying and cooking without significant deterioration. In addition, far less of these saturated fats are absorbed into food while cooking–half as much, according to studies by the US Food and Drug Administration. This means that food that is deep fried in animal fat, such as fish and chips, contains less fat and have better fat than is the case if these are cooked in standard frying oils of hydrogenated vegetable origin.

In India, mostly people use animal butter oil, also known as desi ghee and butter in cooking which are discussed as under.

I. Desi Ghee

Ghee is produced by heating butter. Heating evaporates water present in the latter. As the temperature continues to rise, the initial white sediment of milk protein and salt turns brown. This imparts an irresistible nutty flavour to ghee. Since ghee is derived from milk, it is essentially an animal product. Therefore, it contains a certain amount of saturated fat and cholesterol.

Desi ghee (butter oil) used to be the conventional cooking oil of the Indians. There was nothing wrong with this most favourite cooking medium of Indian households. But the problems started with the change in our eating and living habits. Desi ghee being rich in saturated fats has the tendency to increase total cholesterols including HDL (so called "good cholesterols") and LDL and VLDL (so called "bad cholesterols"). Excessive consumption of saturated fat elevates blood cholesterol level while the contribution of dietary cholesterol per se is not so significant.

As such consumption of desi ghee coupled with fibre rich diet which reduces LDL bad cholesterol and physical activity which reduces VLDL bad cholesterol brings about a favourable lipid profile. In the good olden days, our forefathers used to take fibre rich diet such as chapattis made out of flour of whole grains and lots of leafy vegetables along with desi ghee and the nature of work involved lots of physical labour. All this used to neutralize the adverse effects of desi ghee on LDL and VLDL while retaining its positive effects on HDL and thereby this favourite cooking medium used to bring about a favourable lipid profile. But with the lack of physical activity in the recent years coupled with intake of diet devoid of fibre such as chapattis and other snack foods made from flour of decorticated food grains, consumption of desi ghee started raising total cholesterol levels.

Although saturated fats increase the level of cholesterol in the blood, not all have the same effect. In desi ghee, only a few fatty acids have the cholesterol-raising effect. About 65 per cent of the fat in ghee is saturated and as much as 32 per cent is MUFA (mono-unsaturated fatty acids). MUFA is a highly desirable form of dietary fat, the kind that olive oil is rich in. It is perhaps more desirable than PUFA (poly-unsaturated fatty acids). In this respect, desi ghee scores over many PUFA-rich oils like sunflower, safflower, corn and cottonseed oils, whose MUFA content is dismally poor.

Ghee besides being a concentrated source of energy (9 Kcals/ g) is also rich in vitamins A, D and riboflavin as well as minerals such as calcium, magnesium, phosphorus, and potassium. Vitamin A helps in maintaining good vision, healthy glowing skin and acts as an important antioxidant too. Vitamin D, calcium, magnesium and phosphorus form important constituents of the skeletal structure and also play important roles in other physiological functions like nerve conduction, blood-clotting etc. Potassium is needed to maintain the delicate fluid and electrolyte balance within cells, to keep heartbeat regular and to maintain normal blood pressure.

Another good point about desi ghee is that it has an ideal linoleic / alpha linoleic acid (LA/ALA) ratio. This ratio is unusually high in most PUFA oils, which is undesirable. It is now recognized that the consumption of oils with ideal LA/ALNA ratio is crucial for prevention of coronary heart disease. Excessive consumption of PUFA-rich oils may depress HDL cholesterol (the kind that protect the heart) level, thereby increasing the risk of coronary heart disease. Desi ghee, unlike refined oils, is heated to very high temperatures while cooking. This helps it retain its original nutritional properties.

Cholesterophobia exaggerated fear of cholesterol is now making Indians dump one of the most essential components of their kitchens, the desi ghee. These fears of cholesterol and saturated fat have virtually driven out the most revered cooking ingredients in the Indian kitchen- desi ghee. The negative impression of desi ghee because of several factors including an exaggerated fear of cholesterol (cholesterophobia) is not justified particularly in the Indian vegetarian setup which rarely meets the upper limit of 300 mg per day. Condemning it as a culprit for blocking arteries and replacing it with refined hydrogenated vegetable oils is cause for concern. Other factor was the saturated fat and cholesterol hypothesis of Professor Ancel Keys around the 1960s leading to demonising saturated fats irrespective of what type they were. Both these suited vegetable oil manufacturers who were quick to take advantage of these findings.

While concerns about oils and fats are justified both with respect to their amounts and types, simplistic conclusions drawn on research hypothesis can be hasty and even dangerous. It would do them good if they did some re-thinking before replacing desi ghee with new-age substitutes such as cholesterol-free margarines and unsaturated refined oils. A closer look reveals that such a negative view about this highly nourishing food-ghee does not stand the test of scientific logic. More so, in the traditional Indian texts including Ayurveda desi ghee has been prized for its health promoting properties.

Therefore, the search started for an alternative cooking oil which could reduce the cholesterol levels. Short-term scientific studies conducted in this regard found that vegetable oils rich in polyunsaturated fats had the ability to reduce total cholesterols as such the recommendations tilted in favour of PUFA rich oils such as safflower oil.

In due course of time evidence began to accumulate establishing that although polyunsaturated fats were effective in reducing LDL cholesterol, very high content of polyunsaturated fats had the undesirable effect of reducing HDL cholesterol as well. It further came to light that since oils with high levels of polyunsaturated fats oxidize faster than those with MUFA or SFA profiles, therefore, the excessive intake of these oil could impair the ability of the anti-oxidants in the human system to control free radicals and thereby enhance the risk of certain cancers, cataracts, rheumatoid arthritis, Parkinson's disease and contribute to the ageing problem. All these findings have led to a change with respect to the earlier recommendations and a delicate balance between cholesterol balancing (instead of cholesterol lowering) properties and oxidative stability has become an important concern now a days.

An excess of desi ghee like any other fat is clearly undesirable due to its calorie content. But all those who thought it is higher in calories or fat compared to oils need to think again. Oils / ghee are in the range of 90-95 per cent fat. An excess of desi ghee like any other fat is clearly undesirable due to its calorie density. However, this certainly does not mean that desi ghee is harmful for children and adults even with high cholesterol and heart disease, when taken in right amounts. Also no one cooking medium is ideal, a combination is the best. So desi ghee as the sole cooking medium is not recommended rather a blend of cold pressed / sesame, mustard and olive oil is desirable.

Current research suggests that the real villain in our diet may be hydrogenated vegetable oils and not *desi ghee*. There is little scientific evidence that a low fat diet is beneficial. While fat restriction is advisable to combat undesirable weight gain, it is more important to be concerned about fat quality. It is more important to avoid potato chips, hamburgers, pizzas, French fries, *samosas, namkeens* and other commercial foods prepared in vanaspati or margarines like patties, biscuits, cookies rather than curtailing ghee. Also it is essential to be physically active. Drawing conclusions on a few research findings in the West and applying them in larger contexts in India is not valid. Indians have unique risk factors for developing coronary artery disease, quite distinct from the western world. It is important to analyze these to conduct our own research to formulate special guidelines for Indians, rather than simply applying Western guidelines. Desi ghee should perhaps take the lead!

II. Butter

Butter has long been prized as a high quality food. Health scares about saturated fats of animal origin have frightened a great many people off butter in recent decades but quite wrongly so. All those people who have switched to margarines (mostly based on hydrogenated vegetable oils) have actually been consuming a far less healthy alternative and one that tastes far less good as well. Of course, it makes sense to limit how much butter you eat if you need to cut back on the calories, as butter is a rich source of energy. But given that we all have to eat some fat, indeed fat is an essential part of our diets and butter is a good choice.

Butter is one of the most highly concentrated forms of fluid milk. Twenty litres of whole milk are needed to produce one kilogram of butter. Butter is the product made from churning fresh cream. Commercial butter is 80–82 per cent milk fat, 16–17 percent water, and 1–2 per cent milk solids other than fat (sometimes referred to as curd). It may contain salt, added directly to the butter in concentrations of 1 to 2 per cent. Butter also contains protein, calcium and phosphorus (about 1.2 per cent) and fat-soluble vitamins A, D and E. Although there are over 120 different compounds that contribute to butter's unique flavor, the five primary factors responsible for butter's flavor include fatty acids, lactones, methyl ketones, diacetyl and dimethyl sulfide.

Chemically butter fat consists essentially of a mixture of triglycerides, particularly those derived from fatty acids, such as palmitic, oleic, myristic, and stearic acids. The fatty acid composition of butter fat varies according to the producing animal's diet. It mainly consists of saturated fat.

Table 19.1: Nutrient Composition of Butter

Nutrients per100g	*Salted*	*Unsalted*
Energy (kcal)	717	717
Water (g)	15.87	17.94
Protein (g)	0.85	0.85
Total Lipids (g)	81.11	81.11
Saturated Fat (g)	51.37	51.37
Monounsaturated Fat (g)	21.02	21.02
Polyunsaturated Fat (g)	3.04	3.04
Trans Fat (g)	2.98	2.98
Cholesterol (mg)	215	215
Total Carbohydrates (g)	0.06	0.06
Ash (g)	2.11	0.04

Source: USDA National Nutrient Database for Standard Reference, Release 20 (2007).

Butterfat also contains small amounts of lauric acid, a uniquely health-promoting fat that is also found in coconut oil and mother's milk. It is also a good natural of conjugated linoleic acid (CLA)–a natural polyunsaturated trans fat with anti-cancer properties. CLS is the common name of a group of fatty acids found in dairy products. However, over the last 50 years, changes in livestock feeding practices, have largely removed naturally occurring CLA from our diets. It seems that eating the right butter from cows that are relaxed, content and grazing on green grass (where the CLA comes from) can actually help our body reduce its body fat and increase its lean muscle. Whereas, eating butter from high production cows that never munch away, but are fed stock grains while hooked up to milking equipment, lined up in overcrowded stalls, and leading anything but content lives well, the milk they produce has little or no CLA. In turn, it makes us fatter, particularly in the belly, which is associated with chronic disease.

In several recent studies, CLA has received considerable attention due to its apparent metabolic and other health benefits and anti-cancer properties in animals, as well as some similar, initial results in humans. The effects seen in animals include reduced body fat content, improved serum lipid profiles, decreased aortic lipid deposition, improved glucose control and delayed onset of diabetes.

Now a days there is a growing use of 'butter fat' as an ingredient of processed foods. This is mostly derived from 'surplus' butter, by removing the water, protein etc, then sold cheaply (compared to butter, anyway) as a bulk ingredient to the food industry. As a semi-hard fat, it substitutes directly for hydrogenated oil. Without the water and protein it also has good keeping properties, good enough that, for example, Tesco is happy to use it in its own-brand dark chocolate. Nestlé also uses butterfat in Kit-Kat bars, presumably for the cream filling. Its fatty acid composition is roughly half saturates, and half monounsaturates.

B. Vegetable Oils

The most important and regular consumption of fat is through the cooking oil in our daily diets. There are so many types of edible vegetable oils available in the market for cooking purposes. These include sunflower, safflower, soybean, corn, sesame, cottonseed, groundnut, rice bran, olive, flaxseed, palm oils etc. (Table 19.3). They contain varying amount of different fatty acids. The fatty acid composition of these oils has been given in Table 19.3. Generally, vegetable oils except coconut oil contain unsaturated fatty acids.

Table 19.2: Plant and Animal Sources of Oil

☆ Almond oil	☆ Babassu oil
☆ Avocado oil	☆ Blackcurrant oil
☆ Borrage oil	☆ Coconut oil
☆ Cocoa butter	☆ Cottonseed oil
☆ Corn oil	☆ Fish oils
☆ Evening primrose oil	☆ Jojoba oil
☆ Grapeseed oil	☆ Linseed oil (flaxseed oil)
☆ Hard butter – illipe butter (Borneo tallow), sal fat and shea butter	☆ Groundnut (Arachis or peanut oil)
☆ Hazelnut oil	☆ Macadamia oil
☆ Lard	☆ Palm kernel oil
☆ Olive oil	☆ Pistachio nut oil
☆ Palm oil	☆ Sesame seed oil
☆ Rice bran	☆ Mustard and rapeseed oil
☆ Canola oil	☆ Soybean
☆ Safflower oil	☆ Whale
☆ Sunflower oil	☆ Walnut oil
☆ Tallow	

The nutrient composition, fatty acid composition and health benefits of some of the commonly available and consumed vegetable oils are detailed out as below.

I. Rice Bran Oil

Rice bran a by-product of the rice milling industry is a good source of edible oil in which the country is not yet self-sufficient. Rice bran – both full fat and defatted is a rich source of nutrients and can serve as a source of nutrient supplement. The bran fraction, which includes the germ or embryo in most commercial milling operations, represents only about 8 per cent of paddy weight but contains about three-fourths of

Table 19.3: Fatty Acid Composition of some Common Edible Fats and Oils (Percent by weight of total fatty acids)

Type of Oil	Unsat./ Sat. Ratio	Saturated Fatty Acids					MUFA		PUFA
		Capric Acid C10:0	Lauric Acid C12:0	Myristic Acid C14:0	Palmitic Acid C16:0	Stearic Acid C18:0	Oleic Acid C18:1	Linoleic Acid (ω6) C18:2	Alpha Linolenic Acid (ω3) C18:3
Almond Oil	9.7	–	–	–	7	2	69	17	–
Butterfat (cow)	0.5	3	3	11	27	12	29	2	1
Butterfat (goat)	0.5	7	3	9	25	12	27	3	1
Butterfat (human)	1.0	2	5	8	25	8	35	9	1
Canola Oil	15.7	–	–	–	4	2	62	22	10
Cocoa Butter	0.6	–	–	–	25	38	32	3	–
Cod Liver Oil	2.9	–	–	8	17	–	22	5	–
Coconut Oil	0.1	6	47	18	9	3	6	2	–
Corn Oil	6.7	–	–	–	11	2	28	58	1
Cottonseed Oil	2.8	–	–	1	22	3	19	54	1
Flaxseed Oil	9.0	–	–	–	3	7	21	16	53
Grape seed Oil	7.3	–	–	–	8	4	15	73	–
Olive Oil	4.6	–	–	–	13	3	71	10	1
Palm Oil	1.0	–	–	1	45	4	40	10	–
Palm Olein	1.3	–	–	1	37	4	46	11	–
Palm Kernel Oil	0.2	4	48	16	8	3	15	2	–
Peanut Oil	4.0	–	–	–	11	2	48	32	–
Safflower Oil*	10.1	–	–	–	7	2	13	78	–
Sesame Oil	6.6	–	–	–	9	4	41	45	–
Soybean Oil	5.7	–	–	–	11	4	24	54	7
Sunflower Oil*	7.3	–	–	–	7	5	19	68	1
Walnut Oil	5.3	–	–	–	11	5	28	51	5

* Not high-oleic variety.

Percentages may not add to 100 per cent due to rounding and other constituents not listed. Where percentages vary, average values are used.

the total oil (Juliano and Bechtel, 1985; Lu and Luh, 1991). Containing about 15-20 per cent oil, rice bran is commercially feasible for oil extraction. The high oil content of bran makes it subject to rancidification, one of the reasons that is often separated from the grain before storage or further processing. The bran itself can be heat-treated to increase its longevity. Appearance of rice bran oil ranges from cloudy to clear depending on the degree of dewaxing and winterization process applied.

Rice bran oil is extensively used in Japan, Korea, China, Taiwan and Thailand as 'Premium Edible Oil'. India, China, Japan and Myanmar are important producers of rice bran oil constituting more than 95 per cent of the global production. India is the largest importer of rice bran oil followed by Japan. It is the conventional and the most favourite cooking medium of the Japanese, the longest living human beings on this earth and is popularly known as "Heart Oil" in Japan.

Production in India

India produces 120 million tonnes of paddy annually which contain 5-6 per cent of rice bran, leading to production of 6-7 million tonnes of rice bran. Rice bran contains 16 per cent oil, hence there is a potential for production of 1- 1.2 million tonnes of rice bran oil in the country but the actual production of rice bran oil is only 0.7-0.9 million tonnes. India has a vast rice bran potential, occupying the second place in the world, next only to China.

India is the second largest producer of crude rice bran oil in the world. At present, only about half of the potential source of rice bran is exploited for oil. There is a need to utilise the full potential of the available rice bran in the country, both as a source of healthy edible oil and as a food supplement for promoting our population's nutrition and health. The modern rice mills and huller-cum- shellers are helping in recovering good quality rice bran for oil extraction. The industry believes that rice bran oil production could multiply in the coming years if more awareness could be generated about its nutritional properties.

About 75 per cent of crude oil is used for edible purposes for manufacture of vanaspati and rest goes to industrial sector for manufacture of soap. As India is the second largest producer of crude rice bran oil in the world, some of the leading national and multi-national players in this field are having an eye over this largely untapped potential and are planning to enter in a big way in the branded refined rice

Facts about production of RBO

Global Scenario

- Global production of rice bran oil fluctuates between 10–14 lakh tons depending on rice production.
- Rice Bran Oil is extensively used in Japan, Korea, China, Taiwan and Thailand as 'Premium Edible Oil'.
- India, China, Japan and Myanmar are important producers of rice bran oil constituting more than 95 per cent of global production.
- India is the largest importer of rice bran oil followed by Japan.

Indian Scenario

- India produces around 7 – 9 lakh tons of rice bran oil.
- India imports around 40,000 – 45,000 tons of rice bran oil.
- In normal scenario, India has a capacity to process 12 lakh tons of rice bran oil.
- India exports 20,000 – 30,000 tons of rice bran oil.

bran oil segment. Only recently some of the Indian markets too have started witnessing some brands of pure refined rice bran oil. M/s A.P. Solvex, has launched its pure refined rice bran oil brand "Ricela" in northern India, especially in Himachal Pradesh, Punjab and Jammu and Kashmir. The time is not very far when the leading brands of refined rice bran oil will be available in all the markets of India and consumers in India too could enjoy the benefits of this unique gift from the Mother Nature. The technology for refining of rice bran has been standardised recently by Council of Scientific and Industrial Research (CSIR) and has already been tested.

Moreover, as India imports considerable quantity of edible oil, use of domestic rice bran oil will help in import substitution, thus saving valuable foreign exchange. However, proper promotion of rice bran oil as health oil remains the most important factor in increasing its acceptability as cooking oil among the masses.

Nutrient Composition of Rice bran and RBO

Carbohydrate

The carbohydrate of bran is a mixture of complex carbohydrates and starch. Although starch is absent in true bran, commercial bran obtained on rice milling contains starch derived from the rice kernel, the content of which may range from 10 to 25 per cent depending on the extent of polishing. Rice bran with low levels of available carbohydrate (25 per cent) and high level of fat (20 per cent) can be considered as a good source of energy when used as a supplementary food for diabetics.

Protein, Fat and Micronutrients

Rice bran is a rich source of proteins, fats, minerals and micronutrients, such as B-vitamins and trace elements. The protein of rice bran has higher lysine content and a lower glutamic acid content than rice and wheat and it has a better balance of essential amino acids with an amino acid score of 80 per cent with respect to lysine, and 90 per cent with respect to threonine. It is reported to have a Protein Energy Ratio (PER) value of nearly 2.0. It contains certain unique micro-nutrients which are important for promotion and maintenance of good health. Rice bran with 15 to 20 per cent oil can serve as a good source of energy and essential fatty acids (EFA) (Narasinga Rao, 2000).

The typical composition of crude rice bran oil is 81.3-84.3 per cent triglycerides, 2-3 per cent diglycerides, 5-6 per cent monoglycerides, 2-3 per cent free fatty acids, 0.3 per cent waxes, 0.8 per cent glycolipids, 1.6 per cent phospholipids, 4 per cent unsaponifiables. Oleic and linoleic fatty acids constitute more than 80 per cent of the fatty acids of the glycerides. Rice bran oil is similar to peanut oil in fatty acid composition with a saturation level that is slightly higher than that of conventional soybean oil. The much lower linolenic acid content of rice bran oil makes it more stable to oxidation than soy oil. In comparison with other vegetable oils, crude rice bran oil tends to contain higher levels of non-triglyceride components, most of which are removed during further refining processes. The quality characteristics of properly refined rice bran oil include a maximum free fatty acid levels (as oleic acid) of 0.1 per cent, a maximum peroxide value of 1.0 meq/kg, 0.05 per cent moisture, an iodine value of 99–108, saponification value of 180-195, and a Lovibond color value of 3.5R.

The free fatty acids, monoglycerides and diglycerides in rice bran oil are associated with enzymatic hydrolysis. The phospholispids predominantly include phosphatidylcholine, phosphatidylethanaolamine, and phosphatidylinositol. The wax content of rice bran oil can be somewhat variable, depending upon cultivar and processing parameters. Various sterols constitute the principal portion of the unsaponifiable fraction of nutraceutical interest.

Table 19.4: Comparison of Fatty-Acid Composition of Selected Oils with Rice Bran Oil

Fatty Acid (per cent)	*Percentage Rice Bran*	*Percentage Peanut*	*Percentage Soybean*	*Percentage Cottonseed*
Myristic ((14:0)	0.2	0	0.2	0.8
Palmitic (16:0)	15.0	8.1	10.7	27.3
Stearic (18:0)	1.9	1.5	3.9	2.0
Oleic (18:1)	42.5	49.9	22.8	18.3
Linoleic (18:2)	39.1	35.4	50.8	50.5
Linolenic (18:3)	1.1	0	6.8	0
Arachidic (20:0)	0.5	1.1	0.2	0.3
Behenic (22:0)	0.2	2.1	0.1	0

Source: Young (1996), Sipos and Szuhaj (1996), and Jones and King (1996). Data for rice bran oil are from Riceland Foods, Inc.

Table 19.5: Fatty Acid Composition of Rice Bran Oil, Palm Oil, Palmolein and Groundnut Oil

Fatty Acid	*Rice Bran Oil*	*Palm Oil*	*Palmolein Oil*	*Groundnut Oil*
Myristic	0.60	0-15.00	1.00	–
Palmitic	21.50	41-46.80	39.80	14.40
Stearic	2.90	4-05.10	4.40	3.10
Oleic	38.40	37-40.80	42.50	42.60
Linoleic	34.40	9-11.00	11.20	35.90
Linolenic	2.20	0-0.60	0.40	–
PUFA: MUFA*	0.95	0.37	0.27	0.84

Table 19.6: Comparison of Smoke Point and Balance of Fats in some Commonly Used Oils

Oil Type	*Smoke Point*	*MUFA*	*PUFA*	*Saturated Fat*
Rice Bran Oil	490º	47 per cent	33 per cent	20 per cent
Olive	360º	77 per cent	9 per cent	14 per cent
Canola	450º	61 per cent	33 per cent	7 per cent
Soybean	440º	24 per cent	61 per cent	15 per cent
Grape seed	485º	14 per cent	77 per cent	9 per cent

Fatty Acid Composition of RBO

- ☆ Rice bran Oil contains more than 75 per cent unsaturated fatty acid of which essential fatty acid in the form of linoleic acid (PUFA) constitutes about 35 per cent.
- ☆ Chemically the composition of rice bran oil is very close to groundnut oil containing 34-36 per cent linoleic acid and 2 per cent linolenic acid, the essential fatty acids.
- ☆ The stearic acid content of rice bran oil is 3 per cent compared to about 4 per cent of palm oil. Oleic acid content is almost comparable to palm oil/Palmolein while linolenic acid content is higher (2.2 per cent) as compared to 0.06 per cent in palm oil.
- ☆ According to the recommendations of the National Research Council, Washington DC, the PUFA/MUFA content should be nearly 1.0. The ratio of PUFA/MUFA is nearly this value in rice bran oil while it is of the order of 0.27-0.37 in Palmolein/palm oil. The PUFA/MUFA ratio is considered to be the most important factor in controlling atherosis problem.

Micronutrients

The rice bran oil is characterized by certain micro-nutrients which contribute to its exceptional nutritional qualities as summarized below:

Micronutrient	*Amount %*	*Advantage*
Tocopherol	0.02-0.08	Antioxidant, free radical scavenger, reduces risk of cardiovascular diseases, arthritis, cancer, cataract, antitumour.
Tocotrienol	0.025-0.17	Cholesterol reduction, antithrombetic, anticancer, and anti-ageing properties, tumour suppression, antioxidant.
Oryzanol	1.2-1.7 (physically refined RBO)	Increases good (HDL) cholesterol, decreases bad (LDL) cholesterol, treats nerve imbalance and menopause disorder, retards aging effects, antidandruff and anti-itching agent. Effective in treating a broad range of gastrointestinal disorders including stress-induced gastric and duodenal ulcers.
Squalene	0.3-0.4	Antioxidant, improves skin tone, and anti- wrinkle properties.

Antioxidants

It contains various antioxidants that impart beneficial effects on human health. It is well known that a major rice bran fraction contains 12 per cent -13 per cent oil and highly unsaponifiable components (4.3 per cent). This fraction contains tocotrienol, gamma-oryzanol, and beta-sitosterol; all these constituents may contribute to the lowering of the plasma levels of the various parameters of the lipid profile. Both the bran and oil from rice bran have a range of bioactive phytochemicals with potential for reducing the risk of chronic degenerative diseases.

Table 19.7: Total Natural Antioxidants in Rice Bran and other Cooking Oils

Oil Type	*Tocopherol (ppm*)*	*Tocotrienol (ppm*)*	*Oryzanol (ppm*)*	*Total Natural Antioxidants (ppm*)*
Rice bran oil	81	336	2,000	2,417
Olive oil	51	0	0	51
Canola	650	0	0	650
Sunflower oil	487	0	0	487
Soybean oil	1,000	0	0	1,000
Palm oil	256	149	0	405

* ppm. stands for parts per million

Cooking Application of RBO

Rice bran oil is extremely light, versatile and delicious. It is quickly becoming a favourite in commercial frying to replace hydrogenated oils that contain trans fat. Despite its similarities to other common vegetable oils, rice bran oil offers several unique properties that make it very interesting as specialty oil in niche markets. It has a very appealing nut-like delicate flavour and once extracted is very stable with good fry-life. It has no aftertaste and has a pleasant scent.

This trans fat free rice bran oil has a very mild flavour and high smoke point, so it is ideal for many types of cooking and baking. Rice bran oil also has a very high smoke point, which means the oil can be used to cook at very high temperatures. Rice bran oil's smoke point is 490°F compared to olive oil with a smoke point of 360°F and canola with a 450°F smoke point. This high cooking temperature makes it excellent for deep frying, sautéing and stir frying. The high smoke point prevents fatty acid breakdown at high temperatures. It possesses good storage stability and fry life without hydrogenation, due to its moderate level of naturally occurring saturated fatty acids and at least in part to its low linolenic acid content. It mixes better in salad dressings and improves the taste of baked goods, providing cholesterol reduction, nutritional and anti-oxidant value. It has a light viscosity and foods cooked in rice bran oil absorb less fat (upto 20 per cent) than with many other types of oil. Less oil absorbed also makes it more economical. Rice bran oil creates less polymers than other oils meaning better flavour and easier clean-up.

When processed to retain high levels of tocols, rice bran oil may be used as a natural antioxidant source for topically coating a wide range of products such as crackers, nuts, and similar snacks to extend shelf life. This use is further enhanced by the highly desirable flavour of rice bran oil. The fatty acid composition of rice bran oil and peanut oil are similar and either oil works well at a high temperature, however, while peanut oil has an earthy flavour, rice bran oil is nutty, enhancing the flavour of fried foods. In addition, rice bran oil gives an ideal colour and desirable texture to all types of fried foods. Alternatively, as described in a patented process (Taylor *et al.*,

1996), this specially processed rice bran oil may be blended with less-stable oils (such as soy with a high linolenic acid content) to improve their stability in food systems.

Health Benefits of RBO

Rice bran oil is vastly superior to traditional cooking oils and can be considered nutraceutical (food as medicine) oil that is perfect for all the healthy cooking needs. This is due to health, flavour and performance benefits of rice bran oil. Anti-oxidants of vitamin E group are naturally occurring in rice bran oil. But perhaps its most notable feature is its high level of components with nutraceutical value such as gamma-oryzanol and tocotrienols. Rice bran oil is truly "The World's Healthiest" edible oil, containing vitamins, antioxidants, nutrients and trans fat free. It can help lower cholesterol, fight diseases, enhance the immune system, fight free radicals and more.

Rice bran oil has been proved to be the only edible vegetable oil with the fatty acid profile that is closest to the recommendations made by organisations like the WHO and the American Heart Association. A lot of research has been carried out on this oil by National Institute of Nutrition, Hyderabad, Central Food Technological Research Institute, Mysore and Council of Scientific and Industrial Research, New Delhi. The Research Institutes in India and abroad have found this oil to be a Heart Friendly- Health Oil'.

Recent research shows that a specific component of rice bran has heart-healthy effects. It is the oil and not the fibre that helps to lower cholesterol. Previous research has also pointed to the heart-healthy effects of rice bran and rice bran oil, which is most commonly available in Japan and India. Although the PUFA content of rice bran oil is much lower than the other conventional oils, but it has higher cholesterol reduction power than even the PUFA rich oils. In recent years, U.S. Scientists have also shown a tremendous interest in the cholesterol lowering properties of rice bran oil and this oil has acquired the status of "Health Food" with the Americans. Rice bran oil reportedly has a ratio of saturated, monounsaturated, polyunsaturated and essential fatty acids (omega3 and omega 6 fatty acids) that is close to the ideal ratio recommended by American Heart Association. It also has significant cholesterol and triglyceride reducing properties.

In a recent study, 14 participants followed two different diets for five weeks each. During the first 5-week period, study participants consumed one third of their total daily dietary fat in the form of a blend of peanut oil, olive oil, corn oil, canola oil, palm oil and butter with a fatty acid composition similar to that of rice bran oil. During the second 5-week period, the oil blend was replaced with rice bran oil. At the end of the study, researchers found that participants' cholesterol levels were the lowest when their diet consisted of rice bran oil.

Human trials conducted by the National Institute of Nutrition, Hyderabad, have confirmed significant reduction in total cholesterols particularly the triglyceride levels by using rice bran oil as compared to conventional cooking oils. In this study 21 subjects with high total cholesterols (>225 mg/dl) or high triglycerides (>190 mg/dl)

Benefits of Rice Bran Oil

- ☆ A source of vitamin E complex, antioxidants and other micronutrients to help fight free radicals and combat the effects of aging. Rice bran oil has more of these components than other cooking oils. The components of rice bran oil give it an outstanding shelf life.
- ☆ It contains three categories of natural anti-oxidants as against one in conventional oils.
- ☆ Rice bran oil is a naturally occurring source of many antioxidants such as Tocopherols, Tocotrienols, Gamma Oryzanol, Phytosterols, Polyphenols and Squalene.
- ☆ Research had proved the effectiveness of rice bran oil in reducing cholesterol. It's the oil of choice for improving serum cholesterol levels and preventing cardiovascular diseases.
- ☆ It is good for skin. It contains squalene which improves skin tone and delays wrinkle formation.
- ☆ It has 4 hydroxy 3 methoxy cinnamic acid which stimulates hormonal secretion and rejuvenates health.
- ☆ It has tocopherol which helps in maintaining balance of nervous system.
- ☆ It has tocotrienol which has antithrombotic and anticancer properties.
- ☆ Rice bran oil has the best balance of saturated, monounsaturated and polyunsaturated fats as recommended by the American Heart Association and the World Health Organization.
- ☆ The viscosity of oil is very light and the flavour delicate. Foods cooked with Rice bran oil absorb up to 20 per cent less oil. Less oil absorbed results in reduced calories, better, lighter tasting food and enhanced flavour and palatability.
- ☆ Rice bran oil is hypoallergenic. For those who have intolerance to other cooking oils, this is an excellent alternative.
- ☆ Rice bran oil has a very high smoke point, making it perfect for deep frying, pan or stir frying and is an ideal choice for replacement of hydrogenated oil containing trans fat.
- ☆ Rice bran oil creates less polymers than other oils meaning better flavour and easier clean-up.

were randomly divided into experimental and control groups. Twelve subjects, who constituted experimental group, were instructed to use rice bran oil in place of their usual cooking oil which they were using earlier. The remaining nine who served as controls, were allowed to continue the use of their habitual edible oil. There was a significant reduction in total cholesterol and triglyceride levels 15 and 30 days after the use of rice bran oil. However, in control subjects there were no changes in serum lipids.

Table 19.8: Serum Lipids in Control and Experimental Subjects

	Subjects	*Cholesterol (mg/dl)*	*Triglycerides (mg/dl)*
1.	Control Group Basal	244.0 ± 14.0	295.5 ± 33.0
	After 30 days	249.6 ± 16.1	286.3 ± 34.9
	% change from Basal	2.3	–3.1
2.	Experimental group Basal	247.3 ± 10.5	349.8 ± 42.4
	15 days after RBO	204.0 ± 6.6	236.5 ± 31.9
	30 days after RBO	182.7 ± 8.4	212.9 ± 20.0
	% change from Basal after 15 days	–17.5	–32.4

Similar findings have been reported in the animal studies coupled with the human clinical trials recently completed and published by the University of Lowell, USA. These studies have confirmed that rice bran oil has the ability to reduce blood cholesterol levels up to 40 percent and has significantly better cholesterol lowering than the popular olive oil. Experiments conducted by the Human Nutrition Research Centre., Washington showed a greater reduction in the total and LDL cholesterol in animals fed with the RBO diet than those consuming Canola oil diet. All these studies conducted in India and abroad have attributed the cholesterol reducing properties of rice bran oil to the presence of a unique component in this oil known as "Oryzanol" which is not found in any other edible oil. This fact has been re-confirmed in a most recent study conducted by the Central Food Technological Research Institute, Mysore. In this study it was observed that although the fatty acid composition of groundnut oil and rice bran oil is almost similar but use of rice bran oil significantly raises good cholesterol and reduces bad cholesterol due to "Oryzanol" present in the rice bran oil. Serum lipid levels of rats fed with diet containing 10 per cent groundnut oil and refined rice bran oil containing about 10,000 ppm of oryzanol produced through the latest techniques of refining were reported as under after 11 weeks of feeding:

Table 19.9: Effect of Groundnut Oil and Refined Rice Bran Oil on Serum Lipid Profile

Parameters mg/100 ml	*Groundnut Oil (Control) (mg/dl)*	*Refined Rice Bran Oil (mg/dl)*
HDL Cholesterol (Good cholesterol)	33.8 + 6.69	50.57 + 3.57
LDL + VLDL (Bad cholesterol)	23.48 + 8.51	15.75 + 6.68
Triglycerides	272.8 + 59.7	118.7 + 34.55

The hypocholesterolemic activity of rice bran oil vis-à-vis other vegetable oils is recorded in Table 19.10.

Besides beneficially influencing the lipid profile, oryzanol is also known to have anti-itching, anti-dandruff and anti-ageing properties. It is effective in treating a broad range of gastrointestinal disorders including stress-induced gastric and duodenal ulcers. Oryzanol is also sold abroad as an agent for body building in humans and for treatment of nerve imbalance and disorders of menopause.

Table 19.10: Hypocholesterolemic Activity of Various Edible Oils

Edible Oil	*Linoleic Acid per cent*	*Cholesterol Level*
Safflower	77.1	–16
Sunflower	61.4	–12
Cottonseed	58.0	0
Soybean	50.2	+3
Sesame	45.9	+2
Corn	43.0	–15
Rice bran	36.0	–17
Groundnut	35.0	+5

Rice bran oil is also an abundant source of the primary antioxidants (Vitamin E) including alpha, beta, gamma and delta tocopherol isomers as well as the most active of all antioxidants – the tocotrienols. Tocotrienol is highlighted as the most precious and powerful vitamin E existing in nature and is said to have an anti-cancer effect. As a vitamin-E source, rice bran has the highest amount of tocotrienol in liquid form vegetable oils.

Tocotrienols found only in rice bran oil and in no other conventional Indian oil, besides being a cholesterol reducing agent and a powerful antioxidant are also known to have anti-thrombotic, anti-cancer and anti-ageing properties. Compared to other edible oils, rice bran oil has high content of squalene which is reported to be a quencher of singlet oxygen and a free radical scavenger and it has been shown to maintain the texture of skin. It is well known for its anti-wrinkle properties.

High content of natural antioxidants present in the rice bran oil, impart higher oxidative stability and a longer shelf life as compared to other edible oils. In a study conducted by the Central Food Technological Research Institute, Mysore, oxidative stability of natural antioxidants enriched refined rice bran oil has been found to be five times more than the groundnut oil.

With the population in the country being increasingly prone to lifestyle-induced diseases, including cardiovascular problems, efforts should be made to promote heart-friendly cooking oils such as rice bran oil, speakers at the 10th National Seminar on Rice Bran Oil said. Minister of State for Social Justice and Empowerment Ms Subbulakshmi Jagadeesan said that though average life expectancy had increased, but India lagged behind developed nations in healthy food habits. As the largest producer of rice bran oil, India could emerge as a market leader in its production and consumption, she said. Efforts made by associations like the Solvent Extractors' Association, which organised the conference, have helped to increase the acceptability of the oil in several households (The Hindu, July 1, 2007).

To sum up, the rice bran oil is the only oil which, besides having almost balanced fatty acid composition and linoleic to linolenic (Omega6/Omega3) ratio closest to the recommendation of the nutritionists, contains three categories of natural anti-oxidants namely, tocopherols, tocotrienols and oryzanol as against only one category, *i.e.*

tocopherols found in all other conventional oils. In fact rice ban oil is gaining acceptance as the 'health oil' by virtue of the desirable fatty acid composition with higher oxidative stability along with better cholesterol reducing power than all other edible oils. It contains certain unique micro-nutrients which are important for promotion and maintenance of good health.

II. Olive Oil

Civilisations based in the Mediterranean region have always known about the innate goodness of olive oil, either by instinct or through traditions. For thousands of years, people in Crete, Greece, Italy, French, Spain, and Morocco have centred their diets around olives and the oil they produce, resulting in a uniquely healthy lifestyle. Olive oil has been and still is a staple in the diet of many Mediterranean countries. Today, much of the commercial cultivation of olive oil is still centered in the Mediterranean region in such countries as Spain, Italy, Greece, Portugal and Turkey. Olive oil consumption is also equated with a lowered risk of obesity and improved blood pressure. Recently, scientists have been able to encapsulate pharmaceutical-grade olive oil in a blend with vitamins, minerals and herbals.

The recent discovery that the Mediterranean diet, which features this prized oil, may be linked to a reduced risk of heart disease and other health conditions has caused olive oil to become very popular. Anyone coming from the Mediterranean region of the world would tell about the health benefits, as well as the wonderful flavour, of a good dose of olive oil on salads, pasta, fish and almost anything else. Fortunately, it is available throughout the year to satisfy taste buds and promote good health.

Different Grades of Olive Oil

Olive oil is made from the crushing and then subsequent pressing of olives. The fact that olives are rich in oil is reflected in the botanical name of the olive tree-Olea europea- since the word "oleum" means oil in Latin. Olive oil is available in a variety of grades, which reflect the degree to which it has been processed. Extra virgin olive oil derived from the first pressing of the olives, having the most delicate flavour and most antioxidant benefits is recommended to the customers. Though it is the most expensive yet it has the maximum health benefits. Different grades of olive oil and their properties have been described as under.

Nutrient Composition of Olive Oil

Many research studies have reported that olive oil like other vegetable oils is made up of triglycerides and minor components and its composition greatly depends, among others, on climatic conditions, soil quality and fruit variety. The fatty acids that make up TGs of olive oil just like micro components vary depending on what region the oil is from. Olive oils therefore, around the Mediterranean Basin are not the same and may not have the same effect on the human body as Greek Olive Oil. Research has shown that Greeks despite poor health care had a longer life expectancy (over 80 years) and the world's lowest rates of heart disease and cancer as well as the lowest mortality rate due to cardiovascular illness. In simple words, Greeks seemed

Different Grades of Olive Oil

When you shop for olive oil, you will notice a host of different grades are available, including extra-virgin, fine virgin, refined and pure. Olive oil is "graded" according to its flavour, colour, aroma, as well as its acidity, which is the most important element in determining grade.

- ☆ Extra-virgin is the unrefined oil derived from the first pressing of the olives and has the most delicate flavour. It is characterized by an acidity level of less than one percent. It is considered the finest and fruitiest olive oil and is therefore also the most expensive. It can range from pale champagne to greenish-gold to bright green in colour. In general, the deeper the colour, the more intense the olive oil flavour.
- ☆ Virgin is also derived from the first pressing of the olives but has a higher acidity level (between one and two per cent) than extra virgin olive oil (as well as less phytonutrients and a less delicate taste). Although its flavour varies in intensity, this oil is milder than extra virgin olive oil.
- ☆ Chemically, the difference between extra virgin olive oil and virgin olive oil involves the amount of free oleic acid, which is a marker for overall acidity. According to the standards adopted by the International Olive Oil Council, "virgin" can contain up to 2 per cent free oleic acid, while "extra virgin" can contain up to 0.8 per cent of free oleic acid.
- ☆ Olive oil has an acidity level of no more than 1.5 per cent. It is obtained by blending refined oil with 1-15 per cent extra virgin olive oil. It is much lighter in taste and colour.
- ☆ Pure olive oil is a bit of a misnomer. Don't be fooled if you see the term "pure" on the label; it means the oil is a blend of refined and virgin olive oils. It has an acidity level of no more than 1.5 per cent.
- ☆ Refined olive oil is all virgin olive oil, extracted by cold pressing, which does not conform to the International Oleical Council standards, is refined to correct the taste and lower the acidity level to 0.3 per cent. It has very low nutritional value and lacks all antioxidants and other ingredients that the true 100 per cent extra virgin olive oil has.
- ☆ Another term that you may see on a bottle of olive oil is "cold pressed." This term means that minimal heating was used when mechanically processing the olives to make oil.

to live longer and healthier lives. Today's scientific research on nutrition has recognized the Greek diet as among the healthiest in the world. Scientists tried to pinpoint what was that made Greeks so special health wise. Olive oil, rich in monounsaturated fats, is largely responsible for excellent health of Greeks.

Olive oil is 75 per cent oleic acid, the stable mono-unsaturated fat, along with 13 per cent saturated fat, 10 per cent omega-6 linoleic acid and 2 per cent omega-3 linoleic acid. Rich presence of oleic acid makes olive oil ideal for salads and cooking at moderate temperatures. Extra virgin olive oil is also rich in antioxidants. It should be cloudy, indicating that it has not been filtered, and have a golden yellow colour, indicating that it is made from fully ripened olives. Olive oil has withstood the test of time and it is now considered the safest vegetable oil you can use. The longer chain fatty acids, found in olive oil, are more likely to contribute to the build up of body fat than the short- and medium-chain fatty acids could in butter and coconut oil.

Health Benefits of Olive Oil

In many parts of the world, a high fat intake is associated with degenerative diseases such as atherosclerosis, diabetes, asthma, colon cancer, and arthritis. But in some parts of the world, a high fat intake is actually associated with lower rates of these conditions. A closer look at the foods eaten in these places reveals that the high fat intake is actually due to the generous use of olive oil. Comparing these areas, such as the Mediterranean, where olive oil is the main fat used, to other regions, like the United States, where other fats such as animal fats, hydrogenated fats and vegetable oils like corn oil dominate, turns up some very interesting data. It turns out that people who use olive oil regularly, especially in place of other fats, have much lower rates of heart disease, atherosclerosis, diabetes, colon cancer, and asthma. Olive oil is rich in monounsaturated fat, a type of fat that researchers are discovering has excellent health benefits.

Protection against Heart Diseases

Virgin olive oil, a much richer source of polyphenols than refined olive or other refined oils, is the best vegetable oil for heart health, shows the results of the Eurolive study, published in the September 2006 issue of Annals of Internal Medicine. A review of the research by noted olive oil researcher Maria Covas strongly suggests that diets in which olive oil is the main source of fat can be a useful tool against a wide variety of risk factors for cardiovascular disease.

The researchers have concluded the exclusive use of olive oil during food preparation seems to offer significant protection against coronary heart disease, irrespective of various clinical, lifestyle and other characteristics of the participants. Relying only on olive oil may cut risk of coronary heart disease almost in half, show results from the CARDIO2000 case-control study, published in Clinical Cardiology (Kontogianni *et al.*, 2007). Consuming other fats or oils as well as olive oil, however, conferred no protection.

Studies have shown that olive oil may lower heart disease risk by lowering the levels of bad cholesterol (LDL-low density lipoprotein) in the blood and leaving the good cholesterol (HDL-high density lipoprotein) intact. It slashes the risk of heart disease because it breaks down the plaque in clogged arteries and reduces the risk of hardened arteries.

Research studies on olive oil and atherosclerosis have revealed that the particles of LDL cholesterol of a person whose diet is high in olive oil will primarily contain oleic acid, the fatty acid that predominates in this oil. These particles of LDL cholesterol are more resistant to free radical or oxidative damage. And not only will the LDL of a person whose dietary fat is primarily olive oil produces LDL that is more resistant to free radical damage, but that individual's LDL will be further protected by olive oil's supplies of vitamin E and phenols with antioxidant activity, further lessening the likelihood of its being oxidized. By protecting LDL against oxidation, olive oil short circuits the process through which atherosclerotic plaques form. Since only oxidized cholesterol sticks to artery walls, eventually forming the plaques that can lead to a heart attack or stroke, preventing the oxidation of cholesterol is a good way to help prevent atherosclerosis. Simply put, olive oil reduces the risk of heart disease by lowering LDL cholesterol (bad cholesterol) which contributes to the build up of fatty deposits in the arteries. In turn, it leaves HDL (good cholesterol) which works to actually remove any build up in the arteries that has occurred.

Prevention of Hypertension

By reducing both inflammation and free radical damage to cholesterol, dietary olive oil protects the endothelium, the lining of blood vessels, helping to maintain its ability to relax and dilate, thus preventing high blood pressure. In men from Northern and Central Europe who do not typically eat a Mediterranean diet, daily consumption of 25 ml of olive oil resulted in a 3 per cent decrease in systolic blood pressure.

Theodora Psaltopoulou and colleagues from the University of Athens, Greece investigated whether the Mediterranean diet as a whole, or just olive oil, is responsible for the reduction in blood pressure associated with this way of eating. Their finding was that while the diet as a whole reduces blood pressure, olive oil, by itself, is largely responsible. The Greek team examined the ability of the total diet and of olive oil alone to reduce arterial blood pressure. Their study included over 20,000 Greek participants who were free of hypertension (high blood pressure) when the study began. Food frequency questionnaires were completed and systolic and diastolic blood pressures were taken. Diet was evaluated by a 10 point score that reflected the extent to which study participants followed the Mediterranean diet and also provided scores for individual components of the diet, including olive oil. Data analysis confirmed that the Mediterranean diet as a whole was significantly associated with lower systolic and diastolic blood pressure as were olive oil, vegetables and fruit. On the other hand, consumption of cereals, meat and meat products, and alcohol intake was associated with higher blood pressure. When the effects of olive oil and vegetables were compared, olive oil was found to be responsible for the dominant beneficial effect on blood pressure.

Rich Source of Antioxidants and Protective Effects

Olive oil is a functional food that is also rich in antioxidants and phenolic compounds with a variety of protective effects. "Olive oil is more than a monounsaturated fat. Its phenolic content can also provide benefits for plasma lipid levels and oxidative damage," concluded the researchers. Research studies have suggested that such heart-healthy effects from olive oil are due not only to its high content of monounsaturated fats, but also to its hefty concentration of antioxidants, including chlorophyll, carotenoids and the polyphenolic compounds tyrosol, hydrotyrosol and oleuropein-all of which not only have free radical scavenging abilities, but protect the vitamin E (alpha-tocopherol) also found in olive oil.

The 6 research centre study, led by Maria-Isabel Covas, Head of the Research Group in Oxidative Stress and Nutrition at the Lipids and Cardiovascular Epidemiology Unit of the Municipal Institute of Medical Research in Barcelona, Spain assigned 200 healthy men from 5 European countries including Spain, Denmark, Finland, Italy and Germany to one of three sequences of daily consumption of olive oil. The men replaced their normal dietary fats with olive oil (25 ml) containing either 2.7 (refined), 164 (virgin), or 366 (extra virgin) mg/kg of phenols for 3 weeks. This was followed by 2 weeks without any olive oil and then a cross-over to each of the other 2 remaining interventions. Blood samples were taken before and after each intervention to measure blood sugar, total and HDL (good) cholesterol, triglycerides, free radical damage to cholesterol, and antioxidant levels. The data revealed a linear increase in HDL cholesterol levels as the phenolic content of the olive oil increased, with increases of 0.025, 0.032, and 0.045 mmol/L for the low, medium and high polyphenol containing olive oils. Oxidized LDL (the form in which LDL is involved in atherosclerosis) decreased linearly, dropping from 1.21 U/L, to -1.48 U/L, to -3.21 U/L for the low-, medium-, and high-polyphenol olive oil, respectively. And the ratio of total to HDL cholesterol, considered the most specific cholesterol-associated risk factor for cardiovascular disease, also decreased linearly as the phenolic content of the olive oil rose. Virgin olive oil, a much richer source of polyphenols than refined olive or other refined oils, is the best vegetable oil for heart health, shows the results of this Eurolive study, published in the September 2006 issue of Annals of Internal Medicine.

Greek scientists at the University of Athens reporting their research in the Journal of Agriculture and Food Chemistry believe the synergy of all these beneficial nutrients is what is responsible for olive oil's contribution to the health benefits of the Mediterranean diet, a hypothesis supported by Italian research published in the Journal of Nutrition. In this study, scientists found that the phenols in olive oil have very potent antioxidant effects. The protective effects exerted by extra virgin olive oil biophenols, namely, protocatechuic acid and oleuropein, against LDL oxidation included:

- ✰ Completely preventing LDL's oxidation when placed in a medium containing macrophage-like cells (in the arteries, arteriosclerosis begins when macrophages damage LDL, starting the development of foam cells that infiltrate the lining of the artery and begin plaque formation)
- ✰ Inhibiting the production of two powerful oxidants that would normally have been produced and would have damaged LDL, thus preventing the expected decrease in glutathione, a powerful antioxidant the body produces to disarm oxidants (also called free radicals)
- ✰ Restoring to normal levels the protective activities of two free radical-disarming enzymes that contain glutathione: glutathione reductase and glutathione peroxidase
- ✰ Inducing higher than normal production and activity of both of these glutathione-containing enzymes.

Helps in Losing Body Fat

A study published in the British Journal of Nutrition suggests that substituting olive oil, a monounsaturated fat or MUFA, for saturated fat in the diet can translate into a small but significant loss of both body weight and fat mass without changing anything else about diet or increasing physical activity. One of the most interesting facts about this research is that it was conducted on eight overweight or obese men, ranging in age from 24 to 49 years. All the men followed one of two diets for 4 weeks each. The first, saturated fat-rich diet provided 24 per cent of calories from saturated fat, 13 per cent from monounsaturated fat, and 3 per cent from polyunsaturated fat, while in the second MUFA-rich diet, 11 per cent of calories came from saturated fats, 22 per cent from monounsaturated fat and 7 per cent from polyunsaturated fat. At the end of the MUFA-rich diet, despite the fact that no significant differences were detected in caloric intake, energy expenditure or physical activity, the men were 2.1 kg lighter and their fat mass had decreased by 2.6 kg.

Additional support for olive oil's fat burning effects comes from another study published in the British Journal of Nutrition, which suggests that the monounsaturated fats found in olive oil cause an increase in the breakdown of fats in adipocytes. In this study, 45 laboratory animals were divided into three groups, each of which was fed a diet supplying normal energy but a different type of fat: olive oil, palmitic acid or soybean oil + palmitic acid. At the end of the study, a number of indicators of fat metabolism were measured including body weight, plasma leptin, tissue concentration of fatty acids, fat-cell size, fat cell lipolytic activity, and the capacity of insulin to inhibit fat breakdown. In the animals receiving monounsaturated fats, not only was fat breakdown greater, but insulin's ability to block it was lower. Interestingly, in rats given polyunsaturated fat in the form of soybean oil, the opposite effect was noted in adipose tissue.

Diabetes

Compared to diets high in saturated fat and low fat, high carbohydrate diets, a number of studies have shown that olive oil-rich diets not only reduce LDL cholesterol levels, but also lower blood sugar levels and decrease insulin requirements in persons with type 2 diabetes.

Olive oil has also been reported to prevent abdominal fat and improve insulin sensitivity. Abdominal fat is associated with insulin resistance, which leads to further weight gain and increases risk of type 2 diabetes. When researchers fed type 2 diabetic patients different diets *i.e.* a high carbohydrate diet, or a diet rich in either saturated fat or olive oil (Mediterranean diet), it was observed that the high carbohydrate diet increased abdominal fat compared to the fat-rich diets. Of the three diets, the diet rich in olive oil did best, preventing not only abdominal fat accumulation, but also improved the sensitivity to insulin resistance. A drop in adiponectin was seen after the high carbohydrate diet meals. Adiponectin, a hormone produced and secreted by fat cells (adipocytes), regulates sugar and fat metabolism, improves insulin sensitivity, and has anti-inflammatory effects on the cells lining the blood vessel walls. Low blood levels of adiponectin are a marker for metabolic syndrome, are common in obesity, and are also associated with increased heart attack risk.

A few studies in diabetic patients have shown that healthy meals that contained some olive oil had better effects on blood sugar even than healthy meals that were low in fat. When olive oil is used to enhance a low-saturated fat, high carbohydrate diabetic diet, the diet still has beneficial effects on blood sugar control. In addition to this, a good diabetic diet with some olive oil added helps to keep triglyceride levels low. Triglyceride levels tend to be high in diabetic patients, which is a problem since high levels also contribute to the development of heart disease. So a high in complex carbohydrate, healthy diabetic diet with some olive oil added in can help for several reasons.

Ability to Reduce Breast Cancer Risk

Published studies link judicious use of olive oil to reducing the effect of a growing list of ailments. For example, Greek women have a 42 per cent lower rate of breast cancer than women in USA. Olive oil may be the key reason that eating a Mediterranean diet reduces breast cancer risk in humans, suggests a laboratory study published in the Annals of Oncology. Results of this two-year long study involving 755 women in the Canary Islands suggest that monounsaturated fat and, specifically, olive oil exerts a protective effect against breast cancer.

Study participants consuming the most monounsaturated fat were found to have a 48 per cent lower risk of breast cancer compared to women whose intake of monounsaturated fat was the lowest. Among women consuming the most olive oil, specifically, the risk of breast cancer was even lower. Compared to those consuming the least olive oil, women whose daily intake of olive oil was at least 8.8 grams, had a 73 per cent lower risk of breast cancer risk.

Oleic acid, the main monounsaturated fatty acid in olive oil, has been shown to reduce the expression of the Her-2/neu oncogene, which is associated with the aggressive growth of breast cancer tumours. High levels of Her-2/neu are found in one-fifth of breast cancers, especially those that are resistant to treatment. In this study, when Menendez and his colleagues from Northwestern University in Chicago exposed two strains of aggressive breast cancer cells to oleic acid, levels of Her-2/neu dropped to 46 per cent. When they combined oleic acid with lower levels than are normally used of Herceptin, a drug used to treat breast cancer, oleic acid greatly enhanced the effectiveness of the drug, dropping Her-2/neu expression as much as 70 per cent. The end result was that oleic acid promoted the apoptotic cell death (suicide) of aggressive, treatment resistant breast cancer cells.

Protection against Chronic Degenerative Disease

Olive oil also helps fight other illness such as diabetes, rheumatoid arthritis, breast cancer, colon cancer, asthma, constipation, the effects of aging and more according to research studies. Olive oil contains antioxidants such as vitamin E that protect cells from damage. A natural antioxidant, olive oil slows down the natural aging process. It also slows down acid overproduction in the digestive system thereby diminishing the potential for ulcers and other GIT problems. And its rich supply of polyphenols is also known to have anti-inflammatory, antioxidant and anticoagulant actions.

Potent Anti-Inflammatory Compound

In a study published by Pennsylvania biologist Dr. Gary Beauchamp in Nature, he has suggested that in the times to come, someday soon, olive oil can become the new anti-inflammatory standby and doctors may recommend extra-virgin olive oil in the meals to prevent aches and pains, and reduce the risk of cancer. Inspired by a tasting experience at a molecular gastronomy meeting in Sicily, where he noticed that high quality olive oil produced a throat-stinging sensation similar to that caused by ibuprofen, Beauchamp and his team analyzed freshly pressed extra-virgin olive oil and discovered a compound that suppresses the prostaglandin system, the same pain pathway as non-steroidal anti-inflammatory agents, such as ibuprofen. Although its chemical structure is quite different from the anti-inflammatory compounds in non-steroidal drugs, olive oil's anti-inflammatory component, which Beauchamp named "oleocanthal," has a similar effect. A 50 gram dose (about 4 tablespoons) of extra-virgin olive oil supplies enough oleocanthal to produce an effect equivalent to that of about 10 per cent of the ibuprofen dose recommended for adult pain relief. While this amount won't cure a headache (and most people may not have the room in their diet for the calories and fat contained in 4 tablespoons of olive oil), daily consumption of olive oil may prevent inflammation and confer some of the benefits of long term ibuprofen use without the increased risk of intestinal bleeding and damage to the kidneys that long-term use of non-steroidal drugs like ibuprofen also carries.

Scientists believe this finding is significant because inflammation plays a key role in a variety of chronic diseases. "Some of the health-related effects of the Mediterranean diet may be due to the activity of oleocanthal from premium olive oils," said Beauchamp. Dr Paul Breslin, who directed the research with Beauchamp, added: "The Mediterranean diet, of which olive oil is a central component, has long been associated with numerous health benefits, including decreased risk of stroke, heart disease, breast cancer, lung cancer, and some dementias. Now that we know of oleocanthal's anti-inflammatory properties, it seems plausible that oleocanthal plays a causal role in the health benefits associated with diets where olive oil is the principal source of fat." Although oleocanthal should be present in any extra-virgin olive oil, concentrations will vary depending upon a range of factors, including the variety of olive and the age of the olives at pressing.

Due to presence of antioxidants, olive oil provides protection against the following degenerative diseases:

i) Asthma and Rheumatoid Arthritis

Regular use of olive oil has been associated with lower rates of asthma and rheumatoid arthritis. The monounsaturated fats in olive oil are used by the body to produce substances which are relatively anti-inflammatory. By reducing inflammation, these fats can help reduce the severity of arthritis symptoms, and may be able to prevent or reduce the severity of asthma.

ii) Atherosclerosis

Extra-virgin olive oil, which, when properly cold pressed and stored in opaque containers, is naturally high in phenolic compounds with antioxidant properties, may be one of the key reasons for the lower incidence of cancer and cardiovascular disease in the Mediterranean region, suggests a study published in the British Journal of Nutrition.

Minor components of extra virgin olive oil-namely, its squalene, beta-sitosterol and tyrosol may help explain why the Mediterranean diet has shown such beneficial effects on cardiovascular health and cancer prevention, suggests a study published in Free Radical Biology and Medicine. It is generally accepted in the medical community that excessive production of free radicals and inflammatory compounds derived from the body's use of omega-6 fatty acids (found primarily in meats, corn, safflower and sunflower oils) contributes to the development of both cardiovascular disease and cancer. In this study, researchers tested the effects of squalene, beta-sitosterol and tyrosol on a number of free radicals as well as on inflammatory compounds produced from omega-6 fats (arachidonic acid metabolites). In each case, the olive oil compounds either significantly inhibited production of the problem-causing molecules or rendered them harmless.

A recent *in vitro* study also showed that polyphenolic compounds present in olive oil, including oleuropein, inhibit the adhesion of monocyte cells to the blood vessel lining, a process that is involved in the development of atherosclerosis. In addition, when people with high cholesterol levels removed the saturated fat from their diets and replaced it with olive oil, their total cholesterol levels dropped an average of 13.4 per cent, and their LDL cholesterol levels dropped by 18 per cent. These benefits occurred when the subjects used olive oil in place of other fats, rather than simply adding olive oil to a diet high in unhealthy fats.

Normally, after a meal, endothelial function is impaired for several hours. Blood vessels become less elastic, and blood levels of free radicals potentially harmful to cholesterol (lipoperoxides and 8-epi prostaglandin-F2) rise. But when the subjects in this study ate a breakfast containing virgin olive oil with its normal high phenolic content (400 ppm), their endothelial function actually improved, blood levels of nitric oxide (a blood vessel-relaxing compound produced by the endothelium) increased significantly, and far fewer free radicals were present than would normally be seen after a meal. When they ate the same breakfast containing the same type of virgin olive oil with its phenolic content reduced to 80 ppm, the beneficial effects were virtually absent, and concentrations of cholesterol-damaging free radicals increased.

The anti-inflammatory effects of a virgin olive oil-rich diet also result in a vascular environment in which platelets are less likely to clump together and form blood clots. Not only do olive oil's antioxidant compounds lessen the inflammation initiated by free radical damage, but olive oil is rich in inhibitors of a compound called platelet activating factor (PAF). PAF begins the clotting process by causing platelets to aggregate and is also involved in the activation of immune cells and their binding to the endothelial wall.

iii) Colon Cancer

While most other fats are associated with an increased risk of colon cancer, olive oil is actually associated with a reduced risk of this disease. The incidence of colon cancer is lower in Mediterranean countries compared with those in northern Europe, a benefit believed to be due to the central role of olive oil in the Mediterranean diet. Laboratory research published in the International Journal of Cancer further supports this hypothesis, showing that phenolic compounds in virgin olive oil protect against several stages of colon cancer development. To investigate olive oils' protective mechanisms of action, researchers at the University of Ulster in Northern Ireland extracted phenols from virgin olive oil and used them in a series of *in vitro* (lab test) experiments modeling important stages of colon carcinogenesis. In one cell culture experiment, colon cells incubated with olive phenols for 24 hours were protected from hydrogen peroxide-induced DNA damage. The higher the level of olive oil phenols, the better the protection. In a second cell culture, at 48 hours, olive phenols at a concentration of 50 μg/ml or more had significantly improved the barrier function of colon epithelial cells (the cells that form the lining of the colon), suggesting that the phenols might be exerting an anti-promoter effect in the carcinogenesis pathway. A third cell culture showed significant inhibition of HT115, a highly invasive human colorectal cancer cell line, at phenol concentrations of 25, 50, 75 and 100 μg/ml, indicating that olive oil phenols might also reduce the invasiveness of colon cancer cells.

One reason for olive oil's protective effect may be its ability to reduce the amount of carcinogenic heterocyclic amines (HAs) formed when meats are cooked, suggests a study published in Food Chemistry Toxicology. The addition of foods containing antioxidants to recipes containing meat has previously been shown to decrease the amount of HAs produced during cooking. In this study, beef burgers were fried in both virgin and refined olive oils as well as virgin olive oil with rosemary extract and refined olive oil with rosemary extract. Burgers fried in virgin olive oil had significantly less HAs than those cooked in refined olive oil; however, the longer the oil was stored, the less its HA-reducing effect-a good reason to buy olive oil in small quantities that is used within a month or two. Researchers theorized that adding rosemary to virgin olive oil might help prevent this drop in its protective effects.

iv) Effective against Helicobacter pylori

Helicobacter pylori, bacteria that burrows into the gastric lining causing chronic inflammation and promoting the development of peptic ulcers and gastric cancer, is becoming increasingly resistant to antibiotics. The search is on for other substances able to fight *H. pylori* with researchers increasingly turning not only to herbal extracts and essential oils used in traditional medicines, but to polyphenol-rich foods.

Virgin olive oil, one of the few edible oils that is consumed unrefined, contains a number of active phytonutrients. Having run experiments on food-borne pathogens that showed olive oil polyphenols have a very high level of antimicrobial activity against food-borne pathogens, Concepcion Romero and her colleagues at the University Hospital of Valme, Seville, Spain, decided to in investigate olive oil's effects on *H. pylori*. Using conditions that simulated the human gastric environment, Dr. Romero and her team demonstrated that a significant amount of the polyphenols in the olive oil diffused from the oil into the stomach acid and remained stable for several hours, exerting strong anti-*H. pylori* activity, even against some strains resistant to antibiotics. Also, only very low concentrations of the olive oil extracts were necessary. Among the polyphenols showing anti-*H. pylori* activity, one named Ty-EDA was so effective that only <1.5 μg/mL of this compound was needed to kill *H. pylori* cells in test tube experiments. To put this in practical perspective, Ty-EDA is present in most virgin olive oils in concentrations up to 240 μg/mL.

While these results need confirmation in human studies, they are quite promising, especially given earlier Russian research involving olive oil and gastric ulcer. In this study, when patients with gastric and duodenal ulcers replaced the animal fat in their diet with olive oil, ulcer size was greatly reduced and the percentage of ulcer healing significantly increased as cited in Current Pharmaceutical Design (Taits NS, cited in de la Lastra A, *et al.*, 2001).

v) Osteoporosis

The World Health Organization calls osteoporosis its biggest global healthcare problem with aging populations also beset by obesity, a condition now known to greatly increase inflammation throughout the body, including in bones where it significantly contributes to osteoporosis. Today, a woman's lifetime risk of osteoporotic fracture is 30-40 per cent, and even men face about a 13 per cent risk.

INRA researchers, inspired by epidemiological evidence that people eating a traditional Mediterranean diet were less likely to develop osteoporosis, began investigating the effects of olive oil and different compounds in olive leaves on bone metabolism. Their early studies revealed that two olive polyphenols, oleuropin and hydroxytyrosol, greatly lessen the inflammation-mediated bone loss involved in osteoporosis. Then they published research in the British Journal of Nutrition, showing that both oleuropein and olive oil feeding can prevent inflammation-induced osteopenia (bone thinning) in animals whose ovaries have been removed-an animal model designed to simulate senile osteoporosis, the bone-wasting condition that affects the elderly, as it combines both hormone deficiency with chronic inflammation. Although the animals did not fully recover all their bone density compared to controls, those rats fed oleuropin (0.15g/kg) or olive oil (50 g/kg) daily for 3 months recovered 70-75 per cent of their bone density, a 50 per cent improvement compared to control animals, which were given 25g/kg peanut oil and 25 g/kg rapeseed oil daily.

The INRA team, led by Dr. Veronique Coxam, is developing the protocol for a human study, which, if all goes well, can be started soon. The bone-sparing effects of olive polyphenols revealed in studies conducted by a special team at INRA (France's National Institute for Agricultural Research) are so dramatic that a new Belgium firm, BioActor, has licensed INRA's patents to use olive polyphenols for osteoporosis prevention in food, supplements and herbal medicines.

Recommended Intake of Olive Oil

Extra virgin olive oil is definitely one of the best food oils available today. Simply adding olive oil to an unhealthy diet that is already soaked in saturated fats or vegetable oils will not lead to any of the benefits listed above and may actually cause more harm than good, but when pure, extra virgin olive oil is used as a primary source of fat in a whole foods, healthy eating plan, the potential goodness of this oil prevails.

A study published in the Medical Science Monitor reported that 2 tablespoons a day of olive oil added to an otherwise unchanged diet in 28 outpatients, ranging in age from 64 to 71, resulted in significant drops in total- and LDL cholesterol. Mean concentrations of total cholesterol were lowered by 0.818 mmol/L, and mean concentrations of LDL dropped 0.782 mmol/L. Plus, subjects ratio of HDL: LDL greatly improved; they ended up with higher amounts of protective HDL in relation to lower amounts of dangerous LDL cholesterol.

In November 2004, the Federal Drug Administration (FDA) of the U.S.A permitted a claim on olive oil labels concerning "the benefits on the risk of coronary heart disease of eating about two tablespoons (23 g) of olive oil daily, due to the monounsaturated fat (MUFA) in olive oil." Consuming 25 ml/day of olive oil, in replacement of other fats, did not cause weight gain. A moderate amount of olive oil-a 25 ml dose (1.7 tablespoons) did not promote postprandial oxidative stress (free radical damage to cholesterol) whereas a single olive oil dose of 40 ml (2.7 tablespoons) did.

Olive oil, particularly extra virgin olive oil, provides a number of heart-healthy benefits-increasing HDL "good" cholesterol, improving the ratio of LDL:HDL, and, if one is not already following a Mediterranean diet, may lower systolic blood pressure as well. But don't overdo it. Consuming more than a couple of tablespoons at a meal can increase free radical damage of cholesterol.

Selection and Storage of Olive Oil

Proper storage techniques for olive oil are very important, not only to preserve the delicate taste of the oil, but also to ensure that it does not spoil and become rancid when exposed to light and heat, which will have a negative effect on its nutritional profile.

Research conducted at the University of Lleida in Spain and reported in the Journal of Agriculture and Food Chemistry found that levels of chlorophyll, carotenoids and antioxidant phenols dropped dramatically after virgin olive oil had been in storage 12 months-even under the best controlled conditions. Chlorophyll content dropped by as much as 30 per cent, beta-carotene by 40 per cent, and vitamin E (alpha-tocopherol) by 100 per cent. Phenols, which are not only the main antioxidants in virgin olive oil, but are also responsible for its distinctive rich flavour, also dropped precipitously after 12 months storage.

Research published in New Scientist magazine has confirmed that light destroys many of the antioxidants in olive oil. Researchers at the University of Bari, in southern Italy, compared oils stored in the light or in the dark for 12 months. Oils stored in clear bottles under supermarket lighting lost at least 30 per cent of their tocopherols (vitamin E) and carotenoids. After just two months' exposure to light, peroxide (free radical) levels had increased so much that the olive oil could no longer be classified as extra virgin.

Selection and Storage of Olive Oil

There are some important purchasing criteria which one should follow to ensure buying a better quality product.

- ☆ Since phytonutrients are more concentrated in extra virgin olive oil found in opaque, airtight glass bottles or tins, this is the best bet when purchasing olive oil for both taste enjoyment and health.
- ☆ Even though olive oil's monounsaturated fats are more stable and heat-resistant than the polyunsaturated fats that predominate in other oils, olive oil should be stored properly and used within a few months to ensure its healthy phytonutrients remain intact and available.
- ☆ Purchase only as much as you will use in three to four months and store away from light and heat.
- ☆ In addition, make sure the oil is displayed in a cool area, away from any direct or indirect contact with heat.
- ☆ Look for olive oils that are sold in small dark tinted bottles since the packaging will help protect the oil from oxidation caused by exposure to light.
- ☆ If purchasing oil in tinted glass containers, choose those at the back of the grocery shelf out of direct light. Unless you are certain that turnover is rapid at your grocery.
- ☆ Ask the grocer how long the olive oil has been out on the shelf.
- ☆ Protect olive oil's flavour and antioxidants by transferring a week to 10 days' worth of oil to a smaller bottle to lessen the oxidation that occurs when the oil is exposed to air. Leave this small bottle at room temperature for easy use, but refrigerate the rest.
- ☆ When chilled, olive oil will solidify slightly and turn cloudy, but once restored to room temperature, it will regain its normal appearance, and its quality will be better maintained.
- ☆ Tinted glass containers screen out some light, but non-reactive dark plastic or metal containers are the best choice for preserving olive oil's beneficial compounds.

III. Groundnut Oil/Peanut Oil

History

Groundnuts are considered as one of the best nourishing food of the world. The peanut or groundnut (*Arachis hypogaea*) is a species in the legume family Fabaceae. The peanut, while grown in tropical and subtropical regions throughout the world, is native to the Western Hemisphere. It probably originated in South America and spread throughout the New World as Spanish explorers discovered the peanut's versatility. When the Spaniards returned to Europe, peanuts went with them. Later, traders were responsible for spreading peanuts to Asia and Africa. Thc peanut made its way back to North America on sailing ships in the 1700's. Although there were some commercial peanut farms in the U.S. during the 1700's and 1800's, peanuts were not grown extensively. This lack of interest in peanut farming is attributed to the fact that the peanut was regarded as food for the poor and because growing and harvesting native to South America, techniques were slow and difficult. Until the Civil War, the peanut remained basically a regional food associated with the southern US. After the Civil War, the demand for peanuts increased rapidly. By the end of the nineteenth century, the development of equipment for production, harvesting and shelling peanuts, as well as processing techniques, contributed to the expansion of the peanut industry. The new twentieth century labour-saving equipment resulted in a rapid demand for peanut oil, roasted and salted peanuts, peanut butter and confections.

Peanut oil is a a pale yellow oil pressed from peanuts, which contain between 40 and 50 percent oil. Most peanut oil comes from a specific variety of the peanut plant (*Arachis hypogaea*) that has been bred to produce a healthier oil. Peanut oil is noted to have the slight aroma and taste of its parent legume. This oil was first produced in the early 1900s in the United States. Today, most of the peanuts that are grown in the United States are eaten rather than turned into peanut oil. However, in other areas of the world such as Africa and Asia, peanut oil is especially popular. India and China, the two countries that produce the most peanuts in the world, use 80 to 90 percent of their crops to make peanut oil. In the UK and Asian countries, it is marketed as 'groundnut oil'.

In India, groundnut oil is produced both in crude and refined forms. India produced around 3 lakh tonnes of Groundnut oil in 2011-12. Filtered groundnut/peanut oil has been used in India since generations. Refining of oil was introduced in the 1950s. The first refined groundnut oil was called "Sipahi" but it gained popularity under the brand name "Postman". Ahmedabad, Gondal, Junagadh and Rajkot in Gujarat, Adoni in Rayalseema region of Andhra Pradesh, Mumbai and Delhi are the major trading centres for groundnut oil in India.

Refining and Utilization of Oil

Edible oil is the major product produced from peanuts in the world. About two-third of the world's peanut production is crushed to obtain edible oil. On the basis of cooking and flavour qualities, it is among the three premium oils (peanut, safflower and rapeseed) consumed in India. In India, the major peanut oil is produced by expeller press and consumed in the form of crude oil. In most of the developing countries, a major oilseed produce is crushed to extract edible oil. In India, over 80 per cent of the peanuts are subjected to crushing through traditional screw pressing to extract edible oil, while the western countries including US quality peanuts are processed to other food uses and only the farmers' stock peanuts that do not meet the requirements of food uses after preliminary cleaning are shelled and crushed for oil.

Nutrient Composition

Peanuts

Peanuts are a rich source of protein and monounsaturated fat. Peanuts contain 20 per cent saturated, 50 per cent mono-unsaturated and 30 per cent polyunsaturated fat. Its major fatty acids are palmitic acid, oleic acid and linoleic acid. Recent research on peanuts and nuts in general has found anti-oxidants and other chemicals in them that may provide health benefits. Peanuts are a significant source of resveratrol, a chemical studied for potential anti-aging effects. Because peanuts are considered an incomplete protein, containing relatively low amounts of the essential amino acids lysine, cystine, and methionine, it is advised to be sure that a diet or meal with peanuts as a staple should also include complementary foods such as dairy or whole grain. Peanuts are also an unbalanced source of fat because they are devoid of required Omega-3 fats. Some brands of peanut butter are fortified with Omega-3 in the form of flaxseed oil to balance the ratio of Omega-3 to Omega-6.

Peanut Oil

Peanut oil is an excellent source of vitamin E, mono and poly unsaturated fatty acids. It contains about 18 per cent saturated fat, 48 per cent oleic acid and 34 per cent omega-6 linoleic acid. Kamaladevi *et al.* (1984) reported the major fatty acids in peanut oil as: palmitic acid 7.2 per cent, stearic acid 4.8 per cent, oleic acid 65.5 per cent and linoleic acid 22.2 per cent. Some other studies have reported that major fatty acids present in groundnut oil are oleic acid (56.6 per cent) and linoleic acid (26.7 per cent). The oil also contains some 6–8 per cent (total) of palmitic acid, arachidic acid, arachidonic acid, behenic acid, lignoceric acid and other fatty acids. Similar varietal differences in fatty aid composition have been observed by other researchers. The fatty acid composition of peanut oil is also influenced, although to a lesser extent, by geographical location. The oil content of developing kernels increases with maturity of the kernel (Holley and Hammons, 1968). The mature seeds contain more stearic, oleic and less arachidic, behenic and lignoceric acids than the immature seed. Cultivars with as high as 71.3 per cent oleic acid and as low as 11.2 per cent linoleic acid are available. The oils having high levels of linoleic acid have been found to be highly susceptible to oxidative rancidity. The wider ratio of oleic acid to linoleic acid has been considered by several investigators as an indicator of more stable oils (Salunkhe *et al.*, 1992).

Groundnut oil also contains natural antioxidants like tocopherol and tocotrionols as well as sterols, which are of nutritional importance. The adequacy of oil as a source of vitamin E is determined by the ratio of alpha tocopherol to the total content of PUFA. A ratio of 0.2 was suggested to be satisfactory as an indicator of vitamin E adequacy (Bieri and Evarts, 1973). On this basis, peanut oil is a good source of vitamin E. Amount of these substances present in filtered oil is 137-827 ppm of tocopherols, 38-474 ppm of tocotironols and 900-2856 ppm of sterol. One should note however, that about 50 per cent of these components are retained after the refining process.

Healthy Effects

By summarising recent research data, it is recommended that dietary fat should provide about 25-35 per cent of the total calories in the daily diet. Higher intake of fat may increase the risk of obesity, CVD, hypertension, immune disorders, etc. At the same time, if less than 15 per cent energy is from fat, it may lead to PEM related degenerative diseases, poor brain growth, neuro-disorders and poor immunity. As far as type of fat is concerned, the present consensus among the scientific community is for consumption of fats with high percentage of MUFA like groundnut oil, rice bran oil or canola oil (FnBnews, 2009).

Unfortunately, in the last two decades, the general opinion of eating less fat in an attempt to reduce degenerative diseases like CVD, hypertension and diabetes has resulted in labelling of certain foods as "bad" simply due to their fat content. Peanuts were one of these casualties. However, recent epidemiological and clinical studies have revealed that regular consumption of these nuts actually reduces heart disease. It also provides protection against cancer, obesity and Type II diabetes. Another adverse claim against peanut oil was the development of allergic reactions to peanuts. It is important to note that while allergic reactions are caused by proteins in a substance, during processing of peanuts to produce oil, all proteins are completely removed. Moreover, peanut is not actually a nut, but a legume. It is a member of the pea and bean family. A person with nut allergy (which is relatively common) may not necessarily suffer an allergic reaction to peanuts or peanut oil. If at all there is an undesirable reaction, it could be due to aflatoxin contamination of peanuts.

It is easily digestible and serves as a fair source of linoleic and other unsaturated fatty acids necessary for proper growth and nutrition. The primary dietary essential fatty acid for man is linoleic acid. An intake of 1 per cent of dietary calories in the form of linoleic acid has been found to be adequate for several animal species, including man. However, the higher intake of PUFA may cause possible health problems (FAO, 1977). Hence, less than 10 per cent of dietary energy as PUFA is advised now. Peanut oil due to its lower linoleic acid content (33.2 per cent of total fatty acids) than corn oil (58 per cent), safflower oil (79.5 per cent) or mixtures of soybean oil and cottonseed oil (46.7 per cent) (Carpenter *et al.*, 1974) satisfies the recommendation of the Committee on Dietary Allowances.

Keeping in mind all above factors, groundnut oil seems to be a good choice for the Indian market. It is readily available at an affordable price as compared to the other two recommended oils, *viz.* rice bran and canola. However, while following a diet consisting of groundnut oil as the main source of fat, care should be taken to obtain 1-3 gm of omega-3 essential fatty acids, which are not present in groundnut oil. These can be obtained from other food sources like fish oil, flaxseed oil, green leafy vegetables, walnuts, cereals etc (www.FnBnews.com, 2009).

Heart Disease

New research on the type of fat in the diet has shown that unsaturated fat, mono- and polyunsaturated fat can actually be beneficial for health. The evidence is so convincing that the American Heart Association now says that a high-monounsaturated fat diet can be an alternative to the recommended 30 per cent fat diet to reduce the risk of heart disease (Kris-Etherton, 1999). A higher monounsaturated fat diet can help the heart, so long as saturated fat intake (mainly from animal products) is low and overall energy needs are balanced. Consumers should substitute foods high in monounsaturated fat like peanuts, peanut butter, peanut oil and olive oil for saturated fats in the diet from meat and full-fat milk and cheese.

A landmark study published in the December 1999 issue of the American Journal of Clinical Nutrition found that diets high in monounsaturated fat from foods like peanuts, peanut butter, peanut oil and olive oil are superior to low-fat diets for heart health. The researchers found that diets containing peanuts, peanut butter or peanut oil are as effective as diets high in olive oil in protecting against heart disease. In fact, the results indicated diets containing peanut products are more effective in protecting against heart disease than are very low-fat diets (Food insight, 1998).

Studies have shown that groundnut oil is just as effective in protecting against heart disease, as is olive oil. This is because it has similar properties and a similar fatty acid composition, as does olive oil. Just like the sunflowers used to make sunflower oil, the peanut plant has been genetically bred until its peanuts produce oil with a higher level of monounsaturated fatty acids. This made the oil healthier because monounsaturated fatty acids have been shown to reduce cholesterol levels. The peanut oil made from these plants contains about 45 per cent monounsaturated fatty acids, 38 per cent polyunsaturated fatty acids, and 17 per cent saturated fatty acids. One newer notable variety developed several years ago in Florida is called "SunOleic 97R". This variety has over 80 per cent monounsaturated fatty acids, making it comparable to olive oil and sunflower oil. They contain heart-friendly MUFA that lower the levels of bad cholesterol in our body without lowering the levels of good cholesterol.

To determine whether the lipid lowering effects of diets high in monounsaturated fatty acid (MUFA) from peanut/peanut butter (P/PB) or peanut oil (PO) are comparable to those of diets high in MUFA from olive oil (OO), the effects of five different diets on serum lipids in 22 healthy adults (9 men and 13 women, age 21-54 y) many of whom who had slightly elevated blood cholesterol levels at the beginning of the study, was studied. A randomized, double-blind, five-period crossover design was used to evaluate the following diets: average American (35 per cent fat, 15 per cent saturated fat (SFA)), low-fat (25 per cent fat, 7 per cent SFA), OO (35 per cent fat, 6 per cent SFA), P/PB (35 per cent fat, 7 per cent SFA), and PO (35 per cent fat, 7 per cent SFA). Each participant was randomized into one of five diets: low-fat, olive oil, peanuts plus peanut butter, peanut oil and a typical American diet with 35 percent fat. All the participants were studied for a total of 125 days *i.e.* 25 days on each diet and they maintained their starting weight. The peanut diets had relatively small amounts of peanut products but they were consumed daily, for instance, peanuts as a snack or some peanut butter on a bagel for breakfast. Those who were randomized to the peanut, peanut butter and olive oil diets all had lower total and LDL ("bad") cholesterol and triglyceride levels, yet their HDL ("good") cholesterol levels were not lowered. The participants on the low-fat diet had lower LDL levels, but also lower HDL levels and increased triglycerides.

Dr. Penny Kris-Etherton, distinguished Professor of Nutrition at Penn State University notes that, "What is important about these findings is that we have another food option beyond olive oil – peanuts, peanut butter and peanut oil – for increasing monounsaturated fats in the diet. These options may be preferable than low fat diets for some individuals. Inclusion of peanut products will add variety, flexibility and eating satisfaction to heart healthy diet planning." According to Dr. Tom Pearson, Kaiser Professor, Department of Community and Preventive Medicine at the University of Rochester, and a co-investigator on this study, "The positive effects from peanuts and peanut products may go beyond their content of beneficial fatty acids. The antioxidant Vitamin E, folic acid, phytochemicals, fiber, vitamins, minerals and plant protein may all somehow contribute to heart disease protection." Hence, these researchers speculated that antioxidant vitamin E, folic acid, phytochemicals, fiber, minerals and plant protein contained in peanut products may have all contributed to heart disease protection (Food Insight, 1998). In summary, OO, P/PB, and PO can be used interchangeably in high-MUFA, low-SFA diets, creating additional diet planning options for the development of diets designed to lower TC and LDL-C. Moreover, these diets are all superior to low-fat, low-SFA diets because they do not elevate TG (Food Insight, 1998).

According to a new animal study, fat-free peanut flour, whole peanuts and peanut oil all may have cardio-protective properties. Agricultural Research Service scientists presented these findings at the Institute of Food Technologists 2008 Annual Meeting in New Orleans, La. For the study, male hamsters were randomly divided into four groups. Each group of nearly 20 hamsters was fed one of four different diets, all of which were high-fat and high-cholesterol. Each diet consisted of nearly equal percentages of fats, carbohydrates and proteins. For three of the four test diets, equivalent amounts of food component were substituted with fat-free peanut flour, peanut oil or peanuts without skins. The fourth diet contained no peanut product and served as the control group. After the hamsters had been on the test diets for six months, the researchers tested their blood lipid chemistry. Compared to hamsters in the no-peanut control group, those in each of the three peanut groups were found to have significantly lower total cholesterol and LDL "bad" cholesterol. Also positive, HDL "good" cholesterol levels held steady (Bliss, 2008). Other blood chemistry research has been published that links reduced heart disease risk factors in humans with consuming peanut butter and peanut oil, but this is the first animal study to exhibit such an effect from consuming the fat-free portion of peanuts. While it is still unknown if the effect would translate to humans, additional research studies with peanut components continue.

A study of oils based on their composition reveals that rapeseed oil, olive oil, groundnut oil and rice bran oil have the highest amount (> 50 per cent) of mono-unsaturates. However, only rice bran oil and groundnut oil has a ratio of SFA, MUFA and PUFA closest to WHO recommendations.

Diabetes

Reports are available on the effect of groundnut oil on normal and high-fat diets (Srinivasan and Pugalendi, 2000) and myocardial infarction (Nageswari *et al.*, 1999). Not many investigations have been carried out to study the effect of groundnut oil on glycemic control in diabetic rats. Since groundnut oil contains 46 per cent of MUFA and 32 per cent of PUFA (USDA, 1997), an interest arose in exploring the role of groundnut oil in diabetes by the scientists.

Rasmussen *et al.* (1993) noted a reduction in peak plasma glucose concentration with the consumption of a monounsaturated fatty acid-rich diet. In diabetes, hyperglycemia resulted in the generation of free radicals (Giardino *et al.*, 1996) due to autoxidation of glucose (Hunt and Wolff, 1991) and glycosylation of proteins (Gillery *et al.*, 1988).

The effect of groundnut oil on blood glucose, lipid profile, lipid peroxidation, and antioxidant status in streptozotocin-diabetic rats was investigated and compared with diabetic and drug-treated rats by Ramesh *et al.* (2006). Normal and diabetic rats were fed an oil-free diet containing 2 percent oil supplemented with groundnut oil (6g per 94g diet), to give 8 percent oil content, for 42 days. When diabetic rats were fed groundnut oil, a significant reduction in glucose (244.04 ± 11.66), glycosylated hemoglobin (HbA1c), thiobarbituric acid reactive substances (TBARS), lipid hydroperoxides (HP) levels, and glucose-6-phosphatase and fructose-1, 6-bisphosphatase activities and an elevation in Hb, vitamin E, GSH levels, and hexokinase activity were observed. Diabetic rats had elevated total cholesterol (TC), VLDL-cholesterol, LDL-cholesterol, and triglycerides (TG) and decreased HDL-cholesterol. Diabetic rats fed groundnut oil showed a small but significant reduction in TC, VLDL-C, LDL-C, and TG and an elevation in HDL-C. Groundnut oil consumption slightly but significantly decreased the blood glucose, HbA1c, lipid peroxidation, and lipid profile and increased antioxidant levels in diabetic rats (Ramesh *et al.*, 2006).

Uses in Cooking

Groundnut oil is available in refined form as well as filtered form. Raw oil extracted from peanut kernel contains mucilage and albuminous matter, producing turbidity and free fatty acids in varying amounts. The cold-drawn raw oil may contain some A and D vitamins, which are often removed during refining.

Although the filtered oils are nutritionally superior, they often contain toxic compounds or adulterants. Hence, it is better to buy refined groundnut oils of reputed brands. The oil is suitable for all types of cooking- frying, grilling and seasoning. It is often used in Chinese, South Asian and Southeast cuisine much as olive oil is used in the Mediterranean.

One of the major benefits of peanut oil is that it has a high smoke point of over 450 ° F relative to many other cooking oils. It is most commonly used for deep and stir-frying of foods. Foods fried in peanut oil exhibit an excellent flavour and keeping quality. A moderate proportion of linoleic acid in peanut oil ensures slow deterioration.

Groundnut oil being high in mono-unsaturates, is more stable and usually does not require artificial additives. Like olive oil, peanut oil is relatively stable and therefore, appropriate for stir-frys on occasion. It is considered to be the finest all-round oil for cooking and frying. It is extremely robust and produces fewer flavour defects with long term use as compared with many other oils. This oil is also considered superior in the manufacturing of pourable dressings because of its ability to hold solids in suspension for a longer time. It is therefore extensively used in place of olive oil as a salad oil and in the production of mayonnaise. It is often used in marinades and baked goods too. But the high percentage of omega-6 presents a potential danger, so use of peanut oil should be limited.

Commercial peanut oil will not cause an allergic reaction because the allergen is a protein, not a fat; however, the cold pressed and organic oils will. They are presumably less filtered, retaining some peanut proteins for the sake of flavour and nutrition.

Changes in Oil Quality during Cooking

During frying and heating, many oxidative and hydrolytic changes occur, which decrease functional, sensory and nutritive properties of the oil. Heating increases viscosity, foaming properties, free fatty acid content, refractive index and decreases the iodine value of the oil. Murthi *et al.* (1979) observed that during continuous commercial frying of *sev*, no deleterious changes in the peanut oil were observed at a turnover of 8h. However, with a turnover rate of 13h, free fatty acids and peroxide values increased considerably and colour of the oil changed to very dark. Significant losses in PUFA and iodine value of peanut oil occurred during 12h of intermittent frying of *puri*. These losses were greater when frying was done in an iron rather than an aluminium container. During frying of peanut oil, there was 55 per cent loss of tocopherol (Salunkhe *et al.*, 1992).

Tocopherol losses were observed in peanut oil used for frying both marinated and non-marinated chicken products. The largest losses were seen for γ-tocopherol followed by α-tocopherol and then β- and δ-tocopherols. γ-Tocopherol losses were significantly reduced when hydroxypropylmethylcellulose was applied either as a film or as a breading mix ingredient to pre-fried chicken strips that had been marinated in pickle juice. It is conjectured that the edible film material served as a hydrophilic barrier to migration of the pro-oxidant, acetic acid, from the product to the oil (Holownia *et al.*, 2001).

Storage of Oil

The contents of linoleic acid and other polyunsaturates are inversely proportional to the keeping quality of oil. The ratio of the sum of all PUFA to sum of all saturates for peanut oil is low (1.8) as compared to oil from soybean (2.9), corn (4.3) and safflower (8.7). Hence peanut oil has a better keeping quality than the oil from other oilseeds *e.g.* soybean, corn, and safflower oils. Another criteria often used to evaluate dietary value of an oil is the ratio of the content of linoleic acid to the sum of palmitic and stearic acid (L(P+S)), which for peanut oil is 2.6, soybean oil 2.7, corn oil 4.3 and safflower oil 9.1 (Carpenter *et al.*, 1974). The peanut oil also has a longer shelf life because it contains a smaller amount polyunsaturated fatty acids that are prone to oxidation. It can be kept safe in a dark cupboard for a half year to a year.

The storage stability of peanut oil has been observed to differ among botanical types due to differences in the FA composition. Cultivars having high levels of linoleic acid were found to be highly susceptible to oxidative rancidity. Raw peanut oil stored at ambient temperatures in mild steel and tin containers was stable for 660 days. Peanut oil was found to be more stable while in the kernel at 50°C than when extracted from the seeds (Adnan *et al.*, 1981). The oil was stored in sealed containers and held under cold, hot-humid and hot-dry conditions for 2 y. The oil remained acceptable for 1 y. The losses in the added vitamin A were 17 per cent and 30 per cent after 6 months and 1year, respectively. During storage, both peroxide value and carbonyl contents were increased. The level of hexanal and 2, 4-decadienal was found to be the highest in rancid oil. Among the various antioxidants tested, propyl gallate was found to be the most effective in retarding peroxidation of stored oil and its products (Arya *et al.*, 1980).

Chapter 20

Oil that Matters II

IV. Canola Oil

Christened "Canola" from "Can" (for Canada) and "ola" (for oil low acid), canola is not, strictly speaking, rapeseed. Rapeseed oil is toxic because it contains significant amounts of a poisonous substance called erucic acid. Canola was developed in the early 1970s using traditional plant breeding techniques by Canadian plant breeders to remove the anti-nutritional components (erucic acid and glucosinolates) from rapeseed to assure its safety for human and animal consumption. There is an internationally regulated definition of canola that differentiates it from rapeseed, based upon its having less than two percent erucic acid and less than 30 umoles

Canola Oil: How it is different from Rapeseed Oil

- ☆ Canola was developed through conventional plant breeding from rapeseed, an oilseed plant already used in ancient civilization.
- ☆ The word "rape" in rapeseed comes from the Latin word "rapum," meaning turnip. Turnip, rutabaga, cabbage, Brussels sprouts, mustard and many other vegetables are related to the two canola varieties commonly grown, which are cultivars of Brassica napus and Brassica rapa.
- ☆ The negative associations due to the homophone "rape" resulted in creation of the more marketing-friendly name "Canola".
- ☆ The change in name also serves to distinguish it from regular rapeseed oil, which has much higher erucic acid content.

glucosinolates. Oilseed products that do not meet this standard cannot use the trademarked term "Canola."

Canola oil is widely recognized as the healthiest salad and cooking oil available to consumers. Its unique fatty acid profile, rich in oleic acid and low in saturated fats, makes it particularly beneficial for the prevention of heart disease.

History

Many research studies had reported that excessive use of vegetable oils rich in polyunsaturated fatty acids had adverse effects on health. They reported good effects of Mediterranean diets which included olive oil rich in monounsaturated fatty acids. Therefore, promotion of olive oil, which had a long history of use, seemed more scientifically sound to the health-conscious consumer than the promotion of corn and soy oil, which could only be extracted with modern stainless steel presses. Food industries started facing the problems as there was not enough olive oil in the world to meet its needs. And, like butter and other traditional fats, olive oil was too expensive to use in most processed foods. The industry needed less expensive monounsaturated oil.

Rapeseed oil was a monounsaturated oil that had been used extensively in many parts of the world, notably in China, Japan and India. It contains almost 60 per cent monounsaturated fatty acids (compared to about 70 per cent in olive oil). Unfortunately, about two-thirds of the monounsaturated fatty acids in rapeseed oil are erucic acid, a 22-carbon monounsaturated fatty acid that had been associated with Keshan's disease, characterized by fibrotic lesions of the heart. In the late 1970s, using a technique of genetic manipulation involving seed splitting (Downey, 1964), Canadian plant breeders came up with a variety of rapeseed that produced a monounsaturated oil that was low in 22-carbon erucic acid and high in 18-carbon oleic acid. The new oil was referred to as LEAR oil, for Low Erucic Acid Rapeseed.

Before LEAR oil could be promoted as a healthy alternative to polyunsaturated oils, it needed a new name. Neither "rape" nor "LEAR" could be expected to invoke a healthy image for the new "Cinderella" crop. In 1978, the industry settled on "canola", for "Canadian oil", since most of the new rapeseed at that time was grown in Canada. "Canola" also sounded like "can do" and "payola"–both positive phrases in marketing lingo. However, the new name did not come into widespread use until the early 1990s. It was granted GRAS status in 1985. Since unprocessed canola oil

Canola Oil: Its History

- ☆ Plant breeders in Canada, where rapeseed had been grown (mainly in Saskatchewan) since 1936, worked to improve the quality of the plant.
- ☆ In 1968 Dr Baldur Stefansson of the University of Manitoba used selective breeding to develop a variety of rapeseed low in erucic acid.
- ☆ In 1974 another variety was produced low in both erucic acid and glucosinolates; it was named Canola, from Canadian oil, low acid.

contains not only lots of monounsaturated fatty acids, but also a significant amount of omega-3, it shows up in most of the book's recipes.

The canola industry's approach–scientific conferences, promotion to upscale consumers through books like The Omega Diet, and articles in the health section of newspapers and magazines -was successful. Canola oil began to appear in the recipes of cutting-edge health books, such as those by Andrew Weil and Barry Sears. The technique was to extol the virtues of the Mediterranean diet and olive oil in the text, and then call for "olive oil or canola oil" in the recipes. By the late 1990s, canola use had soared, and not just in the United States, today China, Japan, Europe, Mexico, Bangladesh and Pakistan all buy significant amounts. Canola does well in arid environments such as Australia and the Canadian plains, where it has become a major cash crop.

Genetically Engineered/ Modified Canola

- ☆ The first seed oil to be created through genetic manipulation, canola is also the focus of a variety of genetic engineering/modification (GE/GM) projects in which genetic material from other species is inserted into the seeds in order to magnify certain traits in the resultant plant.
- ☆ Herbicide-resistant GE canola now comprises a large portion of the total canola crop. Apologists point to endorsement by the FDA and the American Dietetic Association that GE canola is nutritionally and environmentally safe and claim that the GE variety means less spraying of herbicides, less chemical runoff and a boon to farmers.
- ☆ Meanwhile, genetic engineers are involved in projects to make canola oil "even more nutritious" by further reducing the amount of saturates in the fatty acid profile and raising the levels of monounsaturates. This, they claim, will make it possible to reduce the amount of trans fats in the processed oil, presumably because levels of omega-3 fatty acids, which need to be deodorised, will also be lowered.
- ☆ Should the genetic engineers be successful, it might be possible to create a diet in which the vast majority of fatty acids is monounsaturated–something that does not exist in any traditional diet anywhere in the world.

(*Source*: Eric Peters, "Let them eat canola", Washington Times, April 29, 2002)

Processing of Canola Oil

Canola oil is the main product of canola seed since about 43 percent of the seed is oil. The canola oil is removed by a combination of high temperature mechanical pressing and solvent extraction. Traces of the solvent (usually hexane) remain in the oil, even after considerable refining. Like all modern vegetable oils, this oil also goes through the process of caustic refining, bleaching and degumming, all of which involve high temperatures or chemicals of questionable safety. And because canola oil is high in omega-3 fatty acids, which easily become rancid and foul-smelling when subjected to oxygen and high temperatures, it must be deodorized. The standard deodorization process removes a large portion of the omega-3 fatty acids by turning them into trans fatty acids. Trans content of canola is permitted to be at a minimal of 0.2 per cent as per regulations of Canadian government. But research at the University of Florida at Gainesville found trans levels as high as 4.6 per cent in commercial liquid oil (O'Keefe *et al.*, 1994). The consumer has no clue about the presence of trans fatty acids in canola oil because they are not listed on the label.

Canola Oil Extraction

- ☆ The first stage in processing canola is to roll or flake the seed. This ruptures cells and makes the oil easier to extract.
- ☆ Next the flaked or rolled seeds are cooked and subjected to a mild pressing process which removes some of the oil and compresses the seeds into large chunks called "cake fragments."
- ☆ The cake fragments undergo further processing to remove most of the remaining oil. The oil extracted during each step is combined. The oil is then subjected to processing according to the end product requirements. Different treatments are used to process salad oils, margarines, and shortenings.

A large portion of canola oil used in processed food is hardened through the hydrogenation process, which introduces levels of trans fatty acids into the final product as high as 40 per cent (Sebedio and Christie, 1998). In fact, canola oil hydrogenates beautifully, better than corn oil or soybean oil, because modern hydrogenation methods hydrogenate omega-3 fatty acids preferentially and canola oil is very high in omega-3s. Higher levels of trans mean longer shelf life for processed foods, a crisper texture in cookies and crackers and more dangers of chronic disease for the consumer.

Physical Properties of Canola Oil

Table 20.1 describes the various physical properties of canola oil.

Table 20.1: Physical Properties of Canola Oil

Properties Parameter	*Value*
Relative Density (g/cm³, 20°C/water at 20°C)	0.914–0.917
Refractive Index (nD 40°C)	1.465 – 1.467
Crismer Value	67–70
Viscosity (Kinematic at 20°C, mm2/sec)	78.2
Cold Test (15 Hrs at 4°C)	Passed
Smoke Point (°C)	220 – 230
Flash Point, Open Cup (°C)	275–290
Specific Heat (J/g at 20°C)	1.910 – 1.916
Thermal Conductivity (W/m°K)	0.179 – 0.188

Nutrient Composition

Canola oil was bred to contain little, if any, erucic acid and has drawn the attention of nutritionist because of its high oleic acid content. This oil has the lowest amount of saturated fat (7 per cent of total content) of all oils commonly consumed including corn oil (13 per cent saturated fat), olive oil (15 per cent), palm oil (51 per cent), soybean oil (15 per cent), and sunflower oil (12 per cent). With just 7 per cent saturated fat, canola oil is 93 per cent healthy monounsaturated and polyunsaturated fats. The polyunsaturated fats in canola oil include the essential fatty acids alpha linolenic acid, an omega-3 fatty acid, and linoleic acid, an omega-6 fatty acid. It is the richest source of alpha-linolenic acid (ALA) (11 per cent of total content). Its ratio of 2:1 of omega-6 to omega-3 is nutritionally ideal. Omega-3 fatty acids protect against heart attacks and strokes by helping to lower bad cholesterol. Omega-6 fatty acid is important for the brain and essential for the growth and development of infants.

Canola oil helps in the absorption of fat soluble vitamins A, D, E, and K which may help keep the heart healthy. It is also a good source of Vitamins E, K and plant sterols. Vitamin E (1 tbsp provides 2.9 mg of vitamin E) is an antioxidizing agent and may be a valuable tool in fighting cancer and heart disease. Canola oil is also good vitamin K source and helps inhibit thrombosis.

Table 20.2: Fatty Acid Composition of Canola Oil

Compound	*Family*	*Per cent of Total*
Oleic acid	ω-9	61
Linoleic acid	ω-6	21
Alpha-linolenic acid	ω-3	9-11
Saturated fatty acids		7
Palmitic acid		4
Stearic acid		2
Trans fat		4

Vitamin K is vital for blood clotting. Therefore, canola oil is not recommended along with other blood thinning drugs or supplements.

There are some indications that canola oil has its own inherent dangers. It has high sulphur content and goes rancid easily. Baked goods made with canola oil develop mould very quickly.

Health Benefits

The Canola Council of Canada states that it is completely safe and is the healthiest of all commonly used cooking oil. It has well established heart health benefits and is recognized by many health professional organizations including the American Dietetics Association, and American Heart Association, among others. Canola oil has been authorized a qualified health claim from the US Food and Drug Administration based on its ability to reduce the risk of coronary heart disease due to its unsaturated fat content.

Heart Health

Canola oil has very low saturated fatty acid and as high as 60 per cent monounsaturated fatty acid with added goodness of ALA omega-3 fatty acid, making the oil healthier than the other oils. It is considered as the second highest vegetable oil source of omega-3 fatty acids after flaxseed oil. Canola oil like flaxseed oil contains both omega-3 and omega-6 fatty acids, but the ratio is different. The omega-6 to omega-3 ratio of flaxseed oil is 0.3:1 while in canola oil it is 2:1. Canola oil is considered one of the most heart healthy oil as it has the highest ratio of unsaturated to saturated fats. This oil is also believed to decrease the total cholesterol levels, reduce serum triglycerides and prevent the platelets from sticking to each other.

Substitution of canola oil for other fats may greatly increase the intake of alpha-linolenic acid (ALA). New research suggests that ALA, the only omega-3 fatty acid found in appreciable amounts in some vegetable oils may help protect the heart by having beneficial effects on abnormal heartbeats, inflammation and blood clots. Furthermore, most research shows that ALA intake is associated with decreased incidence and mortality from heart disease. In October 2006, its high amount of unsaturated fat earned it authorization from the U.S. Food and Drug Administration (FDA) for a qualified health claim. The claim, which canola oil bottlers and makers of eligible products may use on labels and advertising materials, states:

'Limited and not conclusive scientific evidence suggests that eating about 11D2 tablespoons (19 grams) of canola oil daily may reduce the risk of coronary heart disease due to the unsaturated fat content in canola oil. To achieve this possible benefit, canola oil is to replace a similar amount of saturated fat and not increase the total number of calories one takes in a day. One serving of this product contains [x] grams of canola oil'.

This claim offers a simple, affordable and convenient strategy for consumers to reduce their risk of heart disease.

Some Facts about Health Benefits of Canola Oil

- ☆ Low in saturated fat: Saturated fat raises the bad LDL cholesterol in blood and has been linked to increased risk of coronary heart disease.
- ☆ A source of omega-6 fat: Omega-g fat must be consumed in the diet and is important for the brain and essential for the growth and development of infants.
- ☆ High in omega-3 fat: Omega-3 fat must also be consumed in the diet and helps protect against heart attacks and strokes.
- ☆ High in monounsaturated fat: Monounsaturated fat may reduce the risk of coronary heart disease by lowering bad LDL cholesterol in the blood and helping control blood glucose.
- ☆ Cholesterol and trans fat free: Trans fat raises bad LDL cholesterol and lowers good HDL cholesterol.

Effect of Canola Oil on Cholesterol

High levels of blood cholesterol, specifically LDL cholesterol constitute a major risk factor in the development of coronary heart disease (CHD). More recent studies have demonstrated that oxidation (breakdown) of LDL results in changes to the LDL particle that can ultimately increase its atherogenicity. Diets high in monounsaturated fats (MUFA) have been shown to not only reduce both total and LDL cholesterol, but also have the ability to protect LDL against oxidation. Research has established that canola oil has a more potent total and LDL cholesterol lowering effect when compared to other MUFA containing oils (Castro *et al.*, 2000). Canola oil also protects against LDL oxidation to a greater degree than most commonly used vegetable oils that are high in polyunsaturated fat (PUFA).

In the distant past, the connection between dietary fat, cholesterol, and risk for CHD focused upon saturated (SFA) and PUFA. For nearly 30 years the common belief was that SFAs raised cholesterol levels, PUFAs lowered cholesterol levels, and MUFAs were neutral in their effects. However, in the mid 1980s exciting research was published showing that MUFAs, primarily as oleic acid, were as effective as PUFAs in reducing both total plasma and LDL cholesterol. Good sources of MUFA include olive oil (75 per cent), canola oil (61 per cent), corn oil (29 per cent), soybean oil (23 per cent), sunflower oil (16 per cent), and safflower oil (14 per cent).

As the science in this area evolved, it was found that not all MUFA containing oils are created equal in regard to their effects on cholesterol lowering. In 1998 two scientists, Truswell and Choudhury, compared the results of three separate human clinical trials in which diets high in palmolein (an oil high in SFA and low in MUFA) were compared to those high in MUFAs including olive, canola, and high oleic sunflower. Of significance, canola oil produced the most dramatic reduction in both total and LDL cholesterol values in comparison to palmolein. Surprisingly, olive oil did not lower either total or LDL cholesterol when compared to palmolein.

These results clearly demonstrate that not all MUFA containing oils are the same in terms of health benefits. These findings also demonstrate that once again canola oil comes out on top. An explanation for the favorable effects of canola oil on blood cholesterol levels revolve around the nutritionally beneficial fatty acid profile of canola oil in comparison to other high MUFA oils (McDonald, 1999). Canola oil contains one of the lowest concentrations of saturated fat (7 per cent) of all MUFA containing oils. In addition to canola's high MUFA content mentioned above, it is also a good source of the omega-3 fatty acid alpha-linolenic acid (ALA) (11 per cent). Studies have shown that ALA is equally as effective as oleic acid and linoleic acid in reducing both total plasma and LDL cholesterol levels. Finally, canola oil is a good source of vitamin E in comparison to other high MUFA and common vegetable oils. Vitamin E, along with MUFAs, plays a crucial role in protecting the LDL particle against oxidation, which ultimately reduces its atherogenicity.

Uses

Canola oil is a multi-functional oil with a high heat tolerance, neutral taste and light, smooth texture. Because of neutral flavor, canola oil can be blended with other healthy oils before using for culinary purposes. It can be used for sautéing, frying and baking as well as in marinades, salad dressings, sauces and fondue. This all-purpose oil also has a high smoke point, 440°F, so it is excellent for frying and sautëing. Compared to other vegetable oils it blends well with vinegar and other salad dressings as it is less prone to separation. Moreover, the delicate flavor makes it perfect for dressings and mayonnaise.

It is a commonly used oil in sterol-containing margarines and spreads recommended for cholesterol lowering. When used in place of solid fats or other vegetable oils, canola oil produces dishes and baked goods with less saturated fat and trans fat. Use of hydrogenated canola oil for frying is increasing, especially in restaurants.

The low level of saturated fats and wide range of functionality has made canola oil a popular option for food services looking to decrease trans fats in their food. It is the oil of choice in gourmet and health food markets like Fresh Fields Whole Foods Markets, and shows up in many supermarket items as well. Recently, KFC in Canada, Taco Bell throughout North America and McDonald's in the U.S. have switched to using canola oil or a canola oil blend in their food service operations.

V. Safflower Oil

Safflower (Carthamus tinctorius), a plant in the thistle family is among the oldest crops known. Traditionally, safflower (Carthamus tinctorius L.) crop was grown for its seeds, and used for colouring and flavouring foods, in medicines, and making red (carthamin) and yellow dyes, especially before cheaper aniline dyes became available. Safflower was also known as carthamine in the 19th century. For the last 50 years or so, the plant has been cultivated mainly for the vegetable oil extracted from its seeds.

History

Safflower is thought to be native to Iran and North-Western India, and possibly Africa, and is also found in North America and the Far East. According to some researchers, safflower is believed to be indigenous to South-eastern Asia but has long been cultivated in China, the Near East and Northern Africa. Others believe that this crop had originated in an area bounded by the eastern Mediterranean and the Persian Gulf. It has been identified, as growing in Egypt 4,000 years ago. Safflower has been cultivated in Egypt, the Middle East and India initially for the orange dye obtained from the florets. It is still used as dye in India. It spreads throughout the Mediterranean region and eastwards to China and Japan. It was introduced experimentally as an oil crop in the US in 1925, where it has been grown on a commercial scale since 1950, particularly in California.

It was a relatively insignificant oilseed crop until the early 1950s, when higher yielding oil-bearing varieties were developed and it was established as a source oil for surface coatings. It is a minor crop today, with about 600,000 tons being produced commercially in more than sixty countries worldwide. India, United States, and Mexico are the leading producers, with Ethiopia, Kazakhstan, China, Argentina and Australia accounting for most of the remainder. It is now cultivated for oil in parts of North Africa, India, China, the United States and Australia.

Processing for Oil

Safflower oil is obtained from the seeds by expeller pressing, solvent extraction, or a combination of both. There are two types of safflower that produce different kinds of oil; one high in monounsaturated fatty acid and the other high in polyunsaturated fatty acid. Currently the predominant oil market is for the former, which is lower in saturates than olive oil, for example. Interest in the ability of the unsaturated liquid oil to lower serum cholesterol levels catalysed the development of an edible grade of safflower oil. The amount of safflower oil produced worldwide does not rank among the top ten; however, US 2005-06 production of safflower oil was forecast to rank tenth among edible fat and oil sources, at 56 million pounds (USDA, 2006). Unrefined safflower oil is usually a deep amber yellow colour and has a mild, slightly nutty and earthy flavour. Refined safflower oil is typically a very pale yellow in colour and has a bland taste.

Nutrient Composition

Safflower oil is nutritionally similar to sunflower oil. The oil content of the seeds varies from 20 to 38 per cent. The thinner the hull the greater will be the oil content. The regular safflower oil, with a fatty acid profile of 79 percent polyunsaturates, 13 percent monounsaturates and just 8 percent saturated fats, is the most highly polyunsaturated vegetable oil available.

Table 20.3: Comparison of Percentage of Major Fatty Acids in Edible Vegetable Oils

Fatty Acids		*Safflower*		*Canola**	*Soybean*	*Corn*	*Sunflower*	*Peanut*	*Olive*
Denomination	*Name*	*Oleic*	*Linoleic*						
14:0	–	–	–	0.75	0.1	–	–	0.1	–
16:0	Palmitic	5	5-7	4.0	10.8	11.4	6.0-7.0	10.0	11.0
18:0	Stearic	<1	2	1.6	4.0	1.9	4.0-5.0	2.3	2.2
20:0	–	–	–	0.5	–	–	–	–	–
22:0	–	–	–	0.4	–	–	–	–	–
Total Saturated		7.0	10.4	6-9	15.1	13.3	10.8	17.8	13.5
16:1	–	–	–	0.25	0.2	–	–	0.1	0.8
18.1	Oleic	77	15	61.0	23.8	25.3	17-20	47.1	75.8
20:1	–	–	–	1.5	0.2	–	–	1.4	0.3
22:1	–	–	–	0.2	–	–	–	–	–
otal monounsaturated		77	15	61-64	24.3	25.3	20.4	48.6	77.1
18:2	Linoleic	15	77	19-26	53.3	60.7	68.8	33.6	8.3
18:3	Linolenic	–	–	8-13	7.1	0.7	–	–	0.6
Total polyunsaturated		15	77	27-35	60.6	61.4	68.8	33.6	8.8

Source: Adapted from Smith 1996; Ackman 1990; Dorrell 1978.

Note: Figures are rounded or are estimates. Ranges represent various cultivars and locations.

* Average of several types.

Safflower oil is extremely rich (approximately 77-79 per cent) in polyunsaturated linoleic acid (omega-6 Essential Fatty Acids), and also contains 8-10 per cent saturated fats and 13 per cent oleic acid (omega-9s–monosaturates). This oil has the highest18:2 percentage of any known native oil, not considering modern genetic fatty acid modifications of certain oils. A recent study reported slightly greater amounts of 18:2 in a Korean safflower oil, with the fatty acid distribution as 16:0, 5.53 per cent; 18:0, 1.62 per cent; 18:1, 11.00 per cent; 18:2, 81.5 per cent; and 18:3, 0.40 per cent (Lee *et al.*, 2004). For this reason, most safflower oil is used by health conscious individuals as a high polyunsaturated oil even though it is expensive (Chow, 2000). Hence the composition of safflower oil is largely made up of linoleic fatty acid with a very low level of linolenic acid, which results in very nearly drying oil. The oil also contains high levels of Vitamin E (43mg/100g), alpha-tocopherol (34.1mg/100g) and phytosterols (444mg/100g). This oil can be used to prevent and treat EFA deficiencies in the diet.

Health Benefits

Hypocholesterolemic Effect

Monounsaturated safflower oil, high in oleic acid, is used as a heat-stable cooking oil and is very shelf stable. Polyunsaturated oil, high in linoleic acid, is used as cold oil. Like other products high in oleic acid, monounsaturated safflower oil is not terribly beneficial to human health. Polyunsaturated oil, on the other hand, has a great deal of nutritional value. The chief interest in edible safflower oil lies in the fact that it contains about 75 per cent linoleic acid, with total unsaturated acids of about 94 per cent. A number of medical research organizations have reported that the principle ingredient of edible safflower oil, linoleic glyceride, is beneficial in controlling or perhaps preventing arteriosclerosis. Like sunflower oil, safflower oil rich in polyunsaturated linoleic fatty acid has an appeal to health-conscious consumers as it is useful in lessening the threat of human arteriosclerosis.

Linoleic, the principal fatty acid of safflower oil, is an essential fatty acid that cannot be synthesized by the human body. It is required for ensuring the integrity of plasma membranes and for growth, reproduction, skin maintenance, and general body functioning. The health benefits of conjugated linoleic fatty acids are also attracting interest. The potential therapeutic properties are that it is anti- carcinogenic, anti-atherosclerotic, growth promoting, and lean body mass enhancing. It is a natural raw material for the production of conjugated linoleic fatty acid. The medicinal value of linoleic acid came into prominence in the later 1960s following the publication of the findings of researchers in a series of medical and scientific journals. These findings proved that this fatty acid was highly beneficial in lowering serum cholesterol levels in laboratory animals and humans. From virtual obscurity safflower oil became a best-seller within a few years. This is no wonder, with its very high linoleic acid content. Safflower oil has proved beneficial in lowering blood cholesterol. Hence it can be used liberally by persons suffering from cardiovascular disorders. Dr. James Duke in The Green Pharmacy notes one study that found that switching from other oils to safflower oil for eight weeks reduced total serum cholesterol levels by 9 to 15 percent and LDL cholesterol by 12-20 percent.

Improved Calcium Availability

It has also been discovered that linoleic acid promotes and improves availability of calcium to the body's cells, thereby virtually acting as a vitamin. Some scientists refer to it as vitamin F.

Obesity Control

Safflower's ability to help form prostaglandins is just one of its virtues. Cis-linoleic acid, the omega-6 fatty acid in safflower oil responsible for prostaglandin production, is also a catalyst for burning brown fat. Brown fat is the inner body fat that surrounds vital organs and acts as a fat-burning factory, using calories for heat rather than storing them as white fat. During normal metabolism, cis-linoleic acid converts to GLA (gamma linolenic acid). GLA then stimulates the body's brown fat into a flurry of calorie-burning activity.

Fat researchers like Dr. George Bray at the University of California at Los Angeles theorized that brown fat becomes less active with age, making weight control more difficult. Bray also believes that brown fat becomes prematurely sluggish in some people, while staying active in others well into their old age. Heredity may be to blame in this case, but safflower oil with its high levels of omega-6 can help to correct the problem of obesity.

Uses

Safflower oil has multiple abilities, when used correctly. This oil is a good all-purpose oil as it is fairly light in weight and colour. This oil is used in food preparations where a high PUFA content is desired. Its smoking point is high (440-480°F) which makes it suitable for deep fat frying. It is used mainly as a cooking oil, in salad dressing, mayonnaise and for the production of liquid margarine. It may also be taken as a nutritional supplement.

Safflower oil with high linoleic fatty acid content and a low level of natural antioxidants is not particularly stable.

Ill Effects

Safflower oil, taken as a part of a well balanced diet, does not cause any side effects. However, researchers now understand that an excess of omega-6 EFAs in the diet increases the incidence of cardiovascular diseases, hypertension, non-insulin-dependent diabetes mellitus and obesity. All of these diseases are associated with hyperinsulinemia (HI) and insulin resistance (IR) and are grouped together as the insulin resistance syndrome or syndrome X. There is also an increased cancer incidence and mortality rate, especially in women. Researchers conclude that, high omega-6 linoleic acid consumption might aggravate HI and IR; such diets, rather than being beneficial, may have some long-term side effects within the cluster of hyperinsulinemia, atherosclerosis and tumorigenesis. Excesses of omega-6 EFAs also promote high blood levels of estradiol. High circulating estrogen levels in the blood tend to increase insulin levels and this reduces blood sugar. Low blood sugar leads to irritability and this is one of the main problems with PMS. Thus, excess omega-6

EFA in the diet is linked to estrogen dominance, hyperinsulinemia, PMS and many other diseases.

Hence, for culinary purposes, safflower oil should be combined with omega-3-rich oils as this does not contain omega-3 EFAs and too much omega-6 in the absence of adequate omega-3 favours the production of pro-inflammatory prostaglandins which fuel inflammatory diseases. One study showed that safflower oil, when given to animals exposed to toxic chemicals, increased the formation of abnormal growths whereas flaxseed oil prevented the formation of any abnormal growths, followed closely by fish oil and evening primrose oil.

Suggested Amount

Take one to two tablespoons of oils rich in essential fatty acids per day. It is best to take safflower oil blended with flaxseed oil or other oils rich in omega-3 EFAs in order to have an EFA-balanced oil for the diet.

Storage

Monounsaturated safflower oil is very shelf-stable, although it should still be stored in a cool dry place out of the light to prevent it from going rancid. Polyunsaturated safflower oil, which is also colourless and tasteless, needs to be handled much more carefully, because it goes rancid very easily. Polyunsaturated oil should not be used in high-heat cooking, because it will become rancid, developing chemical compounds which will add an unpleasant taste to the food. Some people even recommend storing it in the refrigerator.

VI. Corn Oil

Corn or maize (Zea mays.), is a cereal crop belonging to the grass family of 'Gramineae'. It is one of the most successful cereal grasses of all time which is grown around the world and is one of the globe's most widely used food staples which is consumed both by humans and industries. Corn varieties are directly used for food and animal feed or processed to make food and feed ingredients. Corn flour, corn oil, cornflake, corn syrup, popcorn, rice corn and corn soup are some popular examples of corn products.

History

The origin of corn remains a mystery. Discoveries in the Tehuacán Valley of southern Mexico have yielded evidence that wild corn existed there 7000 years ago and was not much different in fundamental botanical characteristics from the modern corn plant. There are some reports which indicate that Indians living in what is now Mexico about 10,000 years ago, first used corn gathered from wild plants as a food source. Near 5000 B.C., they learned how to grow corn themselves and it came to be called Indian corn. Today the term usually refers to corn varieties with multicoloured kernels.

Conclusive evidence exists, from archaeological and paleobotanical discoveries that cultivated corn has existed in the south-western U.S. for at least 3000 years. It is native to America and was the staple grain of the region for many centuries before

Europeans reached the New World. It is now a principal cereal crop of tropical and sub-tropical regions throughout the world.

Production

In 2005, the U.S. produced 42 percent of the world's corn and over 58 percent of the U.S. corn crop was used for feed. The remaining U.S. crop was split between exports (25 percent) and food, seed or industrial uses such as ethanol production (17 per cent). Other major corn producing countries include China, Brazil, Mexico and the 25 countries that make up the European Union.

Processing for Oil

One bushel of corn contains 704 g of corn oil (2.8 per cent by weight). The first commercial corn oil for cooking purposes was extracted from corn kernel in 1898 and 1899 by machinery invented by Theodore Hudnut and Benjamin Hudnut of the Hudnut Hominy Company of Terre Haute, Indiana, and called "mazoil." There are two basic methods employed in processing corn kernels. They are known as 'dry milling' and 'wet milling'. Dry milling is the process in which corn is separated into flour, corn meal, grits and other products by soaking corn kernels in water, then removing the germ for processing into oil. The remaining parts of the kernel are ground and sieved into various fractions. Wet milling is the process by which corn is separated into starch (syrup, ethanol, corn starch), germ (oil), and fiber and gluten (animal feed) by soaking corn kernels in water (and often sulfur dioxide) before separating them into the components above by grinding and centrifuge.

Crude corn oil extracted from corn germ has a dark reddish amber colour. The unrefined oil contains relatively large amounts of phosphatides and other non-oil substances (often in excess of 2 per cent) and its free fatty acid content (usually above 1.5 per cent) is higher than that found in most vegetable oils. It is further refined by applying strong bleaching treatments and is subjected to stringent deodorization action to obtain pale yellow, tasteless and odourless oil having higher degree of polyunsaturated fats and oxidative stability. Even after refining, this oil is considerably darker than many other vegetable oils. By removing free fatty acids and phospholipids from crude corn oil, the oil refining process gives corn oil one of the qualities consumers value most *i.e.* its excellent frying quality and resistance to smoking or discoloration. This edible oil having a milder taste is less expensive than other types of vegetable oils. The refined oil contains small amounts of waxes which cause a precipitate of cloud to form in oil held at refrigerator temperatures unless the wax is selectively removed by the process called winterization. The keeping quality of this oil is fairly good.

Nutrient Composition

Refined corn oil contains 99 per cent triglyceride, with proportions of approximately 59 per cent polyunsaturated fatty acid, 24 per cent monounsaturated fatty acid, and 13 per cent saturated fatty acid.

The PUFA is linoleic acid (C18:2n-6) primarily, with a small amount of linolenic acid (C18:3n-3) giving a n-6/n-3 ratio of 83. Corn oil contains a significant amount of ubiquinone and high amounts of alpha- and gamma-tocopherols (vitamin E) *i.e.* approximately 45 mg per 100g that protect the oil from oxidative rancidity. Compared to other vegetable oils, corn oil has the highest phytosterol content.

It is a concentrated source of energy, is very digestible, provides essential fatty acids and vitamin E and is a rich source of polyunsaturated fatty acids which help regulate blood cholesterol levels and lower elevated blood pressure. It has good sensory qualities for use as a salad and cooking oil.

Uses

Its main use is in cooking, where its high smoke point makes refined corn oil a valuable frying oil. It is extensively used in baking, salad dressings and frying. Laboratory frying tests show that corn oil performed close to parity with cottonseed oil when used to fry frozen potatoes.

In addition to snack food applications, corn oil can be an effective component in reducing trans fats in restaurant settings. Corn oil has replaced a significant amount of saturated fat in numerous food products. It can be inter-esterified with fully hydrogenated vegetable oil to produce trans free margarines. It is also a top choice for trans fat reduction.

Health Effects

Corn oil is regarded highly for its functionality, exceptional flavour, economy and health benefits. This oil distinguishes itself from other vegetable oils through its high content in essential fatty acids (56 per cent), vitamin E, phytosterols and other important minor components such as coenzymes Q9 and Q10. Essential fatty acids *i.e.* omega-6 linoleic and omega-3 alpha-linolenic acids are essential biological elements that must be absorbed through food as the body itself is unable to synthesize them. Corn oil has been reported to have the following health effects:

Hypocholesterolemic Effect

i) PUFA

Corn oil is a highly effective food oil for lowering serum cholesterol. Because of its low content of saturated fat content (SFAs) which raises cholesterol and its high content of polyunsaturated fatty acids (PUFAs) which lowers cholesterol, consumption of corn oil can replace SFAs with PUFAs, and the combination is more effective in lowering cholesterol than simple reduction of SFA. PUFA primarily lowers low-density-lipoprotein cholesterol (LDL-C) which is atherogenic. Research shows that PUFA has little effect on high-density-lipoprotein cholesterol (HDL-C) which is protective against atherosclerosis. PUFA generally improves the ratio of LDL-C to HDL-C. Recommendations for minimum PUFA intake to prevent gross essential fatty acid deficiency are about 3 per cent of energy (en per cent). Recommendations for prevention of heart disease are 8-10 en per cent. The use of corn oil to contribute to a PUFA intake of 10 en per cent in the diet would be beneficial to heart health. In fact, the Food and Drug Administration of USA has acknowledged the unsaturated fat benefits of corn oil in reducing the risk of heart disease.

In a study carried by Nalbone *et al.* (1989) in France, they supplemented rats with a low-fat diet (2.2 per cent lard plus 2.2 per cent corn oil), a corn oil diet (17 per cent), a salmon oil diet (12.5 per cent) plus 4.5 per cent corn oil, or a lard diet (15 per cent) plus 2 per cent corn oil for eight weeks to investigate the effect of various types of fats on heart lipid peroxidation status and on blood lipid parameters. All these diets contained 1 per cent cholesterol. They found that when compared with the low-fat diet, the salmon oil-diet intake resulted in a lower blood cholesterol, triglyceride and phospholipid concentrations (–50, –56 and –30 per cent, respectively). Corn oil only tended to lower blood lipids; this decrease was significant for triglycerides only (–40 per cent).

ii) Phytosterols

Vegetable oils are the richest dietary source of phytosterols; corn oil contains 0.77 per cent phytosterols by weight. According to the U.S. Department of Agriculture, corn oil contains 968 milligrams of phytosterols per 100 grams of oil. It has one of the highest phytosterol levels of the refined vegetable oils. Corn oil is the only product that contains a natural mixture of free phytosterol, phytosterol esters and phytostanol esters.

Besides PUFA, research has shown that phytosterols present in corn oil may also play an important role in reducing blood cholesterol by inhibiting its absorption from the intestines. Phytosterols and their derivatives have been reported to markedly decrease the intake of bad cholesterol (LDL), thereby reducing the chances of heart and vascular disease. Phytosterols also decrease the risk of colon cancer.

Ostlund *et al.* (2002) have concluded that phytosterols comprising less than 1 per cent of commercial corn oil could substantially reduce cholesterol absorption and this might account for part of the cholesterol-lowering activity of corn oil from a study of healthy subjects with a mean serum cholesterol level of 5.1 mmol/L. They found that the cholesterol absorption was 38 per cent higher after consumption of the sterol-free corn oil than after consumption of commercial corn oil with an identical fatty acid content in a study of 10 healthy subjects. And, when corn oil phytosterols were added back to sterol-free corn oil at a concentration of 150 mg/test meal, cholesterol absorption was reduced by 12 per cent after inclusion of 300 mg phytosterols. They concluded that phytosterols comprising <1 per cent of commercial corn oil substantially reduced cholesterol absorption and may account for part of the cholesterol-lowering activity of corn oil previously attributed solely to unsaturated fatty acids.

Effect on Blood Pressure

Numerous human studies show that diets enriched in polyunsaturated fatty acids can significantly lower elevated blood pressure in individuals with high blood pressure. Corn oil was used in many of these studies. Corn oil diets have shown blood pressure lowering of about 12 percent in men and 5 percent in women who had elevated blood pressure (mild hypertension). No significant effect of polyunsaturates has been noted in persons with normal blood pressure.

Healthy Effects of Essential Fatty Acids

Corn oil is a rich source of linoleic acid, which is a dietary essential for integrity of the skin, cell membranes, the immune system, and for synthesis of eicosanoids. Eicosanoids are necessary for reproductive, cardiovascular, renal, and gastrointestinal functions and resistance to disease. It has been reported that the essential fatty acids in corn oil can help to:

- ☆ Prevent high blood pressure
- ☆ Slow down diabetic effects
- ☆ Combat obesity
- ☆ Keep up the immune system

Antioxidant Activity

Corn oil is recognized as an excellent source of tocopherols. The four major tocopherols found in corn oil are alpha-tocopherol, beta-tocopherol, gammatocopherol and delta-tocopherol. In commercially available corn oil, gamma-tocopherol is most abundant, followed by alpha-tocopherol and delta-tocopherol. The tocopherol that exhibits the greatest antioxidant effect is delta-tocopherol and alpha-tocopherol has the highest vitamin E activity.

Vitamins E present in corn oil is a major antioxidant responsible for actively capturing free radicals and protect the cell membranes. The antioxidant activity of tocopherols is important not only in health terms, but also in terms of quality of the product because it helps to retard the development of rancidity.

Side Effects of Corn Oil

Animal studies have shown that supply of polyunsaturated fatty acid is one of the requirements for cancer growth. However, the amount of polyunsaturated fatty acid required for cancer growth is considered to be larger than that needed of the host. At this time there is no indication from epidemiological studies that PUFA intake is associated with increased risk of breast or colon cancer, which have been suggested to be promoted by high-fat diets in humans.

Wu *et al.* (2004) from Saga Medical School, Japan investigated whether long-term dietary corn oil promotes colon cancer by inhibiting the tumour suppressor gene p53-mediated mitochondria-dependent apoptosis in azoxymethane (AOM)-treated rats. They found that long-term dietary corn oil increased colonic aberrant crypt foci (ACF) in AOM-treated rats at 12 weeks and promoted colon cancer invasion at 48 weeks. Cancer invasion was not observed in the AOM-treated rats without dietary corn oil, although colon adenomas and cancers were detected. Apoptosis was decreased and cell proliferation was increased in the AOM-treated rats with dietary corn oil, compared with the AOM-treated rats with dietary basal diet. Results suggest that long-term dietary corn oil promotes AOM-induced colon cancer development partly by inhibiting the tumour suppressor gene p53-mediated mitochondria-dependent apoptosis.

A high consumption of omega-6 polyunsaturated fatty acids, which are found in most types of vegetable oil including corn oil, may increase the likelihood that postmenopausal women will develop breast cancer (Sonestedt *et al.*, 2008). Similar effect was observed for prostate cancer (Berquin *et al.*, 2007). Other analysis suggested an inverse association between total polyunsaturated fatty acids and breast cancer risk (Pala *et al.*, 2001). Thus, excessive intake of corn oil is not recommended.

VII. Soybean Oil

Soybean (Glycine max), a species of legume native to East Asia is an important source of vegetable oil and protein worldwide. It is sown during June-July period and harvested by October. Though the direct consumption of soybean is limited, the consumption of soy products is very high in India as well as overseas markets. Soybean oil is the main product of soybean which is widely consumed by humans whereas its meal is mainly used in animal feed industry. According to the Soybean Research Advisory Institute, one-fourth of the world's supply of oil comes from soybeans. After palm oil, soybean oil in its crude form is the most traded oil in international market. Today, soybean oil–together with palm oil–accounts for over half of all oil consumed in the world. And a recent report from market analysts Business Communications Company suggests that US production of major crude vegetable oils was about 8.6 million metric tons in 2008, with soybean oil accounting for nearly 87 per cent of the major vegetable oil production at 7.4 million metric tons.

History

Soybeans were a crucial crop in eastern Asia long before written records. The origins of the soybean plant are obscure, but many botanists believe it to have derived from Glycine ussuriensis, a legume native to central China. According to the ancient Chinese, in 2853 BC the legendary Emperor Shennong of China proclaimed that five plants (soybeans, rice, wheat, barley, and millet) were sacred. Cultivation of soybeans was long confined chiefly to China, but gradually spread to other countries.

From about the first century AD to the Age of Discovery (15-16th century), soybeans were introduced into several countries such as Japan, Indonesia, the Philippines, Vietnam, Thailand, Malaysia, Burma, Taiwan, Nepal and India. Soy was introduced to Africa from China in the late 19th Century and is now widespread across the continent.

By the 17th century, soybeans were being planted in Europe. Soybean was introduced in United States in 1765, where it was first grown for hay. Benjamin Franklin wrote a letter in 1770 mentioning sending soybeans home from England.

Production

The main producers of soybean are the United States, Brazil, Argentina, China and India. The countries like USA (38 per cent), Brazil (25 per cent) and Argentina (19 per cent) contribute estimated 82 per cent of the world soybean production. In India, soybean is one of the most important and largest oilseed crops. Madhya Pradesh, the central state of India, produces estimated 53 per cent of the country's soybean followed by Maharashtra (34 per cent) and Rajasthan (8 per cent), thus these 3 states contributing 95 per cent of the total local production.

Soybean oil accounts for around 8 million tons of the estimated 33 million tons of vegetable oil traded in international market. Though U.S. is the biggest producer and exporter of soybeans in the world, Argentina leads the export charts for oil and meal. The major exporters for soybean oil are Argentina (27-37 per cent of the total world exports), Brazil (13-18 per cent), United States (9-18 per cent) and European Union (12-14 per cent). India' contribution is 3.5 per cent of the total production in world while China produces 7 per cent of it.

Asian countries like India, China, Pakistan, Bangladesh, South and Central American countries (Peru, Venezuela, Bolivia, Dominican Republic) and Africa (Egypt, Morocco) are considered as major buyers in world market. Soybean oil is one of the most important edible oil used in our country. India is a biggest importer of edible oil in world and soy oil import is next only to palm oil in country. India's major import of crude soybean oil is from Argentina and Brazil.

Processing

The oil content in soybeans is normally 18 per cent and is basically used in cooking as edible oil. Crude soybean oil can be obtained from the bean by pressing but more normally by the hexane extraction. More than 95 percent of the soybeans are processed by solvent-extraction plants. When arriving at the processing plant, the soybeans are checked for quality. The soybeans then are processed to extract the oil and meal. In processing soybeans for oil extraction and subsequent soy flour production, selection of high quality, sound, clean, dehulled yellow soybeans are very important. From 100 pounds of soybeans, the soybean-crushing process produces 18 pounds of soybean oil and 80 pounds of soybean meal.

There are several steps in the soybean-crushing process involving cracking, adjusting for moisture content, rolling into flakes, solvent extraction with commercial hexane, refining etc

i) Dehulling

First, the soybeans are cracked and the hull is removed.

ii) Soaking

The soybeans then are flaked in special machines and moved to towers or tanks where they are soaked in a chemical solution. This solvent removes about 99 percent of the pure, crude soybean oil from the flake.

iii) Refining

The crude soybean oil may be refined further depending on how it is to be used. In the refining process, crude oil can be degummed, bleached, deodorized or hydrogenated with hydrogen gas.

In "degumming," the fatty acid content of the oil is neutralized with a caustic acid to produce some products (like soap). The oil also may be "bleached" by treating it with an absorbent clay material before it is "deodorized" through a vacuum steam-distillation process.

iv) Toasting and Grinding

After the oil is removed, the soybean flake then is cleaned, toasted and ground to improve its nutritional value. This produces the soybean meal, which consists of 48 percent protein. The residual meal is a major source of animal feed and is being increasingly used in human nutrition.

Good quality oil is light amber in colour with a free fatty acid content of 0.5 per cent. It has a neutral taste and does not impart any colour or flavour to the foods cooked. It is a liquid at room temperature with a high smoking point of 440°F. Oil from damaged beans is darker, higher in free fatty acids and modified lipids and is more difficult to bleach.

Hydrogenated Soybean Oil

The oil has a tendency to oxidative flavour with the linolenic acid in the oil. Its stability for edible purposes is enhanced by partial hydrogenation. Hydrogenation is applied to solidify soybean oil for the manufacture of margarine. This process increases stability of oil and raises the melting point of soybean oil shortening so that it can be used in products that require a certain level of solid fat.

Hence, hydrogenation changes the chemical composition and physical properties of soybean oil and affects the nutritional value. The degree of change in nutritional value depends upon the amount of hydrogenation necessary to produce the final product and the reduction of polyunsaturates that occur.

Nutrient Composition

Like other edible oils, besides culinary roles, soy oil provides us calories, essential fatty acids and fat soluble vitamins. It is also a healthy oil, comparing favourably with canola oil and other highly unsaturated oils.

Table 20.4: Nutrient Composition of Crude and Refined Soybean Oil

Components	*Crude oil*	*Refined oil*
Triglycerides (per cent)	95-97	>99
Phosphatides (per cent)	1.5-2.5	0.003-0.045
Free fatty acids (per cent)	0.3-0.7	0.05
Unsaponifiable matter (per cent)	1.6	0.3
Plant sterols (per cent)	0.33	0.13
Tocopherols (per cent)	0.15-0.21	0.11-0.18
Hydrocarbons (per cent)	0.014	0.01
Trace metals		
Iron (ppm)	1-3	0.1-0.3
Copper (ppm)	0.03-0.05	0.02-0.06

Source: Pryde (1980).

Soybean oil, the world's leading source of edible oil, shows a wide variation in nutrient composition. It is low in saturated fat, with a content of about 15 per cent, high in unsaturated fat, with 61 per cent polyunsaturated and 24 per cent monounsaturated fat. It contains no trans fat and cholesterol.

The five major fatty acids in soybean oil are palmitate, stearate, oleate, linolenate, and linoleate. This oil is a good source of both linoleic (omega-6) and linolenic acids (omega-3), which are essential for humans. The highest percentage of fatty acids in soybean oil is linoleic acid (more than 50 per cent of the fat) followed in decreasing order by oleic, palmitic, linolenic, and stearic acid. Soybean also contains some minor fatty acids, including arachidic, behenic, palmitoleic and myristic acid. When soybean oil is hydrogenated, the percentages of these polyunsaturated fats decrease.

Strong interrelationships exist between the fatty acids. Linolenic and linoleic acids are directly correlated; linolenic and oleic acids are negatively correlated. Saturated acids range from 1 to 26 per cent and are virtually independent of the

Fatty Acid Profile of Soybean Oil

- *Palmitate*: It is made up of 16 carbon atoms and a full set of hydrogen atoms, which makes it a saturated fatty acid. Palmitate has a negative impact on human nutrition. It has desirable characteristics for making margarine and shortening.
- *Stearate*: It is made up of 18 carbon atoms and a full set of hydrogen atoms. Stearate is a saturated fatty acid that does not have the same negative effect on human nutrition as does palmitate. It has desirable characteristics for making margarine and shortening.
- *Oleate*: It is made up of 18 carbon atoms, two of which each lack a hydrogen atom. The absence of a full set of hydrogen atoms make it an unsaturated fatty acid. Oleate is referred to as a monounsaturate. It is desirable for human nutrition and for frying oils.
- *Linoleate*: It is made up of 18 carbon atoms, four of which each lack a hydrogen atom. Linoleate is an unsaturated fatty acid that is referred to as a polyunsaturate. It is desirable for nutrition, but can lead to off-flavors in food products that are not hydrogenated.
- *Linolenate*: It is made up of 18 carbon atoms, six of which each lack a hydrogen atom. Linolenate is an unsaturated fatty acid that is described as a polyunsaturate. It is desirable for nutrition, but it is the fatty acid most responsible for the off-flavours in food products that are not hydrogenated.

To improve the nutritional characteristics of soybean oil, it is desirable to reduce the content of the saturated fatty acids, particularly palmitate, and lower the content of linolenate to eliminate the need for hydrogenation. Both of these changes have been accomplished in soybeans by developing genes that alter the fatty acid content.

iodine value. There is a large genetic variation in fatty acid composition of soybean oil, mainly resulting from plant breeding.

The fatty acids differ in the number of carbon and hydrogen atoms they contain, which causes differences in the nutritional value of each and their influence on the characteristics of food products.

Soybean oil obtained from the extraction of oil from its seed is fairly rich in glycerides of the unsaturated fatty acids particularly linoleic and linolenic with few oleic fatty acids, which do not oxidize readily because they contain natural antioxidants (Naz *et al.*, 2005; Naz *et al.*, 2004). Before processing, soybeans are very high in the fat soluble vitamin E, as both alpha and gamma tocopherols. Processing removes over 30 per cent of the vitamin E which then becomes a valuable by-product used to make vitamin E supplements. The processed oil is still considered a good source of vitamin E because one serving (1 teaspoon) provides more than 10 per cent of the minimum daily requirement. Soybean oil also contains phytosterols which could lower LDL cholesterol.

Uses

Soybean oil is the world's most widely used edible oil. As soybean oil is the most abundant, almost all margarine and shortenings contain it. Soybean oil has little flavour, which is an advantage because it won't interfere with the taste of the food. Most oils sold as "vegetable oil" are soybean oil, but not all.

Food manufacturers have selected soybean oil for its versatility and competitive pricing. It is widely used in various food products including salad dressings, shortening, vegetable margarine, frozen foods, sandwich spreads, imitation dairy and meat products, non-dairy coffee creamers and commercial baked goods such as breads and crackers. Soybean oil is used in prepared foods such as whipped toppings, potato chips and battered and breaded snacks and vegetables. Compared to other vegetable oils, soybean oil has good emulsifying ability. This makes it an appropriate ingredient in mayonnaise, and the first choice of the general food industry. It has a high smoking point (440°F), making it an excellent option for frying foods quickly and easily.

Health Benefits

Soybean oil is a very healthy food ingredient despite the bad publicity regarding fats and oils in general. Soybean oil is low in saturated fats and high in unsaturated fats, especially essential fatty acids, linoleic acid (Ù-6) and alpha-linolenic acid (Ù-3). Like all other oils from vegetable origin, soybean oil contains no cholesterol. Saturated fat and cholesterol cause heart diseases and mainly found in products from animal origin. Appearing as either polyunsaturated or monounsaturated fat, consumption of soybean oil is reported to provide following health benefits:

1. It may reduce "bad" LDL cholesterol and keep "good" HDL cholesterol unchanged when replacing saturated fats in the diet which reduces the risk of heart disease and cancer.
2. Soybean oil provides an excellent source of ALA, as do leafy greens, some nuts and flax.

This oil contains 7 per cent of the omega-3 fatty acid, alpha-linolenic acid, and 50 per cent of the omega-6 fatty acid, linoleic acid, both of which are essential fatty acids and are the precursors of prostaglandins, the hormone like substances that have a variety of functions in the human body like contraction and relaxation of smooth muscles, contraction and dilation of the blood vessels, controls blood pressure, reducing pain and inflammation etc. Scientists now believe that ALA decreases C-reactive protein (CRP), a marker of inflammation strongly associated with heart disease. Two new studies shed light on the power of alpha-linolenic acid (ALA) to reduce heart disease risk.

3. Soybean oil is one of the few non-fish sources of omega-3 fatty acids. These polyunsaturated fatty acids positively affect overall cardiovascular health, including reducing blood pressure and preventing heart disease. Omega-3 fatty acids also reduce the risk of autoimmune diseases and cancers, act as a blood thinner and prevent the formation of clots and improve depression. They may prevent osteoporosis also.
4. Soybean oil is a good source of phytosterols which act as antioxidants along with vitamin E which remain in the oil even after extraction. These antioxidants help to prevent the oxidative rancidity and help to remove the harmful free radicals from the body and maintain the integrity of cell membrane. Also has high amount of vitamin K, which prevents internal and external bleeding.

Storage

Soybean oil has normally a shelf life of 1 year but it is better to store this oil only for a few months at room temperature. Soybean oil should be stored in a dry and dark place. It should be stored away from heat and if you want to keep soybean oil for longer periods it should be kept refrigerated. Oils high in polyunsaturated fatty acids must not be heated.

Future Researches

Researchers are trying to develop soybeans that have increased omega-3 traits. These are expected to be used as an additive to fortify traditional oils.

Soybean oil is often hydrogenated to increase its shelf life or to produce a more solid product. In this process, unhealthy trans fats are produced which may raise blood cholesterol levels and increase the risk of heart disease. Food manufacturers are now trying to remove trans fats from their product. For this purpose, scientists are breeding new varieties of soybeans containing oil that does not need to be hydrogenated. A new variety of soybean oil that has twice the amount of oleic acid found in conventional soybean oil and only 1 percent of linolenic acid is being tested by researchers.

New varieties of soybean oil including low linolenic oil, and low linolenic–high oleic oil are quickly coming of stream to meet the demand of the food industry that requires healthy fats that can be used for frying and for shelf stable products.

VIII. Mustard Oil

Mustard, an oil seed and also an annual crop known throughout the world is a member of the Brassica family. Global annual production of mustard seed is estimated to be around 40 million tonne. China, European Union, Canada and India are leading producers of mustard seed.

Global mustard seed trade is estimated around 5-6 million tons per annum. Mustard seeds are well known for smell, strong flavour and pungency. They were used by the ancient Chinese and Greeks because of their medicinal properties, but it was likely the Romans who first ground mustard seeds into a paste similar to modern mustard sauce. Mustard seeds can also be used to garnish or spice food directly, as well as pressed into oil.

India is the fourth largest oilseed producing country in the world, with mustard seed having major percentage of this. The role of mustard in country's edible oil sector is vital as it contributes about 40 per cent of total edible oil production. The country is self sufficient in mustard production and there is no exportable surplus. It needs fewer inputs as compared to other oilseed crops. About 4 crore to 5 crore (40 million to 50 million) farmers grow mustard in India. This is a winter crop, usually planted in October and harvested in March, and mostly in the cooler north, particularly in the states of Rajasthan, Uttar Pradesh, Haryana, West Bengal, Madhya Pradesh, Gujarat, and Assam. Rajasthan leads the production with estimated 2.9 million tonne followed by Uttar Pradesh with about 8.8 lakh tonne and other states produce about 2.0 million tonne. Most popular varieties grown in Indian subcontinent are *Brassica juncea, Braassca campestris* and *Brassica napus* L.

Mustard oil is used every day in Indian households. In some parts of India, mustard used is used for massages. Research has shown that massage with mustard oil improves blood circulation, enhances muscular development texture gives good texture to skin. Mustard seed oil has very low saturated content. Experts have proved that mustard oil is healthy cooking oil. It has immense nutritional benefits and is far more superior to other oils. It is one of the wisest health investments.

History

Black mustard is a native of Eurasia. It has been in cultivation in, Europe, Belgium, China, India and Japan for a long time. This was the first species to provide table mustard for use as a condiment. It has been used by Romans, Greeks and Indians since ancient times.

The French have used mustard seeds as a spice since 800 AD, and it was amongst spices taken by the Spanish on explorations throughout the 1400s. Pope John XXII was particularly fond of mustard, and created a new position in the Vatican, 'grand moutardier du pape', or 'mustard maker to the pope.'

Its English name, mustard, is derived from a contraction of the Latin mustum ardens meaning burning wine. This is a reference to the spicy heat of the crushed mustard seeds and the French practice of mixing the ground seeds with must, the young, unfermented juice of wine grapes.Our ancient holy literatures *i.e.* Veds,

Upnishads, Charak Sanhita etc. had emphasized the medicinal values of mustard oil apart to their unparallel use in cooking, pickles and massage

Production

Mustard/Rapeseed oil is the third largest edible oil produced in the world after soy oil and palm oil. At a production level of 13-14 million tons, it accounts for about 12 per cent of the total World's edible oil production. However the export trade has come down, due to the dominance of other oils like palm and soya, which have become comparatively cheaper. The share has come down to almost 3 per cent from the earlier figures of about 5 per cent (of the total 30 million tons of edible oils traded in the export market annually). The production and consumption of this oil has been growing at the rate of 4.65 per cent and 5.03 per cent, respectively (compound growth over the last decade). Canada is the major exporter of seed and oil. Other major producers like China, India and EU are large consumers themselves. On crushing rapeseed or mustard, oil and meal are obtained. The average oil recovery from the seed is about 33 per cent. The remaining is obtained as cake, which is rich in proteins and is used as an animal feed ingredient.

Production of Mustard Seed and Oil: Global and Indian Scenario

Global Scenario

- ☆ The global production of rapeseed and its oil is around 38-42 and 12-14 million tons.
- ☆ China (11-12 million tons), EU (10-13 million tons), Canada (6-7 million tons) and India (4-7 million tons) are the world's major producers.
- ☆ 4.5-6, 1.5 and 2.5 million tons of seed, oil and meal are traded globally.
- ☆ Canada (2.5-3.5 million tons) and Australia (1.5 million tons) are major exporters, while Japan (2 million tons) and Mexico (1 million tons) are the major importers of seed.
- ☆ Canada is the major exporter of oil too. US is the major importer of oil.

Indian Scenario

- ☆ India produces 4-7, 1-2, 2-4 million tons of seed, oil and meal.
- ☆ India does not export or import seed and oil. Meal is exported.
- ☆ The major growing states are Rajasthan (40 per cent), UP (16 per cent), Haryana/Punjab (15 per cent).
- ☆ The oil content varies between 36-42 per cent, with average oil recovery of 34-35 per cent. The remaining is used as rapeseed meal cake.

Table 20.5: India in World Rapeseed Industry

(Rounded figs.)	*India*	*World*	*Per cent Share*
		(In million tons)	
Annual Seed Production	6	40	15
Annual Oil Production	1.5	13	11.5
Annual Oil Consumption	1.5	13	11.5

India was the world's fifth-largest producer of major oilseeds in 2005–2006, producing around 3.066 crore (30.66 million) metric tons, or 8 percent of the world total, behind the United States, Brazil, China, and Argentina (USDA 2006). Mustard-rapeseed (grouped together in most agricultural statistics) accounted for about 22 percent of India's oilseed production in that period. Mustard-rapeseed is produced almost entirely domestically, with imports typically accounting for less than 1 percent of production. In 2005–2006, imports accounted for just 17,000 MTs of a total harvest of 6.5 crore (65 million) MTs, an increase of more than 350 percent since 1964. However, the dramatic increase in production has been due more to acreage expansion than to yield improvements. For mustard-rapeseed yield per hectare in India is only about one-half the world average (Dohlman *et al.*, 2003).

Processing

Around 90 percent of the mustard seed grown in India is used to make oil. Oil is extracted from seeds by crushing and then pressing them slowly. In ascending order of efficiency and yield, mustard oil is produced in the home using a mortar and pestle; in small village-based mills, known as ghanis, for personal consumption and local sale; in small-scale expeller facilities; and in large factories. Though no reliable estimates exist about the extent of home production, anecdotally, quite a bit is processed in this ghanis are the most numerous processing facility (about 1,50,000), but they accounted for less than 5 percent of total oil output in the 1990s because of their low yield. Crushing time is from 2 to 5 hours, with a yield of oil of only about 30 percent. Ghanis have an average output of 60 kg per day, often operating at just 10 percent capacity. The Technology Mission on Oilseeds, Pulses and Maize in the Department of Agriculture and Cooperation is implementing a program to modernize processing and replace ghanis with mechanical expellers to get fuller recovery of oil from the seed and reduce labour time. However, one attraction of hand-milled oil for consumers is its pungency, in addition to the low capital costs for the ghani operator. Natural unrefined mustard oil extracted through cold process is quite pungent. The consumers of traditional product prefer pungent oil. Till now the extraction of pungent oil could be possible only by Rotary Ghani due to mustard seed moisture range of 10-12 per cent, low temperature of extraction in wooden bowl wherein the pungent principle *i.e.* allyl isothiocyanate does not evaporate and consumers of especially rural area prefer it (Singh, 2006). However, the expeller made of metallic components and high compression ratio raises the seed temperature up to 80-100°C resulting in loss of pungent principles. The "Modern" oil expeller provides high pungency mustard oil by low temperature crushing through incorporation of a water cooled chamber and processing at critical moisture levels of oilseed. Mustard oil is extracted at a low pressure at low temperature (40-60°C). It contains 0.30-0.35 per cent essential oil (Allyl Iso Thiocynate) which acts as preservative. The Kachchi Ghani oil considered as a nutritious oil used by common man is cold pressed mustard oil expelled by rotor ghani; it is also rich in both monounsaturated fats and anti-oxidant beside most beneficial omega 3 fatty acid.

Large manufacturers with solvent extractors operate primarily in Rajasthan, Uttar Pradesh, Haryana, and Punjab. The large mills operating in these states account for around 75 percent of mustard oil production (Singh, 2006). In these larger mills, large stone crushers (kolus) enable cold pressing production, which produces oil and a kolu cake. The cakes are then fed through expellers, which use solvents to get the rest of the oil. The first-pressed oil is the purest and most expensive, but most oil in the market is a combination of the two methods.

Even though large manufacturers are more efficient, small-scale expellers and ghanis dominate mustard oil processing. This is largely because of government regulatory and trade policies, including plant scale restrictions, movement and storage restrictions, credit controls, taxes and tax incentives, and restrictions on futures trading (Dohlman *et al.*, 2003; USDA 2006).

The crude mustard oil is dark brown in colour with a pungent odour. Refined mustard oil is used mainly for cooking as it is slightly more viscous and has a lower saponification value and a higher refractive index compared to other vegetable oils.

Consumption

Consumption of mustard oil has grown about 5 percent per year for the past 40 years and currently stands at some 2.3 MTs annually. Across many northern states of India, average consumption exceeds 30g per person per month, but this statistic masks both large differences between states and differences within them. The pattern of consumption across classes suggests that mustard oil is a fairly integral part of many Indian households, regardless of income, though at higher income levels there seems to be a switch to more expensive oils (Dohlman *et al.*, 2003).

Although consumption of mustard oil is typically more prevalent in rural areas, total consumption is usually higher in urban areas. Despite being called the "poor man's oil," mustard oil is roughly double the cost of other oils, such as palm, rice bran, or soybean. This higher price, combined with its pungency, also makes it fairly easy for producers to adulterate it with other, less costly oils (Singh, 2006). The government has made a push toward more packaged oil since 1998, when loose mustard oil was adulterated with argemone, a poisonous additive, causing a number of illnesses (Shiva, 2001).

Nutrient Composition

Fatty Acids

The basic composition of mustard oil is monounsaturated fatty acids (erucic acid, oleic acid), polyunsaturated fatty acids (linolenic and linoleic), proteins (30 per cent), isothiocyanates, phenolics, phytin and dithiol thiones. Mustard oil has about

60 per cent monounsaturated fatty acids of which 42 per cent erucic acid and 12 per cent oleic acid, it has 21 per cent polyunsaturates of which 6 per cent is the omega-3 alpha-linolenic acid and 15 per cent omega-6 linoleic acid and it has 12 per cent saturated fats.

Table 20.6: Fatty Acid Composition of Mustard Oil

Sl.No.	Fatty Acid	Range (per cent)
1.	Palmitic	1-3
2.	Stearic	0.4-3.5
3.	Arachidic	0.5-2.4
4.	Behenic	0.6-2.1
5.	Lignoceric	0.5-1.1
6.	Oleic	12-24
7.	Eicosenoic	3.5-11.6
8.	Erucic	40-55
9.	Linoleic	12-16
10.	Linolenic	7-10

In Table 20.7, fatty acid composition of mustard oil has been compared with that of other edible oils which reveals that mustard oil has less amount of saturated fatty acids when compared to other edible oils and fats like ghee, vanaspati, red palm oil and soybean oil. The MUFA content of soybean oil is lower, with a high amount of linoleic acid (disturbing the prescribed ratio of n-6 to n-3 acids), PUFA being the predominant fatty acid. Mustard oil contains a high amount of MUFA as compared to its PUFA and SFA contents (having the desired ratio of n-6 to n-3 fatty acids). The red palm oil is deficient in alpha-linolenic acid, which is an essential fatty

Table 20.7: Approximate Fatty Acid Composition of Mustard Oil and other Common Fats and Oils (g/100g)

Fats/Oils	SFA	MUFA	Linoleic	α-Linolenic	Predominant Fatty Acids
Mustard Oil	8	70	12	10	MUFA
Soybean	15	27	53	5	PUFA
Palm Oil	45	44	10	<0.5	SFA+MUFA
Red Palm Oil	50	40	9	<0.5	SFA+MUFA
Olive Oil	13	76	10	<0.5	MUFA
Groundnut	24	50	25	<0.5	MUFA
Sunflower	13	27	60	<0.5	PUFA
Safflower	13	17	70	<0.5	PUFA
Cottonseed	22	25	52	1	PUFA
Palm Kernel	82	15	2	<0.5	SFA
Coconut oil	90	7	2	<0.5	SFA
Sesame	15	42	42	1	PUFA+MUFA
Ghee	65	32	2	<1	SFA
Vanaspati	24	19	3	<0.5	SFA
Rice bran	22	41	35	1.5	MUFA+PUFA
Corn Oil	12	32	55	1	PUFA
Canola Oil	4	62	22	10	MUFA+PUFA

acid. Olive oil contains comparatively lesser amount of essential fatty acids as compared to mustard oil. Moreover, sunflower and safflower oils also have a very high percentage of linoleic acid whereas linolenic acid content is very low. However, the ratio of omega fatty acids, n-6 to n-3 (close to 10:1) is within desirable proportions in mustard oil. The relatively high level of oleic acid and the favourable balance between linolenic and linoleic acids is present in mustard oil, therefore, it is good for heart. Least amount of saturated fatty acids in this oil further makes it safe for heart patients.

Erucic Acid

Erucic acid in mustard oil varies between 22 per cent to 50 per cent of the total fatty acid content. The erucic acid gives the strong pungent smell and can cause allergic reactions. Heating the oil to the smoking point can mild the pungency.

The effects of erucic acid from edible oils on human health are controversial. However no negative health effects have ever been documented in humans. Mustard oil was once considered unsuitable for human consumption in the western countries due to the high content of erucic acid. This is because of flawed studies in rats. Subsequent studies on rats have shown that they are less able to digest vegetable fats (whether they contain erucic acid or not) than humans and pigs. Charlton *et al.* (1975) suggested that inefficient activation of erucic acid to erucyl-CoA in rats and a low level of activity of triglyceride lipase and enzymes of betaoxidation for erucic acid probably contribute to the accumulation and retention of cardiac lipid. Before this process was fully understood, it led to the belief that erucic acid and mustard oil were both highly toxic to humans. Feeding a high erucic acid rapeseed oil, with 20 per cent, 22:1, n-9 has been reported to cause an even greater platelet reduction and increased platelet size throughout the 4 wk trial (Kramer *et al.*, 1998).

Epidemiological studies suggest that, in regions where mustard oil is still used in a traditional manner, mustard oil may afford some protection against cardiovascular diseases. In this sense "traditional" means that the oil is used fresh and vegetable fats count only as a small percentage of the total caloric intake. Whether this effect is due to the nature of erucic acid per se to make the blood platelets less sticky, or to the presence of a reasonably high percentage of α-linolenic acid, or to a combination of properties of fresh unrefined oil, is as yet uncertain. Care needs to be taken with such epidemiological studies in order to exclude the possibility of early deaths from other causes skewing the results. The fact that early asymptomatic coronary disease is readily detectable post mortem and is absent in the mustard oil cohorts tends to add weight to the hypothesis that mustard oil is protective.

Some researchers have reported that erucic acid is very beneficial in the genetic disease Adrenoleukodystrophy (ALD) which occurs among male children linked to X-chromosome. To treat this disorder "Oleic-Erucic Acid" formulation (A four-to-one mixture of erucic acid and oleic acid) is used. Intake of erucic acid in large amount can produce ill effects on heart too.

In United States, Canada and European Unions, oils exceeding 5 per cent erucic acid (Percentage of total fatty acid) are deemed to be non-edible, and unsuitable for human consumption. To this end, many packers sell a blend of mustard oil and soybean oil.

Glucosinolate and Isothiocyanates

Glucosinolate, the pungent principle in mustard oil, has anti bacterial, anti-fungal and anti-carcinogenic properties, which account for many medicinal utilities of the oil. High content of glucosinolate is desirable in mustard, as they are precursors of flavour components, also called 'essential oil'. When mustard seeds are crushed, exposed to water, vinegar, or grape juice, an enzyme called myrosinase (thioglucoside gluochydrolase) hydrolyses glucosinolates to isothiocyanates. Isothiocyanates give pungency to mustard oil. Both allyl isothiocyantes from *B.juncea* and aromatic PHBIT (parahyroxy benzyl isothiocyanate) from *S.alba* are quiet effective antifungals. However, PHBIT is more effective. Allyl isothiocyanates destroys mycotoxin-producing moulds like *Aspergillus flavus, Pencillium citrinum* and *Fusarium graminarium* and Neurosproa yeast. An antibacterial activity and an anticarcinogenic activity are also exhibited. Dithiol thiones are also present which are anti mutagenic agents.

Antioxidants

Antioxidants are compounds that protect against oxidation and peroxidation caused by free radicals. Free radicals cause damage to the nuclear material, cell death and tumour formation. High doses of antioxidants are required for scavenging free radicals. Antioxidants are crucial for healthier life and to prevent disorders like atherosclerosis, dementia, skin disorder, arthritis and neurological disorders. Diets rich in PUFA increase the requirement for antioxidants. Mustard oil contains adequate amount of alpha tocopherol and phenolic compounds, thus acts as a potent antioxidant for human health.

Phytins

It is present in mustard oil (2.3 per cent) and has cariostatic property.

Minerals

Mustard oil also contains 490 mg calcium per 100g. Presence of calcium and zinc and absence of trans fatty acid in mustard oil make it ideal for heart. It is better for heart but not a cure.

Health Benefits

Our ancient holy literatures *i.e.* Veds, Upnishads, Charak sanhita etc. had emphasized the medicinal values of mustard oil. Mustard oil in addition to being an important oil is superior also because of its balanced fatty acids profile in terms of SFA, MUFA, Linoleic and alpha linolenic acid in comparison to other oils like palm oil, red palm oil, sunflower, safflower, palm kernel oil, coconut oil, ghee, vanaspati and corn oil etc. Mustard oil has a lower amount of SFA *i.e.* 8 per cent which is good and prescribed clinically for healthy heart. Mustard oil contains a higher amount of MUFA as compared to its PUFA and SFA content with a desired ratio of n-6: n-3 fatty acids.

A ratio of n-6:n-3(4:5) is effective in reducing the risk of heart diseases and this ratio may be met through mustard oil. The American Heart Association has suggested that the ratio of monounsaturated fatty acids to polyunsaturated fatty acids should be 1.5 and mustard oil adheres to this ratio.

Mustard oil is found to have very low levels of artery clogging saturated fatty acid and rich in alpha linolenic acid which has been shown to reduce cholesterol levels and reduce the risk of heart diseases. Moreover, this oil has an ideal ratio of omega 3 and omega 6 fatty acids which is good for heart. A recent study by Harvard school of medicine, AIIMS and St. Johns Hospital, Banglore concluded that chances of heart disease drop by nearly 70 per cent on use of mustard oil as cooking medium.

Professsor Manchanda, eminent cardiologist and senior consultant at Sir Ganga Ram Hospital and ex-HOD of AIIMS has considered mustard oil as good oil for heart due to its fatty composition rich in mono saturated fats and Omega -3 essential oil which ultimately soften the arteries walls and regulate good cholesterol to control and maintain blood pressure. While speaking at a Mustard Research Promotion Consortium, he said that coronary heart disease is emerging as a leading cause of death worldwide and South Asians are especially prone to this. While deaths due to infections and other causes are coming down, heart-relate diseases are registering an upsurge. Unhealthy cooking oil brings home harmful higher levels of cholesterol, saturated fats and trans-fatty acid which when combined with an unhealthy diet, stress, smoking and lack of exercise causes hypertension, diabetes and heart diseases. As far as use of different cooking oils is concerned, he said that cardiologists comparing the nutritional benefits of mustard oil with olive oil have come to a conclusive proof of its superiority (The Hindu, March 26, 2007).

According to a survey by American Heart Association also, mustard oil is better than olive oil from the health point of view. It is not only good for healthy people but is also good for heart patients. The reason behind the fact is that this oil comprises of 12 per cent omega-3 (alpha linolenic fatty acid) as compared to olive oil (only 0.6 per cent).

Some cancer specialists have suggested that unplanned growth of cells is controlled by omega-3 fatty acids and metallic Zn as well as allylisothiocynate which are present in mustard oil. Rapeseed oil contains isothiocynate, which inhibits ATP, a chemical in the body that keeps us young and healthy. Linolenic acid present in rapeseed oil also increases one of the essential Omega-3 fatty acids called EPA in human tissues which actually reduces the stickiness of red blood cells and thereby, reduces blood clotting tendencies.

Others health benefits of mustard oil reported are as under:

- ☆ It can be used as an antibacterial oil.
- ☆ Helps to detoxify human body.
- ☆ Stimulates digestion, circulation and excretory system.
- ☆ Helps preventing fungal growth, thus it can be used as anti-fungal.
- ☆ Helps making immune system strong.

- Organic mustard oil helps preventing cancer and is also helpful for slowing down the ageing process. Kachi ghani mustard oil has more oxidants and vitamins as compared to normal oil which prevent early ageing.
- Helps stimulating sweat glands and helps lowering body temperature.
- Helps in controlling Crohn's disease, curing asthma, arthritis, cramps, adult diabetes and smooth skin.

Use in Cooking

Mustard-rapeseed oil has long been one of the most consumed edible oils in India and currently is third, after palm and soybean oil. It is the popular cooking oil in Northern, Central, Eastern and North Eastern Region of India. Mustard oil is most preferred for medicinal and culinary usages. In India, the vast majority of mustard seed is consumed as oil in cooking or pickling or as seasoning. It is also used for flavouring western foods and Indian recipes.

Storage

Mustard oil has a shelf life of up to one year but is seldom kept for that long before consumption. Instead, it is distributed quickly along the supply chain from processor to market. The annual pickling season takes place from July to August, during which demand is the highest. Mustard oil moves rapidly from processor to market because of the high demand during these two months. Processors typically keep the oil after extraction for a maximum of four to five days because they lack sufficient storage capacity. The shelf life of mustard oil is very good and it is observed that up to 3 years it remains intact because the oleic acid is resistant against rancidity.

In fact, Dr. Narender Saini, a world renowned cardiologist, claims that Mustard Oil's oxidative stability is unmatched. No other edible oil is more stable than that of Mustard Oil's intrinsic potential to remain unaffected by storage conditions, the processing environment and the concept of shelf life.

Future Research

A newer type of mustard oil called ($^{2}00^{2}$) rapeseed oil has been extracted from a bioengineered variety of mustard. The good thing about this variety is that it has a very low amount of erucic acid (less than 2 per cent). The low erucic acid varieties are called LEAR (Low Erucic Acid Rapeseed). These also have a lower glucosinolate content *i.e.* <30 micro moles/g. Increased oleic acid and decreased linoleic acid in *B.juncea* has been controlled by a single gene and is highly heritable.

Chapter 21

Dietary Oils and their Blending for Good Health

Since cooking oils serve as the major source of fat in the Indian diet, the dietary fatty acid profile can be manipulated to a large extent simply by switching the type of cooking oil used. The optimal balance of saturated, polyunsaturated and monounsaturated fatty acids makes ideal oil. Therefore, it is very important that one should select a cooking oil or blend of oils that contain an optimum ratio of above mentioned fatty acids.

The latest trend in edible oil industry is blended oils to attain optimum ratio of saturated, MUFA and PUFA. The "Sundrop Heart" available in market is a blend of sunflower and rice bran oils (refined rice bran oil 80 per cent and sunflower oil 20 per cent). Saffola has also started marketing sunflower and safflower refined oils blended with rice bran oil.

Since cooking oils serve as the major source of fat in the Indian diet, the dietary fatty acid profile can be manipulated to a large extent simply by switching the type of cooking oil used. No one oil or fat except canola and olive oil contains the optimum ratio of saturated, unsaturated and monosaturated fatty acids which can be considered healthy for the human beings. Earlier many studies reported the ill effects of saturated fats like desi ghee and hydrogenated fats on blood cholesterol levels. They were reported to be not healthy for heart and doctors started advising heart patients to take vegetable oils rich in PUFA to lower blood cholesterol levels.

Now there has been concern that long-term consumption of PUFA-rich diets may have adverse health effects such as increased risk to cancer (Braden and Carroll, 1986), cholelithiasis (Sturdevant *et al.*, 1973), immunosuppression (Ring *et al.*, 1974;

McHugh *et al.*, 1977) and reduction of the protective high density lipoprotein cholesterol (Sheperd *et al.*, 1978). More recently, linoleic and MUFA, contrary to expectation, have also been shown to be thrombogenic, *i.e.* elevate the plasma levels of fibrinogen and factor VII coagulant activity (Sanders, 1996). High intakes of PUFA would also augment lipid peroxidation in vivo, thus imposing an increased demand for dietary antioxidant nutrients, especially vitamin E.

Since the use of polyunsaturated vegetable oils or their blends is necessary for diets containing 10 per cent kcal linoleic acid, it is noteworthy that such PUFA-rich vegetable oils are susceptible to oxidation during frying. The oxidation products or "polar materials" formed in these polyunsaturated vegetable oils, being non-volatile, tend to accumulate in the frying medium, get absorbed into fried foods, and can have deleterious effects on health.

In the pathogenesis of cancer, the adverse influence of PUFA is due primarily to the linoleic acid component and impacts mainly in the development phase, *i.e.* enhance the metastatic spread of tumour cells (Klurfeld, 1995). Studies on mammary tumorigenesis in rats fed 20 per cent ω/ω or 40 per cent kcal fat (Carroll *et al.*, 1981; Ip *et al.*, 1985) have indicated that the critical level for the tumour-promoting effect of linoleic acid (acting as EFA) was about 3.0-4.4 per cent ω/ω or 6.0-8.8 per cent kcal. Thus, it would be premature to consider that the adverse effects of linoleic acid in humans are only significant when dietary levels exceed 10 per cent kcal, although a critical level of 12 per cent kcal was cited by the British Nutrition Foundation (1992). In contrast to the effects of linoleic acid, most studies with ù-3 FA have shown an inhibitory effect on tumour growth (Kort *et al.*, 1987; Karmali *et al.*, 1984; Karmali *et al.*, 1987). Thus, ω-6/ω-3 FA ratio may have a vital influence on tumour cell growth.

In the light of above research findings, it is quite evident that no single source of oil or fat is ideal in itself. Some contain more of saturated fat and others may contain more of PUFA or imbalanced ratio of saturated, PUFA and MUFA. But ideal ratio of these three types of fatty acids can be obtained through blending of various cooking oils available in the market. Therefore, it is very important for the consumer to know what kind of fat source he or she should buy from the market for blending to obtain ideal fatty acid ratios as recommended recently (Table 21.1) for keeping good health.

Table 21.1: Recommended Fat and Fatty Acid Intake

Nutrient	*Recommended Intake as Percent of Total Calories*
Total Fat	25-35 per cent
Saturated fat	Less than 7 per cent
Polyunsaturated fat	Up to 10 per cent
Monounsaturated fat	Up to 20 per cent
Carbohydrate	50-60 per cent of total calories
Protein	Approx. 15 per cent
Cholesterol	Less than 200mg/day
Total calories	Balance energy intake and expenditure to maintain desirable body weight and prevent weight gain

Quality of Fat and its Food Sources Available in the Market

Meats, baked goods, and full-fat dairy products are the main sources of saturated fats in most diets. Coconut, palm, and palm kernel oils also contain saturated fats. Healthy people should consume less than 10 per cent of calories from saturated fats daily.

Monounsaturated and polyunsaturated fatty acids are unsaturated fats. Polyunsaturated fats are further distinguished by the position of the double bonds in their structure. Designated by "omega" (*e.g.*, omega-3, omega-6), this term indicates the position of the beginning of the first double bond starting from the methyl end of the fatty acid. Two examples of omega-3 fatty acids include eicosapentaenoic acid (EPA) and docosahexaenoic acid (DHA). Oily fish from cold waters, such as salmon, mackerel, tuna, and trout are especially rich in EPA and DHA.

When unsaturated fats replace saturated fats in the diet, they help reduce blood cholesterol levels and thus, lower the risk of heart disease. It is recommended that keeping total fat intake between 20 and 35 percent of calories, these should be derived from most of the fats coming from sources of polyunsaturated and monounsaturated fatty acids such as fish, nuts, and vegetable oils. From the previous chapters, it must have become clearer to the reader that canola, olive, peanut, high oleic safflower and sunflower oils, and nuts are rich in monounsaturated fats. Sources of alpha-linolenic and linoleic acids, which are unsaturated fats and essential, include vegetable oils,

Table 21.2: Sources of Saturated and Unsaturated Fats

Systematic Name	*Common Name*	*Typical Fat Source*
Common Saturated Fatty Acids		
Hexanoic Acid	Caproic Acid	Butterfat
Octanoic Acid	Caprylic Acid	Coconut Oil
Decanoic Acid	Capric Acid	Coconut Oil
Dodecanoic Acid	Lauric Acid	Coconut Oil
Tetradecanoic Acid	Myristic Acid	Butterfat, Coconut Oils
Hexadecanoic Acid	Palmitic Acid	Palm, Cottonseed Oils
Octadecanoic Acid	Stearic Acid	Cocoa Butter, Animal Fat
Eicsanoic Acid	Arachidic Acid	Peanut Oil
Common Unsaturated Fatty Acids		
Hexadecenoic Acid	Palmitoleic Acid	Some Fish Oils, Beef Fat
9-Octadecenoic Acid	Oleic Acid	Olive, Canola Oils
9, 12 Octadecadienoic Acid	Linoleic Acid	Soybean, Corn Oils
9,12,15 Octadecatrienoic Acid	Alpha-Linolenic Acid	Soybean, Canola Oils
5, 8,11,14 Eicosatetraenoic Acid	Arachidonic Acid	Lard
5, 8, 11, 14, 17 Eicosapentaenoic Acid	EPA	Some Fish Oils
Docosohexaenoic Acid	DHA	Some Fish Oils

walnuts, and flaxseed. Flax (linseed) oil has 55 per cent plant-based omega-3 but is uncommon as a table or cooking oil.

In Table 21.2, sources of various types of fatty acids have been indicated.

Predominant Fatty Acids of Various Fat and Oil Sources

In order to help out the consumers, it is essential for scientists to make them aware of the benefits and/or the harms of different components of edible oils. For blending of oils also, the consumer must know the predominant fatty acids of various fats and oil sources (Table 21.3).

Table 21.3: Predominant Fatty Acids of Common Fats and Oils (g/100g)

Fats/Oils	*SFA*	*MUFA*	*Linoleic*	*α-Linolenic*	*Predominant Fatty Acids*
Mustard Oil	8	70	12	10	MUFA
Soybean	15	27	53	5	PUFA
Palm Oil	45	44	10	<0.5	SFA+MUFA
Red Palm Oil	50	40	9	<0.5	SFA+MUFA
Olive Oil	13	76	10	<0.5	MUFA
Groundnut	24	50	25	<0.5	MUFA
Sunflower	13	27	60	<0.5	PUFA
Safflower	13	17	70	<0.5	PUFA
Cottonseed	22	25	52	1	PUFA
Palm Kernel	82	15	2	<0.5	SFA
Coconut oil	90	7	2	<0.5	SFA
Sesame	15	42	42	1	PUFA+MUFA
Ghee	65	32	2	<1	SFA
Vanaspati	24	19	3	<0.5	SFA
Rice bran	22	41	35	1.5	MUFA+PUFA
Corn Oil	12	32	55	1	PUFA
Canola Oil	4	62	22	10	MUFA+PUFA

Coconut oil is a rich source of saturated fatty acids. Mono-unsaturated fatty acids (MUFA) are found mainly in vegetables oils such as mustard, canola, olive, groundnut, rice bran oil etc. Polyunsaturated fatty acids (PUFA) are found mainly in vegetable oils such as safflower, sunflower, corn, cottonseed, soybean oil etc. Trans fatty acids (TFA) are mostly found in margarine, hydrogenated vegetables oil or vegetable shortening. They also occur naturally in some animal products and also in few dairy products.

The edible oils and fats like ghee, vanaspati, red palm oil and soybean oil are very high in SFA. Olive oil has a higher amount of SFA as compared to mustard oil. The MUFA content of soybean oil is lower, with a high amount of linoleic acid (disturbing the prescribed ratio of n-6 to n-3 acids); PUFA being the predominant fatty acid. The red palm oil is deficient in alpha-linolenic acid, which is an essential fatty acid. Olive oil contains comparatively lesser amount of essential fatty acids as compared to mustard oil. Sunflower and safflower oils have a very high percentage of linoleic acid whereas linolenic acid content is very low. Mustard oil is a good source of MUFA. The ratio of omega fatty acids, n-6 to n-3 is within desirable proportions in mustard oil but erucic acid can pose problem if consumed in excess for a very long time.

Canola oil, and olive oil are thought to be beneficial but are not used due to certain limitations. Canola oil is not easily available in India. Olive oil is expensive and Indians donot have acceptability for its flavour in cooked dishes.

Buying Vegetable Oils for making Ideal Oil Blends

In Tables 21.3 and 21.4, amount of various fatty acids and their ratio in various commonly used vegetable oils has been compared with that of the recommended ratio.

Table 21.3: Comparison of fatty acid composition of various commonly used vegetable oils with the recommended values

Name of Oil	*Fatty Acids Per cent Weight*			*Essential Fatty Acids*	*Antioxidants*
	SFA	*MUFA*	*PUFA*	*Omega6/ Omega3*	
MustardOil/Rapessed Oil	6	67	27	2	Tocopherols
Sunflower Oil	12	38	50	57	Tocopherols
Safflower Oil	10	15	75	69	Tocopherols
Soybean Oil	16	24	60	10	Tocopherols
Groundnut Oil	20	50	30	32	Tocopherols
Rice Bran Oil Recommended	20	45	35	15	Tocopherols Tocotrienols and Oryzanol
Soybean Oil	16	24	60	10	Tocopherols
Recommended	Less than 7%	Up to 20%	Up to 10%		

Some of commercially available oil brands of soybean, sunflower, mustard, olive, rice bran oil, groundnut etc in the Indian market have been given in Table 21.5. If we compare the PUFA/Saturated fatty acids and Omega6/Omega 3 fatty acid compositions of commonly available vegetable oils with that of their WHO recommended values, it is noticed that no single oil can be considered the best (Table 21.5).

Choice of a healthy cooking oil is a controversial subject. What kind of fat or oil, we should select for our daily use, the ideas keep on changing as new evidence accumulates. Moreover, in the light of above facts, and on the basis of composition of commonly available vegetable oils available in the market (Tables 2,3,4 and 5), it is

Table 21.4: Ratio of Various Fatty Acids in Commonly Used Vegetable Oils

Name of Oil	*Saturated Fatty Acids (SFA)*	*Poly-Unsaturated Fatty Acids (PUFA)*	*Mono-Unsaturated Fatty Acids (MUFA)*	*SFA/MUFA/PUFA Ratio as against Ideal Ratio 1: 1.5: 1*
Rapeseed Oil	6	27	67	0.09: 0.4: 1
Groundnut Oil	22	36	43	0.51:0.84: 1
Rice Brain Oil	25	37	38	0.65: 0.95: 1
Soybean Oil	16	60	40	0.66: 2.50: 1
Safflower Oil	10	75	15	0.66: 5.0: 1
Sunflower Oil	12	67	21	0.57: 3.20: 1
Palmolein Oil	45	12	43	1.06: 0.27: 1
Cotton Seed Oil	28	50	22	1.27: 2.27: 1

Table 21.5: How Good is our Oil on WHO Recommendations

Brand	*PUFA/SFA (WHO: 0.8-1)*	*Omega 6/Omega 3 (WHO: 5-10)*
Fortune – Soybean	4.1	8.6
Nature Fresh Soybean	3.1	2.1
Sweekar – Sunflower	1.7	76.3
Sundrop – Sunflower	4.0	65.3
RR Primio- Groundnut	1.8	7.5
Dhara refined – Mustard	6.8	4.1
Fortune kachi ghani–Mustard	4.6	1.4
Saffola – Safflower	5.9	88.2
Saffola gold – Blend	2.2	117.3
Figaro – Olive	0.6	0
Shalimar – Rice bran	1.2	4
Ruchi gold – Palm oil	0.2	23

quite clear that no one source of fat or oil contains the right kind of fatty acid composition which is good for us. No oil is the best oil. Every oil has some components which are harmful and some which are helpful. Under the present findings and recommendations by WHO, various researchers have recommended blending of various vegetable oils. The mantra today by the experts is 'blending oils' rather than 'éxclusive oils', for maximum health benefits. Oil blends help to attain the healthy n-6 and n-3 ratio, PUFA, MUFA requirements by the body which significantly affect lowering of LDL (bad cholesterol), triglycerides and subsequent increase in HDL (good cholesterol).

In practice, given the scientific evidence what would work best is a mixture of oils. Different oils have different qualities and quantities of different types of fatty acids. Some oils are high in n6 and others in n3. So it is a good idea to blend oils to get optimum health benefits.

Either buy different oils every month or cook different foods items in different oils. Blending oil means cooking the entire day's meal in a variety of oils, balancing them in a way, which would complement the requirements of human body and the meal being prepared. For instance not every dish can be prepared in mustard oil given to its pungent flavour, at the same time it has a very good balance of MUFA (monounsaturated fatty acid) and PUFA (polyunsaturated fatty acid; n-6 and n-3).

I. Research Studies Carried out on Blending of Oils from Health Point of View in India

It is increasingly recognized now that a balanced intake of saturated, poly and mono unsaturated fatty acids as well as n-3 and n-6 fatty acids is essential for good health. There is a need for improving consumer awareness on amounts and types of oil consumption which are associated with low risk of cardiovascular diseases. As it is evident that as no single oil has the appropriate proportion of fatty acids (Saturated, mono- and poly- unsaturated with appropriate n-3:n-6 ratio), the nutritionists have suggested the following two alternative methods for improving balanced consumption of edible oils:

1. Using a variety of cooking oils at the household level,
2. By commercially making available the blended oils with appropriate fatty acid composition so that the people have appropriate fatty acid composition in the oil they regularly use.

Getting balanced fatty acid intake by selecting appropriate combination of oils at the household level gives an option to the consumers to select oils according to their availability, cost, culinary practices and dietary preferences. However, in India, there are substantial regional variations in the type of oils used, thereby making one kind of blending unviable. Moreover, the common populace may not be aware of the nutritional composition (P/S, SFA: MUFA: PUFA, n-6/n-3) of each kind of oil. Also the issues of availability of oils in the local market and purchasing power limitations may further stand in the way of this option being used widely and appropriately at the household level.

Under these circumstances we need to take appropriate stand in regard to different kinds of formulations for commercial blending of oils, as also the possibilities of incorporating other nutritionally important constituents like antioxidants, cholesterol lowering molecules, vitamin A precursors etc. based on regional tastes and dietary diversifications. We also need to know the adverse aspects of blending, if any known.

Optimum Combinations Based on Studies Done at NIN, India

A.

Dr. Ghafoorunissa, former Deputy Director, National Institute of Nutrition, India has recommended the following:

1. Moderation in linoleic acid intake (LA (n-6) from visible fat, increase in alpha linolenic acid (ALNA (n-3), reduction in saturated fatty acid (SFA) and trans fatty acids (TFA) in the total diet (visible and invisible fat). For achieving this, she recommended the use of preferred vegetable oil(s) along with ALNA containing oil(s) or vegetable oil(s) containing high LA (n-6) along with moderate LA (n-6) or low LA (n-6) containing oil(s). However, she added that the latter combination would ensure moderation in LA intake only and is therefore recommended when fish is consumed or when other dietary components provide adequate ALNA (n-3).
2. She emphasized that balancing fatty acid intake by selecting appropriate combination of 2 or more vegetable oils at household level, gives option to the consumer to select oils according to availability, cost and culinary practice.
3. She stated that according to PFA (Prevention of Food Adulteration Act) 4th Amendment Rules 1992, blending of any two vegetable oils (wherein the component oil used in the admixture is not less than 20 per cent) has been permitted so as to increase the overall availability of oils of consumers' choice.
4. On the basis of her research carried out at NIN, she suggested blending of vegetable oils as per the combinations presented below in order to ensure optimal health benefits and prevent diet related chronic diseases in Indian population.
5. Among the most appropriate combinations suggested in the NIN table include combining in the 1:1 ratio groundnut, or sesame oil with one of the following three for optimum food value: canola, soybean, mustard oil.

Table 21.6: Recommended Oil Combinations (1:1) in Indian Diets

$\downarrow$*LA (n-6)* $\uparrow$*ALNA (n-3)*	$\downarrow$*LA (n-6)*
Groundnut/Sesame/Rice bran oil + Mustard oil	Sunflower/Safflower oil + Palmolein/Olive oil
Groundnut/Sesame/Rice bran oil + Canola oil	Safflower/Sunflower oil + Groundnut/Sesame/ Rice bran oil
Groundnut/Sesame/Rice bran + Soybean oil	
Palmolein/Olive oil + Soybean oil	
Safflower/Sunflower oil +Palmolein/Olive oil+ Mustard oil	
Additional advantage other than phytosterols and vitamin E: Sesame -Lignans;	
Ricebran-T3 and Oryzanol; RPO/Palmolein -Carotenes/T3; Olive oil – polyphenols	
In view of the regional preferences, choose combinations of oils and fats, that are able to provide the prescribed ratios of n-6 and n-3 fatty acids	
Use low PUFA containing oils with natural anti-oxidants for deep frying	

Source: Ghafoorunissa, 2005.

Dr. Ghafoorunissa reiterated that the minor components of fats and oils have hypocholesterolemic and antioxidant properties. She pointed out the recent studies that have demonstrated synergism in the beneficial effects of minor components of vegetable oils. Therefore, she suggested that use of more than one oil provides this additional advantage. She made her recommendation to ensure optimal quantity and quality of fat in total diet throughout life, which may significantly contribute to decreased incidence of low birth weight and chronic under-nutrition, at one end of socioeconomic spectrum and diet related chronic diseases in late adult life at the other, in the Indian population.

B.

According to Dr. Mahtab S. Bamji, Dangoria Charitable Trust, Hyderabad, most Indian oils are very high in n-6 fatty acid -linoleic (lin) acid and very low in n-3 fatty acid linolenic acid (len) (Also called omega -6 and omega-3, respectively). The ratio lin/len should not exceed 10. This can be achieved by mixing oils like sunflower, saffola etc with high len oils like soybean, mustard and canola. Also it is advisable to reduce the degree of unsaturation present in oils like saffflower, sunflower, etc. by mixing with groundnut or palm oil. He suggested to mix soybean oil and palm oil. Unfortunately both imported, but it provides a good blend of saturated/unsaturated fatty acid and lin/len ratio. Len acid can also be derived from the bound fat contained in green leafy vegetables, nuts etc. The richest source of long chain n-3 fatty acid is fish. He further reported that he understands that the ban on blending oils has been lifted, and in future it may be possible to get designer oils with some other nutraceuticals added.

C.

Some of the recommended oil combinations for optimal health benefits as reported by other researchers are:

- ☆ Groundnut: Soybean oil:: 2:1
- ☆ Mustard: Sesame oil:: 3:1
- ☆ Sunflower: Groundnut oil:: 1:1
- ☆ Sesame: Soybean oil:: 2:1
- ☆ Ground nut oil/sesame/RBO: Mustard oil 3:1
- ☆ Groundnut oil/sesame/RBO: Canola oil 2:1
- ☆ Groundnut oil/sesame/RBO: soybean oil 2:1
- ☆ Palmolein: soybean oil 1:1
- ☆ Safflower: Mustard: Palmolien oil 1:1:1

Source: Dr. B. Sesikeran, Director, NIN, Hyderabad

Commercially available Blended Oils

Some of the food industries have launched blended oils in the Indian market which are mentioned as under:

1. *Sundrop Heart* is a brand of commercially blended oil that is a blend of 80 per cent rice bran oil and 20 per cent sunflower oil manufactured by Agro Tech Foods ltd, Secunderabad. Their label claims 21 per cent saturates 46

per cent monounsaturates, and 33 per cent poly unsaturates. As per the fatty acid composition in the Nutritive Value of Indian foods, the composition works out to be slightly different with lower MUFA, about 36 per cent and higher PUFA, about 39 per cent. While this blend provides a better balance in the SAFA, MUFA and PUFA, it has practically no n-3 fatty acid. A combination of this blended oil with soybean oil at home level in the proportion of 2:1, provides n-6 to n-3 fatty acid in the ratio of 14:1.

2. MARICO Industries has launched Saffola Gold, a blend of ricebran and safflower oil (Kardi oil) in a 70:30 ratio, claiming the formulation has dual benefits of lowering cholesterol and enabling food cooked in it to absorb lesser oil. Apart from reducing bad cholesterol, Saffola Gold possesses other health benefits, the company claims in a statement adding it is fortified with vitamin E to boost immunity and contains Lobsorb, which ensures that food cooked in this oil absorbs less oil.

II. Research Studies Carried out on Blending of Oils from Health Point of View in Abroad

i) Plasma Cholesterol-Lowering Potential of Edible-Oil Blends Suitable for Commercial Use

Nestel et. al. (1992) tested semi-hardened blends of edible oils, suitable for commercial food manufacture, with a lower than conventional saturated fatty acid content, for their effects on plasma cholesterol. Twenty-six mildly hypercholesterolemic men took part in a double-blind crossover experiment in which two test blends were compared with two control dietary periods [which resembled the Australian fat intake: proportions of polyunsaturated, monounsaturated, and saturated fatty acids (PMS) 0.4:0.9:1]. PMS in the test diets was approximately 0.8:1.3:1 and resulted in significantly lower LDL-cholesterol concentrations (reductions of less than or equal to 7.7 per cent). HDL cholesterol and plasma triglyceride were unchanged. The trans fatty acid (mainly elaidic) content of the blends was 16 per cent, raising its contribution to energy by 4 per cent but without apparent effect on LDL and HDL concentrations. They reported that provided the overall ratio of linoleic acid to palmitic acid in commercial edible- oil blends exceeds that in the prevailing national diet, partial hydrogenation will not negate the LDL-lowering potential.

A study on lipid profile of rats fed blends of rice bran oil in combination with sunflower and safflower oil was undertaken (Sunitha *et al.*, 1997). Rats fed RBO + SNO/SFO at 70:30 ratio for a period of 28 days showed significantly ($p < 0.05$) lower levels of total cholesterol (TC), triglycerides (TG) and low density lipoprotein (LDL) cholesterol and increased high density lipoprotein (HDL) cholesterol in animals fed a high cholesterol diet (HCD) and cholesterol free diet (CFD). Liver total cholesterol (TC) and triglycerides (TG) were also reduced. Fecal excretion of neutral sterols and bile acids was increased with use of RBO blends. RBO, which is rich in tocopherols and tocotrienols, may improve the oxidative stability of the blends. Tocotrienols are known to inhibit 3-hydroxy, 3-methyl, glutaryl CoA (HMG-COA) reductase (rate limiting enzyme in cholesterol biosynthesis), resulting in hypocholesterolemia. In addition to improving the lipid profile by lowering TC, TG and LDL-C and increasing HDL-C, blending of RBO with other oils can result in an economic advantage of lower prices.

Blended oils comprising coconut oil (CNO) and rice bran oil (RBO) or sesame oil (SESO) with saturated fatty acid/monounsaturated fatty acid/polyunsaturated fatty acid at a ratio of 1:1:1 and polyunsaturated/ saturated ratio of 0.8-1 enriched with nutraceuticals were prepared. Blended oils (B) were subjected to interesterification reaction using sn-1, 3 specific lipase from *Rhizomucor miehei*. Fatty acid composition and nutraceutical contents of the blended oil were not affected by interesterification reaction. Male Wistar rats were fed with AIN-76 diet containing 10 per cent fat from CNO, RBO, SESO, CNO+RBO blend (B), CNO+SESO(B), CNO+RBO interesterified (I), or CNO+SESO(l) for 60 days. Serum total cholesterol (TC), low-density lipoprotein cholesterol, and triacylglycerols (TAGs) were reduced by 23.8, 32.4, and 13.9 per cent, respectively, in rats fed CNO+RBO(B) and by 20.5, 34.1, and 12.9 per cent, respectively, in rats fed CNO+SESO(B) compared to rats given CNO (Malongil and Lokesh, 2007). Rats fed interesterified oils showed a decrease in serum TC, low-density lipoprotein cholesterol (LDL-C), and TAGs in CNO+RBO(l) by 35, 49.1, and 23.2 and by 33.3, 47, and 19.8 per cent in CNO+SESO(l), respectively, compared to rats given CNO. Compared to rats fed CNO+RBO blended oils, rats on CNO+RBO interesterified oil showed a further decrease of 14.6, 24.7, and 10 per cent in TC, LDL-C, and TAG. Rats fed CNO+SESO interesterified oils showed a decrease in serum TC, LDL-C, and TAG by 16.2,19.6, and 7.8 per cent, respectively, compared to rats given blended oils of CNO+SESO (B). Liver lipid analysis also showed significant change in the TC and TAG concentration in rats fed blended and interesterified oils of CNO+RBO and CNO+SESO compared to the rats given CNO. This study suggested that feeding fats containing blended oils with balanced fatty acids lowers serum and liver lipids. Interesterified oils prepared using lipase have a further lowering effect on serum and liver lipids even though the fatty acid composition of blended and interesterified oils remained same. These studies indicated that the atherogenic potentials of a saturated fatty acid containing CNO can be significantly decreased by blending with an oil rich in unsaturated lipids in appropriate amounts and interesterification of blended oil.

A range of human and animal studies have shown that rice bran oil (RBO) is an edible oil of preference for improving serum cholesterol levels and lipoprotein profiles with similarity to the more commonly used vegetable oils such as corn oil and safflower oil. Of particular interest is the observation that blending RBO with safflower oil at a definite proportion (7:3, wt/wt) magnifies the hypocholesterolemic efficacy, compared with the effect of each oil alone. Although the mechanism underlying this effect is not apparent at present, the blending may have a practical significance. The blending effect was reproduced in rats fed a cholesterol-enriched diet, and there was also a decrease in liver cholesterol. The occurrence of peculiar components such as -oryzanol and tocotrienols could be responsible for the hypocholesterolemic effect of RBO (Sugano and Tsuji, 2008).

ii) Effects of Fish Oil Substitution with a Mix Blend Vegetable Oil on Nutrient Digestibility in Murray Cod, *Maccullochella peelii peelii*

The replacement of fish oil with vegetable based oils is a strategy which is increasingly being adopted by the aquafeed industry as an essential component to reduce the reliance on a limited supply of a natural resource, which in turn also provides cost benefits. The aim of the present investigation was to evaluate the lipid and fatty acid digestibility of a mix blend vegetable oil in juvenile Murray cod; an emerging species of increasing interest in the Australian aquaculture sector. Five semi purified experimental diets were formulated with 17 per cent lipid originating from fish oil (FO) which was substituted in 25 per cent increments by blended vegetable oil (VO), formulated using olive oil (12 per cent), palm oil (43 per cent) and linseed oil (45 per cent) to match the major fatty acid classes of the FO (David *et al.*, 2007).

Significant differences between the dietary treatments with regard to the lipid and individual fatty acid digestibility were recorded. This study clearly demonstrated that in Murray cod fatty acid digestibility decreases with chain length, and inversely increases relative to the degree of unsaturation. The combination of chain length, degree of unsaturation and the melting point of individual fatty acids resulted in the digestibility of PUFA > MUFA > SFA and short chain > longer chain fatty acids. Therefore, the inclusion of a mixed blend vegetable oil resulted in significantly reduced lipid digestibility in juvenile Murray cod.

iii) Effect of Blending Dietary Oils on Growth Performance, Total and Individual Fatty Acid Absorption by the Growing Chick

Crick *et al.* (1988) blended canbra oil (6.1 per cent erucic acid) with sunflower oil or lard in the ratio of 1:1 (w/w). They blended canola oil (0.55 per cent erucic acid) with sunflower oil in ratios of 9:1, 8:2, 7:3, 6:4 and 5:5 (w/w). Influence of blending of dietary oils on growth performance, digestibility of total lipids and absorbability of individual fatty acids was studied using growing chicks fed lipids at 8 per cent in practical diets. Results indicated significant differences ($P<0.05$) in final body weight, weight gain, feed consumption and feed conversion ratio among chicks fed various oils and oil blends. There was however no clear case of synergism in growth performance of chicks fed blended oils. There were significant differences ($P<0.05$) in digestibility of lipids and absorbability of individual fatty acids (but not of total fatty acids). Fatty acid absorption was not significantly different in blended and unblended canbra oils. This trend was however reversed among the canola-sunflower blends in which fatty acid absorption from the 7:3 and 5:5 blends was superior to that from the unblended oils (except soybean oil).

iv) Changes in Lipid Profile by Vegetable Oil Blends Rich in Polyunsaturated Fatty Acids in Rats with Hypercholesterolemia

The objective of this study was to investigate the effect of different blended vegetable oils having different levels and profiles of polyunsaturated fatty acids (PUFA) on hypercholesterolemia by analyzing the changes in lipid profile in high-cholesterol diet fed rats (Ramadan et.al., 2009). Three vegetable oils (soy oil, sunflower oil, and the nonconventional flaxseed oil) were blended to obtain blends rich in PUFA. Thirty albino rats were used over the 2-month period. The animals were divided into five groups, wherein group 5 represents negative control, where rats were fed basal diet, while rats in group 4 received high cholesterol diet and served as positive controls. The other three groups were fed hypercholesterolemic diet (1 per cent cholesterol + 0.25 per cent colic acid) supplemented with blended oils. Generally, rats fed blended oils showed significantly lower levels of total cholesterol (TC), triacylglycerol (TG), and low-density lipoprotein (LDL) cholesterol as well as higher levels of high-density lipoprotein (HDL) cholesterol, in comparison with animals fed high-cholesterol diet and cholesterol-free diet. Thus, oil blends under study may be useful formulations for the treatment of hypercholesterolemia. In addition to improving the lipid profile by lowering TC, total TG, and total LDL and increasing HDL, blending of vegetable oils can result in an economic advantage of lower prices.

III. Blending of Oils from Cooking Point of View

During storage and heat treatment, vegetable oils undergo hydrolysis, oxidation and polymerization, resulting in quality deterioration with respect to their sensory and nutritive value. Although the mechanisms of such processes are essentially the same in different fats, the kinetics of deteriorative reactions may vary. The deep fried flavours are due to degradation products of linoleic acid and their intensity can be lowered if the food is fried in oil of low linoleic acid content. Nutritional advantages have been recognized for oils rich in oleic and other monounsaturated fatty acids with reduced linoleic acid contents and low contents of saturates (Nestel *et al.*, 1994).

Oleic acid (C18:1) is the most abundant mono-unsaturated fatty acid in many common edible oils. Compared with polyunsaturated fatty acids, oleic acid is more resistant toward oxidation, both at ambient storage and at high temperatures that prevail during the cooking and frying of food. Conventionally, soybean, rapeseed, sunflower or peanut oils, with high contents of polyenoic FA, are the main edible oils used for domestic cooking purposes. Pan-frying, however, is not suitable for deep fat frying due to the higher magnitude of thermoxidation at elevated temperatures. Some low-linoleic, high-oleic vegetable oils could be used for deep-frying, *e.g.* canola, olive, or almond oils, as they are quite stable at high frying temperatures. However, their high cost restricts their usage on a major scale.

Therefore, the use of more stable frying oils of comparatively low price would be desirable. To overcome the problem of poor stability of traditional soybean, sunflower and rapeseed oils, ways of reducing the unstable polyunsaturated fatty acid content have been studied by some scientists. One way to improve the stability of these oils is by blending with oils of high-oleic acid contents. Blending of vegetable oils and fats has emerged as an economical way of modifying the physicochemical characteristics of vegetable oils and fats besides enhancement in oxidative stability (Chu and Kung, 1997, Chu and Kung, 1998 and Premavalla *et al.*, 1998).

Proper mixing of high-oleic and high-linoleic oils may result in oil blends with improved stability characteristics. Studies of Padmavathy *et al.* (2001) have shown that the FA profile of the oils can be improved by blending; hence, the need to hydrogenate unsaturated oils is appreciably decreased, thereby eliminating the chances of formation of harmful trans- fatty acids. Some of the studies reviewed in this regard are given as under:

a) Improvements in the Frying Quality of Vegetable Oils by Blending with Palm Olein

Fats and oils are widely used for deep frying. In the normal deep fat frying, the content of linoleic and linolenic acid is kept low to improve the oxidative stability of the oils. Thus it is customary to partially hydrogenate vegetable oils to reduce their linolenic acid content to an acceptable level. An alternative means is to blend vegetable oils with palm olein which has a similar effect to partial hydrogenation in reducing the linoleic and linolenic acid content, but without introducing trans isomers of fatty acids. Plam oil and its products have excellent oxidative and frying stability owing to their inherent composition and to the presence of tocopherols, which are natural antioxidants. By blending vegetable oils with palm olein, the positive effects of palm olein are conferred on the blending during frying. Addition of 30 per cent palm olein to peanut oil and cottonseed oil has been found to improve their frying quality in terms of their primary and secondary oxidation and the formation of free fatty acids, other volatiles and polymers. The cloud points of most vegetable oils are raised slightly (into the range of -10°C to +50°C) by blending with palm olein (Kun, 1998).

Gupta et. al.(2001) studied the oxidative stability of edible grade crude palm oil (CPO) blends with sunflower oil or ground nut oil (GNO) as the deep-frying medium and reported that CPO:SFO had better oxidative stability than had CPO:GNO.

b) Enhancement of the Oxidative Stability of some Vegetable Oils by Blending with *Moringa oleifera* Oil

M. oleifera oil (MOO) is reported to have a high level of oleic acid and different tocopherol isomers (Anwar *et al.*, 2005). Tsaknis and Lalas (2002) reported that MOO has excellent oxidative stability during frying. So, great potential exists for blending of MOO with other high-linoleic oils.

Anwar *et al.* (2006) prepared blends (20 per cent, 40 per cent, 60 per cent, 80 per cent w/w) of Moringa oleifera oil (MOO) with sunflower oil (SFO) and soybean oil (SBO) to evaluate the changes in fatty acid (FA) composition, oxidative and thermal stability of SFO and SBO (Anwar *et al.*, 2007). The blending of MOO with SFO and SBO in proportions of 0–80 per cent resulted in the reduction of linoleic acid (C18:2) content of SFO and SBO from 67.0 per cent to 17.2 per cent and 56.2 per cent to 14.6 per cent and increase in the contents of oleic acid (C18:1) from 26.2 per cent to 68.3 per cent and 21.4 per cent to 65.9 per cent, factors of 0.72, 0.72 and 1.27, 1.33, respectively. A storage ability test (180 days; ambient conditions) showed an appreciable improvement in the oxidative stability of substrate oils with increase of MOO concentration, as depicted by the least oxidative alterations in PV, IV and highest increase in induction period, IP, of the MOO:SBO (80: 20 w/w) blend. Each 20 per cent addition of MOO resulted in decreases of PV and IV by factors of 0.84, 0.85 and 0.89, 0.88, respectively, and increases in IP by factors of 1.45 and 1.37 of SFO and SBO, respectively.

The heating performance test (180 °C for 42 h; 6 h heating cycle per day), as followed by the measurement of polymer contents and total polar contents (TPC), also revealed the MOO: SBO (80:20 w/w) blend to be the most stable. Every 20 per cent addition of MOO in SFO and SBO resulted in reduction of the polymer contents and TPC of SFO and SBO by factors of 0.91, 0.92 and 0.94, 0.94, respectively. On the basis of the present findings, it appears that proper blending of high linoleic oils with MOO can result in oil blends which could meet nutritional needs with improved stability for domestic cooking and deep-frying.

c) Sensory Odour Profiling and Physical Characteristics of Edible Oil Blends during Frying

Oils and fats, apart from providing nutrition, are known to play functional roles during product preparation contributing to the palatability of processed foods. Generally, consumers tend to prefer oil which is produced or is available in the region. Owing to continued culinary use of one particular oil, the consumers develop a liking for its odour and flavour. In India, commonly used edible oils are groundnut oil (GNO), mustard oil (MO) and sunflower oil (SNO). These oils have characteristic odour notes such as nutty odour of GNO, pungent and sulphury odour of MO and seedy odour of SNO. Sensory evaluation of oils is considered a critical test of quality. Sensory odour evaluation of edible oils is governed by three factors, namely, medium in which the oil is dispersed, temperature of oil during testing and panel training for unambiguous understanding of descriptors (Rajalakshmi and Narasimhan, 1996).

In order to have nutritional enrichment and improve frying stability, blending of oils is done. Odour attributes of oil blends that are used as frying media are also important. Edible oil blends containing 80 parts of mustard oil (MO) or groundnut oil (GNO) or sunflower oil (SNO) and 20 parts of sesame oil (SO) or refined red palm oil (RPO) or rice bran oil (RBO) were studied to determine the changes in their physical and sensory characteristics during deep fat frying (Ravi et.al., 2005). This study revealed that odour profiles of common edible oils are modified on blending with other oils in the ratio of 80:20. The present changes in odour profile become more evident on frying; the oils showed subdued notes compared to their inherent

Table 21.7: Some Edible Oils and their Dominant Odours

Oil	*Dominant Odours*
Base oils	
Mustard oil	Sulphury, pungent, sour
Groundnut oil (refined)	Nutty, sweet, fresh, oil-like
Sunflower oil (refined)	Seedy, sweet, fresh, oil-like
Blending oils	
Sesame oil	Nutty, earthy, oil-like
Rice bran oil	Branny, oil-like, husk-like
Refined palm oil	Husk-like, oil-like, beany

characteristic notes. Deep fat frying caused an increase in apparent viscosity for all oil blends.

Intensity of sulphury, pungent and vinegar (sour) notes of MO, nutty and sweet notes of GNO, sweet and seedy notes of SNO, seedy and earthy notes of SO, husk-like note of RPO and beany and branny notes of RBO decreased significantly by end of the 7th frying. Apparent viscosity of the oil blends increased on successive frying. Colour measured in CIE system indicated that the dominant parameters were a+ (redness) in RPO blends, b+ (yellowness) in blend containing SO or MO and a^- (greenness) in RBO blends. The redness component decreased and yellowness increased with successive frying in SNO + RPO blend and GNO and RBO blend, respectively. Applying principal component analysis (PCA) to the data showed seggregation of various oil blends as distinct groups exhibiting their typical and characteristic attributes. PCA also revealed the pathway of change of oils during different frying cycles. MO and blend of MO + RPO were characterised by sulphury, pungent, harsh odour notes and red colour; GNO occupied a quadrant with fresh-oil-like, green and sweet notes, and SNO was characterised by fresh-oil-like, seedy odour and yellow colour. Addition of SO increased earthy note and lightness value, while blends containing RBO had distinct yellow colour, increased heated note and higher apparent viscosity (Ravi *et al.*, 2005). The study has shown that odour profiles of blended oils were distinguishable even after seven fryings.

d) Oil Stability Index and Peroxide Value of Oil Blends

Chu and Kung (1998) used the oil stability index (OSI) and peroxide value (PV) to determine the quality of oil blends. The quality of soybean oil (SBO) blended with other refined, bleached and deodorized (RBD) oils was between the quality of SBO and the RBD oils selected for blending. However, crude peanut oil blended with SBO diminished the quality of SBO while crude sesame oil with unique antioxidants improved the quality of SBO blends. To study the effect of fatty acid composition (FAC) on the oxidative stability of oil blends, 21 oil blends were prepared by using 7 commercial RBD oils which were re-deodorized and followed by tocopherol adjustment. A mathematical model describing the relationship between OSI and FAC of 21 oil blends was obtained as follows: OSI (h) = 7.5123 + per cent C16:0 × (0.2733) + per cent C18:0 × (0.0797) + per cent C18:1 × (0.0159) + per cent C18:2 × (–0.1141) + per cent C18:3 × (–0.3962), $r^2 = 0.911$. The difference between the values of each predicted and measured OSI were within 10 per cent, which indicated that the oxidative stability of oil blends of any ratio from the 7 RBD oils under study could be predicted by using this model.

The physicochemical characteristics and minor component contents of blended oils packed in pouches in relation to starting oils used for blending were studied over a period of 6 mon at two storage temperatures and humidity conditions: 27°C/65 per cent RH and 40°C/30–40 per cent RH. Color, PV, FFA value, β-carotene content, tocopherol content, and oryzanol content of the oils were monitored at regular intervals (Shiela *et al.*, 2004). The color, PV (0.6–20.7 meq O2/kg, FFA value (0.08–2.1 per cent), tocopherol content (360–1700 ppm per cent), oryzanol content (460–2,000 mg per cent), and sesame oil antioxidants (400–2,000 mg per cent) were not changed in either the starting oils or their blends. Oils and oil blends containing a higher initial PV (18.9–20.7 meq O_2/kg) showed a slight reduction in value at 40°C, whereas oils having lesser PV of 5–10 showed a slight increase during the storage period. Among the minor components studied, only β-carotene showed a reduction, 8.9–60.2 per cent at 27°C and 48–71 per cent at 40°C, for the different oil blends studied. The observed results indicated that the packed oil blends studied were stable under the conditions of the study, and the minor components, other than β-carotene, remained unaltered in the package even at the end of 6 mon of storage.

Blends of sunflower oil (SFO) and rice bran oil (RBO) were also evaluated by Samia and Karl (2007) for their stability. Additionally, known amounts of natural antioxidants extracted from RBO were added to SFO, and their protective effect was compared to that of the blends. The results found indicate that by raising the amount of RBO, from 10 to 50 per cent, an increase of OLO, OLP, PPL, OOO, PPO, OPO, 18:1 and 16:0 occurred, followed by a decrease of LLL, LLO, and 18:2. These changes in fatty acid and triacylglycerol (TAG) composition led to an increase of the oil stability index at 120 °C and a reduction of polymer TAG formation in the heated blends at 180 °C during 8 h. A comparable protective effect of natural antioxidants to that of blending was observed in a 50: 50 blend, by remarkably increasing the induction period.

e) Fatty Acid Composition, Oxidative Stability, and Radical Scavenging Activity of Vegetable Oil Blends with Coconut Oil

Coconut (*Cocos nucifera*) contains 55–65 per cent oil, having C12:0 as the major fatty acid. Coconut oil has >90 per cent saturates and is deficient in monounsaturates (6 per cent), polyunsaturates (1 per cent), and total tocopherols (29 mg/kg). However, coconut oil contains medium chain fatty acids (58 per cent), which are easily absorbed into the body. Therefore, blends of coconut oil (20–80 per cent incorporation of coconut oil) with other vegetable oils (*i.e.* palm, rice bran, sesame, mustard, sunflower, groundnut, safflower, and soybean) were prepared (Bhatnagar *et al.*, 2009). Coconut oil + sunflower oil and coconut oil + rice bran oil blends exhibited 36.7–89.7 per cent ($p < 0.0005$) and 66.4–80.5 per cent ($p < 0.0313$) reductions in peroxide formation in comparison to the individual sunflower oil and rice bran oil, respectively. It was concluded that blending coconut oil with other vegetable oils provides medium chain fatty acids and oxidative stability to the blends, while coconut oil will be enriched with polyunsaturates, monounsaturates, natural antioxidants, and a greater radical scavenging activity.

Edible Oil Sector Seeks Nod to Blend More Than Two Oils

At present sale of blends of only two edible oils is allowed that also with a condition that ratio of any oil in the blend should not be below 20 per cent. According to Mr A.R. Sharma, President of Solvent Extractors' Association of India Ltd (Sea), it is impossible to prepare nutritionally desirable blend with just two oils. One needs to use three or more oils to exactly match the desirable fat composition as well as ratio of Omega-6/Omega-3. The ratio of any particular oil in such a blend could be as low as 5 per cent. The edible oil trade and industry should be allowed to sell blends of multiple oils without any condition as to minimum percentage of any particular oil, industry sources said (The Financial Express, Nov. 27, 2009). The proposed amendments in the current rules regarding sale of blended oils would offer both nutritional and economical blends of edible oils to the consumers.

The fat composition of the blend should be required to be mentioned on the label, which in any case is becoming compulsory with effect from August 20, 2007 as per the new labelling regulations. The condition of compulsory Agmark registration for blended oils should also be done away with effect from August 20, 2007 when new labelling regulations came into force. Health authorities will be in a position to monitor the blends in terms of new labelling regulations. Therefore for ease of operations, multiple regulations have to be avoided, sources said.

Problems in Blending and Way Forward

1. Blending with inexpensive imported vegetable oils: RBD (Refined, deodorised and bleached) palmolein rules at Rs. 32,600 a tonne in the domestic edible oil market. In contrast, refined sunflower oil costs Rs 44,500, refined soybean oil Rs 43,000 and refined groundnut oil Rs 55,000 a tonne (Mr. M.R. Subramani, Business Line, The Hindu, Feb. 25, 2009).

   In these circumstances, a consumer will naturally tend to go for an edible oil that costs less. What if an edible oil producer offers groundnut oil at, say, Rs 40,000 a tonne? Surely, it is costlier than RBD palmolein, but given consumers' reservation over the palm group of oils, one would naturally tend to go for groundnut oil that is being offered at Rs 40,000 a tonne. But are you sure that the groundnut oil being sold at a price lower than the one prevailing in the market is a pure one?

   If one were to go by the latest letter of the Solvent Extractors' Association of India to its members, some manufacturers' are resorting to "unethical blending" of edible oils.

   "The price of most of the edible oils is ruling very low. RBD palmolein has become the cheapest oil in the market, pulling down the prices of other oils. The wide price difference between domestically produced oils and RBD palmolein is creating a serious problem, as unofficially it is blended into other oils on a large-scale and sold as domestic oil," said the association President, Mr Ashok Sethia, in the letter."This unethical blending pushes the honest manufacturers to the brink and we should strongly oppose this malpractice as it does not benefit anyone," he said.

   When contacted the association Executive Director, Mr B.V. Mehta, told Business Line that edible oil producers are allowed to blend different oils but they would have to declare how much percentage of blending of other oil has taken place in a particular brand of oil. For example, if a producer sells edible oil as vegetable oil, he has to mandatorily declare in the pack what oils are blended to make up the consumer pack. Usually, RBD palmolein is blended with sunflower, mustard or soybean oil. Industry insiders say the problem with some producers is that they mix oils, for example, say, groundnut oil with RBD palmolein, and then sell it as groundnut oil. "We are concerned over this unethical blending since besides manufacturers, even farmers are affected by this trend," Mr Mehta said. What this "unethical blending" does is that it forces manufacturers, who do not indulge in such practices, to lower their price and face losses.

According to Mr Sethia, the practice could end if the centre brings all edible oils under the duty regime, which could narrow the difference in price of domestic and imported vegetable oils.

Currently, the centre imposes a customs duty of 20 per cent on degummed or crude soybean oil. This duty was imposed in November, 2008 after early last year the Union Government had made it zero to tackle surging inflation and soaring edible oil prices. Until the third quarter of 2008, edible oil prices ruled higher in the global market on supply shortage and raging crude prices, which have now declined by over two-thirds to around $40 a barrel. Interestingly, refined soybean oil attracts only 7.5 per cent duty as also other refined ones such as RBD palmolein, sunflower oil and rapeseed oil.

Other crude vegetable oils such as sunflower and palm oil are still imported at zero duty. Crude palm stearin and crude palm kernel oil, which are imported for industrial purpose, attract 19.57 per cent and 17.37 per cent duty, respectively, while palm fatty acid distillate, palm kernel fatty acid distillate and split palm kernel fatty acid can be imported at 32.76 per cent duty. According to industry sources, the Centre has been urged to raise the duty on imports of vegetable oils, but so far nothing has been heard in this regard.

2. PFA (4th Amendment Rules) 1992 specifies that blending of any two vegetable oils (wherein the component oil used in the admixture is not less than 20 per cent) is permitted. However, very few suitably blended oils are currently being marketed. Available blended oils (80:20 blend of any two oils) cannot provide the optimal ratio of fatty acids.

   The members of Solvent Extractors' Association of India hold the view that scientists can work out an appropriate and affordable combination of oils taking into account regional preferences. It might be possible to add more than two oils in the blend, in proportions other than 20:80 and achieve better fatty acid composition. By choosing appropriate oils, it may also be possible to lower the cost, maintain desirable cooking quality, improve their marketability for direct consumption and even add additional nutrients or phyto-chemicals to have better health implications.

   However, to pave way for such blending of oils, modification of existing PFA Acts would be required. It would be essential to assess the potential problems of contamination and adulteration of blended cooking oil, its possible adverse health consequences, and the feasibility of detection and elimination adulteration in blended oils. Members stated there is also a need for enhancing consumer awareness regarding consumption of fats and oils in right quantities and in proper combinations to minimize the risk of cardiovascular and other diet-related diseases.

References

Abate N, Vega GL, Grundy SM. Variability in cholesterol content and physical properties of lipoproteins containing apolipoprotein B-100. Atherosclerosis. 1993; 104:159-171.

Abe Y, El-Masri B, Kimball KT, *et al.* Soluble cell adhesion molecules in hypertriglyceridemia and potential significance on monocyte adhesion. Arterioscler Thromb Vasc Biol. 1998; 18: 723–731.

Agren JJ, Vaisanen S, Hanninen O, *et al.* Hemostatic factors and platelet aggregation after a fish-enriched diet or fish oil or docosahexaenoic acid supplementation. *Prostaglandins Leukot Essent Fatty Acids.* 1997; 57: 419–421.

Aguilera CM, Ramirez-Tortosa MC, Mesa MD, Gil A. 2001. Protective effect of monounsaturated and polyunsaturated fatty acids on the development of cardiovascular disease. Nutr. Hosp. 16(3):78-91.

Ahlqwist M, Bengtsson C, Lapidus L, *et al.* Serum mercury concentration in relation to survival, symptoms, and diseases: results from the prospective population study of women in Gothenburg, Sweden. *Acta Odontol Scand.* 1999; 57: 168–174.

Alarcon *de la Lastra*, C., Barranco, M.D., Motilva, V. and Herrerias, J. M. 2001. Mediterranean diet and health: biological importance of olive oil. *Current Pharmaceutical Design*, 7 (10), 933-50.

Albert CM, Campos H, Stampfer MJ, *et al.* Blood levels of long-chain n-3 fatty acids and the risk of sudden death. *N Engl J Med.* 2002; 346: 1113–1118.

Albert, C.M.; Willet, W.C.; Manson, J.E.; Hennekens, C.H. 1998. Nut Consumption and the Risk of Sudden and Total Cardiac Death in the Physicians' Health Study. Abstract, American Heart Association. November 9-11, 1998.

Allam, S.H. 2001. Utilization of some untraditional sources of high oleic acid oils for improving vegetable oils stability. Rivista Italiana Delle Sostanze Grasse 78 (6):337–341.

American Diabetes Association. Standards of medical care in diabetes. 2006, *Diabetes Care.* 2006; 29(suppl.1):S4-S42.

Anderson JW, Johnstone BM, Cook-Newell ME. 1995.Meta-analysis of the effects of soy protein intake on serum lipids. *N Engl J Med*, 333: 276-282.

Anderson JW, Story, L *et al.* 1984. Hypocholesterolemic effects of oat-bran or bean intake for hypercholesterolemic men. *Am. J. Clin. Nutr.*, 40: 1146-1155.

Anwar, F., Ashraf, M. and Bhanger, M.I. 2005. Interprovenance variation in the composition of *Moringa oleifera* oilseeds from Pakistan. J. American Oil Chemists Soc. 82: 45–51.

Anwar, F., Hussain, A.I., Iqbal, S. and Bhanger, M.I. 2007. Enhancement of the oxidative stability of some vegetable oils by blending with *Moringa oleifera* oil. *Food Chem.* 103(4): 1181-1191.

AOAC. 1984. In S. William (Ed.), Official methods of analysis of the Association of Analytical Chemist Inc. (4th ed., pp. 516–518). Virginia, USA.

AOCS, Official methods and recommended practices of the American Oil Chemist Society (5th ed.), AOCS Press, Champaign, USA.

Appel LJ, Miller ER3rd, Seidler AJ, *et al.* Does supplementation of diet with 'fish oil' reduce blood pressure? A meta-analysis of controlled clinical trials. *Arch Intern Med.* 1993; 153: 1429–1438.

Aradhey, A. 2009. Annual Report on oilseeds (India). USDA Foreign Agricultural Service. Gain Report No.1N9051. Global Agricultural Information Network.

Archer SL, Green D, Chamberlain M, *et al.* Association of dietary fish and n-3 fatty acid intake with hemostatic factors in the coronary artery risk development in young adults (CARDIA) study. *Arterioscler Thromb Vasc Biol.* 1998; 18: 1119–1123.

Aro, A, Jauhiainen, M, *et al.* Stearic acid, trans fatty acids, and dairy fat: effects on serum and lipoprotein lipids, apolipoproteins, lipoprotein(a), and lipid transfer proteins in healthy subjects. Am J Clin Nutr. 1997; 65: 1419-26

Arya, S.S., Vidya sagar, K., Premavalli, K.S. and Parihar, D.B. 1980. Chemical changes in refined groundnut oil during storage and frying operations. In Fats and oils in Relation to Food Products and Their Preparation. Trop. Oil Seeds Abstr. 5: 71-75.

Ascherio A, Rimm EB, Giovannucci EL, *et al.* Dietary fat and risk of coronary heart disease in men: cohort follow up study in the United States. *BMJ.* 1996; 313: 84–90.

Ascherio A, Rimm EB, Stampfer MJ, *et al.* Dietary intake of marine n-3 fatty acids, fish intake, and the risk of coronary disease among men. *N Engl J Med.* 1995; 332: 977–982.

ASCN/AIN Task Force on Trans Fatty Acids. Position paper on trans fatty acids. Am J Clin Nutr. 1996; 63: 663-70

Austin MA, Edwards KL. Small, dense low-density lipop5oteins, the insulin resistance syndrome and noninsulin-dependent diabetes. *Curr Opin Lipidol.* 1996; 7: 167-171.

Baigent C, Keech A, Kearney PM, *et al.* Cholesterol Treatment Trialists' (CTT) Collaborators. Efficacy and safety of cholesterol-lowering treatment prospective meta-analysis of data from 90,056 participants in 14-randomized trials of statins. *Lancet.* 2005; 366: 1267-1278.

Balasekaran R, Porter JL, Santa Ana CA, *et al.* Positive results on tests for steatorrhea in persons consuming Olestra potato chips. *Ann Intern Med.* 2000; 132: 279–282.

Bao W, Srinivasan SR, Wattigney WA, Berensoin GS. Usefulness of childhood low-density lipoprotein cholesterol level in predicting adult dyslipidemia and other cardiovascular risks. The Bogalusa Heart Study. *Arch Intern Med.* 1996; 156: 1315-1320.

Bao W, Srinivasan SR, Wattigney WA, Berenson GS. Persistence of multiple cardiovascular risk clustering related to syndrome X from childhood to young adulthood. The Bogalusa Heart Study. *Arch Intern Med.* 1994; 154: 1842-1847.

Barcelli U, Glas-Greenwalt P, Pollak VE. Enhancing effect of dietary supplementation with omega-3 fatty acids on plasma fibrinolysis in normal subjects. *Thromb Res.* 1985; 39: 307–312.

Barrett-Connor E, Bush TL. Estrogen and coronary heart disease in women. *JAMA.* 1991; 265: 1861-1867.

Bass KM, Newschaffer CJ, Klag MJ, Bush TL. Plasma lipoprotein levels as predictors of cardiovascular death in women. *Arch Intern Med.* 1993; 153: 2209-2216.

Bayon Y, Croset M, Daveloose D, *et al.* Effect of specific phospholipid molecular species incorporated in human platelet membranes on thromboxane $_{A2}$/ prostaglandin $_{H2}$ receptors. *J Lipid Res.* 1995; 36: 47–56.

Beauchamp GK, Keast RS, Morel D, Lin J, Pika J, Han Q, Lee CH, Smith AB, Breslin PA. 2005. Phytochemistry: ibuprofen-like activity in extra-virgin olive oil. Nature. 437(7055):45-6.

Bemelmans WJ, Broer J, Feskens EJ, *et al.* Effect of an increased intake of alpha-linolenic acid and group nutritional education on cardiovascular risk factors: the Mediterranean Alpha-linolenic Enriched Groningen Dietary Intervention (MARGARIN) study. *Am J Clin Nutr.* 2002; 75: 221–227.

BerquinBerquin IM, Min Y, Wu R, Wu J, Perry D, Cline JM, Thomas MJ, Thornburg T, Kulik G, Smith A, Edwards IJ, D'Agostino R, Zhang H, Wu H, Kang JX, Chen YQ.2007. Modulation of prostate cancer genetic risk by omega-3 and omega-6 fatty acids. J. Clin. Invest. 117 (7): 1866-75.

Bhatnagar, S., Prasanth Kumar, P. K., Hemavathy, J. and Gopala Krishna, A. G. 2009. Fatty acid composition, oxidative stability, and radical scavenging activity of vegetable oil blends with coconut oil. J. American Oil Chemists' Soc. 86(10): 991-999.

Billman GE, Kang JX, Leaf A. Prevention of ischemia-induced cardiac sudden death by n-3 polyunsaturated fatty acids in dogs. *Lipids*. 1997; 32: 1161–1168.

Bingwin, L, *et al.* 1981. Effect of bean meal on serum cholesterol and TGs. *Chinese Med. J.*, 94: 455-458.

Black KL, Culp B, Madison D, *et al.* The protective effects of dietary fish oil on focal cerebral infarction. *Prostaglandins Med.* 1979; 3: 257–268.

Boden WE. High-density lipoprotein cholesterol as an independent risk factor in cardiovascular disease: assessing the data from Framingham to the Veterans Affairs High-Density Lipoprotein Intervention Trial. Am J. Cardiol. 2000;86:19L-22L.

Bonanome A, Biasia F, De Luca M, *et al.* n-3 fatty acids do not enhance LDL susceptibility to oxidation in hypertriacylglycerolemic hemodialyzed subjects. *Am J Clin Nutr.* 1996; 63: 261–266.

Bondia-Pons I, Schroder H, Covas MI, Castellote AI, Kaikkonen J, Poulsen HE, Gaddi AV, Machowetz A, Kiesewetter H, Lopez-Sabater MC. 2007. Moderate consumption of olive oil by healthy European men reduces systolic blood pressure in non-Mediterranean participants. J Nutr. 137(1):84-87.

Bonna KH, Njolstad I, Ueland PM, Schirmer H, Tverdal A, Steigen T, Wang H, Nordrehaug, JE, Arnesen, E and Rasmussen, KRl. 2006. Homocystseine lowering and cardiovascular events after acute myocardial infarction. *N Engl J Med* 2006, 354.

Boren J.,Gustafasson M,Skalen K,Food C, Innerarity TL. Role of extracellular retention of low density lipoproteins in atherosclerosis. *Curr Opin Lipidol.* 2000;11:451-456.

Boskou D, Elmadfa I: Frying of Food. Oxidation, Nutrient and Non-Nutrient Antioxidants, Biologically Active Compounds and High Temperatures. Boca Raton, CRC 2OO9; in press.

Brude IR, Drevon CA, Hjermann I, *et al.* Peroxidation of LDL from combined-hyperlipidemic male smokers supplied with omega-3 fatty acids and antioxidants. *Arterio Thromb Vasc Biol.* 1997; 17: 2576–2588.

Bucher HC, Hengstler P, Schindler C, *et al.* N-3 polyunsaturated fatty acids in coronary heart disease: a meta-analysis of randomized controlled trials. *Am J Med.* 2002; 112: 298–304.

Burdge GC, Calder PC: Alpha-linolenic acid me- tabolism in adult humans: the effects of gen- der and age on conversion to longer-chain polyunsaturated fatty acids. Eur J Lipid Sci Technol 2005a. 107:426–439.

Burdge GC, Calder PC: Conversion of alpha-linolenic acid to longer-chain polyunsaturated fatty acids in human adults. Reprod Nutr Dev 2005b; 45: 581–597.

Burke AP, Farb A, Malcom GT, Liang Y, Smialek J, Virmani R. Effect of risk factors on the mechanism of acute thrombosis and sudden coronary death in women. *Circulation*. 1998;97:2110-2116.

Burr ML, Fehily AM, Gilbert JF, *et al.* Effects of changes in fat, fish, and fibre intakes on death and myocardial reinfarction: diet and reinfarction trial (DART). *Lancet*. 1989; 2: 757–761.

Burr ML, Sweetham PM, Fehily AM. Diet and reinfarction. *Eur Heart J*. 1994; 15: 1152–1153.

Cairns JA, Gill J, Morton B, *et al.* Fish oils and low-molecular-weight heparin for the reduction of restenosis after percutaneous transluminal coronary angioplasty. The EMPAR Study. *Circulation*. 1996; 94: 1553–1560. 51.

Calorie Control Council. Fat replacers: food ingredients for healthy eating. Available at: http://www.caloriecontrol.org/fatreprint.html.

Canner PL, Furberg CD, Terrin ML, McGovern ME. Benefits of niacin by glycemic status in patients with healed myocardial infarction (from the Coronary Drug Project). *Am J Cardiol*. 2005; 95: 254-257.

Cannon CP, Braunwald E, McCabe CH, *et al.* Pravastatin or Atorvastatin Evaluation and Infection Therapy-Thrombolysis in Myocasrdial Infaarction 22 Investigators. Intensive versus moderate lipid lowering with statin after acute coronary syndromes. *N Engl J Med*. 2004; 350: 1495-1504.

Caponio F, Bilancia MT, Pasqualone A, Sikorska E, Gomes T. 2005. Influence of the exposure to light on extra virgin olive oil quality during storage. European Food Research and Technol. 221(1-2):92-98.

Carpenter, D., Lehmann, J., Mason, B.S. and Solver, H.T. 1974. Lipid composition of selected vegetable oils. J. Am. Oil Chem.Soc. 51: 287A.

Castro, P. and others. 2000. Consumption of and oleic acid enriched-diet vs NCEP-I diet on LDL susceptibility of oxidative modifications. Eur. J. Clin. Nutr. 54:61-67.

Center for Food Safety and Applied Nutrition, US Food and Drug Administration. Consumer advisory: an important message for pregnant women and women of childbearing age who may become pregnant about the risks of mercury in fish. March 2001. Available at: http://www.cfsan.fda.gov/~dms/admehg.html.

Chand Ramesh. 2007. Trade competitiveness in oilseeds. In: Hegde, D.M. 2007. Changing global vegetable oil scenario: Issues and challenges before India. Indian Society of Oilseeds Research, Hyderabad. P (465-470).

Chang NW, Huang PC. Effects of dietary monounsaturated fatty acids on plasma lipids in humans. J Lipid Res 1990; 31.

Charlton K.M., Corner A.H., Davey K., Kramer, J.K., Mahadevan, S. and Sauer, F.D. (1975). Cardiac lesions in rats fed rapeseed oils. Can. J. Comp. Med. 39 (3): 261-69.

Che Man, Y.B., Liu, J.L., Jamilah, B. and Rahman, R.A. 1999. Quality changes of refined-bleached-decolorized (RBD) palm olein, soybean oil and their blends during deep-fat frying. J. Food Lipids. 6: 181–193.

Cheng GS. Cardiac events increased in first two years of HRT. *Intern Med News.* 2000; 33: 1-2.

Chin JP, Dart AM. How do fish oils affect vascular function? *Clin Exp Pharmacol Physiol.* 1995; 22: 71–81.

Chow, C. K. 2000. Fatty acids in foods and their health implications. 2nd Edition. CRC Press

Christensen JH, Gustenhoff P, Korup E, *et al.* Effect of fish oil on heart rate variability in survivors of myocardial infarction: a double blind randomised controlled trial. *BMJ.* 1996; 312: 677–678.

Christensen JH, Korup E, Aaroe J, *et al.* Fish consumption, n-3 fatty acids in cell membranes, and heart rate variability in survivors of myocardial infarction with left ventricular dysfunction. *Am J Cardiol.* 1997; 79: 1670–1673.

Chu, Y.H. and Kung, Y.H. 1997. A study on oxidative stability of vegetable oil blends. Shipin Kexue 24 (4):389–397.

Chu,Y.H. and Kung,Y.L. 1998. A study on vegetable oil blends. Food Chem. 62 (1): 191–195.

Colhoun HM, Betteridge DJ, Durrington FN, *et al.* CARDS investigators. Primary prevention of cardiovascular disease with atorvastatin in type 2 diabetes in the Collaborative Atorvastatin Diabetes Study (CARDS): multicentre randomized placebo-controlled trial. *Lancet.* 2004; 364: 685-696.

Colhoun HM, Betteridge DJ, Durrington FN, *et al.* CARDS investigators. Primary prevention of cardiovascular disease with atorvastatin in type 2 diabetes in the Collaborative Atorvastatin Diabetes Study (CARDS): multicentre randomized placebo-controlled trial. *Lancet.* 2004; 364: 685-696.

Collins R, Armitage J, Parish S, Sleigh P, Peto R. Heart Protection Study Collaborative Group. MRC/BHF Heart Protection Study of cholesterol-lowering with simvastatin in 5963 people with diabetes: a randomized placebo-controlled trial. *Lancet.* 2003; 361: 2005-2016.

Collins R, Armitage J, Parish S, Sleigh P, Peto R. Heart Protection Study Collaborative Group. MRC/BHF Heart Protection Study of cholesterol-lowering with simvastatin in 5963 people with diabetes: a randomized placebo-controlled trial. *Lancet.* 2003; 361: 2005-2016.

Connor WE. Importance of n-3 fatty acids in health and disease. *Am J Clin Nutr.* 2000; 71 (1 Suppl): 171S–175S.

Cooper DA, Webb DR, Peters JC. Evaluation of the potential for Olestra to affect the availability of dietary phytochemicals. *J Nutr.* 1997; 127: 1699S–1709S.

Covas MI. 2007. Olive oil and the cardiovascular system. Pharmacol Res. 55(3):175-86.

Cowie CC, Howard BV, Harris MI. Serum lipoproteins in African Americans and whites with non-insulin-dependent diabetes in the US population. *Circulation.* 1994; 90: 1185-1193.

Crick, D.C., Nwokolo, E.N. and Sim, J.S. 1988. Effect of blending dietary oils on growth performance, total and individual fatty acid absorption by the growth chick. Nutr. Res. 8(6): 643-651.

Crouse JR, Morgan T, Terry JG, Ellis J, Vitolins M, Burke GL. 1999. A randomized trial comparing the effects of casein with that of soy protein containing varying amounts of isoflavones on plasma concentrations of lipids and lipoproteins. *Arch Intern Med*; 159: 2070-2076.

CSE Report 2009. Fat of the matter An analytical study on the fatty acid profile of the oils we eat and its health and policy implications. Pollution Monitoring Laboratory, Centre for Science and Environment www.cseindia.org for full laboratory study. 2141–2147.

Cui Y, Blumenthal RS, Flaws JA, *et al.* Non-high-density lipoprotein cholesterol level as a predictor of cardiovascular disease mortality. Arch Intern Med. 2001:161:1413-1419.

Dandona P, Aljada A, Chaudhuri A, Mohanty P, Garg R. Metabolic syndrome: a comprehensive perspective based on interactions between obesity, diabetes, and inflammation. *Circulation.* 2005; 111: 1448-1454.

Dansinger ML, Gleason, JA, Griffith JL, Selker HP, Schaefer EJ. 2005. Comparison of the Atkins, Ornish, Weight Watchers, and Zone diets for weight loss and heart disease reduction, a randomized clinical trial. *JAMA*, 293: 43-53.

David S. Francis, Giovanni M. Turchini, Paul L. Jonesand Sena S. De Silva. 2007. Effects of fish oil substitution with a mix blend vegetable oil on nutrient digestibility in Murray cod, *Maccullochella peelii peelii.* Aquaculture. 269 (1-4): 447-455.

Daviglus ML, Stamler J, Orencia AJ, *et al.* Fish consumption and the 30-year risk of fatal myocardial infarction. *N Engl J Med.* 1997; 336: 1046–1053.

De Caterina R, Libby P. Control of endothelial leukocyte adhesion molecules by fatty acids. *Lipids.* 1996; 31: S57–S63. 92.

De Caterina R, Liao JK, Libby P. Fatty acid modulation of endothelial activation. *Am J Clin Nutr.* 2000; 71 (1 Suppl): 213S–223S.

de Lorgeril M, Renaud S, Mamelle N, *et al.* Mediterranean alpha-linolenic acid-rich diet in secondary prevention of coronary heart disease. *Lancet.* 1994; 343: 1454–1459.

de Lorgeril M, Salen P, Martin JL, *et al.* Mediterranean diet, traditional risk factors, and the rate of cardiovascular complications after myocardial infarction: final report of the Lyon Diet Heart Study. *Circulation.* 1999; 99: 779–785.

Delmas PD, Bjarnason NH, Mitlak BH, *et al.* Effects of raloxifene on bone mineral density, serum cholesterol concentrations, and uterine endometrium in postmenopausal women. *N Engl J Med.* 1997; 337: 1641-1647.

Denke MA, Sempos CT, Grundy SM. Excess body weight. An under-recognized contributor to dyslipidemia in white American women. *Arch Intern Med.* 1994; 154: 401-410.

Denke MA, Sempos CTm, Grundy SM. Excess body weight. An underrecognized contributor to high blood cholesterol levels in white American men. *Arch Intern Med.* 1993; 153: 1093-1103.

Denke MA. 1995. Cholesterol-lowering diets. A review of the evidence. *Arch Intern Med.*; 155: 17-26.

Denke MA. 1995. Review of human studies evaluating individual dietary responsiveness in patients with hypercholesterolemia. *Am J Clin Nutr.*; 62: 4718-4778.

Department of Health and Human Services: Dietary Guidelines for Americans. 2005. www. healthierus.gov/dietaryguidelines (accessed July 2008).

Department of Health and Human Services, US Food and Drug Administration. Substances affirmed as generally recognized as safe: menhaden oil. *Federal Register*. June 5, 1997. Vol. 62, No. 108: pp 30751–30757.

Despres JP, Lamarche B, Mauriege P, *et al.* Hyperinsulinemia as an independent risk factor for ischemic heart disease. *N Engl J Med.* 1996; 334: 952-957.

Despres P, Moorjani S, Lupien PJ, Tremblay A, Nadeau A, Bouchard C. Regional distribution of body fat, plasma lipoproteins, and cardiovascular disease. *Arteriosclerosis.* 1990; 10: 497-511.

Detrano RC, Wong ND, Doherty TM, *et al.* Coronary calcium does not accurately predict near-term future coronary events in high risk adults. *Circulation.* 1999; 99:2633-2638.

Dietary supplementation with n-3 polyunsaturated fatty acids and vitamin E after myocardial infarction: results of the GISSI-Prevenzione trial. Gruppo Italiano per lo Studio della Sopravvivenza nell'Infarto miocardico. *Lancet.* 1999; 354: 447–455.

Djousse L, Pankow JS, Eckfeldt JH, *et al.* Relation between dietary linolenic acid and coronary artery disease in the National Heart, Lung, and Blood Institute Family Heart Study. *Am J Clin Nutr.* 2001; 74: 612–619.

Dobarganes, M.C. and Perea-Camini, M.C. 1991. Systematic evaluation of heated fats based on quantitative analytical methods. J. Am. Oil Chemists Soc. 65 (1):101–105.

Dolecek TA, Granditis G. Dietary polyunsaturated fatty acids and mortality in the Multiple Risk Factor Intervention Trial (MRFIT). *World Rev Nutr Diet.* 1991; 66: 205–216. 7.

Downey, R.K. 1964. Genetic Control of Fatty Acid Biosynthesis in Rapeseed. J. Am. Oil Chemist' Soc. 41: 475-478.

Dreon DM, Fernstrom HA, Williams PT, Krauss RM. Reduced LDL particle size in children consuming a very-low-fat diet is related to parental LDL-subclass patterns. *Am J Clin Nutr.* 2000; 71: 1611-1616.

Duke, J.A. 1981. Handbook of legumes of world importance. Plenum Press, USA.

Dupont, J., White, P.J., Carpenter, M.P., Schaefer, E.J., Meydani, S.N., Elson, C.E. Woods, M. and Gorbach S.L. 1990. Food uses and health effects of corn oil. *J Am College Nutr* 9 (5): 438-470.

Durrington P. Dyslipidemia. *Lancet.* 2003; 362: 717-731.

Eckel RH, Grundy SM, Zimmet PZ. The metabolic syndrome. *Lancet.* 2005; 365: 1415-1428.

Eitenmiller, RR. Vitamin E Content of Fats and Oils – Nutritional Implications. Food Technology. 1997; 51(5): 78-81

Elam MB, Hunninghake DB, Davis KB,s *et al.* Effect of niacin on lipid and lipoprotein levels and glycemic control in patients with diabetes and peripheral arterial disease: the ADMIT study. A randomized trial. Arterial Disease Multiple Intervention Trial. *JAMA.* 2000; 284: 1263-1270.

Elmadfa I, Schwalbe P: Some aspects of alpha- tocopherol bioavailability. Fat Sci Technol. 1989; 91: 402-407.

Emken EA, Adlof RO, Gulley RM. Dietary linoleic acid influences desaturation and acylation of deuterium-labeled linoleic and linolenic acids in young adult males. *Biochim Biophys Acta.* 1994; 1213: 277–288.

Endres S, von Schacky C. n-3 polyunsaturated fatty acids and human cytokine synthesis. *Curr Opin Lipidol.* 1996; 7: 48–52.

Erickson, D.K. 1996. Production and composition of frying fats. In: *E.G.* Perkins and M.D. Erickson, Editors, Deep frying, AOCS Press, Champaign, IL, USA. pp. 9–28.

Eritsland J, Arnesen H, Gronseth K, *et al.* Effect of dietary supplementation with n-3 fatty acids on coronary artery bypass graft patency. *Am J Cardiol.* 1996; 77: 31–36. 49.

Executive Summary of the Third Report of the National Cholesterol Education Program (NCEP) Expert Panel on Detection, Evaluation, and Treatment of High Blood Cholesterol in Adults (Adult Treatment Panel III). JAMA. 2001; 285:2486-2497.

Fahy E, Subramaniam S, Brown H, Glass C, Merrill JA, Murphy R, Raetz C, Russell D, Seyama Y, Shaw W, Shimizu T, Spener F, van Meer G, Vannieuwenhze M, White S, Witztum J and Dennis E.A. 2005. A comprehensive classification system for lipids. *J. Lipid Res.* 46: 839-861.

Fahy E, Subramaniam S, Murphy R, Nishijima M, Raetz C, Shimizu T, Spener F, van Meer G, Wakelam M and Dennis E.A. 2009. Update of the LIPID MAPS comprehensive classification system for lipids. *J. Lipid Res.* 50: S9-S14.

FAO 2004. Food and Agriculture Organization, FAO Production year Book, 51 (142):104-05.

Farhoosh R, Kenari RM, Hashem Poorazrang H: Frying stability of canola oil blended with palm olein, olive, and corn oils. J Am Oil Chem Soc 2009; 86:71–76.

Farooq Anwar, F., Hussain, A.I., Iqbal, S. and Muhammad Iqbal Bhanger, M.I.2006. Enhancement of oxidative estability of some vegetable oils by blending with *Moringa oleifera* oil. Food Chem. 103 (4): 1181-1191.

Fielding CJ, Havel RJ, Todd KM, Yeo KE, Schloetter M C, Weinberg V and Frost PH. 1995. Effects of dietary cholesterol and fat saturation on plasma lipoproteins in an ethnically diverse population of healthy young men. *J Clin Invest.* 1995; 95: 611-618.

Flegal, KM, Carroll MD, Ogden CL, Johnson CL. Prevalence and trends in obesity among US adults. 1999-2000. *JAMA.* 2002; 288: 1723-1727.

Folsom AR, Jacobs DR Jr, Wagenknecht LE, *et al.* Increase in fasting insulin and glucose over seven years with increasing weight and inactivity of young adults. The CARDIA Study. Coronary Artery Risk Development in Young Adults. *Am J Epidemiol.* 1996; 144: 235-246.

Food Standards Australia, New Zealand (June 2003) Erucic acid in food: A Toxicological Review and Risk Assessment. Technical report series No. 21; Page 4 paragraph 1; ISBN 0 642 34526 0, ISSN 1448-3017.

Foster GD, Wyatt HR, Hill JO, McGuckin BG, Brill C, Mohammed, BS, Szapary PO, Rader, dJ, Edman, JS and Klein, S. 2003. A randomized trial of a low-carbohydrate diet for obesity. *N Engl J Med.*; 348: 2082-2090.

Fraser, G.; Sabate, J.; Beeson, L.W.; Strahan, M.T. 1992. A Possible Effect of Nut Consumption on Risk of Coronary Heart Disease. Archives of Internal Med. 152:1416-24

Freeman DJ, Norrie J, Sattar N, *et al.* Pravastatin and the development of diabetes mellitus: evidence for a protective treatment effect in the West of Scotland Coronary Prevention Study. *Circulation.* 2001; 103: 357-362.

Freston JW, Ahnen DJ, Czinn SJ, *et al.* Review and analysis of the effects of Olestra, a dietary fat substitute, on gastrointestinal function and symptoms. *Regul Toxicol Pharm.* 1997; 26: 210–218.

Friedberg CE, Janssen MJ, Heine RJ, *et al.* Fish oil and glycemic control in diabetes: a meta-analysis. *Diabetes Care.* 1998; 21: 494–500.

Gapinski JP, VanRuiswyk JV, Heudebert GR, *et al.*, Preventing restenosis with fish oils following coronary angioplasty: a meta-analysis. *Arch Intern Med.* 1993; 153: 1595–1601.

Garcia-Segovia P, Sanchez-Villegas A, Doreste J, Santana F, Serra-Majem L.2006. Olive oil consumption and risk of breast cancer in the Canary Islands: a population-based case-control study. Public Health Nutr. 9(1A):163-7.

Garg A, Grundy SM. Nicotinic acid as therapy for dyslipidemia in non-insulin-dependent diabetes mellitus. *JAMA.* 1990; 264: 723-726.

Garg A. Insulin resistance in the pathogenesis of dyslipidemia. *Diabetes Care.* 1996; 19: 387-389.

Giardino I, Edelstein D, Brownlee M. BCL-Z expression or antioxidants prevent hyperglycemia-induced formation of intracellular advanced glycation end products in bovine endothelial cells. *J Clin Invest.* 1996; 46:223–234.

Gill CI, Boyd A, McDermott E, McCann M, Servili M, Selvaggini R, Taticchi A, Esposto S, Montedoro G, McGlynn H, Rowland I.2005. Potential anti-cancer effects of virgin olive oil phenols on colorectal carcinogenesis models *in vitro.* Int J Cancer. 117(1):1-7.

Gillery P, Monboisse JC, Maquat FX, *et al.* Glycation of protein as a source of superoxide. *Diabetes Metab.* 1988;14:25–30

Gilles Nalbone, Jeannie, L., Termine, E., Portugal, H., Lechene, P., Pauli, A.M. and Lafonf, H. 1989. Effects of fish oil, corn oil and lard diets on lipid peroxidation status and glutathione peroxidase activities in rat heart. Lipids. 24 (3): 179-186.

Gillum RF, Mussolino ME, Madans JH. The relationship between fish consumption and stroke incidence: the NHANES I Epidemiologic Follow-up Study (National Health and Nutrition Examination Survey). *Arch Intern Med.* 1996; 156: 537–542.

Glueck CJ, Lang J, Hamer T, Tracy T. Severe hypertriglyceridemia and pancreatitis when estrogens replacement therapy is given to hypertriglyceridemic women. *J Lab Clin Med.* 1994; 123: 59-64.

Glueck CJ, Taylor HL, Jacobs D, Morrison JA, Beaglehole R, Williams OD. Plassma high-density lipoprotein cholesterol: association with measurements of body mass. The Lipid Research Clinics Program Prevalence Study. *Circulation.* 1980; 62(suppl 4): IV61-IV69.

Godsland IF, Crook D, Simpson R, *et al.* The effects of different formulations of oral contraceptive agents on lipid and carbohydrate metabolism. *N Engl J Med.* 1990; 323: 1375-1381.

Goff DC, Shekelle RB, Moye LA, Katan MB, Gotto AM, Stamler J. Does body fatness modify the effect of dietary cholesterol on serum cholesterol? Results from the Chicago Western Electric Study. *Am J Epidemiol.* 1993; 137: 1171-177.

Goldberg RB, Mellies MJ, Sacks FM, *et al.* Cardiovascular events and their reduction with pravastatin in diabetic and glucose-intolerant myocardial infarction survivors with average cholesterol levels: subgroup analyses in the cholesterol and recurrent events (CARE) trial. The Care Investigators. *Circulation.* 1998; 98: 2513-2519.

Goldman L, Goldman PA, Williams LW, Weinstein MC. Cost-effectiveness considerations in the treatment of heterozygous familial hypercholesterolemia with medications. *Am J Cardiol.* 1993; 72: 75D-79D.

Goldschmid MG, Barrett-Connor EL, Edelstein SI, Wingard DL, Cohn BA, Herman WH. Dyslipidemia and ischemic heart disease mortality among men and women with diabetes. *Circulation.* 1994; 89: 991-997.

Goode GK, Garcia S, Heagerty AM. Dietary supplementation with marine fish oil improves in vitro small artery endothelial function in hypercholesterolemic patients: a double-blind placebo-controlled study. *Circulation.* 1997; 96: 2802–2807.

Gotto AM, Whitney E., Stein EA, *et al.* Relation between baseline and on-treatment lipid parameters and first acute major coronary events in the Air Force/Texas Coronary Atherosclerosis Prevention Study (AFCAPS/TexCAPS). Circulation, 2000;101:477-484.

Gotto AM. Jr. Targeting high-risk young patients for statin therapy. *JAMA.* 2004; 292: 377-378.

Grady D, Wenger NK, Herrington D, *et al.* Postmenopausal hormone therapy increases risk for venous thromboembolic disease. The Heart and Estrogen Progestin Replacement Study. *Ann Intern Med.* 2000; 132: 689-606.

Granfone A, Campos H, McNamara JR, *et al.* Effects of estrogen replacement on plasma lipoproteins and apolipoproteins in postmenopausal dyslipidemic women. *Metabolism.* 1992; 41: 1193-1198.

Grimsgaard S, Bonaa KH, Hansen JB, *et al.* Effects of highly purified eicosapentaenoic acid and docosahexaenoic acid on hemodynamics in humans. *Am J Clin Nutr.* 1998; 68: 52–59.

Grimsgaard S, Bonaa KH, Hansen JB, *et al.* Highly purified eicosapentaenoic acid and docosahexaenoic acid in humans have similar triacylglycerol-lowering effects but divergent effects on serum fatty acids. *Am J Clin Nutr.* 1997; 66: 649–659.

Grundy SM, Bazzarre T, Cleeman J, *et al.* Prevention Conference V: Beyond secondary prevention: identifying the high-risk patient for primary prevention: medical office assessment: Writing Group I. Circulation. 2000; 101:E3-E11.

Grundy SM, Benjamin IJ, Burke GL, *et al.* Diabetes and cardiovascular disease: a statement for healthcare professionals from the American Heart Association. *Circulation.* 1999; 100: 1134-1146.

Grundy SM, Cleeman JI, C. Merz CNB, Brewer, Jr HB, Clark LT, Hunninghake DB, Pasternak RC, Sidney C. Smith, Jr SC and Stone NJ. 2004. Implications of Recent Clinical Trials for the National Cholesterol Education Program Adult Treatment Panel III Guidelines. *Circulation.* 110:227-239.

Grundy SM, Cleeman JI, Daniels SR, Donato KA, Eckel RH, Barry A. Franklin BA, Gordon DJ, Krauss RM, Savage PJ, Smith, Jr SC, John A. Spertus JA, Costa F. 2005. Diagnosis and Management of the Metabolic Syndrome. Circulation. 2005;112:2735-2752

Grundy SM, Cleeman JI, Merz CN, *et al.* National Heart, Lung, and Blood Institute; American College of Cardiology Foundation; American Heart Association, Implications of recent clinical trials for the National Cholesterol Education Program Adult Treatment Panel III guidelines. *Circulation.* 2004; 110: 227-239.

Grundy SM, *et al.* (2001). Executive summary of the third report of the National Cholesterol Education Program (NCEP) Expert Panel on Detection, Evaluation, and Treatment of High Blood Cholesterol in Adults (Adult Treatment Panel III). JAMA, 285(19): 2486–2497.

Grundy SM. Non-high-density lipoprotein cholesterol level as potential risk predictor and therapy target. Arch Intern Med. 2001; 161:1379-1380.

Grundy SM. Small LDL, atherogenic dyslipidemia, and the metabolic syndrome. Circulation. 1997; 95:1-4.

Grundy SM. Hypertriglyceridemia, insulin resistance, and the metabolic syndrome. *Am J Cardiol.* 1999; 83: 25F-29F.

Guallar E, Aro A, Jimenez FJ, *et al.* Omega-3 fatty acids in adipose tissue and risk of myocardial infarction: the EURAMIC study. *Arterioscler Thromb Vasc Biol.* 1999; 19: 1111–1118.

Gupta, N., Sinddhu, A. and Sundararaj, P. 2001. Oxidative stability of edible grade crude palm oil blends with sunflower oil or ground oil as deep frying medium. Int. J. Oil Palm. 2 (1): 11–18.

Haban P, Klvanova J, Zidekova E, Nagyova A. 2004. Dietary supplementation with olive oil leads to improved lipoprotein spectrum and lower n-6 PUFAs in elderly subjects. Dietary supplementation with olive oil leads to improved lipoprotein spectrum and lower n-6 PUFAs in elderly subjects. Med Sci Monit. 10(4):PI49-PI54.

Haffner SM, Lehto S, Ronnemaa T, Pyorasla K, Laskso M. Mortality from coronary heart disease in subjects with type 2 diasbetes and in nondiabetic subjects with and without prior myocardial infarction. *N Engl J Med.* 1998; 339: 229-234.

Hallaq H, Smith TW, Leaf A. Modulation of dihydropyridine-sensitive calcium channels in heart cells by fish oil fatty acids. *Proc Natl Acad Sci U S A.* 1992; 89: 1760–1764.

Harper CR, Jacobson TA. 2001. The fats of life. The role of omega-3 fatty acids in the prevention of coronary heart disease. Arch Intern Med; 161:2185-92.

Harris WS, Connor WE, Alam N, *et al.* Reduction of postprandial triglyceridemia in humans by dietary n-3 fatty acids. *J Lipid Res.* 1988; 29: 1451–1460.

Harris WS, Ginsberg HN, Arunakul N, *et al.* Safety and efficacy of Omacor in severe hypertriglyceridemia. *J Cardiovasc Risk.* 1997; 4: 385–391.

Harris WS, Rambjor GS, Windsor SL, *et al.* N-3 fatty acids and urinary excretion of nitric oxide metabolites in humans. *Am J Clin Nutr.* 1997; 65: 459–464.

Harris WS. n-3 Fatty acids and serum lipoproteins: human studies. *Am J Clin Nutr.* 1997; 65 (5 Suppl): 1645S–1654S.

Hashim YZ, Eng M, Gill CI, McGlynn H, Rowland IR. 2005. Components of olive oil and chemoprevention of colorectal cancer. Nutr Rev. 63(11):374-86.

Hau MF, Smelt AH, Bindels AJ, *et al.* Effects of fish oil on oxidation resistance of VLDL in hypertriglyceridemic patients. *Arterioscler Thromb Vasc Biol.* 1996; 16: 1197–1202. 99.

Hayes, K.C. 2002. Dietary fat and heart health: in search of the ideal fat. Review article. Asia Pacific J. Clin. Nutr. 11 (Suppl): S394-S400.

Hegde, D.M and Venkattakumar. R. 2007. Development of oilseeds- a step towards self-sufficiency in India. Souvenir. All India Convention on Oilseeds, Oil trade and Industry. Nagpur. 27-28 October 2007: 41-48.

Hegde, D.M. 2005. Oilseeds: Striving for self-sufficiency. Survey of Indian Agriculture. The Hindu. P (58-63).

Hegde, D.M. 2006. Finding newer niches imperative. Survey of Indian Agriculture. The Hindu.P (66-70).

Hegde, D.M. 2007. An overview of oilseed scenario in India and scope and potential of bio-fuel crops. Paper presented in the Expert Group Discussion on Role of Bio-fuels for Decentralized Application in Agriculture and Allied Activities, May 14-15, 2007 at Administrative Staff College of India, Hyderabad.

Hegde, D.M. 2007. Increasing production area. Survey of Indian Agriculture. The Hindu. P (42-45).

Hegde, D.M. 2007. Agro-ecoregion-specific cropping systems for sustainable oilseeds production. Directorate of Oilseeds Research, Hyderabad. 124p.

Hegde, D.M. 2012. Carrying capacity of Indian agriculture: Oilseeds. Current Sci., 102(6): 25.

Hegsted DM, McGandy RB, Myers ML, Stare FJ. Quantitative effects of dietary fat on serum cholesterol in man. *Am J Clin Nutr.* 1965; 17: 281-295.

Higdon JV, Du SH, Lee YS, *et al.* Supplementation of postmenopausal women with fish oil does not increase overall oxidation of LDL ex vivo compared to dietary oils rich in oleate and linoleate. *J Lipid Res.* 2001; 42: 407–418.

Hilbert G, Lillemark L, Balchen S, *et al.* Reduction of organochlorine contaminants from fish oil during refining. *Chemosphere.* 1998; 37: 1241–1252.

Hill JO, Seagle HM, Johnson SL, *et al.* Effects of 14 d of covert substitution of Olestra for conventional fat on spontaneous food intake. *Am J Clin Nutr.* 1998; 67: 1178–1185.

Hines LM and Rimmb EB. 2001. Moderate alcohol consumption and coronary heart disease: a review. *Postgrad Med J* 2001;77:747-752.

Hjermann I, Enger SC, Helgeland A, Holme I, Leren P, Trygg K. The effect of dietary changes on high density lipoprotein cholesterol. The Oslo Study. Am J Med 1979; 66: 105–109.

Holownia, K. I., Erickson, M. C., Chinnan, M. S. and Eitenmiller, R. R. 2001.Tocopherol losses in peanut oil during pressure frying of marinated chicken strips coated with edible films. Food Research Int. 34 (1): 77-80.

Howard BV. Lipoprotein metabolism in diabetes mellitus. *J Lipid Res.* 1987; 28: 613-628.

Howard G, O'Leary DH, Zaccaro D, *et al.* Insulin sensitivity and atherosclerosis. The Insulin Resistance Atherosclerosis Study (IRAS) Investigators. *Circulation.* 1996; 93: 1809-1817.

Howe PR. Dietary fats and hypertension: focus on fish oil. *Ann N Y Acad Sci.* 1997; 827: 339–352.

Hu FB, Bronner L, Willett WC, *et al.* Fish and omega-3 fatty acid intake and risk of coronary heart disease in women. *JAMA.* 2002; 287: 1815–1821.

Hu FB, Stampfer MJ, Manson JE, *et al.* Dietary intake of alpha-linolenic acid and risk of fatal ischemic heart disease among women. *Am J Clin Nutr.* 1999; 69: 890–897.

Hu FB, Stampfer MJ, Manson JE, *et al.* Trends in the incidence of coronary heart disease and changes in diet and lifestyle in women. *N Engl J Med.* 2000; 343: 530-537.

Hu FB, Stampfer MJ, Rimm EB, Manson JE, Ascherio A, Colditz GA, Rosner BA, Spiegelman D, Frank E. Speizer FE, Frank M. Sacks FM, Hennekens CH and Willett WC. A Prospective Study of Egg Consumption and Risk of Cardiovascular Disease in Men and Women. *JAMA.* 1999;281:1387-1394.

Hubert HB, Feinleib M, McNamara PM, Castelli WP. Obesity as an independent risk factor for cardiovascular disease: a 26-year follow-up of participants in the Framingham Heart Study. *Circulation.* 1983; 67: 968-977.

Hulley S, Grady D, Bush T, *et al.* Randomized trial of estrogen plus progestin for secondary prevention of coronary heart disease in postmenopausal women. Heart and Estrogen/progestin Replacement Study (HERS) Research Group. *JAMA.* 1998; 280: 605-613.

Hunt JV, Wolff SP. Oxidative glycation and free radical production: a casual mechanism of diabetic complication. *Free Radic Res.* 1991;12-13:115–123

Ibrahim, A., Natarajan, S. and Ghafoorunissa. 2005. Dietary trans fatty acids alter adipocyte plasma membrane fatty acid composition and insulin sensitivity in rats. Metabolism. 54: 242-246.

Institute of Medicine (IOM). Dietary Reference Intakes for Energy and Macronutrients. Washington, DC: National Academy Press; 2002.

Iso H, Rexrode KM, Stampfer MJ, *et al.* Intake of fish and omega-3 fatty acids and risk of stroke in women. *JAMA.* 2001; 285: 304–312.

IUPAC, 1987. International Union of Pure and Applied Chemistry (IUPAC) In: C. Paquot and A. Hautfenne, Editors, Standard methods for the analysis of oils, fats and derivatives (7th rev. enlarged ed.), Blackwell Scientific, London.

Jacobs MN, Santillo D, Johnston PA, *et al.* Organochlorine residues in fish oil dietary supplements: comparison with industrial grade oils. *Chemosphere.* 1998; 37: 1709–1721.

Jandacek RJ, Kester JJ, Papa AJ, *et al.* Olestra formulation and the gastrointestinal tract. *J Lipids.* 1999; 34: 771–783.

Jenkins, DJ, Wong, GS, Patten, R *et al.*, 1983. Leguminous seeds in the dietary management of hyperlipidemia. *Am. J. Clin. Nutr.*, 38: 567–573.

Johansen O, Brekke M, Seljeflot I, *et al.*, N-3 fatty acids do not prevent restenosis after coronary angioplasty: results from the CART study. Coronary Angioplasty Restenosis Trial. *J Am Coll Cardiol.* 1999; 33: 1619–1626.

Johansen O, Seljeflot I, Hostmark AT, *et al.* The effect of supplementation with omega-3 fatty acids on soluble markers of endothelial function in patients with coronary heart disease. *Arterioscler Thromb Vas Biol.* 1999; 19: 1681–1686.

Jones DY, Judd JT, Taylor PR, Campbell WS, Padmanabhan PN. Influence of caloric contribution and saturation of dietary fat on plasma lipids in premenopausal women. Am J Clin Nutr 1987; 45:1451–1456

Judd, JT, Clevidence, BA, *et al.* Dietary trans fatty acids: effects on plasma lipids and lipoproteins of healthy men and women. Am J Clin Nutr. 1994; 59: 861-8

Kahlon, T.S., Chow, F.I., Chiu, M.M., Hudson, C.A. and Sayre, R.N. 1996. Cholesterol lowering by rice bran and rice bran oil unsaponifiable matter in Hamsters. Cereal Chem. 73(1): 69-74.

Kang JX, Leaf A. Antiarrhythmic effects of polyunsaturated fatty acids: recent studies. *Circulation.* 1996; 94: 1774–1780.

Kant AK, Graubard BI, Schatzkin A, Ballard- Barbash R: Proportion of energy intake from fat and subsequent weight change in the NHANES I Epidemiologic Follow-up Study. Am J Clin Nutr 1995;61:11–17.

Kaushik, K.K. 1993. Growth and instability of oilseeds production. Indian J. Agri. Eco. 48 (3): 334.

Kaushik, M, Mozaffarian, D, Spiegelman, D, Manson, JE, Willett, WC, and Hu, FB, 2009. Long chain omega-3 fatty acids, fish intake and the rid of type-2 diabetes mellitus. *Am. J. Clin. Nutr.*, 90(3): 613-620.

Keech A. Simes RJ. Barter P, *et al.* for the FIELD study investigators. Effects of long-term fenofibrate therapy on cardiovascular events in 9795 people with type 2 diabetes mellitus (the FIELD study) randomized controlled trial. *Lancet.* 2005; 366: 1849-1861.

Kennedy ET, Bowman SA, Powell R. Dietary-fat intake in the US population. *J Am Coll Nutr.* 1999; 18: 207–212.

Kingman, SM, 1991. The influence of legume seeds in human plasma lipid concentrations. *Nutr. Res. Reviews,* 4: 97–123.

Kinoshita I, Itoh K, Nishida-Nakai M, *et al.* Antiarrhythmic effects of eicosapentaenoic acid during myocardial infarction–enhanced cardiac microsomal (Ca^{2+}-Mg^{2+})-ATPase activity. *Japan Circ J.* 1994; 58: 903–912.

Knapp HR. Dietary fatty acids in human thrombosis and hemostasis. *Am J Clin Nutr.* 1997; 65 (5 Suppl): 1687S–1698S.

Kontogianni MD, Panagiotakos DB, Chrysohoou C, Pitsavos C, Zampelas A, Stefanadis C. 2007. The impact of olive oil consumption pattern on the risk of acute coronary syndromes: The CARDIO2000 case-control study. Clin Cardiol. 30(3):125-9. 2007.

Kornsteiner M, Singer I and Elmadfa I: Very low n–3 long-chain polyunsaturated fatty acid status in Austrian vegetarians and vegans. Ann Nutr Metab 2008; 52:37–47.

Kornsteiner M, Wagner KH, Elmadfa I: Tocoph- erols and total phenolics in 10 different nut types. Food Chem 20006; 98: 381–387.

Kornsteiner, E. M. 2009. Fats and fatty acid requirements for adults. Ann Nutr Metab 2009; 55: 56–75.

Krauss RM, Eckel RH, Howard B, *et al.* AHA Dietary Guidelines: revision 2000: a statement for healthcare professionals from the Nutrition Committee of the American Heart Association. *Circulation.* 2000; 102: 2284–2299.

Krauss RM, Eckel RH, Howard B, *et al.* American Heart Association's Dietary Guidelines: revision 2000: a statement for healthcare professionals from the Nutrition Committee of the American Heart Association. *Circulation.* 2000; 102: 2284–2299.

Kris-Etherton PM, Harris WS, Appel LJ. 2002. American Heart Association Nutrition Committee on Fish Consumption, fish oil, omega-3 fatty acids, and cardiovascular disease. *Circulation.*; 106: 2747-2757.

Kris-Etherton PM, Lichtenstein AH, Howard BV, Steinberg D, Witztum JL. 2004. Nutrition Committee of the American Heart Association Council on Nutrition, Physical Activity, and Metabolism. Antioxidant vitamin supplements and cardiovascular disease. *Circulation.*; 110: 637-641.

Kris-Etherton PM, Taylor DS, Yu-Poth S, *et al.* Polyunsaturated fatty acids in the food chain in the United States. *Am J Clin Nutr.* 2000; 71 (1 Suppl): 179S–188S. 104. USDA Nutrient Data Laboratory.

Kris-Etherton, PM, Pearson TA. Wan Y. Hargrove RL. Moriarty K. Fishell V. Etherton TD. 1999. High-monounsaturated fatty acid diets lower both plasma cholesterol and triacylglycerol concentrations. Am. J. Clin. Nutr. 70 (6):1009-15.

Kris-Etherton, PM, Yu, S. Individual fatty acid effects on plasma lipids and lipoproteins: human studies. Am J Clin Nutr. 1997; 65(suppl): 1628S-1644S

Krolewski AS, Kosinski EJ, Warran JH, *et al.* Magnitude and determination of coronary artery disease in juvenile-onset, insulin-dependent diabetes mellitus. *Am J Cardiol.* 1987; 59: 750-755.

Kromann N, Green A. Epidemiological studies in the Upernavik District, Greenland. *Acta Med Scand.* 1980; 208: 401–406.

Kromhout D, Bloemberg BP, Feskens EJ, *et al.* Alcohol, fish, fibre and antioxidant vitamins intake do not explain population differences in coronary heart disease mortality. *Int J Epidemiol.* 1996; 25: 753–759.

Kromhout D, Bosschieter EB, de Lezenne Coulander C. The inverse relation between fish consumption and 20-year mortality from coronary heart disease. *N Engl J Med.* 1985; 312: 1205–1209.

Kromhout D, Feskens EJ, Bowles CH. The protective effect of a small amount of fish on coronary heart disease mortality in an elderly population. *Int J Epidemiol.* 1995; 24: 340–345.

Kromhout D. Fish consumption and sudden cardiac death. *JAMA.* 1998; 279: 65–66.

Kromhout D., Menotti A., Bloemberg B., Aravanis C., Blackburn H., Buzina R., Dontas A. S., Fidanza F., Giaipaoli S., Jansen A., Karvonen M., Katan M., Nissinen A., Nedeljkovic S., Pekkanen J., Pekkarinen M., Punsar S., Rasanen L., Simic B. and Toshima H.1 995. Dietary saturated and trans fatty acids and cholesterol and 25-year mortality from coronary heart disease: the Seven Countries Study. *Prev Med.*; 24: 308-315.

Kuhn FE, Rackley CE. Coronary artery disease in women. Risk factors, evaluation, treatment, and prevention. *Arch Intern Med.* 1993; 153: 2626-2636.

Kun, T.U. 1998.Improvements in the frying quality of vegetable oils by blending with palm olein. Food Chem. 62(2): 191-195.

Kuusisto J, Mykkanen L, Pyorala K, Laakso M. NIDDM and its metabolic control predict coronary heart disease in elderly subjects. *Diabetes.* 1994; 43: 960-967.

Lahiri, A.K. 2006. Report of the Committee on rationalization of customs and excise duties on edible oils and oilseeds. Deptt. of Economic Affair, Ministry of Finance, Govt. of India.

Lamon-Fava S, Wilson PW, Schaefer EJ. Impact of body mass index on coronary heart disease risk factors in men and women. The Framingham Offspring Study. *Arterioscler Thromb Vasc Biol.* 1996; 16: 1509-1515.

Landmark K, Abdelnoor M, Kilhovd B, *et al.* Eating fish may reduce infarct size and the occurrence of Q wave infarcts. *Eur J Clin Nutr.* 1998; 52: 40–44.

Landmark K, Abdelnoor M, Urdal P, *et al.* Use of fish oils appears to reduce infarct size as estimated from peak creatine kinase and lactate dehydrogenase activities. *Cardiology.* 1998; 89: 94–102. 26.

Lands WE. Biochemistry and physiology of n-3 fatty acids. *FASEB J.* 1992; 6: 2530–2536.

Lawton CL, Blundell JE. The role of reduced fat diets and fat substitutes in the regulation of energy and fat intake and body weight. *Curr Opin Lipidol.* 1998; 9: 41–45.

Leaf A, Jorgensen MB, Jacobs AK, *et al.* Do fish oils prevent restenosis after coronary angioplasty? *Circulation.* 1994; 90: 2248–2257.

Lee RT, Libby P. The unstable atheroma. *Arterioscler Thromb Vasc Biol.* 1997; 17: 1859–1867.[Free Full Text]

Lee, J. H., Shin, J.A., Lee, J. H. and Lee, K. T. 2004. Production of lipase-catalyzed structured lipids from safflower oil with conjugated linoleic acid and oxidation studies with rosemary extracts. Food Res. Int. 37 (10): 967-974.

Lichtenstein AH, Kennedy E, Barrier P, *et al.* Dietary fat consumption and health. *Nutr Rev.* 1998; 56(5 pt 2): S3–S19.

Lopes-Virella MF, Virella G. Immune mechanisms of artherosclerosis on diabetes mellitus. *Diabetes.* 1992; 41 (suppl 2): 86-91.

Loscalzo, J. 2006. Homocysteine trials-clear outcomes for complex reasons. The New England J. Medicine, 354: 1629-1632.

Lottenberg AMP, Nunes VS, Lottenberg SA, McPherson R, Quintao ECR. Plasma cholesteryl ester synthesis, cholesteryl ester transfer protein concentration and activity in hypercholesterolemic women: effects of the degree of saturation of dietary fatty acids in the fasting and postprandial states. Atherosclerosis 1996; 126: 265–275.

Lotufo PA, Gaziano JM, Chae CU, *et al.* Diabetes and all-cause and coronary heart disease mortality among US male physicians. *Arch Intern Med.* 2001; 161: 242-247.

Luepker RV, Perry CL, McKinlay SM, *et al.* Outcomes of a field trial to improve children's dietary patterns and physical activity. The Child and Adolescent Trial for Cardiovascular Health. CATCH collaborative group. *JAMA.* 1996; 275: 768-776.

Malongil B. R. and Belur R. L. 2007. Hypolipidemic effect of oils with balanced amounts of fatty acids obtained by blending and interesterification of coconut oil with rice bran oil or sesame oil. J. Agri. Food Chem. 55 (25): 10461-10469.

Manson JE, Colditz Stampfer MJ, *et al.* A prospective study of naturally-onset diabetes mellitus and risk of coronary heart disease and stroke in women. *Arch Intern Med.* 1991; 151: 1141-1147.

Manson JE, Stampfer MJ, Hennekens CH, Willett WC. Body weight and longevity. A reassessment. *JAMA.* 1987; 257: 353-358.

Manson JE, Willett WC, Stampfer MJ, *et al.* Body weight and mortality among women. *N Engl J Med.* 1995; 333: 677-685.

Marchioli R, Barzi F, Bomba E, *et al.* Early protection against sudden death by n-3 polyunsaturated fatty acids after myocardial infarction: time-course analysis of the results of the Gruppo Italiano per lo Studio della Sopravvivenza nell'Infarto Miocardico (GISSI)-Prevenzione. *Circulation.* 2002; 105: 1897–1903.

Marckmann P, Bladbjerg EM, Jespersen J. Dietary fish oil (4 g daily) and cardiovascular risk markers in healthy men. *Arterioscler Thromb Vasc Biol.* 1997; 17: 3384–3391.

Marckmann P, Grønbæk M. Fish consumption and coronary heart disease mortality: a systematic review of prospective cohort studies. *Eur J Clin Nutr.* 1999; 53: 585–590.

Mariod, A., Matthaus, B., Eichner, K. and Hussain, I.H. 2005. Improving the oxidative stability of sunflower oil by blending with *Sclerocarya birrea* oil and *Aspongopus viduatus* oils. J. Food Lipids. 12: 150–158.

McDonald, B. 1999. Canola oil: nutritional properties. Canola Council of Canada Website www.canola-council.org.

McGill HC, McMahan CA, Zieske AW, *et al.* Association of coronary heart disease risk factors with the intermediate lesion of atherosclerosis in youth. The Pathobiologic Determinants of Atherosclerosis in Youth (PDASY) Research Group. *Arterioscler Thromb Vasc Biol.* 2000; 20: 1998-2004.

McGill HC, Mcmahan CA, Zieske, AW, Trachy RE, Malcom GT, Herderick, EE and Strong, JP. 2000. Association of Coronary Heart Disease Risk Factors with microscopic qualities of coronary atherosclerosis in youth. *Circulation* 2000, 102:374-379

McGinely, L. 1991. Analysis and quality control for processing and processed fats. In: J.B. Rossell and J.L.R. Pritchard, Editors, Analysis of oilseeds, fats and fatty foods, Elsevier Applied Science, New York, USA. pp. 460–470.

McRorie J, Zorich N, Riccardi K, *et al.* Effects of Olestra and sorbitol consumption on objective measures of diarrhea: impact of stool viscosity on common gastrointestinal symptoms. *Regul Toxicol Pharmacol.* 2000; 31: 59–67.

McVeigh GE, Brennan GM, Cohn JN, *et al.* Fish oil improves arterial compliance in non-insulin-dependent diabetes mellitus. *Arterioscler Thromb.* 1994; 14: 1425–1429.

Mehta, B.V. 2007. India's edible oil demand/ supply and future projection. In: Hegde, D.M. 2007. Changing global vegetable oil scenario: Issues and challenges before India. Indian Society of Oilseeds Research. Hyderabad. P (445-450).

Mekki N, Christofilis MA, Charbonnier M, *et al.* Influence of obesity and body fat distribution on postprandial lipemia and triglyceride-rich lipoproteins in adult women. *J Clin Endocrinol Metab.* 1999; 84: 184-191.

Menendez JA, Vellon L, Colomer R, Lupu R. 2005. Oleic acid, the main monounsaturated fatty acid of olive oil, suppresses Her-2/neu (erbB-2) expression and synergistically enhances the growth inhibitory effects of trastuzumab (HerceptinTM) in breast. Ann Oncol. PMID: 15642702.

Mensink, RP, Katan, MB. Effect of dietary trans fatty acids on high density and low densitylipoprotein cholesterol levels in healthy subjects. N Engl J Med. 1990; 323: 439-445

Meropi D. Kontogianni, Panagiotakos, D.B., Chrysohoou, C., Pitsavos, C., Zampelas, A. and Stefanadis, C. 2007. The impact of olive oil consumption pattern on the risk of acute coronary syndromes: the cardio2000 case-control study. Clinical Cardiol. 30 (3): 125-129.

Metrohm, A. G. 1993.Oxidative stability of oils and fats- Rancimat method. Metrohm application bulletin No. 204/le: Metrohm AG, Herisau, Switzerland, pp. 1–4.

Meyer BJ, Mann NJ, Lewis JL, Milligan GC, Sin- clair AJ, Howe PR: Dietary intakes and food sources of omega-6 and omega-3 polyunsat- urated fatty acids. Lipids 2003; 38: 391–398.

Mielke, T. 2008. Global impacts on India: oilseeds and products. Paper presented on the AGM of the SEA on Sept. 26, 2008 in Mumbai.

Mizushima S, Moriguchi EH, Ishikawa P, *et al.* Fish intake and cardiovascular risk among middle-aged Japanese in Japan and Brazil. *J Cardiovasc Risk.* 1997; 4: 191–199.

Mokdad AH, Serdula MK, Dietz WH, Bowman BA, Marks JS, Koplan JP. The spread of the obesity epidemic in the United States, 1991-1998. *JAMA.* 1999; 282: 1529-1522.

Moller DE, Chang PY, Yaspelkis BB, Flier JS, Wallberg-Henriksson H, Ivy JL. Transgenic mice with muscle-specific insulin resistance develop increased adiposity, impaired glucose tolerance, and dyslipidemia. *Endocrinology.* 1997; 137: 2397-2405.

Monika, H., Franciszek, S., Stanislaw, Z. and Stanislaw, B. 2002. Frying performance of rapeseed–palm oil blends, Polish J. Food Nutr. Sci. 11: 65–71.

Montori VM, Farmer A, Wollan PC, *et al.* Fish oil supplementation in type 2 diabetes: a quantitative systematic review. *Diabetes Care.* 2000; 23: 1407–1415.

Morello JR, Motilva MJ, Tovar MJ, Romero MP.2004. Changes in commercial virgin olive oil (cv Arbequina) during storage, with special emphasis on the phenolic fraction. J Agric Food Chem. 85(3):357-364.

Moreno DA, López-Berenguer C, García-Viguera C. 2007. Effects of stir-fry cooking with different edible oils on the phytochemical composition of broccoli. J Food Sci. 72(1):S064-8.

Mori TA, Beilin LJ, Burke V, *et al.* Interactions between dietary fat, fish, and fish oils and their effects on platelet function in men at risk of cardiovascular disease. *Arterioscler Thromb Vasc Biol.* 1997; 17: 279–286.

Mori TA, Watts GF, Burke V, *et al.* Differential effects of eicosapentaenoic acid and docosahexaenoic acid on vascular reactivity of the forearm microcirculation in hyperlipidemic, overweight men. *Circulation.* 2000; 102: 1264–1269.

Morris MC, Manson JE, Rosner B, *et al.* Fish consumption and cardiovascular disease in the Physicians' Health Study: a prospective study. *Am J Epidemiol.* 1995; 142: 166–175.

Morris MC, Sacks F, Rosner B. Does fish oil lower blood pressure? A meta-analysis of controlled trials. *Circulation.* 1993; 88: 523–533.

Mosca L, Appel LJ, Benjamin EJ, *et al.* Evidence-based guidelines for cardiovascular disease prevention in women. *Circulation.* 2004; 109: 672-693.

Moser GA, McLachlan MA. A non-absorbable dietary fat substitute enhances elimination of persistent lipophilic contaminants in humans. *Chemosphere.* 1999; 39: 1513–1521.

Mruthyunjaya. 2007. Technical efficiency in vegetable oilseeds in India. In: Souvenir. National Seminar on changing global vegetable oils scenario: Issues and challenges before India. January 29-31, 2007. Indian Society of Oilseeds Research. Hyderabad. P (4-8).

Mustad VA, Etherton TD, Cooper AD, Mastro AM, Pearson TA, Jonnalagadda SS, Kris-Etherton PM. Reducing saturated fat intake is associated with increased levels of LDL receptors on mononuclear cells in healthy men and women. J Lipid Res 1997; 38: 459–468.

Murao K, Wada Y, Nakamura T, Taylor AH, Mooradian AD, Wong NC. Effects of glucose and insulin on rat apolipoprotein A-I gene expression. *J Biol Chem.* 1998; 273: 18959-18965.

Must A, Spadano J, Coakley EH, Field AE, Colditz G, Dietz WH. The disease burden associated with overweight and obesity. *JAMA.* 1999; 282: 1523-1529.

Nabulsi AA, Filsom AR, White A, *et al.* Association of hormone-replacement therapy with various cardiovascular risk factors in postmenopausal women. The Atherosclerosis Risk in Communities Study Investigators. *N Engl J Med.* 1993; 328: 1069-1075.

Nageswari K, Banerjee R, Menon VP. Effect of saturated, w-3 and w-6 polyunsaturated fatty acids on myocardial infarction. *J Nutr Biochem.* 1999;10:338–343.

Narasinga Rao, B.S. 2000. Nutritive value of rice bran. NFI.

Natarajan, S., Ibrahim, A. and Ghafoorunissa. 2005. Dietary trans fatty acids alter diaphragm phospholipid fatty acid composition, triacylglycerol content and glucose transport in rats. British J.Nutr. 93: 1-6.

Natarajan, S., Nasreen, Z.E. and Ghafoorunissa. 2005. Differential effects of dietary trans fatty acids expression of genes associated with insulin sensitivity in rat adipose tissue: molecular basis of insulin resistance Eur. J.Endoc. 153: 1-8.

Nathan DM, Cleary PA, Backlund JY, *et al.* For the Diabetes Control and Complications Trial/Epidemiology of Diabetes Interventions and Complications (DCCT/EDIC) Study Research Group. Intensive diabetes treatment and cardiovascular disease in patients with type 1 diabetes. *N Engl J Med.* 2005; 353: 2643-2653.

National Health and Medical Research Council: Dietary guidelines for Australian adults. Canberra, NHMRC, 2003.

Natvig H, Borchgrevink CF, Dedichen J, *et al.* A controlled trial of the effect of linolenic acid on the incidence of coronary heart disease. *Scand J Clin Lab Med.* 1968; 105 (suppl): 1–20.

NCEP Resources Page. National Heart, Lung, and Blood Institute National Institutes of Health Web site. Third Report of the National Cholesterol Education Program (NCEP) Expert Panel on Detection, Evaluation, and Treatment of High Blood Cholesterol in Adults (Adult Treatment Panel III). Executive Summary. Available at http://www.nhlbi.nih.gov guidelines cholesterol atp3xsum pdf Accessed April 3, 2006.

Neels JG, Olefsky JM. Inflammed fat, what starts the fire? *J Clin Invest.* 2006; 116: 33-35.

Nelson GJ, Schmidt PC, Kelley DS. Low-fat diets do not lower plasma cholesterol levels in healthy men compared to high-fat diets with similar fatty acid composition at constant caloric intake. Lipids 1995; 30: 969–976.

Nestel, P. Clifton and Noakes, M.1994. Effects of increasing dietary palmoleic acid compared with palmitic and oleic acids on plasma lipids of hypercholesterolemic men. J. Lipid Res. 35: 656–662.

Nestel, PJ, Noakes, M., Belling, G.B., McArthur, R. Clifton, R.M. and Abbey, M. 1992. Plasma cholesterol-lowering potential of edible oil blends suitable for commercial use. Am. J. Clin. Nutr, 55: 46-50,

Nigam S.N. and Reddy L.J. 1994. *Genetic Enhancement in groundnut,* Prasad (Eds), Sustainability in Oilseeds, Indian Society of Oil Seeds Research, Hyderabad.

Niinikoski H, Viikari J, Ronnemaa T, *et al.* Prospective randomized trial of low-saturated fat, low-cholesterol diet during the first 3 years of life. The STRIP baby project. *Circulation.* 1996; 94: 1386-1393.

Nilsen DW, Albrektsen G, Landmark K, *et al.* Effects of a high-dose concentrate of n-3 fatty acids or corn oil introduced early after an acute myocardial infarction on serum triacylglycerol and HDL cholesterol. *Am J Clin Nutr.* 2001; 74: 50–56.

Noakes, M., Nestel, P.J. and Clifton, P.M. 1996. Commercial frying fats and plasma lipid-lowering potential. Australian J. Nutr. Dietet. 53 (1): 25–30.

Office of Nutritional Products, Labeling, and Dietary Supplements, Center for Food Safety and Applied Nutrition, US Food and Drug Administration. Letter responding to a request to reconsider the qualified claim for a dietary supplement health claim for omega-3 fatty acids and coronary heart disease. Docket No. 91N-0103. February 8, 2002. Available at: http://www.cfsan.fda.gov/~dms/ds-ltr28.html.

Office of Water, US Environmental Protection Agency. Consumption Advice Fact Sheet. National advice on mercury in fish caught by family and friends: for women who are pregnant or may become pregnant, nursing mothers, and young children. January 2001. EPA-823-F-01-004.

O'Keefe, S. and others. 1998. Levels of Trans Geometrical Isomers of Essential Fatty Acids in Some Unhydrogenated US Vegetable Oils. J. Food Lipids. 1:165-176.

Olshansky SJ, Passaro DJ, Hershow RC, *et al.* A potential decline in the life expectancy in the United States in the 21st century. *N.Engl J Med.* 2005; 352: 1138-1145.

Oomen CM, Feskens EJ, Rasanen L, *et al.* Fish consumption and coronary heart disease mortality in Finland, Italy, and The Netherlands. *Am J Epidemiol.* 2000; 151: 999–1006.

Oomen CM, Ocke MC, Feskens EJ, *et al.* Alpha-Linolenic acid intake is not beneficially associated with 10-y risk of coronary artery disease incidence: the Zutphen Elderly Study. *Am J Clin Nutr.* 2001; 74: 457–463.

Orchard TJ, Eichner J, Kuller LH, Becker DJ, McCallum LM, Grandits GA. Insulin as a predictor of coronary heart disease: interaction with apolipoprotein E phenotype. A report from the Multiple Risk Factor Intervention Trial. *Ann Epidemiol.* 1994; 4: 40-45.

Orencia AJ, Daviglus ML, Dyer AR, *et al.* Fish consumption and stroke in men: 30-year findings of the Chicago Western Electric Study. *Stroke.* 1996; 27: 204–209.

Ou J, Tu H, Shan B, *et al.* Unsaturated fatty acids inhibit transcription of the sterol regulatory element-binding protein-Ic (SREBP-Ic) gene by antagonizing ligand-dependent activation of the LXR. *Proc Natl Acad Sci USA.* 2001; 98: 6027-6032.

Padmavathy, A., Siddhu, A. and Sundararaj, P. 2001. Effect of blending edible grade crude palm oil with refined groundnut or sunflower oils on storage stability and sensory attributes. JOTAI. 33 (3): 93–103.

Paniagua JA, Gallego de la Sacristana A, Romero I, Vidal-Puig A, Latre JM, Sanchez E, Perez-Martinez P, Lopez-Miranda J, Perez-Jimenez F.2007. Monounsaturated fat-rich diet prevents central body fat distribution and decreases postprandial adiponectin expression induced by a carbohydrate-rich diet in insulin-resistant subjects. Diabetes Care. 30(7):1717-23.

Patalay M, Lofgren IE, Freake HC, Koo SI, Fernandez ML. The lowering of plasma lipids following a weight reduction program is related to increased expression of the LDL receptors and lipoprotein lipase. *J Nutr.* 2005; 135: 735-739.

Patil, B.N., Bhonde, S.R. and Khandikar, D.N. 2009. Trends in area, production and productivity of groundnut in Maharashtra. Financing Agri.-A National J. Agri. And Rural Dev. March-April issue: 35-39.

Patterson RE, Kristal AR, Peters JC, *et al.* Changes in diet, weight, and serum lipid levels associated with Olestra consumption. *Arch Intern Med.* 2000; 160: 2600–2604.

Paul, AA and Southgate, DAT, 1978. McCance and Widdowson's The Composition of Foods. Her Majesty's Stationery Office, London.

Pawlosky RJ, Hibbeln JR, Novotny JA, *et al.* Physiological compartmental analysis of alpha-linolenic acid metabolism in adult humans. *J Lipid Res.* 2001; 42: 1257–1265.

Pepe S, McLennan PL. Dietary fish oil confers direct antiarrhythmic properties on the myocardium of rats. *J Nutr.* 1996; 126: 34–42

Perry IJ, Wannamethee SG, Whincup PH, Shaper AG, Walker MK, Albert KG. Serum insulin and incident coronary heart disease in middle-aged British men. *Am J Epidemiol.* 1996; 144: 224-234.

Peterson S, Sigman-Grant M, Eissenstat B, *et al.* Impact of adopting lower-fat food choices on energy and nutrient intake of American adults. *J Am Diet Assoc.* 1999; 99: 177–183.

Peterson S, Sigman-Grant M. Impact of adopting lower-fat food choices on nutrient intake of American children. *Pediatrics.* 1997; 100: E4.

Pietinen P, Ascherio A, Korhonen P, *et al.* Intake of fatty acids and risk of coronary heart disease in a cohort of Finnish men: the Alpha-Tocopherol, Beta-Carotene Cancer Prevention Study. *Am J Epidemiol.* 1997; 145: 876–887.

Premavalla, K.S., Madhura, C.V. and Arya, S.S. 1998. Storage and thermal stability of refined cottonseed oil: mustered blend. J. Food Sci, Technol. 35 (6): 530–532.

Pronczuk A, Hayes KC. Ideal LDL/HDL ratio requires precise balance in dietary saturates (SFA) and polyunsaturates (PUFA). FASEB J 1999; 13: A561.

Psaltopoulou T, Naska A, Orfanos P, Trichopoulos D, Mountokalakis T, Trichopoulou A. 2004. Olive oil, the Mediterranean diet, and arterial blood pressure: the Greek European Prospective Investigation into Cancer and Nutrition (EPIC) study. Am J Clin Nutr. 80(4):1012-8.

Pyorala K, Pedersen TR, Kjekshus J, Faergeman O, Olsson AG. Thorgeirsson G Cholesterol lowering with simvastatin improves prognosis of diabetic patients with coronary heart disease. A subgroup analysis of the Scandinavian Simvastatin Survival Study (4S). *Diabetes Care.* 1997; 20: 614-620.

Rai. T. and Narayanan, K.M. 1984. Effect of intermittent frying on the physico-chemical and constants of ghee and refined groundnut oil. J. Food Sci. Technol. 21:400-402.

Rajalakshmi, D. and Narasimhan, S. 1996. Food antioxidants: source and methods of evaluation In: D.L. Madhavi, S.S. Deshpande and D.K. Salunkhe, Editors, Food antioxidants – technological toxicological and health perspectives, Marcel Dekker Inc, New York. pp. 65–157.

Ramadan, M.F., Afify Amer, M.M., El-Saadany, S.S., Abd El-Fatah El-Masry, R. and Awad, A. El. 2009. Food Sci. Technol. Int. 15(2): 119-130.

Ramesh, B., Saravanan, R. and Pugalendi, K.V. 2006. Effect of dietary substitution of groundnut oil on blood glucose, lipid profile, and redox status in streptozotocin-diabetic rats. Yale J Biol Med. 79(1): 9–17.

Rao, K.P.C. 2007. Can India achieve self-sufficiency in edible oils once again? In: Souvenir. National Seminar on changing global vegetable oils scenario: Issues and challenges before India. January 29-31, 2007. Indian Society of Oilseeds Research. Hyderabad. P (9-15).

Rasmussen OW, Thomsen C, Hansen KW, Vesterlund M, Winter E, Hermansen K. Effects on blood pressure, glucose, and lipid levels of a high-monounsaturated fat diet compared with a high-carbohydrate diet in NIDDM subjects. *Diabetes Care.* 1993;16:1565–1571.

Ravi, R., Prakash, M. and Bhat, K.K. 2005. Sensory odour profiling and physical characteristics of edible oil blends during frying. *Food Res. Int. 38 (1):* 59-68.

Reiser, S, 1987. Metabolic effects of dietary pectins related to human health. Food Technol., 41(2): 71-80.

Report of the Expert Panel on Blood Cholesterol Levels in Children and Adolescents. National Cholesterol Education Program. US Department of Health and Human Services. NIH Publication No. 91-2732 September, 1991.

Report of the expert panel on trans fatty acids and coronary heart disease. Trans fatty acids and coronary heart disease risk. Am J Clin Nutr. 1995; 62(suppl): 655S-708S

Reynhout, G. 1991. The effect of temperature on induction time of stabilized oil. J. Am. Oil Chemists' Soc. 68 (12): 983–984.

Ribaya-Mercado JD, Maramag CC, Tengco LW, Dolnikowski GG, Blumberg JB, Solon FS: Carotene-rich plant foods ingested with minimal dietary fat enhance the total-body vitamin A pool size in Filipino schoolchil- dren as assessed by stable-isotope-dilution methodology. Am J Clin Nutr 2007; 85: 1041–1049.

Richard D. O'Brien. 2004. Fats and oils: formulating and processing for applications. 3rd Edition. CRC Press.

Richard E Ostlund, R.E. Jr, Racette, S.B., Okeke, A. and William F Stenson, W.F. 2002. Phytosterols that are naturally present in commercial corn oil significantly reduce cholesterol absorption in humans. Am. J. Clin. Nutr. 75 (6): 1000-1004.

Rifkind BM, Schucker B, Gordon DJ. When should patients with heterozygous familial hypercholesterolemia be treated? *JAMA*. 1999; 281: 180-181.

Rimm EB, Willeztt WC, Hu FB, Sampson, L, Colditz, GA, Manson, JE, Hennekens, C and Stampfer, MJ. 1998. Folate and vitamin B6 from diet and supplements in relation to risk of coronary heart disease among women. *JAMA*. 1998; 279: 359-364.

Rissanen T, Voutilainen S, Nyyssonen K, *et al.* Fish oil-derived fatty acids, docosahexaenoic acid and docosapentaenoic acid, and the risk of acute coronary events: the Kuopio ischaemic heart disease risk factor study. *Circulation*. 2000; 102: 2677–2679.

Robins SJ, Targeting low high-density lipoprotein cholesterol for therapy: lessons from the Veterans Affairs High-Density Lipoprotein Intervention Trial. *Am J Cardiol.* 2001; 88: 19N-23N.

Roche HM, Gibney MJ. Postprandial triacylglycerolaemia: the effect of low-fat dietary treatment with and without fish oil supplementation. *Eur J Clin Nutr.* 1996; 50: 617–624.

Romero C, Medina E, Vargas J, Brenes M, Castro AD. 2007. *In Vitro* Activity of Olive Oil Polyphenols against Helicobacter pylori. J Agric Food Chem. 55(3):680-6.

Ross R. Atherosclerosis-an inflammatory disease. *N Engl J. Med.* 1999;340:115-126.

Ruano J, López-Miranda J, de la Torre R, Delgado-Lista J, Fernández J, Caballero J, Covas MI, Jiménez Y, Pérez-Martínez P, Marín C, Fuentes F, Pérez-Jiménez F.2007. Intake of phenol-rich virgin olive oil improves the postprandial prothrombotic profile in hypercholesterolemic patients. Am J Clin Nutr. 86(2):341-6.

Rubins HB, Robins SJ, Collins DF, *et al.* Gemfibrozil for the secondary prevention of coronary heart disease in men with low levels of high-density lipoprotein cholesterol. Veterans Affairs High-Density Lipoprotein Cholesterol Intervention Trial Study Group. *N Engl J Med.* 1999; 341: 410-418.

Rukmini, C, Raghuram, TC, 1991. Nutritional and biochemical aspects of the hypolipidemic action of rice bran oil: A review. *J. Am. Coll. Nutr.,* 10: 593-601.

Sacks FM, Pfeffer MA, Moye LA, *et al.* The effect of pravastatin on coronary events after myocardial infarction in patients with average cholesterol levels. Cholesterol and Recurrent Events Trial investigators. *N Engl J Med.* 1996; 123: 18-19.

Sacks FM, Stone PH, Gibson CM, *et al.* Controlled trial of fish oil for regression of human coronary atherosclerosis. HARP Research Group. *J Am Coll Cardiol.* 1995; 25: 1492–1498.

Sacks FM, Stone PH, Gibson CM, Silverman DI, Rosner B, Pasternak RC, for the HARP Research Group. Controlled trial of fish oil for regression of human coronary atherosclerosis. *J Am Coll Cardiol.* 1995; 25: 1492-1498.

Salonen JT, Seppanen K, Lakka TA, *et al.* Mercury accumulation and accelerated progression of carotid atherosclerosis: a population-based prospective 4-year follow-up study in men in eastern Finland. *Atherosclerosis.* 2000; 148: 265–273.

Salunkhe, D.K., Adsule, R.N., Chavan, J.K. and Kadam, S.S. 1992. World oilseeds: chemistry, technology and utilization. An AVI book published by Van Nostrand Reinhold, 115, Fifth Avenue, New York.

Samia, M. and Karl, E.2007. Evaluation of the stability of blends of sunflower and rice bran oil. European J. Lipid Sci. Technol. 109 (5): 531-535.

Sanders TA, Oakley FR, Miller GJ, *et al.* Influence of n-6 versus n-3 polyunsaturated fatty acids in diets low in saturated fatty acids on plasma lipoproteins and hemostatic factors. *Arterioscler Thromb Vasc Biol.* 1997; 17: 3449–3460.

Sanders TAB: Fat and fatty acid intake and metabolic effects in the human body. Ann Nutr Metab 2OO9;55:162–172.

Schaefer EJ, Levy RI, Ernst ND, Van Sant FD, Brewer HB. The effects of low-cholesterol, high polyunsaturated-fat, and low-fat diets on plasma lipid and lipoprotein cholesterol levels in normal and hypercholesterolemic subjects. Am J Clin Nutr 1981; 34: 1758–1763.

Schlagheck TG, Riccardi KA, Zorich NL, *et al.* Olestra dose response on fat-soluble and water-soluble nutrients in humans. *J Nutr.* 1997; 127 (suppl 8): 1646S–1665S.

Schwandt P, Janetschek P, Weisweiler P. High density lipoproteins unaffected by dietary fat modification. Atherosclerosis. 1982; 44: 9–17.

Sebedio, J. L. and Christie, W.W. 1998. Trans fatty acids in human nutrition, The Oily Press, Dundee, Scotland. Pp. 49-50.

Seljeflot I, Arnesen H, Brude IR, *et al.* Effects of omega-3 fatty acids and/or antioxidants on endothelial cell markers. *Eur J Clin Invest.* 1998; 28: 629–635.

Shahar E, Folsom AR, Wu KK, *et al.* Associations of fish intake and dietary n-3 polyunsaturated fatty acids with a hypocoagulable profile. The Atherosclerosis Risk in Communities (ARIC) Study. *Arterioscler Thromb.* 1993; 13: 1205–1212.

Sheard NF. Fish consumption and risk of sudden cardiac death. *Nutr Rev.* 1998; 56: 177–179.

Shekelle RB, Missell L, Paul O, *et al.* Fish consumption and mortality from coronary heart disease. *N Engl J Med.* 1985; 313: 820.

Shenoi, P.V. 2007. Strategy for the oilseed sector. In: Souvenir. National Seminar on changing global vegetable oils scenario: Issues and challenges before India. January 29-31, 2007. Indian Society of Oilseeds Research. Hyderabad. P (16-19).

Shiela, P. M., Sreerama, Y. N. and Gopala Krishna, A. G. 2004. Storage stability evaluation of some packed vegetable oil blends. J. American Oil Chemists' Soc. 81(12): 1125-1129.

Shimomura I, Matsuda M, Hammer RE, Bashmakov Y, Brown MS, Goldstein JL. Decreased IRS-2 and increased SREBP –Ic lead to mixed insulin resistance and sensitivity in livers of lipodystrophic and ob/ob mice. *Mol Cell.* 2000; 6: 77-86.

Shiota, M., Konishi, H. and Tatsumi, K. 1999. Oxidative stability of fish oil blended with butter. J. Dairy Sci. 82: 1877–1881.

Shlipak MG, Simon JA. Vittinghoff E, *et al.* Estrogens and progestin, lipoprotein(s) and the risk of recurrent coronary heart disease events after menopause. *JAMA.* 2000; 283: 1845-1852.

Shutter, SM, Bircher, GM, Tredger, JA, Morgan, LM, Walker, AF and Low, AG, 1989. The effect of daily baked bean consumption on the plasma lipid level of young normo-cholesterolemic men. *Brit. J. Nutr.*, 61: 257-265.

Sibley C, Stone NJ. Familial hypercholesterolemia: a challenge of diagnosis and therapy. *Cleve Clin J Med.* 2006; 73: 57-64.

Siddhuraju, P. and Becker, K. 2003. Antioxidant properties of various solvent extracts of total phenolic constituents from three different agroclimatic origins of drumstick tree (*Moringa oleifera* Lam.). J. Agri. Food Chem. 51: 2144–2155.

Sigman-Grant M. Can you have your low-fat cake and eat it too? The role of fat modified products. *J Am Diet Assoc.* 1997; 97 (suppl 7): S76–S81.

Simon JA, Fong J, Bernert JT Jr, *et al.* Serum fatty acids and the risk of stroke. *Stroke.* 1995; 26: 778–782.

Simon, JA, Fong, J, *et al.* Serum fatty acids and the risk of stroke. Stroke. 1995; 26: 778-782

Simopoulos AP. Evolutionary aspects of omega-3 fatty acids in the food supply. *Prostaglandins Leukot Essent Fatty Acids.* 1999; 60: 421–429.

Singh RB, Niaz MA, Sharma JP, *et al.* Randomized, double-blind, placebo-controlled trial of fish oil and mustard oil in patients with suspected acute myocardial infarction: the Indian experiment of infarct survival-4. *Cardiovasc Drugs Ther.* 1997; 11: 485–491.

Singh, N.B.2007. Role of public sector in increasing oilseeds production. In: Souvenir. National Seminar on changing global vegetable oils scenario: Issues and challenges before India. January 29-31, 2007. Indian Society of Oilseeds Research. Hyderabad. P (1-3).

Siscovick DS, Raghunathan TE, King I, *et al.* Dietary intake and cell membrane levels of long-chain n-3 polyunsaturated fatty acids and the risk of primary cardiac arrest. *JAMA.* 1995; 274: 1363–1367.

Sivakumar, S. 2007. New models for transfer of technology and empowerment of soybean farmers: Experience of ITC e Choupal initiative. In: Hegde, D.M. 2007. Changing global vegetable oil scenario: Issues and challenges before India. Indian Society of Oilseeds Research. Hyderabad. P (433-444).

Smith SC, Greenland P, Grundy SM. AHA Conference Proceedings. Prevention conference V: Beyond secondary prevention: Identifying the high risk patient for primary prevention: executive summary, American Heart Association. Circulation, 2000; 101:111-116.

Sniderman AD, Dagenais GR, Cantin B, Despres JP, Lamarche B. High apolipoprotein B with low high-density lipoprotein cholesterol and normal plasma triglycerides and cholesterol. Am J Cardiol. 2001; 87:792-793, A8.

Sniderman AD. Counterpoint: to (measure apo) B or not to (measure apo) B: a critique of modern medical decision-making. Clin Chem. 1997;4 3:1310-1314.

Solfrizzi, V., Panaza, F., Torres, F., Mastroianni, F., Del-Prigi, A. and Venezia, A.1999. High monounsaturated fatty acid intake protects against age-related cognitive decline. Neurology 52 (8):1563–1569.

Sonestedt, E., Ericson, U., Gullberg, Bo, Skog, K., Håkan Olsson, H. and Wirfält, E. (2008). Do both heterocyclic amines and omega-6 polyunsaturated fatty acids contribute to the incidence of breast cancer in postmenopausal women of the Malmö diet and cancer cohort? The International J. Cancer 123(7): 1637-1643.

Sorensen NS, Marckmann P, Hoy CE, *et al.* Effect of fish-oil-enriched margarine on plasma lipids, low-density-lipoprotein particle composition, size, and susceptibility to oxidation. *Am J Clin Nutr.* 1998; 68: 235–241.

Sosenko JM, Breslow JL, Miettinen OS, Gabby KH. Hyperglycemia and plasma lipid levels: a prospective study of young insulin-dependent diabetic patients. *J Engl J Med.* 1980; 302: 650-654.

Srinivasan KN, Pugalendi KV. Effect of excessive intake of thermally oxidized sesame oil on lipids, lipid peroxidation and antioxidants' status in rats. *Ind J Exp Biol.* 2000;38:777–780.

Stamler J, Daviglys ML. Garside DB, Dyer AR. Greenland P, Neaton JD. Relationship of baseline serum cholesterol levels in 3 large cohorts of younger men to long-term coronary cardiovascular, and all-cause mortality and to longevity, *JAMA* 2000;284:311-318.

Stamler J. Epidemic obesity in the United States. *Arch Intern Med.* 1993; 153: 1040-1044.

Steel, R.G.D. and Torrie, J.H. 1980. Principles and procedures of statistics, McGraw-Hill, London.

Stefanick ML, Mackey S, Sheehan M, Ellsworth N, Haskell WL, Wood PD. Effects of diet and exercise in men and postmenopausal women with low levels of HDL cholesterol and high levels of LDL cholesterol. N Engl J Med 1998; 339: 12–20.

Stein EA, Illingworth DR, Kwiterovich PO, *et al.* Efficacy and safety of lovastatin in adolescent males with heterozygous familial hypercholesterolemia: a randomized controlled trial. *JAMA.* 1999; 281: 137-144.

Stern L, Iqbal N, Seshadri P, Chicano, KL, Daily, DA, McGrory, JM, Williams, M., Gracely, EL and Samaha, FF. 2004. The effects of low-carbohydrate versus conventional weight loss diets in severely obese adults: one-year follow-up of a randomized trial. *Ann Intern Med.*; 140: 778-785.

Stevens J, Cai J, Pamuk ER, Williamson DF, Thun MJ, Wood JL. The effect of age on the association between body-mass index and mortality. *N Engl J Med.* 1998; 338: 1/7.

Stone NJ. Estrogen-induced pancreatitis: a caveat worth remembering. *J Lab Clin Med.* 1994; 123: 18-19.

Stone NJ. Fish consumption, fish oil, lipids, and coronary heart disease. *Circulation.* 1996; 94: 2337–2340.

Strong JP, Malcom GT, McMahan CA *et al.* Prevalence and extent of atherosclerosis in adolescents and young adults implications for prevention from the pathobiological Determinants of Atherosclerosis in Youth Study. *JAMA.* 199; 218:727-735.

Subramanian, A.N. 2007. Oilseeds and their products- what steps to be in the realms of becoming a front-runner? In: Souvenir. National Seminar on changing global vegetable oils scenario: Issues and challenges before India. January 29-31, 2007. Indian Society of Oilseeds Research. Hyderabad. P (20-26).

Sugano, M. and Etsuko Tsuji, E. 1997. Rice bran oil and cholesterol metabolism. The J. Nutr. 127 (3): 521S-524S.

Suh I, Oh KW, Lee KH, Psaty BM, Nam CM, Kim SI, Kang HG, Cho SY, Shim WH: Moderate dietary fat consumption as a risk factor for ischemic heart disease in a population with a low fat intake: a case-control study in Ko- rean men. Am J Clin Nutr 2OO1;73:722–727.

Sun Yat-sen University, 2007.Optimal Dietary Fat Pattern to Prevent Cardiovascular Disease among Type 2 Diabetes. Clinical Trials. Gov Identifier (NCT00467168-on line journal).

Sundram K, Hayes KC, Siru OH. A balance between dietary 18:2 and 16:0 may be required to improve the serum LDL/HDL cholesterol ratio in normocholesterolemic men. J Nutr Biochem 1995; 6: 179–187.

Sundram K, Ismail A, Hayes KC. *Trans* (elaidic) fatty acids adversely affect the lipoprotein profile relative to specific saturated fatty acids in humans. J Nutr 1997; 127: 514S–520S.

Sunitha, T., Manorama, R. and Rukmini, C. 1997. Lipid profile of rats fed blends of rice bran oil in combination with sunflower and safflower oil. Plant Foods for Human Nutr. 51(3): 219-230.

Taira K, Hikita M, Kobayashi J, *et al.* Delayed post-prandial lipid metabolism in subjects with intra-abdominal visceral fat accumulation. *Eur J Clin Invest.* 1999; 29: 301-308.

Talati, R, Pharm, D, Baker, WL, *et al.*, 2009. The effects of barley-derived soluble fibre on serum lipids. *Ann. Fam. Med.*, 7(2): 157-163.

Talwar, S (2003), Peanut in India, History, Production and Utilization. Sustainable Human Ecosystem Laboratory, University of Georgia, Athens, Georgia, U.S.A. ppA-38.

Taskinen MR, Puolakka J, Pyorala T, *et al.* Hormone replacement therapy lowers plasma Lp(a) concentrations. Comparison of cyclic transdermal and continuous estrogen-progestin regimens. *Arterioscler Thromb Vasc Biol.* 1996; 16: 1215-1221.

The DCCT Research Group. Lipid and lipoprotein levels in patients with IDDM. Diabetes Control and Complications Trial experience. *Diabetes Care.* 1992; 15: 886-894.

The Diabetes Control and Complications Trial (DCCT) Research Group. Effect of intensive diabetes management on macrovascular and risk factors in the Diabetes Control and Complications Trial. *Am J Cardiol.* 1995. 75: 894-903.

The Heart Outcomes Prevention Evaluation (HOPE) 2 Investigators. 2006. Homocysteine lowering with folic acid and B vitamins in vascular disease. *N Engl J Med.*; 354. Article published at www.nejm.org on March 12, 2006.

The USDA Nutrient Database for Standard Reference. August. Washington: USDA; 1997.

The Writing Group for the DISC Collaborative Research Group. Efficacy and safety of lowering dietary intake of fat and cholesterol in children with elevated low-density lipoprotein cholesterol. The Dietary Intervention Study in Children (DISC). *JAMA.* 1995; 273: 1429-1435.

Thomas JL, Braus PA, Coronary artery disease in women. A historical perspective. *Arch Intern Med.* 1998; 158: 333-337.

Tietyen, JL, Nevins, DL, Shoemaker, CF and Schneeman, BO, 1995. Hypocholesterolenic potential of oat bran treated with an endo-β-d-glucanase from *B. subtitis. J. Food Sci.*, 60: 558-560.

Traven ND, Kuller LH. Lves DG Rutan GH. Perper JA. Coronary heart disease mortality and sudden death: trends and patterns in 35- to 44-year-old white males. 1970-1990. *Am Epidemtol*, 1995;145:45-52.

Truswell, A.S. 1998. Monounsaturated oils do not all have the same effect on plasma cholesterol. Eur. J. Clin. Nutr. 52:312-315

Tsaknis, J. and Lalas, S. 2002. Stability during frying of *Moringa oleifera* seed oil variety "Periyakulam 1". J. Food Composition and Analysis 15: 79–101.

Tuomilehto J, Lindstrom J, Eriksson JG, Valle TT, Hamalainen H, Ilanne-Parikka P, Keinanen-Kiukaanniemi S, Laakso M, Louheranta A, Rastas M, Salminen V, Uusitupa M. 2001. Finnish Diabetes Prevention Study Group. Prevention of type

2 diabetes mellitus by changes in lifestyle among subjects with impaired glucose tolerance. *N Engl J Med.* 2001; 344: 1343-1350.

Uauy R, Mena P, Valenzuela A. Essential fatty acids as determinants of lipid requirements in infants, children and adults. *Eur J Clin Nutr.* 1999; 53 (Suppl 1): S66–S77.

Uchara Y, Engel T, Li Z. *et al.* Polyunsaturated fatty acids and acetoacetate downregulate the expression of the ATP-binding cassette transporter A1. *Diabetes.* 2002; 51: 2922-2928.

Ullmann D, Connor WE, Hatcher LF, Connor SL, Flavell DP. Will a high-carbohydrate, low-fat diet lower plasma lipids and lipoproteins without producing hypertriglyceridemia? *Arterioscler Thromb.* 1991; 11" 1059-1067.

US Food and Drug Administration, Center for Food Safety and Applied Nutrition, Office of Seafood. Mercury Levels in Seafood Species. May 2001. Available at: http://www.cfsan.fda.gov/~frf/sea-mehg.html.

US Food and Drug Administration. Mercury in fish: cause for concern? *FDA Consumer.* 1994;28(September). Revised May 1995. Available at: http://www.fda.gov/fdac/reprints/mercury.html.

USDA National Nutrient Database for Standard Reference, Release 21 (2008)

USDA, 2012. Annual report on oilseeds (India). USDA Foreign Agricultural Service, Gain Report, Global Agricultural Information Network.

USDA, 2013. Annual report on oilseeds (India). USDA Foreign Agricultural Service, Gain Report, Global Agricultural Information Network.

Vaccaro O, Ruth KJ, Stamler J. Relationship of postload plasma glucose to mortality with 19-year follow-up. Comparison of one versus two plasma glucose measurements in the Chicago Peoples Gas Company Study. *Diabetes Care.* 1992; 15: 1328-1334.

Van Horn L, Obarzanek E, Friedman LA, Gernhofer N. Barton B Children's adaptations to a fat-reduced diet: the Dietary Intervention Study in Children (DISC). *Pediatrics.* 2005; 115: 1723-1833.

Vedin I, Cederholm T, Freund Levi Y, Basun H, Garlind A, Faxén Irving G, Jönhagen ME, Vessby B, Wahlund LO, Palmblad J: Effects of docosahexaenoic acid-rich n–3 fatty acid supplementation on cytokine release from blood mononuclear leukocytes: the Ome- gAD study. Am J Clin Nutr 2008; 87: 1616–1622.

Vidyasagar (1980), Decomposition of Growth Trends and Centain Related Issues, Indian Journal of Agricultural economics, 35 (2), pp. 42-59.

Visioli F, Galli C. Alpha-linolenic acid and cardiovascular disease. *Am J Clin Nutr.* 2002; 75: 1121.Letter. 32. Keli SO, Feskens EJ, Kromhout D. Fish consumption and risk of stroke: the Zutphen Study. *Stroke.* 1994; 25: 328–332.

Vivekanathan DP, Penn MS, Sapp SK, Hsu A, Topol EJ. 2003. Use of antioxidant vitamins for the prevention of cardiovascular disease: meta-analysis of randomized trials. *Lancet.*; 361: 2017-2023.

von Schacky C, Angerer P, Kothny W, *et al.* The effect of dietary omega-3 fatty acids on coronary atherosclerosis: a randomized, double-blind, placebo-controlled trial. *Ann Intern Med.* 1999; 130: 554–562.

Von Schacky C, Angerer P, Kothny W, Theisen K, Mudra H. The effect of dietary omega-3 fatty acids on coronary atherosclerosis. A randomized, double-blind, placebo-controlled trial. *Ann Intern Med.* 1999; 130: 554-562.

Walsh BW, Sacks FM. Effects of low dose oral contraceptives on very low density and low density lipoprotein metabolism. *J Clin Invest.* 1993; 91: 2126-2132.

Warner, K. and Knowlton, S.1997. Frying quality and oxidative stability of high-oleic corn oils. J. Am. Oil Chemists' Soc. 74: 1317–1321.

Waters DD, Edwin L. Alderman, Judith Hsia, Barbara V. Howard, Frederick R. Cobb, William J. Rogers, Pamela Ouyang, Paul Thompson, Jean Claude Tardif, Lyall Higginson, Vera Bittner, Michael Steffes, David J. Gordon, Michael Proschan, Naji Younes, and Joel I. Verter 2002. Effects of hormone replacement therapy and antioxidant vitamin supplements on coronary atherosclerosis in postmenopausal women: a randomized controlled trial. *JAMA.* 2002; 288: 2432-2440.

Weisweiler P, Janetschek P, Schwandt P. Influence of polyunsaturated fats and fat restriction on serum lipoproteins in humans. Metabolism 1985; 34: 83–87.

Westerveld HT, van Lennep JE, ven Lennep HW, *et al.* Apolipoprotein B and coronary artery disease in women: a cross-sectional study in women undergoing their first coronary angiography. Arterioscler Thromb Vaso Biol, 1998; 18:1101-1107.

Whiteley L, Padmanabhan S, Hole D, Isles C. Should diabetes be considered a coronary heart disease risk equivalent? Results from 25 years of follow-up in the Renfrew N Paisley survey. *Diabetes Care.* 2005; 28: 1588-1593.

Wiegman A, Hutten BA, de Groot E, *et al.* Efficacy and safety of statin therapy in children with familial hypercholesterolemia: a randomized controlled trial. *JAMA.* 2004; 292: 331-337.

Wilson PW, Kannel WB, Silbershatz H, D'Agostino RB. Clustering of metabolic factors and coronary heart disease. Arch Intern Med. 1999;159:1104-1109.

Wingard DL, Barrett-Connor EL, Ferrara A. Is insulin really a heart disease risk factor? *Diabetes Care.* 1995; 18: 1299-1304.

Wolk, A, *et al.*, 1998. A prospective sludge association of mono-unsaturated fat and other types of fat with risk of breast cancer. *Arch. Intern. Med.*, 158: 41-45.

Wong, R., Patel, J. D., Grant, I., Parber, J., Charne, D., Ethalwagy, M. and Sys, E. 1991. In I. Mc. Gregor (Ed.), Proceedings of the rapeseed congress, programme and abstract, Sasbatoom, p. 53.

Wylie-Rosett, J. 2002. Fat substitutes and health: An advisory from the nutrition committee of the American Heart Association. Circulation. 105: 2800-2804.

Yeghiazarians Y. Braunstein JB. Askari A, Stone PH Unstable angina pectoris *N Engl J Med.* 2003:342:1101-114.

Zhang J, Sasaki S, Amano K, *et al.* Fish consumption and mortality from all causes, ischemic heart disease, and stroke: an ecological study. *Prev Med.* 1999; 28: 520–529.

Zock, PL, Katan, MB. Butter, margarine, and serum lipoproteins. Atherosclerosis. 1997; 131(1): 7-16

Zorich NL, Jones MB, Kesler JM, *et al.* A randomized, double-blind study of the effect of Olestra on disease activity in patients with quiescent inflammatory bowel disease. Olestra in IBD Study Group. *Am J Med.* 1997; 103: 389–399.